Minimally Invasive Approaches to Colon and Rectal Disease

Howard M. Ross • Sang W. Lee
Matthew G. Mutch • David E. Rivadeneira
Scott R. Steele
Editors

# Minimally Invasive Approaches to Colon and Rectal Disease

## Technique and Best Practices

Springer

*Editors*
Howard M. Ross, MD, FACS, FASCRS
Division of Colon and Rectal Surgery
Department of Surgery
Temple University Health System
Philadelphia, PA, USA

Sang W. Lee, MD, FACS, FASCRS
Division of Colon and Rectal Surgery
Department of Surgery
Weill-Cornell Medical College
New York Presbyterian Hospital
New York, NY, USA

Matthew G. Mutch, MD, FACS, FASCRS
Department of Surgery
Washington University School of Medicine
St. Louis, MO, USA

David E. Rivadeneira, MD, MBA, FACS, FASCRS
North Shore-LIJ Health System, Huntington Hospital
Hofstra University School of Medicine
Huntington, NY, USA

Scott R. Steele, MD, FACS, FASCRS
Department of Colon and Rectal Surgery
Madigan Army Medical Center
Olympia, WA, USA

Videos to this book can be accessed at http://www.springerimages.com/videos/978-1-4939-1580-4

ISBN 978-1-4939-4748-5 ISBN 978-1-4939-1581-1 (eBook)
DOI 10.1007/978-1-4939-1581-1
Springer New York Heidelberg Dordrecht London


Softcover reprint of the hardcover 1st edition 2015


Printed on acid-free paper

Springer is part of Springer Science+Business Media (www.springer.com)

# Foreword

This is an exciting and urgently needed text that takes a comprehensive, critical approach to the latest developments in minimally invasive surgery for colon and rectal diseases, and does so in a highly practical fashion. The book highlights the important ideas of many of the most experienced and well-respected leaders in the field from the USA and adds perspective from internationally respected surgeons from Japan and Europe. Drs. Ross, Lee, Mutch, Rivadeneira, and Steele form an all-star team of editors and contributors. They have clearly been leaders in colon and rectal surgery who continue to search for better outcomes for their patients and patients everywhere.

The book provides the reader with a format that will be of practical use on a day-by-day or case-by-case basis, since each chapter stands alone independently, and provides important technical details and highly useful illustrations and videos on procedures, as well as "pearls and pitfalls" at the conclusion of each chapter.

Important and controversial new techniques such as use of robotics and single-incision laparoscopic surgery (SILS) are addressed head on by experts in these techniques, and "standard" laparoscopic methods are also presented in various forms by surgeons who have performed many hundreds of these procedures in their practice.

I have had the pleasure of watching many of the authors and editors of this important book hone their skills and judgment over many years. We are fortunate to experience their collective wisdom on tackling some of the most difficult intestinal surgical problems in a format that is easy to use and enjoyable.

This book is certain to find an important place on the shelves of surgeons around the world who wish to keep current with the rapidly evolving field of minimally invasive surgery for colon and rectal diseases. The editors should prepare themselves for future editions, as we readers will be looking for them to continue to define the field!!

New York, NY, USA — Jeffrey Milsom, MD

# Preface

> "We should strive to welcome change and challenges, because they are what help us grow."
>
> H.G. Wells

Change is most often simply a matter of time, and in surgery that is no different. Large incisions have frequently been replaced by small, and hands by graspers. The surgeon may now find themselves away from the operative table, as open surgery is steadily transitioning to laparoscopic and robotic techniques. Even traditional approaches to anorectal lesions have witnessed a new paradigm. That is not to say that all changes are needed, or even welcome. Yet, the changes witnessed in the evolution of minimally invasive colorectal surgery have played a large role in both minimizing morbidity and maximizing outcomes. Change also brings certain challenges, and specifically, colorectal surgery presents its own unique set of trials. It is within this context that *Technique and Best Practices* examines the considerations, drawbacks, and advancements minimally invasive techniques have provided in the evaluation, management, and outcomes across a broad range of colorectal disease and procedures.

For some readers of this book, a minimally invasive approach to colorectal disease may add a new dimension to the management of these patients. For others, it is the opportunity to learn helpful tips, specifics about a certain procedure, or to fine-tune what has already become a routine part of their practice. Even if you have successfully overcome many of the technical challenges of minimally invasive surgery, the preoperative evaluation, perioperative decision-making, and management of postoperative complications can be demanding and consuming. Wherever you may be on this spectrum, *Technique and Best Practices* has something to offer. The underlying focus throughout the text is on providing pragmatic advice and reproducible techniques that can be readily implemented by surgeons of varying experience to successfully treat complex colorectal problems through minimally invasive methods.

Our author experts have years of experience with minimally invasive approaches to colorectal disease, and in some cases, have been the pioneers in this field. Despite extensive training and a wealth of clinical experience, many surgeons do not have the resources or volume to garner the skills and experience to feel completely comfortable with, or in some cases, master these techniques. In this text, our authors have cogently and equitably provided a unique, practical guide that covers the evaluation, step-by-step technical approach, and detailed management techniques. Within each chapter, they focus on the details to help overcome the issues that make these procedures and disease processes challenging. Yet, this is more than a "how to" manual or an algorithm-based guide.

Our other aim with *Technique and Best Practices* was to understand the intricate thought process behind each author's proposed technique and describe their personal insight as to why they approach a particular colorectal disease process or minimally invasive procedure a certain way. This abundant practical advice allows a concise depiction of a methodical, understandable approach to both straightforward and complex cases. Additionally, by providing separate chapters on the procedure and the disease process, we systematically provide both an overview as well as detailed portrayal of how a minimally invasive approach aids in the management of these patients.

Since its conception, it has been our privilege and pleasure to work with this expert cohort of authors, as their individual contributions have come together to make a combined effort where the sum is definitely greater than the parts. We would like to personally thank each one of them for taking time away from their busy practices and families to share their knowledge, skill, and valuable insights regarding minimally invasive colorectal surgery. We are grateful for their candor in discussing both the positive aspects as well inherent limitations. It is our wish that *Technique and Best Practices* serves as a valuable resource for surgeons of all ages and expertise, and hope you will find this as intriguing and helpful as we have.

## Internet Access to Video Clip

The owner of this text will be able to access these video clips through Springer with the following Internet link: http://www.springerimages.com/video/978-1-4939-1580-4.

Philadelphia, PA, USA — Howard M. Ross, MD, FACS, FASCRS
New York, NY, USA — Sang W. Lee, MD, FACS, FASCRS
St. Louis, MO, USA — Matthew G. Mutch, MD, FACS, FASCRS
Huntington, NY, USA — David E. Rivadeneira, MD, MBA, FACS, FASCRS
Olympia, WA, USA — Scott R. Steele, MD, FACS, FASCRS

# Acknowledgements

The completion of this textbook has been a dream of mine, but its production is truly the work of so many. I would like to thank my wife, who has always helped me to become everything I always wanted, my children, who make all work worthwhile, and my parents, uncle, in laws and teachers who were so generous with their love, time and support. Further, I would like to thank my many colleagues, friends and mentors in the American Society of Colon and Rectal Surgery who strive so hard to improve the care of those with colon and rectal disease.

Howard M. Ross, MD

I would like to acknowledge and thank many colleagues and friends for volunteering their precious time and expertise. I would like to thank our Developmental Editor at Springer, Elektra McDermott, for encouraging us throughout the writing of the textbook. I also would like to thank my mentors, Jeff Milsom and Larry Whelan for guiding and supporting me throughout my career. To my coeditors, Howard, David, Scott, and Matt, thank you for your hard work and friendship.

Finally, and most importantly, I would like to thank my wife, Crystal, for her support, encouragement and unwavering love; and my sons, Eric and Ryan, for making me a better person and making everything worthwhile.

Sang W. Lee, MD

To my parents for the giving me everything I needed to realize my goals. To my wife, Jennifer, for her unconditional love and support and to my children, Megan and Adam, for showing me the most important thing in life is family. To my coeditors for their dedication and tireless effort that has made my participation rewarding. To all of the authors for their contributions and mentorship to constantly improve the quality of our specialty.

Matthew Mutch, MD

To my parents, Eduardo and Manuela for teaching me to dream. To my wife, Anabela, for teaching me to love. And to my children, Sophia and Gabriella, for teaching me to laugh. To my fellow coeditors H.R., M.M., S.L., S.S., and surgical mentors throughout my career "If I have seen further it is by standing on the shoulders of giants"—Isaac Newton.

David E. Rivadeneira, MD

I would first like to thank our outstanding Developmental Editor, Elektra McDermott, for her extraordinary efforts in overseeing this edition and ensuring its timely completion and thoroughness. I personally would like to thank my fellow editors for their tremendous vision and hard work throughout this entire process, as well as all of my mentors in colorectal surgery for guiding me and giving me such incredible opportunities. Finally, and most importantly, thank you to Michele and Marianna for supporting and encouraging me throughout this endeavor.

Scott R. Steele, MD

# Contents

**Part I Preoperative**

1 **Perioperative Assessment** ... 3
Charlotte Kvasnovsky and Andrea Chao Bafford

2 **Patient Positioning, Instrumentation, and Trocar Placement** ... 15
Mehraneh Dorna Jafari, Michael J. Stamos, and Steven Mills

3 **Surgical Anatomy** ... 25
Todd D. Francone and Ron G. Landmann

**Part II Procedures**

4 **Right Colectomy: Straight Laparoscopic** ... 53
Steven Robert Hunt

5 **Right Colectomy: Hand-Assist** ... 61
Kirk A. Ludwig and Timothy Ridolfi

6 **Laparoscopic Sigmoidectomy/Left Colectomy** ... 71
Toyooki Sonoda

7 **Hand-Assisted Left Colectomy** ... 81
Steven Lee-Kong and Daniel L. Feingold

8 **Total Abdominal Colectomy: Straight Laparoscopic Approach** ... 89
Amanda V. Hayman and Eric J. Dozois

9 **Total Abdominal Colectomy: Hand-Assisted Approach** ... 103
Kiyokazu Nakajima, Tsunekazu Mizushima, and Riichiro Nezu

10 **Operative Details of Laparoscopic Rectal Resection for Cancer** ... 111
Martin R. Weiser

11 **Laparoscopic Hand-Assisted Low Anterior Resection** ... 119
Govind Nandakumar and Sang W. Lee

12 **Laparoscopic Abdominoperineal Resection** ... 131
Jennifer S. Davids and Justin A. Maykel

13 **Laparoscopic Proctocolectomy** ... 143
David A. Etzioni and Tonia M. Young-Fadok

14 **Laparoscopic Rectopexy** ... 155
Mia DeBarros and Scott R. Steele

15 **Minimally Invasive Approach for Stoma Creation** ... 169
Seth I. Felder, Zuri Murrell, and Phillip Fleshner

16 **Laparoscopic Stoma Reversal** ... 179
Emre Gorgun

17 **Laparoscopic Parastomal Hernia Repair** ... 189
Joshua A. Tyler and Matthew G. Mutch

**Part III Technical Challenges and Tips**

18 **Overcoming Technical Challenges: The Abdomen** ... 201
Eric K. Johnson

19 **Overcoming Technical Challenges: The Pelvis** ... 213
M. Shane McNevin

20 **Overcoming Technical Challenges: Reoperative Surgery** ... 221
Brian R. Englum, M. Benjamin Hopkins, and John Migaly

21 **Overcoming Technical Challenges: Prevention and Managing Complications** ... 235
Bradley R. Davis

**Part IV New Horizons**

22 **Single-Incision Laparoscopic Approaches to Colorectal Disease** ... 249
Virgilio George

23 **Natural Orifice Surgery (NOTES)** ... 263
Mark H. Whiteford

24 **Robotic Surgery** ... 273
Mehraneh Dorna Jafari, David E. Rivadeneira, and Alessio Pigazzi

25 **Transanal Minimally Invasive Surgery (TAMIS): Operative Technique, Pitfalls, and Tips** ... 283
Francisco Quinteros, Kumaran Thiruppathy, and Matthew R. Albert

26 **Combined Endo-Laparoscopic Surgery (CELS)** ... 293
Kelly A. Garrett and Sang W. Lee

**Part V Special Situations**

27 **Emergent Laparoscopic Colorectal Surgery** ... 303
Rodrigo Pedraza and Eric M. Haas

28 **Laparoscopy in the Elderly Patient** ... 309
Joshua I. S. Bleier and Brian R. Kann

29 **Laparoscopic Colectomy in the Obese Patient** ... 321
Arida Siripong and H. David Vargas

30 **Minimally Invasive Surgery in Crohn's Disease Patients** ... 337
Chang Sik Yu

31 **Minimally Invasive Surgery in Ulcerative Colitis Patients** ... 345
Marco E. Allaix and Alessandro Fichera

32 **Minimally Invasive Approaches to Colon and Rectal Diseases: Technique and Best Practices—Pediatrics** ... 357
Eric J. Krebill and Daniel J. Robertson

**33 Laparoscopy in Pregnant Patients** ........ 373
Melissa M. Alvarez-Downing and David J. Maron

**34 Economics of Laparoscopic Colectomy** ........ 381
Anthony J. Senagore

**35 Outcomes of Laparoscopic Surgery** ........ 385
Jennifer Leahy and Rocco Ricciardi

**Part VI Conclusions**

**36 Future Directions in Minimally Invasive Surgery** ........ 399
Howard M. Ross and Matthew Miller Philp

**Index** ........ 407

# Contributors

**Matthew R. Albert, MD, FACS, FASCRS** Department of Colorectal Surgery, Center for Colon and Rectal Surgery, Orlando, FL, USA

**Marco E. Allaix, MD** Department of Surgery, University of Pritzker School of Medicine Chicago, Chicago, IL, USA

**Melissa M. Alvarez-Downing, MD** Department of Colorectal Surgery, Cleveland Clinic Florida, Weston, FL, USA

**Andrea Chao Bafford, MD, FACS** Section of Colon and Rectal Surgery, Division of General and Oncologic Surgery, Department of Surgery, University of Maryland School of Medicine, Baltimore, MD, USA

**Joshua I.S. Bleier, MD, FACS, FASCRS** Division of Colon and Rectal Surgery, Pennsylvania Hospital, University of Pennsylvania, Philadelphia, PA, USA

**Jennifer S. Davids, MD** Division of Colorectal Surgery of Colon and Rectal Surgery, University of Massachusetts Memorial Hospital Center, Worcester, MA, USA

**Bradley R. Davis, MD** Department of Surgery, University of Cincinnati Medical Center, Cincinnati, OH, USA

**Mia DeBarros, MD** Department of Surgery, Madigan Army Medical Center, Fort Lewis, WA, USA

**Eric J. Dozois, MD** Division of Colon & Rectal Surgery, Department of Surgery, Mayo Clinic, Rochester, MN, USA

**Brian R. Englum, MD** Department of Surgery, Duke University Medical Center, Durham, NC, USA

**David A. Etzioni, MD, MSHS** Division of Colon and Rectal Surgery, Mayo Clinic College of Medicine, Phoenix, AZ, USA

**Daniel L. Feingold, MD** Department of Surgery, New York Presbyterian Hospital, Columbia University, New York, NY, USA

**Seth I. Felder, MD** Department of Colon and Rectal Surgery, Cedars-Sinai Medical Center, Los Angeles, CA, USA

**Alessandro Fichera, MD** Department of Surgery, University of Washington Medical Center, Seattle, WA, USA

**Phillip Fleshner, MD** Department of Colon and Rectal Surgery, Cedars-Sinai Medical Center, Los Angeles, CA, USA

**Todd D. Francone, MD, MPH** Department of Colon and Rectal Surgery, Lahey Health and Medical Center, Lahey Hospital and Medical Center, Tufts University Medical Center, Burlington, MA, USA

**Kelly A. Garrett, MD, FACS, FASCRS** Section of Colon and Rectal Surgery, Department of General Surgery, New York Presbyterian Hospital, Weill Cornell Medical College, New York, NY, USA

**Virgilio George, MD** Associate Professor of Surgery, Indiana University School of Medicine, Department of Surgery, Richard L. Roudebush VA Medical, Center, Indianapolis, IN, USA

**Emre Gorgun, MD, FACS** Department of Colon and Rectal Surgery, Digestive Disease Institute, Cleveland Clinic, Cleveland, OH, USA

**Eric M. Haas, MD, FACS, FASCRS** Division of Minimally Invasive Colon and Rectal Surgery, Department of Surgery, The University of Texas Medical School at Houston, Houston, TX, USA

**Amanda V. Hayman, MD, MPH** Division of Colon & Rectal Surgery, Department of Surgery, Mayo Clinic, Rochester, MN, USA

**M. Benjamin Hopkins, MD.** Department of Surgery, Duke Raleigh Hospital, Raleigh, NC, USA

**Steven Robert Hunt, MD** Department of Surgery, Barnes-Jewish Hospital, St. Louis, MO, USA

**Mehraneh Dorna Jafari, MD** Department of Surgery, University of California, Irvine School of Medicine, Orange, CA, USA

**Eric K. Johnson, MD, FACS, FASCRS** Associate Professor of Surgery, Uniformed Services University of the Health Sciences and Madigan Army Medical Center, Joint Base Lewis-McChord, WA, USA

**Brian R. Kann, MD, FACS, FASCRS** Division of Colon and Rectal Surgery, Pennsylvania Hospital, University of Pennsylvania, Philadelphia, PA, USA

**Eric J. Krebill, MD** Department of General Surgery Residency, Michigan State University, Grand Rapids, MI, USA

**Charlotte Kvasnovsky, MD, MPH** Department of Colorectal Surgery, King's College Hospital, University of Maryland School of Medicine, Baltimore, MD, USA

**Ron G. Landmann, MD, FACS, FASCRS** Department of Colon and Rectal Surgery, Mayo Clinic, Jacksonville, FL, USA

**Jennifer Leahy, BA, MS** Department of Colon and Rectal Surgery, Lahey Clinic, Burlington, MA, USA

**Sang W. Lee, MD, FACS, FASCRS** Division of Colon and Rectal Surgery, Department of Surgery, Weill-Cornell Medical College, New York Presbyterian Hospital, New York, NY, USA

**Steven Lee-Kong, MD** Department of Surgery, New York Presbyterian Hospital, Columbia University, New York, NY, USA

**Kirk A. Ludwig, MD** Division of Colorectal Surgery, Department of Surgery, Medical College of Wisconsin, Milwaukee, WI, USA

**David J. Maron, MD, MBA** Department of Colorectal Surgery, Cleveland Clinic Florida, Weston, FL, USA

**Justin A. Maykel, MD** Division of Colorectal Surgery of Colon and Rectal Surgery, University of Massachusetts Memorial Hospital Center, Worcester, MA, USA

**M. Shane McNevin, MD** Sacred Heart Hospital, Spokane, WA, USA

**John Migaly, MD** Department of Surgery, Duke University Medical Center, Durham, NC, USA

**Steven Mills, MD** Department of Surgery, Division of Colorectal Surgery, University of California, Irvine School of Medicine, Orange, CA, USA

**Jeffrey Milsom, MD** Center for Advanced Digestive Care, New York Presbyterian Hospital/Cornell, Weill Cornell Medical College, New York, NY, USA

**Tsunekazu Mizushima, MD, PhD** Department of Gastroenterological Surgery, Osaka University Graduate School of Medicine, Suita, Osaka, Japan

**Zuri Murrell, MD** Department of Colon and Rectal Surgery, Cedars-Sinai Medical Center, Los Angeles, CA, USA

**Mathew G. Mutch, MD, FACS, FASCRS** Section of Colon and Rectal Surgery, Barnes-Jewish Hospital, Washington University of Medicine, St. Louis, MO, USA

**Kiyokazu Nakajima, MD, FACS** Department of Gastroenterological Surgery, Osaka University Graduate School of Medicine, Suita, Osaka, Japan

**Govind Nandakumar, MD** Division of Colon and Rectal Surgery, Department of Surgery, Weill Cornell Medical School, New York, NY, USA

**Riichiro Nezu, MD, PhD** Department of Surgery, Nishinomiya Municipal Central Hospital, Nishinomiya, Hyogo, Japan

**Rodrigo Pedraza, MD** Division of Minimally Invasive Colon and Rectal Surgery, Department of Surgery, The University of Texas Medical School at Houston, Houston, TX, USA

**Matthew Miller Philp, MD** Division of Colon and Rectal Surgery, Department of Surgery, Temple University Hospital, Philadelphia, PA, USA

**Alessio Pigazzi, MD, PhD** Colorectal Surgery, University of California, Irvine Medical Center, Orange, CA, USA

**Francisco Quinteros, MD** Department of Colorectal Surgery, Center for Colon and Rectal Surgery, Orlando, FL, USA

**Rocco Ricciardi, MD, MPH** Department of Colon and Rectal Surgery, Lahey Clinic, Burlington, MA, USA

**Timothy Ridolfi, MD** Division of Colorectal Surgery, Department of Surgery, Medical College of Wisconsin, Milwaukee, WI, USA

**David E. Rivadeneira, MD, MBA, FACS, FASCRS** North Shore-LIJ Health System, Huntington Hospital, Hofstra University School of Medicine, Huntington, NY, USA

**Daniel J. Robertson, MD** Department of Pediatric Surgery, Helen Devos Children's Hospital, Grand Rapids, MI, USA

**Howard M. Ross, MD, FACS, FASCRS** Division of Colon and Rectal Surgery, Department of Surgery, Temple University Health System, Philadelphia, PA, USA

**Anthony J. Senagore, MD, MS, MBA** Department of Surgery, Central Michigan University, School of Medicine, Saginaw, MI, USA

**Arida Siripong, MD** Department of Colon and Rectal Surgery, Ochsner Clinic, New Orleans, LA, USA

**Toyooki Sonoda, MD** Section of Colon and Rectal Surgery, New York Presbyterian Hospital, Weill College of Cornell University, New York, NY, USA

**Michael J. Stamos, MD** Department of Surgery, Division of Colorectal Surgery, University of California, Irvine School of Medicine, Orange, CA, USA

**Scott R. Steele, MD, FACS, FASCRS** University of Washington, Seattle, WA, USA

Department of Surgery, Madigan Army Medical Center, Fort Lewis, WA, USA

**Kumaran Thiruppathy, FRCS, MBBS, MPhil, BSc** Department of Colorectal Surgery, Center for Colon and Rectal Surgery, Florida Hospital Orlando, Orlando, FL, USA

Department of Colorectal Surgery, Colchester General Hospital, UK

**Joshua A. Tyler, MD** Chief, Colon and Rectal Surgery, Department of General Surgery Keesler Medical Center, MS, USA

**H. David Vargas, MD, FACS, FASCRS** Department of Colon and Rectal Surgery, Ochsner Clinic, New Orleans, LA, USA

**Martin R. Weiser, MD** Department of Surgery, Memorial Sloan Kettering Cancer Center, Cornell Weill Medical College, Cornell University, New York, NY, USA

**Mark H. Whiteford, MD, FACS, FASCRS** Gastrointestinal and Minimally Invasive Surgery Division, The Oregon Clinic, Portland, OR, USA

Providence Cancer Center, Portland, OR, USA

Oregon Health & Science University, Portland, OR, USA

**Tonia M. Young-Fadok, MD, MS, FACS, FASCRS** Division of Colon and Rectal Surgery, Mayo Clinic College of Medicine, Phoenix, AZ, USA

**Chang Sik Yu, M.D, PhD** Department of Colon & Rectal Surgery, Asan Medical Center, University of Ulsan College of Medicine, Seoul, South Korea

# Part I

# Preoperative

# Perioperative Assessment

# 1

Charlotte Kvasnovsky and Andrea Chao Bafford

**Key Points**

- Pneumoperitoneum leads to increased cardiac preload and afterload, hypotension, increased airway pressures, increased end-tidal $CO_2$, and decreased urine output.
- Laparoscopic colorectal surgery is associated with decreases in postoperative pain, ileus, length of hospital stay, and wound complications, and improved cosmesis when compared to open surgery.
- Oncologic outcomes and IBD recurrence rates are similar after laparoscopic and open colectomy.
- Routine laboratory studies are recommended prior to laparoscopic colorectal surgery. More intensive cardiopulmonary testing should be reserved for symptomatic patients and those with significant risk factors.
- Laparoscopic surgery can be safely performed in elderly and obese patients as well as in certain cases of emergency and reoperative surgery.
- Bowel preparation should generally be used in order to improve maneuverability of the bowel and to allow for intraoperative endoscopy.
- Colorectal tumors should be localized with 4-quadrant tattooing and Crohn's lesions with imaging and endoscopy prior to surgery.
- Patients should be securely positioned with arms tucked and legs apart (for left colon and rectal procedures).
- Judicious fluid administration, early feeding and mobilization, and minimization of narcotics should be part of postoperative care.

**Electronic supplementary material:** Supplementary material is available in the online version of this chapter at 10.1007/978-1-4939-1581-1_1. Videos can also be accessed at http://www.springerimages.com/videos/978-1-4939-1580-4.

C. Kvasnovsky, M.D., M.P.H.
Department of Colorectal Surgery, King's College Hospital, University of Maryland School of Medicine, Baltimore, MD, USA
e-mail: ckvasno@gmail.com

A.C. Bafford, M.D., F.A.C.S. (✉)
Section of Colon and Rectal Surgery, Division of General and Oncologic Surgery, Department of Surgery, University of Maryland School of Medicine, 29 S. Greene St., Suite 600, Baltimore, MD 21201, USA
e-mail: abafford@smail.umaryland.edu

## Physiologic Effects of Laparoscopy

Pneumoperitoneum is the sine qua non of laparoscopic surgery. Insufflation of the abdomen has both mechanical and physiologic effects. These changes become especially relevant in colorectal surgery, where positioning varies steeply over the course of operations. Colorectal operations may also be prolonged, which can further amplify effects.

Although less than ideal, carbon dioxide ($CO_2$) is currently the primary gas being used in laparoscopic surgery. The ideal gas would be noncombustible, colorless, and have limited physiologic effects. Because electrocautery is commonly used in laparoscopic surgery, combustible gases are absolutely contraindicated [1]. This precludes the use of oxygen, room air (which is 21 % oxygen), and nitrous oxide. Meanwhile, helium and argon as inert gases would fulfill the requirement of nonflammability; however, they have lower thresholds for toxicity. $CO_2$ remains the gas of choice. Transperitoneal absorption of $CO_2$ results in increased dissolved $CO_2$ in the blood, which can create a mild acidosis and hypercapnia.

Pneumoperitoneum causes further physiologic effects that may influence decision-making in colorectal surgery. The majority of these changes will be well tolerated in ASA I and II patients (Table 1.1). For those with higher ASA grades, the effect is highly variable and often more problematic.

### Cardiovascular Effects

There are many cardiovascular and hemodynamic changes during laparoscopic surgery as well as concomitant changes with positioning (Table 1.2). These do not usually affect

H.M. Ross et al. (eds.), *Minimally Invasive Approaches to Colon and Rectal Disease: Technique and Best Practices*, DOI 10.1007/978-1-4939-1581-1_1, © Springer Science+Business Media New York 2015

**Table 1.1** American Society of Anesthesiologists (ASA) grades

| ASA grade | Status | Absolute mortality (%) |
|---|---|---|
| 1 | Normal healthy patient | 0.1 |
| 2 | Mild systemic disease or patient over 80 years old | 0.2 |
| 3 | Systemic disease that causes definite functional limitation on life | 1.8 |
| 4 | Severe systemic disease that is a constant threat to life | 7.8 |
| 5 | Moribund patient unlikely to survive 24 h without surgery | 9.4 |

**Table 1.2** Summary of physiologic effects with pneumoperitoneum and positioning

| | Pneumoperi-toneum | Magnified in Trendelen-burg | Magnified in reverse Trendelenburg |
|---|---|---|---|
| *Cardiovascular changes* | | | |
| Systemic vascular resistance (SVR) | Increases | Yes | |
| Central venous pressure (CVP) | Increases | Yes | |
| Mean arterial pressure (MAP) | Decreases | Yes | |
| Cardiac output (CO) | Decreases | | Yes |
| *Respiratory changes* | | | |
| Airway resistance | Increases | | |
| Pulmonary capillary wedge pressure (PCWP) | Increases | Yes | |
| Functional residual capacity (FRC) | Decreases | Yes | |
| Chest wall compliance | Decreases | | |
| *Renal changes* | | | |
| Renal function | Decreases | | |
| Urine output | Decreases | | |
| *Acid–base changes* | Respiratory acidosis | | |

cardiac output in healthier patients but can be important in patients with preexisting cardiovascular disease [2]. Important changes include hypotension, decreased preload, and increased afterload. Pneumoperitoneum results in decreased venous return, decreased right-sided heart filling, and decreased cardiac output, resulting in the potential for hypotension if systemic vascular resistance cannot compensate.

## Pulmonary Effects

The respiratory changes seen in laparoscopic surgery result from a combination of the mechanical effects of pneumoperitoneum, patient positioning, and carbon dioxide absorption. Mechanical effects relate to displacement of the lungs due to increased intra-abdominal pressure. As the diaphragm is elevated, increases in peak inspiratory pressure, plateau pressures, and end-tidal $CO_2$ are seen [3]. Lung compliance may decrease by as much as half during laparoscopy [4].

Carbon dioxide is continually added during insufflation; therefore, it continuously dissolves in blood, increasing arterial and alveolar $CO_2$. This increase in alveolar carbon dioxide is routinely monitored intraoperatively by following end-tidal carbon dioxide levels. Hypercarbia can usually be counteracted by an increasing respiratory rate; however, with prolonged cases, steep positioning, and underlying pulmonary disease, it can be difficult to manage.

## Renal Effects

Laparoscopic surgery is associated with decreased urine output. In part, this is secondary to the negative effect of pneumoperitoneum on renal blood flow. This can be exacerbated by bowel preparation, which depletes intravascular volume even before the operation begins. While a normal goal for urine output is 1–2 ml/kg/h, this should be halved in laparoscopy [5]. This decrease, does not affect renal function postoperatively. It is important to ensure that anesthesia providers (especially those in training) are aware of this effect, such that excess intraoperative fluid administration which may cause untoward effects postoperatively can be avoided.

## Benefits of Laparoscopy

Laparoscopic colorectal surgery has grown in prevalence since the first described laparoscopic colectomy in 1991. As of 2006, approximately one in three elective colorectal operations is being performed laparoscopically [6] and likely approaching 50 % currently.

Evidence now shows that laparoscopic surgery is safe in benign disease. Patients have faster recoveries, shorter length of hospital stay, decreased ileus [7], and lower morbidity following laparoscopic surgery [7–10]. This is true for such varied operations as rectopexy for rectal prolapse [10] and elective resection for diverticular disease. Indeed, in a randomized controlled trial of elective surgery for diverticulitis, patients undergoing laparoscopic surgery had lower incidence of major complications, such as anastomotic leak, intra-abdominal bleeding, abscess, and evisceration [11]. Biomarker studies have also pointed to decreased surgical trauma following laparoscopic compared to open colectomy [12].

Patients with inflammatory bowel disease are also ideal candidates for laparoscopic surgery, though these procedures may be some of the most technically challenging. Benign conditions do not require extended lymphadenectomy or wide mesenteric excision. Furthermore, patients are often young and undergo multiple procedures over their lifetime. They are highly likely to benefit from the decreased adhesions and improved cosmesis following laparoscopic surgery. This has been borne out in laparoscopic ileocecal resection for Crohn's disease [13], where a meta-analysis showed decreased morbidity and shorter hospital stay. Randomized trials have shown similar rates of recurrent disease and better body image in patients postoperatively [14]. A Cochrane review of laparoscopic ileal pouch-anal anastomosis (IPAA) for ulcerative colitis, however, found little difference with regard to overall morbidity [15]. Operative times were longer when IPAA was performed laparoscopically, and unlike all other laparoscopic colorectal operations, hospital stays were the same as in open surgery.

There is now level 1 evidence to support laparoscopy in surgery for colon cancer [16]. The COST non-inferiority randomized trial demonstrated similar overall survival and recurrence rates between open and laparoscopic surgery [17]. In addition to equivalent oncologic outcomes, multiple clinical trials have now also consistently shown lower perioperative mortality, fewer wound complications, less blood loss, and reduced postoperative pain scores with a reduction in narcotic requirements after laparoscopic surgery [18–21]. In spite of early concerns over port-site metastasis, cancer recurrence in wounds is similar to the 0–1 % seen in open surgery [17, 19].

Laparoscopic surgery for rectal cancer is often even more technically challenging and may be best recommended only in a clinical trial setting until we await further data [22]. Several trials are ongoing to provide more high-quality data on outcomes following laparoscopic rectal surgery for cancer (COLOR II, JCOG 0404, ACOSOG Z6051). Early data suggests similar oncologic outcomes in experienced hands [23].

In sum, previous concerns over the safety of laparoscopic surgery for both benign and malignant conditions have been dispelled. We anticipate that the rates of laparoscopic surgery will continue to grow over the coming years.

## Preoperative Evaluation for Elective Patients

Proper preoperative patient assessment is the first step in improving outcomes following laparoscopic colorectal surgery. While there are many similarities between the preoperative evaluation of patients for laparoscopic and open surgery, nuances do exist. Decisions for preoperative testing and evaluation should be made in conjunction with the anesthesiology staff, medical physicians, and the surgeon. Laparoscopic colorectal surgery will generally be performed under general anesthesia with endotracheal intubation; patients must therefore be able to tolerate a general anesthetic.

Increasing evidence is supporting laparoscopy in emergency colorectal surgery patients. In these patients, a thorough preoperative evaluation may not be possible (see below—"Special Patient Populations"), yet even a brief evaluation can often identify risk factors for perioperative comorbidity that can be closely monitored and intervened upon.

### Laboratory Testing

Anesthesiologists have mixed opinions regarding the need for specific preoperative laboratory screening, as there is little controlled data to support guidelines [24]. In general, all patients undergoing an abdominal surgery should have routine laboratory tests drawn, including hemoglobin, serum chemistry, and coagulation studies. Women of childbearing age must have a urine pregnancy test. For patients with colorectal malignancies, a CEA level should be drawn prior to definitive surgery as levels may be followed postoperatively to monitor for recurrence.

The American Diabetes Association recommends preoperative screening for diabetes in overweight patients (BMI $\geq$ 25) with one additional risk factor, such as hypertension, family history, or inactivity [25]. Some experts suggest a fasting blood glucose level drawn on the morning of surgery [26]. We prefer to screen patients prior to the day of surgery.

There is some evidence to support checking random hemoglobin A1C levels in patients without diabetes. For instance, one study found that nondiabetic patients with a preoperative hemoglobin A1C above 6.0 were more likely to have complications after major colorectal surgery [27]. Additionally, the stress of surgery may unmask borderline diabetic (i.e., insulin resistant) patients, significantly affecting their ability to control glucose levels, postoperatively.

### Cardiac Evaluation

Cardiac evaluation may be advisable for patients with known cardiac or other systemic diseases. There is limited evidence to support routine preoperative electrocardiogram in patients without documented coronary artery disease or other risk factors for cardiac disease, such as peripheral arterial disease and cerebrovascular disease [25, 28].

All laparoscopic colorectal procedures are considered of intermediate risk. In such cases, the American Heart Association (AHA) recommends stress testing only in patients with an active cardiac condition, designated AHA class I. This includes patients with unstable or severe angina, recent myocardial infarction, decompensated heart failure, significant arrhythmia, or severe valvular disease [25].

Additionally, AHA class II patients may require cardiac stress testing if the testing will change management. This includes patients with intermediate risk factors, such as a history of ischemic heart disease, prior heart failure, cerebrovascular disease, diabetes mellitus, and/or renal insufficiency. For patients in whom the decision for stress testing is unclear, it may be best to discuss planning with the anesthesia staff that will be performing the operation. Although recent evidence shows increasing overuse of preoperative stress testing resulting in higher costs, [29] it is incumbent on the surgery team to identify patients at risk and evaluate them properly.

### Pulmonary Evaluation

Current guidelines do not support preoperative pulmonary function testing in patients without evidence of preexisting lung disease for non-thoracic surgery [30]. Patients with chronic obstructive pulmonary disease (COPD) or other pulmonary disorders should be considered for spirometry prior to surgery. Further testing should be based on the results and degree of dysfunction. Patients on steroid inhalers and bronchodilators should be identified to ensure that these medications are taken as scheduled perioperatively.

## Special Patient Populations

There is no patient population in whom laparoscopic surgery has been proven unsafe. One study even suggests equivalent outcomes in the hemodynamically unstable patient [31], long considered an absolute contraindication to laparoscopy. There are, however, special patient populations and situations to consider.

### The Elderly

Elderly patients may be the least able to tolerate the increased operative times seen in laparoscopic surgery, as they more often have diminished cardiopulmonary reserve. Preoperative cardiovascular evaluation in these patients should be carried out according to the AHA guidelines described above. Noninvasive testing may also be considered in elderly patients with poor functional capacity if it will change management [25]. Studies have shown similar postoperative outcomes in octogenarian patients compared to younger patients following laparoscopic colorectal surgery [32]. We tend to favor laparoscopic surgery for elderly patients as they may especially benefit from decreased postoperative pain and shorter recovery times. Drs. Bleier and Kann present an in-depth discussion on the evaluation, technical aspects, and outcomes for minimally invasive approaches in the elderly in Chap. 28.

### Morbidly Obese Patients

Obesity is a risk factor for worse postoperative outcome, both because surgery is more technically difficult in obese patients and because obese patients often have comorbid conditions, such as hypertension and diabetes. Results of studies examining body mass index (BMI) as a risk factor for poor outcome have been mixed, with some showing higher rates of conversion and postoperative complication [33] and others showing no difference [34]. Given the well-described benefits of laparoscopic colorectal surgery (accelerated recovery of bowel function, decreased postoperative pain, shorter hospital stay, as discussed above) and the fact that surgery in obese patients can be technically challenging regardless of operative technique, we recommend laparoscopy. Surgeons should be prepared for longer operative times in these patients. Also, specialized equipment including footboards, safety straps, large-size operating room tables, and extra-long laparoscopic instruments must be made available. Please see Chap. 29 for a more detailed discussion by Drs. Siripong and Vargas on laparoscopy in the obese patient.

### Emergency Colorectal Surgery Patients

Accumulating evidence also supports laparoscopic surgery in emergency colorectal surgery patients. For instance, Myers et al. [35] demonstrated the feasibility of laparoscopic peritoneal lavage in the treatment of 100 patients with perforated diverticulitis. All eight patients presenting with Hinchey grade 4 diverticulitis were treated with a Hartmann's procedure. The remaining 92 study patients had Hinchey grades 2 and 3 disease and were treated with laparoscopic peritoneal lavage. Only two required postoperative intervention for pelvic abscesses and two represented with diverticulitis after a median follow-up of 36 months. Additional randomized clinical trials evaluating laparoscopic peritoneal lavage for the treatment of complicated diverticulitis are ongoing [36, 37]. Studies have also demonstrated the safe and effective use of laparoscopic colectomy for other emergent indications, including gastrointestinal bleeding, colonic obstruction, and colonic perforation [38]. The preoperative evaluation of emergency colorectal surgery patients is limited to rapid and critical tests, including assessment of cardiovascular vital signs, volume status, hematocrit, electrolytes, renal function, urine analysis, and ECG. These allow the surgeon and anesthesiologist to tailor both operative strategy and perioperative monitoring and resuscitation accordingly. Additional tests and interventions are deferred until after surgery. Dr. Haas and colleagues present an excellent overview of minimally invasive approaches in the emergent setting in Chap. 27.

## Reoperative Surgery

Although Dr. Migaly presents a more comprehensive review of the use of a minimally invasive approach for reoperative surgery in Chap. 20, a few points pertinent to preoperative assessment are warranted. Laparoscopic reoperative surgery can be technically challenging, although reoperation after laparoscopic surgery is often less difficult than after open surgery [39]. Adhesions and dilated bowel may preclude adequate visualization. However, as long as a sufficient field of view can be established and bleeding and contamination can be controlled, laparoscopy is safe in the management of complications, such as postoperative bleeding and anastomotic leak. Peritoneal access via an open (Hasson) technique should be considered in reoperative laparoscopy [40]. Patients must be counseled that there is an increased likelihood of prolonged operative times, conversion to open surgery, and risk for inadvertent enterotomy or other visceral injury. Surgeons preparing for reoperative laparoscopic surgery should obtain previous operative records in order to anticipate such challenges as extensive adhesions and prosthetic meshes. This knowledge may facilitate safe trocar placement and allow for customized preoperative interventions, including placement of ureteral stents.

## Preoperative Management

Our individualized approach to perioperative patient management is multifaceted. Some of the considerations are important for all patients, while others are more specific to certain patient populations or operations.

### Bowel Preparation

Bowel preparation in colorectal surgery remains controversial. Studies have shown no difference in rates of surgical site infection or anastomotic leak with or without bowel preparation [41, 42]. Furthermore, bowel preparation may predispose patients to dehydration and electrolyte abnormalities, particularly in the elderly [43]. However, there are several benefits to bowel preparation specifically for laparoscopic surgery. First, as the bowel is lighter and more compressible after mechanical preparation, manipulation with instruments is easier and more ergonomically favorable. Additionally, laparoscopic colorectal surgery often relies on gravity to serve as a bowel retractor; this is often more effective with an empty colon. A prepared colon also allows for intraoperative endoscopy to localize a tumor if necessary and/or to assess left-sided anastomoses after creation for intactness, leak, and hemostasis. A final benefit is easier specimen extraction, possibly through smaller extraction incisions. In a combined statement, the Society of Alimentary Gastrointestinal Endoscopic Surgeons and the American Society of Colon and Rectal Surgeons endorsed the use of mechanical bowel preparations in laparoscopic colorectal surgery [44].

### Preoperative Fasting

Patients routinely fast for over 8 h prior to surgery in an effort to avoid pulmonary aspiration, in spite of the lack of evidence in support of this practice [45, 46]. The best evidence suggests preoperative fasting should begin 2 h prior to operation for liquids and 6 h for solid foods [45]. An exception to this rule may be diabetic patients with known neuropathy, who are at risk of delayed gastric emptying [47].

### Lesion Localization

Preoperative lesion localization is important in laparoscopic surgery, where tactile feedback is reduced. The site of colorectal tumors should routinely be marked. Colonoscopic tattooing of lesions with India ink is the gold standard [48, 49]. However, in as many as one in five cases, the tattoo will not be evident at surgery [50]. Four-quadrant tattooing may improve the likelihood that the tattoo will be visualized and not hidden on the mesenteric or retroperitoneal side of the colon (Video 1.1) [51].

Preoperative mapping is also important in benign conditions, such as in Crohn's disease, where skip lesions are not uncommon. This is especially true in cases of reoperative surgery, as adhesions may preclude safe running of the bowel. Disease localization can be accomplished using imaging studies, such as enterography, and also via endoscopy.

### Ostomy Marking

Patients undergoing colorectal surgery may require temporary or permanent fecal diversion. Whenever possible, patients should undergo preoperative marking and education by an enterostomal therapist in order to decrease postoperative stoma complications [52]. It is often important to mark not only the primary suggested site but other potential stoma sites as alternative options as well, in case the disease pathology prohibits stoma placement in the optimal location (Figs. 1.1 and 1.2). Of note, there is some evidence that parastomal hernias are more common after laparoscopic surgery, especially when the surgical specimen is extracted through the future ostomy site [53]. We therefore recommend avoiding stoma site specimen extraction in cases of permanent stoma creation.

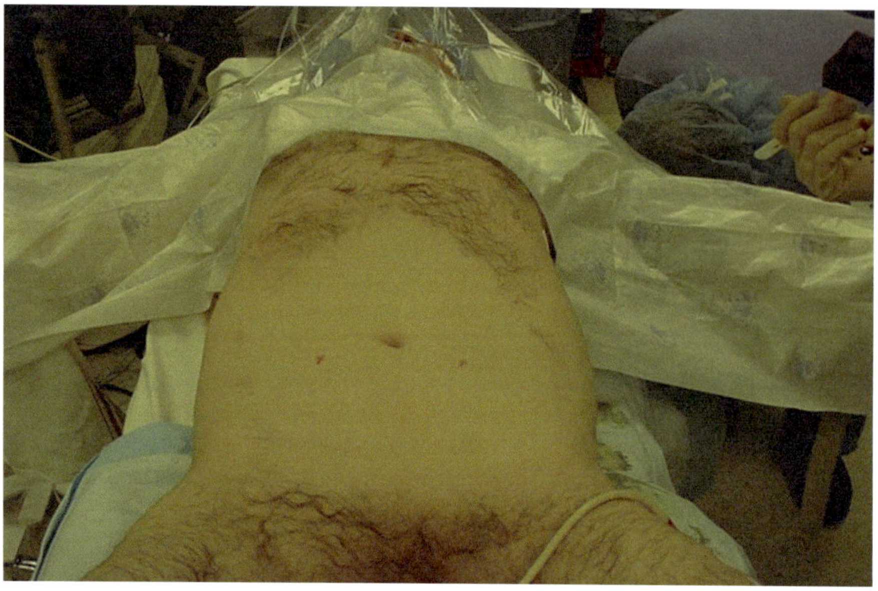

**Fig. 1.1** Preoperative marking of possible stoma sites

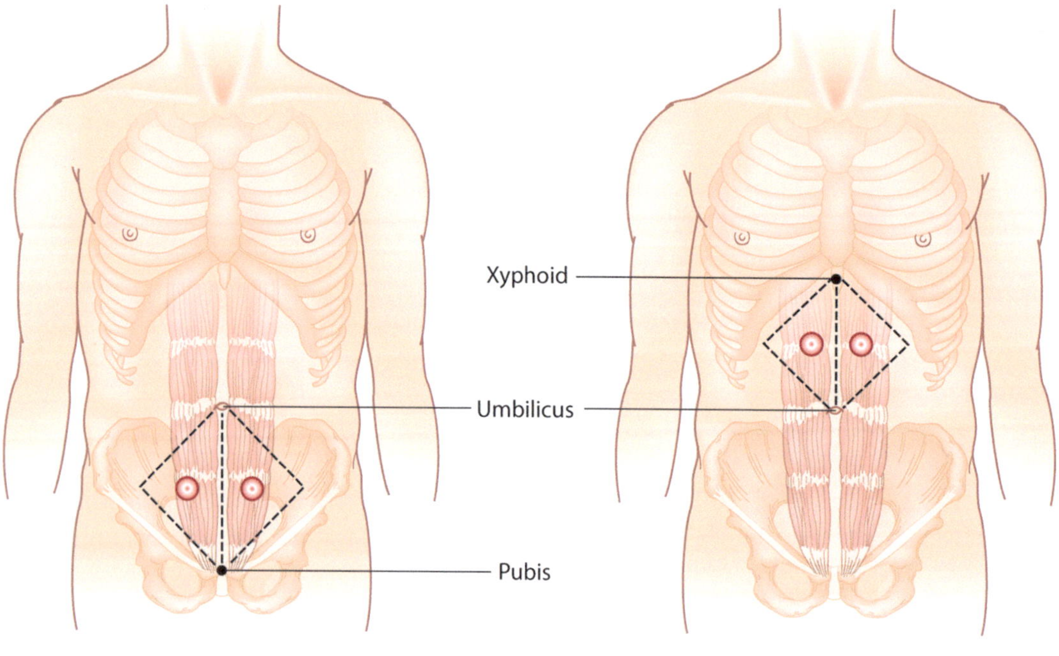


**Fig. 1.2** Ostomy triangle stoma site marking

## Corticosteroids

Previously steroid-dependent IBD patients may exhibit some degree of adrenal insufficiency for up to 1 year after discontinuing therapy [54]. Because of concern for cardiovascular collapse due to surgical stress, patients are often given high-dose steroids perioperatively, with little evidence to support this practice. In fact, recent studies have shown no evidence of hemodynamical instability when low- rather than high-dose corticosteroids are administered around surgery [55, 56]. The exception to this is patients with primary disease of the hypothalamic-pituitary-adrenal axis [56].

A prospective study assessing perioperative steroid dosing in patients with IBD is underway. It is our typical practice to continue steroids at their preoperative dose levels rather than administer "stress" doses perioperatively. Postoperative steroid tapering is then adjusted according to the chronicity of patients' preoperative exposure; most commonly prednisone is used and tapered by 5 mg/week.

## Perioperative Antibiotics

Surgical site infections are the leading cause of postoperative morbidity and mortality in colorectal surgery, whether laparoscopic or open. Prophylactic antibiotics are known to decrease the risk of infection. A single dose administered within 60 min of incision and discontinuation of therapy within 24 h of surgery are generally advised [57]. Second-generation beta-lactam antibiotics, such as cefoxitin and cefotetan, are established choices. The addition of preoperative oral antibiotics to mechanical bowel preparation was once the standard of care following the influential work of Nichols et al. in the 1970s [58]. More recently, however, a move away from mechanical bowel preparation occurred after studies failed to demonstrate an associated improvement in rates of infectious complications [42]. Oral antibiotic administration was similarly abandoned, largely because the efficacy of this practice was not established in uncleansed bowel. New studies show decreased rates of surgical site infection when oral antibiotics are given, with or without concomitant mechanical bowel preparation [59, 60]. Accordingly, our colorectal patients receive erythromycin and neomycin on the day prior to surgery.

## Analgesic Considerations

Though epidural anesthesia appears to improve analgesia and decrease ileus after open colorectal surgery [61], there is a paucity of data assessing the benefits of postoperative analgesic regimens following laparoscopy. In one recent trial, patients with spinal analgesia or patient-controlled analgesia had shorter length of stay and faster return of bowel function as compared to epidural analgesia [62]. We currently do not recommend routine epidural placement prior to laparoscopic colorectal surgery. Epidural anesthesia should be considered, however, in certain circumstances, such as in patients with a history of chronic pain and chronic narcotic use and also those in whom a high likelihood of conversion to open surgery is expected.

## Consent

There are risks specific to laparoscopic surgery that must be included in the informed consent. First is the possibility of conversion to open surgery. Conversion rates depend on patient-specific, surgeon-specific, and procedure-specific factors. Patient-specific factors include older age, male gender, higher ASA, and higher BMI. Low rectal surgery, presence of adhesions, abscess, phlegmon, or fistula and higher T-stage are operation-specific factors that increase conversion. Finally, junior surgeons are more likely to convert to open procedures than their more experienced counterparts. Based on these results, the "Cleveland Clinic Colorectal Laparoscopic Conversion Score" was created to aid surgeons in predicting conversion rates for specific procedures [63]. A meta-analysis found conversion rates from 4.8 to 29.2 % in Crohn's disease [13]. Rates are similar in oncologic surgery, ranging from 11 to 23 % in large series [17, 19]. Consent should also include the increased risk of iatrogenic ureteral injury associated with laparoscopic colorectal surgery, which is around 0.66 % according to one retrospective series [64].

# Intraoperative Management

## Patient Monitoring

Standard intraoperative monitors include a five-lead electrocardiogram, blood pressure cuff, and pulse oximeter. End-tidal $CO_2$ monitors may also be used, as most patients will be endotracheally intubated. Pneumoperitoneum with carbon dioxide likely contributes to intraoperative hypothermia [65]. Therefore, patients should routinely be covered with upper-body forced-air heating devices to maintain normothermia. There is currently insufficient evidence to support heated carbon dioxide insufflation to reduce hypothermia or postoperative pain [66].

Select patients may benefit from more invasive monitoring, such as those with severe cardiopulmonary disease or hemodynamic instability. Arterial lines allow for precise and timely hemodynamic measurements. They also allow for rapid arterial blood gas determinations. Central venous pressure monitoring, Swan-Ganz catheter measurements, and intraoperative transesophageal echocardiography may also be considered for severely ill patients, but are usually not necessary in colorectal surgery patients.

## Patient Positioning

Patient positioning is important both for ease of operation and patient safety. A right hemicolectomy is generally performed in supine position, while the modified lithotomy position is chosen for left-sided or rectal surgery. The latter provides access to the rectum for anastomosis creation and/or intraoperative endoscopy. Trendelenburg positioning facilitates pelvic surgery, as it allows the small bowel to fall out of the pelvis and into the upper abdomen. By tucking the patient's arms, the surgeon is afforded the flexibility to change where he or she stands throughout the procedure. Finally, patients should be properly padded and belted to allow for safe intraoperative position changes. Drs. Mills and Stamos provide a thorough review of patient positioning tips in Chap. 2.

Trendelenburg positioning does not significantly affect intra-abdominal pressure or respiratory compliance [67]. It does, however, lead to increases in both venous return and cardiac preload [68]. Lithotomy position redistributes blood away from the legs, also increasing preload. Meanwhile, reverse Trendelenburg position reduces venous return, leading to decreases in cardiac output and arterial pressure.

## Venous Thromboembolism (VTE) Prevention

Patients undergoing colorectal surgery, whether or not for malignancy, appear to be at higher risk for VTE compared to patients undergoing general or other surgeries [69]. Reasons for this are unclear but may relate to pelvic dissection, patient disease, and/or patient positioning. Pneumoperitoneum has been shown to promote lower extremity venous stasis in gastric bypass patients [70]. Data in colorectal surgery patients, however, is lacking. The American Society of Colon and Rectal Surgeons (ASCRS) recommends that patients undergoing a laparoscopic colorectal procedure receive VTE prophylaxis according to the same risk-based guidelines used by the American College of Chest Physicians (ACCP) for the equivalent open procedure. That is, moderate- to high-risk patients should receive prophylaxis with unfractionated (LDUH) or low-molecular-weight heparin (LMWH), and those at the highest risk should receive both mechanical and heparin prophylaxis [71, 72].

## Urinary Drainage and Ureteral Stenting

Placement of a urinary catheter allows for both bladder decompression and intraoperative monitoring of urinary output. This is helpful both as a marker of volume status and resuscitation. The catheter can generally be removed on postoperative day one with low risk of urinary retention [73]. Longer duration of urinary drainage should be considered after low anterior and abdominoperineal resection, as these procedures may be associated with higher retention rates [74]. Minimizing perioperative fluid resuscitation may decrease the incidence of urinary retention [75].

Laparoscopic colorectal surgery appears to carry a higher risk of iatrogenic ureteral injury compared to open surgery [64]. Preoperative ureteral stent placement attempts to minimize this risk but has been shown to translate more to improved ability for intraoperative identification of injuries rather than a decrease in the overall rate of injury. Stents are typically used in patients with more complicated pathology, including previous pelvic surgery, irradiation, complicated diverticulitis, obesity, invasive malignancy, and closure of Hartmann's colostomy [76]. Lighted ureteral stents may aid in intraoperative visualization (Video 1.2) [77].

## Gastric Decompression

Intraoperative orogastric or nasogastric decompression is routine as increased abdominal pressure in laparoscopy places patients at risk for regurgitation and aspiration [78]. Accumulated data favors tube discontinuation postoperatively in order to enhance return of bowel function and decrease pulmonary complications [79].

## Availability of Endoscopy

Endoscopy has been used for both lesion identification and evaluation of left-sided and low rectal anastomoses. Carbon dioxide is much more rapidly absorbed than air and therefore facilitates intraoperative endoscopy by avoiding persistent dilation of the colon and small bowel during the remaining portion of surgery. We therefore highly recommend that a $CO_2$ insufflation device be made available for laparoscopic colon procedures. If not available, serial clamping of the proximal colon with an atraumatic grasper, such as a Debakey, should be performed to minimize dilation as much as possible. Simultaneous insufflation of $CO_2$ into the peritoneal cavity and the colon lumen was shown to be safe in one pilot study [80].

# Postoperative Care

Postoperative care is a continuation of pre- and intraoperative care. Enhanced recovery after surgery (ERAS) is a widely used comprehensive set of largely evidence-based protocols for surgery [81]. Nevertheless, the care of each patient should be individualized.

## ERAS

Professors Ken Fearon and Olle Ljungqvist assembled the ERAS Study Group in 2001, furthering multimodal surgical care ideas proposed by Professor Henrik Kehlet in the 1990s. Their mission was to improve perioperative care and recovery through the development and implementation of evidence-based practices [82]. Pre- and intraoperative guidelines concerning codified counseling, bowel preparation, fasting, VTE

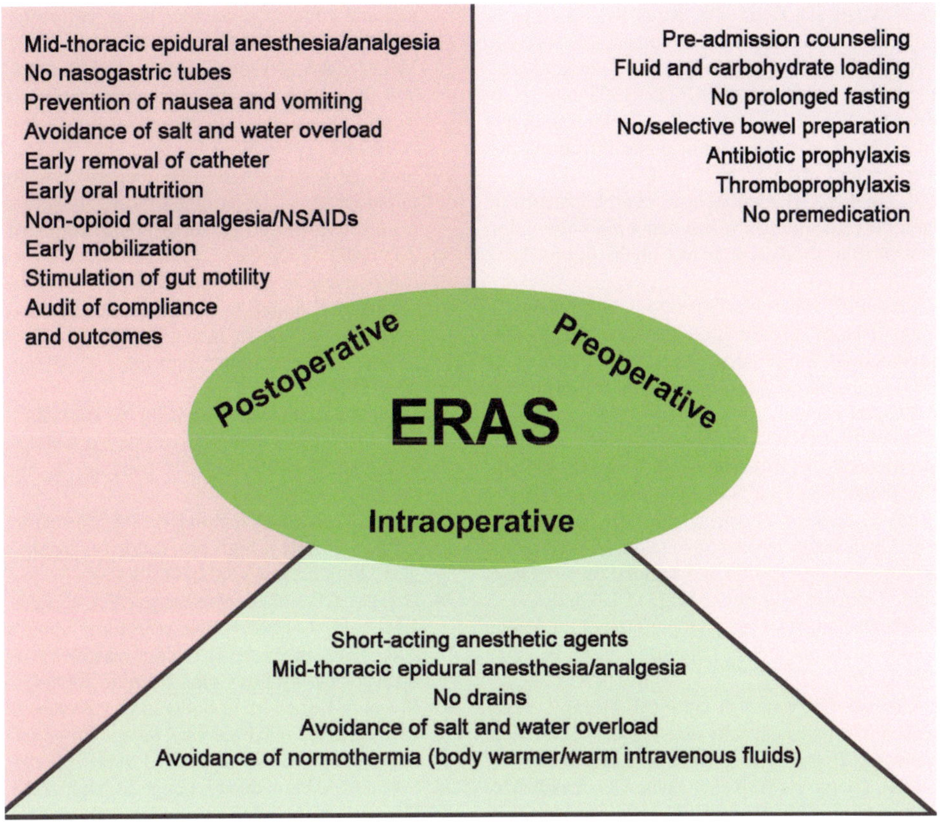


**Fig. 1.3** Components of an enhanced recovery after surgery (ERAS) protocol. Courtesy of Professor O. Ljungqvist and the ERAS Society (www.erassociety.org), with permission

prophylaxis, antimicrobial prophylaxis, anesthetic protocol, prevention and treatment of postoperative nausea and vomiting, nasogastric tube decompression, prevention of intraoperative hypothermia, perioperative fluid management, and peritoneal and urinary drainage are described (Fig. 1.3) [82]. Laparoscopic surgery is advocated to improve short-term outcomes. With regard to postoperative care, the authors recommend (1) the use of narcotic-sparing analgesics, such as acetaminophen and nonsteroidal anti-inflammatory drugs; (2) oral diet at will after surgery, including oral nutritional supplements starting on the day of surgery; and (3) early mobilization beginning 2 h postoperatively.

## Summary

Laparoscopic colorectal surgery begins with careful patient selection and preoperative evaluation. Because of the decreased tactile feedback associated with laparoscopy and to minimize unnecessary abdominal exploration, particularly in the setting of adhesions, preoperative mapping of target anatomy is imperative. Combining these steps with evidence-driven perioperative care allows for optimal patient outcomes following laparoscopic colon and rectal surgery.

## References

1. Neuhaus SJ, Gupta A, Watson DI. Helium and other alternative insufflation gases for laparoscopy. Surg Endosc. 2001;15(6): 553–60.
2. Larsen JF, Svendsen FM, Pedersen V. Randomized clinical trial of the effect of pneumoperitoneum on cardiac function and haemodynamics during laparoscopic cholecystectomy. Br J Surg. 2004; 91(7):848–54.
3. Suh MK, Seong KW, Jung SH, Kim SS. The effect of pneumoperitoneum and Trendelenburg position on respiratory mechanics during pelviscopic surgery. Korean J Anesthesiol. 2010;59(5):329–34.
4. Bardoczky GI, Engelman E, Levarlet M, Simon P. Ventilatory effects of pneumoperitoneum monitored with continuous spirometry. Anaesthesia. 1993;48(4):309–11.
5. Nguyen NT, Perez RV, Fleming N, Rivers R, Wolfe BM. Effect of prolonged pneumoperitoneum on intraoperative urine output during laparoscopic gastric bypass. J Am Coll Surg. 2002;195(4): 476–83.
6. Hedrick T, Turrentine F, Sanfey H, Schirmer B, Friel C. Implications of laparoscopy on surgery residency training. Am J Surg. 2009; 197(1):73–5.
7. Scuderi PE, James RL, Harris L, Mims 3rd GR. Multimodal antiemetic management prevents early postoperative vomiting after outpatient laparoscopy. Anesth Analg. 2000;91(6):1408–14.
8. Benoist S, Panis Y, Beaufour A, Bouhnik Y, Matuchansky C, Valleur P. Laparoscopic ileocecal resection in Crohn's disease: a case-matched comparison with open resection. Surg Endosc. 2003;17(5): 814–8.

9. Kirat HT, Pokala N, Vogel JD, Fazio VW, Kiran RP. Can laparoscopic ileocolic resection be performed with comparable safety to open surgery for regional enteritis: data from national surgical quality improvement program. Am Surg. 2010;76(12):1393–6.
10. Magruder JT, Efron JE, Wick EC, Gearhart SL. Laparoscopic rectopexy for rectal prolapse to reduce surgical-site infections and length of stay. World J Surg. 2013;37(5):1110–4.
11. Klarenbeek BR, Veenhof AA, Bergamaschi R, et al. Laparoscopic sigmoid resection for diverticulitis decreases major morbidity rates: a randomized control trial: short-term results of the Sigma Trial. Ann Surg. 2009;249(1):39–44.
12. Hildebrandt U, Kessler K, Plusczyk T, Pistorius G, Vollmar B, Menger MD. Comparison of surgical stress between laparoscopic and open colonic resections. Surg Endosc. 2003;17(2):242–6.
13. Tan JJY, Tjandra JJ. Laparoscopic surgery for Crohn's disease: a meta-analysis. Dis Colon Rectum. 2007;50(5):576–85.
14. Stocchi L, Milsom JW, Fazio VW. Long-term outcomes of laparo scopic versus open ileocolic resection for Crohn's disease: follow-up of a prospective randomized trial. Surgery. 2008;144(4):622–7.
15. Ahmed Ali U, Keus F, Heikens JT, Bemelman WA, Berdah SV, Gooszen HG, et al. Open versus laparoscopic (assisted) ileo pouch anal anastomosis for ulcerative colitis and familial adenomatous polyposis. Cochrane Database Syst Rev. 2009;(1):CD006267.
16. Liska D, Lee SW, Nandakumar G. Laparoscopic surgery for benign and malignant colorectal diseases. Surg Laparosc Endosc Percutan Tech. 2012;22(3):165–74.
17. Nelson H, The Clinical Outcomes of Surgical Therapy Study Group. A comparison of laparoscopically assisted and open colectomy for colon cancer. N Engl J Med. 2004;350(20):2050–9.
18. Guillou PJ, Quirke P, Thorpe H, Walker J, Jayne DG, Smith AM, et al. Short-term endpoints of conventional versus laparoscopic-assisted surgery in patients with colorectal cancer (MRC CLASICC trial): multicentre, randomised controlled trial. Lancet. 2005;365(9472):1718–26.
19. Lacy AM, Garcia-Valdecasas JC, Delgado S, Castells A, Taurá P, Piqué JM, et al. Laparoscopy-assisted colectomy versus open colectomy for treatment of non-metastatic colon cancer: a randomised trial. Lancet. 2002;359(9325):2224–9.
20. Tjandra JJ, Chan MK. Systematic review on the short-term outcome of laparoscopic resection for colon and rectosigmoid cancer. Colorectal Dis. 2006;8(5):375–88.
21. Veldkamp R, Kuhry E, Hop WC, Jeekel J, Kazemier G, Bonjer HJ, et al. Laparoscopic surgery versus open surgery for colon cancer: short-term outcomes of a randomised trial. Lancet Oncol. 2005;6(7):477–84.
22. Nandakumar G, Fleshman JW. Laparoscopy for colon and rectal cancer. Clin Colon Rectal Surg. 2010;23(1):51–8.
23. Ng SS, Lee JF, Yiu RY, Li JC, Hon SS, Mak TW, et al. Long-term oncologic outcomes of laparoscopic versus open surgery for rectal cancer: a pooled analysis of 3 randomized controlled trials. Ann Surg. 2014;259(1):139–47.
24. American Society of Anesthesiologists Task Force on Preanesthesia Evaluation. Practice advisory for preanesthesia evaluation: a report by the American Society of Anesthesiologists Task Force on Preanesthesia Evaluation. Anesthesiology. 2002;96(2):485–96.
25. Fleisher LA, Beckman JA, Brown KA, Calkins H, Chaikof E, Fleischmann KE, et al. ACC/AHA 2007 guidelines on perioperative cardiovascular evaluation and care for noncardiac surgery: a report of the American College of Cardiology/American Heart Association Task Force on Practice Guidelines (Writing Committee to Revise the 2002 Guidelines on Perioperative Cardiovascular Evaluation for Noncardiac Surgery). Circulation. 2007;116(17):e418–99.
26. Sheehy AM, Gabbay RA. An overview of preoperative glucose evaluation, management, and perioperative impact. J Diabetes Sci Technol. 2009;3(6):1261–9.
27. Gustafsson UO, Thorell A, Soop M, Ljungqvist O, Nygren J. Haemoglobin A1c as a predictor of postoperative hyperglycaemia and complications after major colorectal surgery. Br J Surg. 2009;96(11):1358–64.
28. Van Klei WA, Bryson GL, Yang H, Kalkman CJ, Wells GA, Beattie WS. The value of routine preoperative electrocardiography in predicting myocardial infarction after noncardiac surgery. Ann Surg. 2007;246(2):165–70.
29. Sheffield KM, McAdams PS, Benarroch-Gampel J, et al. Overuse of preoperative cardiac stress testing in medicare patients undergoing elective noncardiac surgery. Ann Surg. 2013;257(1):73–80.
30. Zibrak JD, O'Donnell CR. Indications for preoperative pulmonary function testing. Clin Chest Med. 1993;14(2):227–36.
31. Odejinmi F, Sangrithi M, Olowu O. Operative laparoscopy as the mainstay method in management of hemodynamically unstable patients with ectopic pregnancy. J Minim Invasive Gynecol. 2011;18(2):179–83.
32. Chautard J, Alves A, Zalinski S, Bretagnol F, Valleur P, Panis Y. Laparoscopic colorectal surgery in elderly patients: a matched case-control study in 178 patients. J Am Coll Surg. 2008; 206(2):255–60.
33. Pikarsky AJ, Saida Y, Yamaguchi T, Martinez S, Chen W, Weiss EG, et al. Is obesity a high risk factor for laparoscopic colorectal surgery? Surg Endosc. 2002;16(5):855–8.
34. Delaney CP, Pokala N, Senagore AJ, Casillas S, Kiran RP, Brady KM, et al. Is laparoscopic colectomy applicable to patients with body mass index >30? A case-matched comparative study with open colectomy. Dis Colon Rectum. 2005;48(5):975–81.
35. Myers E, Hurley M, O'Sullivan GC, Kavanagh D, Wilson I, Winter DC. Laparoscopic peritoneal lavage for generalized peritonitis due to perforated diverticulitis. Br J Surg. 2008;95(1):97–101.
36. Swank HA, Vermuelen J, Lange JF, Mulder IM, van der Hoeven JA, Stassen LP, et al. The ladies trial: laparoscopic peritoneal lavage or resection for purulent peritonitis and Hartmann's procedure or resection with primary anastomosis for purulent or faecal peritonitis in perforated diverticulitis (NTR2037). BMC Surg. 2010;10:29.
37. Thornell A, Angente E, Gonzales E, Heath J, Jess P, Läckberg Z, et al. Treatment of acute diverticulitis laparoscopic lavage vs resection (DILALA): study protocol for a randomized controlled trial. Trials. 2011;12:186.
38. Koh FH, Tan KK, Tsang CB, Koh DC. Laparoscopic versus an open colectomy in an emergency setting: a case-controlled study. Ann Coloproctol. 2013;29(1):12–6.
39. McCormick JT, Simmang CL. Reoperation following minimally invasive surgery: are the "rules" different? Clin Colon Rectal Surg. 2006;19(4):217–22.
40. Gersin KS, Heniford BT, Arca MJ, Ponsky JL. Alternative site entry for laparoscopy in patients with previous abdominal surgery. J Laparoendosc Adv Surg Tech A. 1998;8(3):125–30.
41. Contant CM, Hop WC, van't Sant HP, Oostvogel HJ, Smeets HJ, Stassen LP, et al. Mechanical bowel preparation for elective colorectal surgery: a multicentre randomised trial. Lancet. 2007;370(9605):2112–7.
42. Guenaga KK, Matos D, Wille-Jørgensen P. Mechanical bowel preparation for elective colorectal surgery. Cochrane Database Syst Rev. 2011;(9):CD001544.
43. Holte K, Nielsen KG, Madsen JL, Kehlet H. Physiologic effects of bowel preparation. Dis Colon Rectum. 2004;47(8):1397–402.
44. Society of American Gastrointestinal Endoscopic Surgeons (SAGES). SAGES evidence-based guidelines for laparoscopic resection of curable colon and rectal cancer. Los Angeles, CA: Society of American Gastrointestinal Endoscopic Surgeons (SAGES); 2012.
45. Ljungqvist O, Søreide E. Preoperative fasting. Br J Surg. 2003; 90(4):400–6.
46. Practice guidelines for preoperative fasting and the use of pharmacologic agents to reduce the risk of pulmonary aspiration: application to healthy patients undergoing elective procedures: a report by the American Society of Anesthesiologists Task Force on Preoperative Fasting. Anesthesiology. 1999;90(3):896–905.

47. Kong MF, Horowitz M. Diabetic gastroparesis. Diabet Med. 2005;22:13.
48. Beretvas RI, Ponsky J. Endoscopic marking: an adjunct to laparoscopic gastrointestinal surgery. Surg Endosc. 2001;15(10):1202–3.
49. Kim SH, Milsom JW, Church JM, et al. Perioperative tumor localization for laparoscopic colorectal surgery. Surg Endosc. 1997;11(10):1013–6.
50. Conaghan PJ, Maxwell-Armstrong CA, Garrioch MV, Hong L, Acheson AG. Leaving a mark: the frequency and accuracy of tattooing prior to laparoscopic colorectal surgery. Colorectal Dis. 2011;13(1):1184–7.
51. Hyman N, Waye JD. Endoscopic four quadrant tattoo for the identification of colonic lesions at surgery. Gastrointest Endosc. 1991;37(1):56–8.
52. Bass EM, Del Pino A, Tan A, Pearl RK, Orsay CP, Abcarian H. Does preoperative stoma marking and education by the enterostomal therapist affect outcome? Dis Colon Rectum. 1997;40(4):440–2.
53. Randall J, Lord B, Fulham J, Soin B. Parastomal hernias as the predominant stoma complication after laparoscopic colorectal surgery. Surg Laparosc Endosc Percutan Tech. 2012;22(5):420–3.
54. Axelrod L. Perioperative management of patients treated with glucocorticoids. Endocrinol Metab Clin North Am. 2003;32(2):367–83.
55. Marik PE, Varon J. Requirement of perioperative stress doses of corticosteroids: a systematic review of the literature. Arch Surg. 2008;143(12):1222–6.
56. Zaghiyan KN, Murrell Z, Melmed GY, Fleshner PR. High-dose perioperative corticosteroids in steroid-treated patients undergoing major colorectal surgery: necessary or overkill? Am J Surg. 2012;204(4):481–6.
57. Bratzler DW, Houk PM, Surgical Infection Prevention Guidelines Writers Working Group. Antimicrobial prophylaxis for surgery: an advisory statement from the National Surgical Infection Prevention Project. Clin Infect Dis. 2004;38(12):1706–15.
58. Nichols RL, Broido P, Condon RE, Gorbach SL, Nyhus LM. Effect of preoperative neomycin-erythromycin intestinal preparation on the incidence of infectious complications following colon surgery. Ann Surg. 1973;178(4):453–62.
59. Cannon JA, Altom LK, Deierhoi RJ, Morris M, Richman JS, Vick CC, et al. Preoperative oral antibiotics reduce surgical site infection following elective colorectal resections. Dis Colon Rectum. 2012;55(11):1160–6.
60. Englesbe MJ, Brooks L, Kubus J, Luchtefeld M, Lynch J, Senagore A, et al. A statewide assessment of surgical site infection following colectomy: the role of oral antibiotics. Ann Surg. 2010;252(3):514–9.
61. Marret E, Remy C, Bonnet F, Postoperative Pain Forum Group. Meta-analysis of epidural analgesia versus parenteral opioid analgesia after colorectal surgery. Br J Surg. 2007;94(6):665–73.
62. Levy BF, Scott MJ, Fawcett W, Fry C, Rockall TA. Randomized clinical trial of epidural, spinal or patient-controlled analgesia for patients undergoing laparoscopic colorectal surgery. Br J Surg. 2011;98(8):1068–78.
63. Tekkis PP, Senagore AJ, Delaney CP. Conversion rates in laparoscopic colorectal surgery. Surg Endosc. 2005;19(1):47–54.
64. Palaniappa NC, Telem DA, Ranasinghe NE, Divino CM. Incidence of iatrogenic ureteral injury after laparoscopic colectomy. Arch Surg. 2012;147(3):267–71.
65. Ott DE. Laparoscopic hypothermia. J Laparoendosc Surg. 1991;1(3):127–31.
66. Birch DW, Manouchehri N, Shi X, Jadi G, Karmali S. Heated $CO_2$ with or without humidification of minimally invasive abdominal surgery. Cochrane Database Syst Rev. 2011:CD007821.
67. Rauh R, Hemmerling TM, Rist M, Jacobi KE. Influence of pneumoperitoneum and patient positioning on respiratory system compliance. J Clin Anesth. 2001;13(5):361–5.
68. Barker L. Positioning on the operating table. Update Anaesth. 2002;15:1–6.
69. Alizadeh K, Hyman N. Venous thromboembolism prophylaxis in colorectal surgery. Surg Technol Int. 2005;14:165–70.
70. Nguyen NT, Cronan M, Braley S, Rivers R, Wolfe BM. Duplex ultrasound assessment of femoral venous flow during laparoscopic and open gastric bypass. Surg Endosc. 2003;17(2):285–90.
71. Stahl TJ, Gregorcyk SG, Hyman NH, Buie WD, Standards Practice Task Force of the American Society of Colon and Rectal Surgeons. Practice parameters for the prevention of venous thrombosis. Dis Colon Rectum. 2006;49(10):1477–83.
72. Geerts WH, Pineo GF, Heit JA, Bergqvist D, Lassen MR, Colwell CW, et al. Prevention of venous thromboembolism: the Seventh ACCP Conference on Antithrombotic and Thrombolytic Therapy. Chest. 2004;126(3 Suppl):338S–400.
73. Benoist S, Panis Y, Denet C, Mauvais F, Mariani P, Valleur P. Optimal duration of urinary drainage after rectal resection: a randomized controlled trial. Surgery. 1999;125(2):135–41.
74. Delacroix Jr SE, Winters JC. Voiding dysfunction after pelvic colorectal surgery. Clin Colon Rectal Surg. 2010;23(2):119–27.
75. Kin C, Rhoads KF, Jalali M, Shelton AA, Welton ML. Predictors of postoperative urinary retention after colorectal surgery. Dis Colon Rectum. 2013;56(6):738–46.
76. Bothwell WN, Bleicher RJ, Dent TL. Prophylactic ureteral catheterization in colon surgery. A five-year review. Dis Colon Rectum. 1994;37(4):330–4.
77. Chahin F, Dwivedi AJ, Paramesh A, Chau W, Agrawal S, Chahin C, et al. The implications of lighted ureteral stenting in laparoscopic colectomy. JSLS. 2002;6(1):49–52.
78. Ibrahim AA, Abrego D, Issiah IA, Smith DW. Is post-operative proximal decompression a necessary complement to elective colon resection? South Med J. 1977;70(9):1070–1.
79. Nelson R, Edwards S, Tse B. Prophylactic nasogastric decompression after abdominal surgery. Cochrane Database Syst Rev. 2007;(3):CD004929.
80. Trencheva K, Dhar P, Sonoda T, Lee S, Samuels J, Stein B, et al. Physiologic effects of simultaneous carbon dioxide insufflation by laparoscopy and colonoscopy: prospective evaluation. Surg Endosc. 2011;25(10):3279–85.
81. Lassen K, Soop M, Nygren J, Cox PB, Hendry PO, Spies C, et al. Consensus review of optimal perioperative care in colorectal surgery: Enhanced Recovery After Surgery (ERAS) group recommendations. Arch Surg. 2009;144(10):961–9.
82. History of the ERAS Society. http://www.erassociety.org/index.php/about-us/history. Accessed 29 May 2013.

# Patient Positioning, Instrumentation, and Trocar Placement

# 2

Mehraneh Dorna Jafari, Michael J. Stamos, and Steven Mills

**Key Points**

- Position patients in a manner to pad all pressure points and maximize gravity's effects, while avoiding nerve damage and undue traction.
- Appropriate abdominal access should be based on patient factors and surgeon preference.
- Avoid complications by understanding the limitations and strengths of laparoscopic instruments.

## Introduction

The utilization of laparoscopy in general surgery became popularized over the decade following its introduction by Erich Mühe in 1982 [1]. The observation of decreased postoperative pain and length of stay following laparoscopic cholecystectomy, when compared to the conventional Kocher incision for an open cholecystectomy, further supported this approach [1]. The improved outcomes, in conjunction with the advent of new technology, led many surgeons to rapidly apply these approaches to their practice, resulting in laparoscopic cholecystectomy becoming the standard of care in a relatively short time span. Yet, this has not always translated to all operative procedures. Consider that the first laparoscopic colectomy was reported by Moises Jacobs and J. C. Verdeja in Miami, Florida, in 1990. Furthermore, Joseph Uddo performed the first sigmoid resection utilizing a circular end-to-end anastomotic stapler in 1990 [2]. Yet, here we are almost 25 years later, and still less than 50 % of colon resections are being performed via a laparoscopic approach. In part, the technical difficulties of laparoscopic colectomies, combined with the fear of port-site recurrence and the possibility of poor oncological outcomes for cancer, initially hindered the wide acceptance of this approach [2]. These concerns were subsequently dissipated by numerous multicenter randomized control trials that concluded that no differences between conventional open colectomy and minimally invasive colectomy exist in terms of long-term survival, disease-free survival, and local and distant recurrence [3].

## Laparoscopic Instrumentation

Since the introduction of laparoscopy in 1902, minimally invasive surgery has been evolving and has expanded dramatically over the past two decades [4]. This expansion can mainly be attributed to the exponential growth in technology over this period of time. The evolution of laparoscopic instrumentation and, most importantly, the laparoscope have allowed for the growth of this approach.

### Trocars

There are a variety of precision-engineered laparoscopic trocars available on the market. Most institutions will have a set of available trocars, each of which will have advantages and disadvantages to their use. The design of trocars has been evolving since their introduction in 30 AD (Fig. 2.1) [5].

---

**Electronic supplementary material:** Supplementary material is available in the online version of this chapter at 10.1007/978-1-4939-1581-1_2. Videos can also be accessed at http://www.springerimages.com/videos/978-1-4939-1580-4.

M.D. Jafari, M.D.
Department of Surgery, University of California, Irvine School of Medicine, 333 City Blvd. West, Suite 850, Orange, CA 92868, USA
e-mail: Jafarim@uci.edu

M.J. Stamos, M.D. • S. Mills, M.D. (✉)
Department of Surgery, Division of Colorectal Surgery, University of California, Irvine School of Medicine, 333 City Blvd. West, Suite 850, Orange, CA 92868, USA
e-mail: mstamos@uci.edu; sdmills@uci.edu

H.M. Ross et al. (eds.), *Minimally Invasive Approaches to Colon and Rectal Disease: Technique and Best Practices*,
DOI 10.1007/978-1-4939-1581-1_2, © Springer Science+Business Media New York 2015

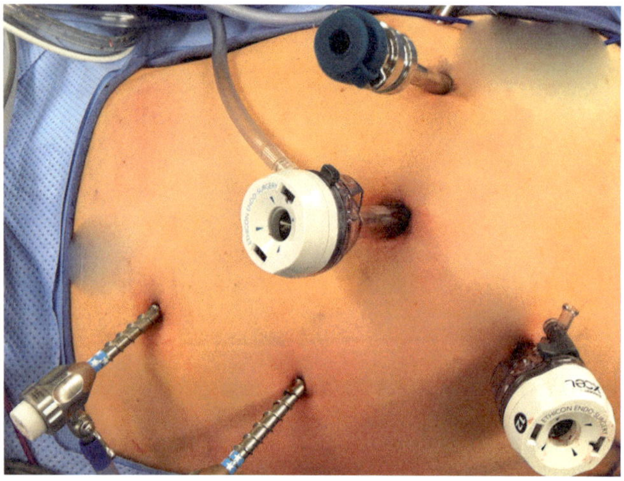

**Fig. 2.1** Outer port/cannula of a 10 mm dilating/non-cutting trocar

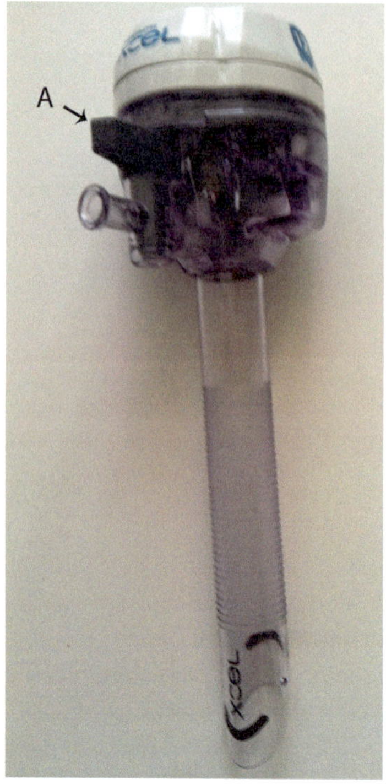


**Fig. 2.2** Multiple ports used in one case: robotic ports and two varieties of laparoscopic non-cutting dilating trocars

All modern trocars generally include a gas-tight valve, which allows for removal and introduction of instruments without the loss of pneumoperitoneum. In addition, new valveless trocars have been introduced that use the pressurized curtain of gas at the top of the instrument to reduce carbon dioxide leakage. There exists a variety of single-use and reusable laparoscopic trocars. Although reusable trocars may have advantages in terms of cost, with use their tips may become blunt and valves may become incompetent.

Trocar sizes range from 3 mm to 30 mm, with the size referring to the inside diameter. The 5, 8, 10, and 12 mm trocars are the most commonly used in advanced laparoscopic and robotic colorectal surgery. The trocar itself is made of an inner, removable obturator and outer port or cannula (Fig. 2.2), which remains in place for the passage of instruments. The sleeve may be metal, plastic, smooth, and/or threaded. The transparent trocars have the advantage of allowing the laparoscope to monitor the trocar as it passes through the abdominal wall. While metal trocars are more durable, they run the risk of capacitive coupling, resulting in unintentional thermal spread and injury, with improper use of energy devices such as the electrocautery.

The trocar can be further categorized into cutting or dilating trocars. Cutting trocars can be metal or plastic and cut through the tissue as force is applied. There are designs that include a spring-loaded plastic shield that are intended to automatically cover the blade as it enters the abdominal cavity. The dilating trocars use a blunt, tapered tip that separates and dilates the tissue as it is inserted. The cutting trocars can decrease the amount of force required to enter the abdomen compared to the blunt-tipped dilating trocar. Although easy to insert, these bladed trocars were initially associated with occasional vascular and visceral complications, as well as abdominal wall hematoma, trocar site pain, and hernia. The newer-generation retracting tips seem safer but have not been proven to have a better safety profile [5]. Blunt tip/dilating trocars require a smaller skin incision and stretch the remaining abdominal wall, rather than incising, which may result in improved retention. The dilating trocars have been associated with decreased postoperative pain, port-site bleeding, smaller scars, and increased patient satisfaction. In summary, radially dilating trocars require an increased insertion force and have a smaller defect size compared to cutting trocars [6, 7]. Our preference for colorectal surgery is a variety of blunt tip/dilating 5, 10, and 12 m trocars to minimize risk to bowel and abdominal wall.

## Instruments

Laparoscopic instrumentation is continuously evolving with new technology allowing for better ergonomics and tissue handling. Multiple companies manufacture the laparoscopic instruments; however, the principles remain uniform.

### Camera/Laparoscope

Adequate visualization is an essential aspect of laparoscopic surgery. There is a wide range of available laparoscopes with regard to diameter and viewing angles. There are also flexible tip laparoscopes, which are advantageous in providing versatility in the angle viewed. Laparoscopes can be classified as a telescopic rod lens system, which are connected to a video camera, or a digital laparoscope with an integrated

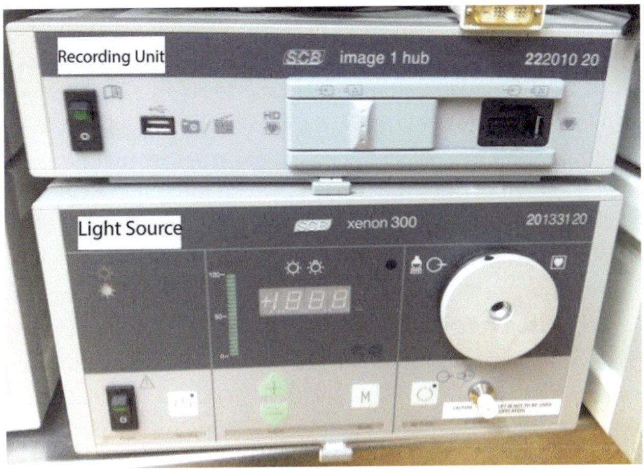


**Fig. 2.3** Camera light source and video unit

light source. Camera processor unit, light source, recording device, and monitors with articulating arms should be available (Fig. 2.3). Recently, high-definition scopes have become available. Individual choice of cameras is often dictated by surgeon preference and the hospital purchasing body or Value Analysis Committee. Regardless of which camera is used, it is important to test the camera and light source prior to gaining access to the abdomen as well as to "white balance" the camera for optimal color resolution. Typically, the surgeon stands on the opposite side of the abdomen from the pathology (and thus the expected resection segment), and the laparoscope points toward the pathology. A laparoscopic warmer and antifog solution should be available to allow for enhanced visualization. In many cases, the most junior member of the operative team is charged with "driving the camera." Unfortunately, this often results in unnecessary confusion in the anatomy, lack of unity during the case (i.e., focusing in on a different viewpoint), prolonged operations, poor ergonomics, and overall increased frustration. The traditional guidance to "keep the camera buttons toward the ceiling" is ill advised and incorrect in colorectal surgery. Rather, proper education regarding recognition of the horizon and maintaining camera orientation to identify the correct field of view is crucial for colorectal operations, especially when transitioning between the various abdominal quadrants.

## Insufflator

Once abdominal access is gained, pneumoperitoneum is essential in providing adequate visualization and space to perform the operation. This is achieved via an insufflator. At the beginning of each case, prior to the incision, assure that the insufflator is working. Turn the insufflator on and check carbon dioxide cylinders to ascertain that adequate gas is available for the case. Always have an extra available container, as inevitably the tank will run out at a crucial moment

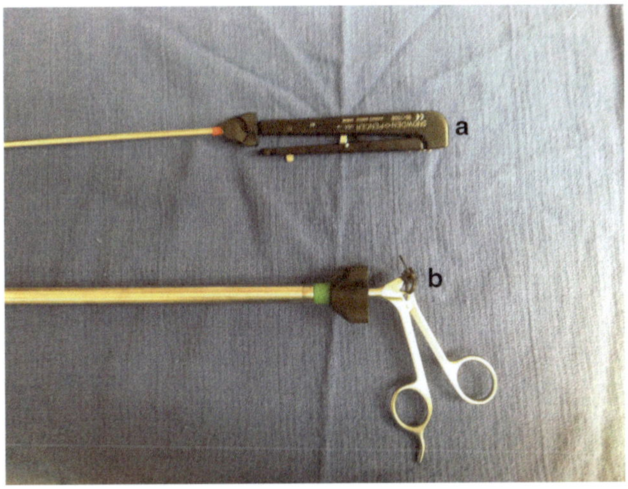


**Fig. 2.4** Handles of different instruments, demonstrating that ring handle offers a greater precision (**a**) secondary to the pincer grip compared to handles (**b**) that allow for a greater form of a palm grip can be used for tasks involving power over precision

if not prepared. Advanced, integrated surgical rooms will often have carbon dioxide lines directly attached to the insufflator, thus obviating the need for a tank. The insufflator will display the intra-abdominal pressure and contain an adjustable pressure selector and digital flow and volume displays. Once pneumoperitoneum is established, the setting should be placed on high flow (20–40 L/min), typically to achieve a steady 15 mmHg pneumoperitoneum. Select patients with cardiopulmonary issues may require lower levels of abdominal pressure to be maintained. The anesthesiologist will monitor the patient's hemodynamics during insufflation, and it is important to continue good communication.

## Graspers

Laparoscopic graspers represent the most varied yet most used type of instrument in laparoscopic colon surgery. They can be reusable or disposable and can have various types of handles, insulated shafts, and tips. Some versions can also have attachments for monopolar cautery. Diameters range from 1.8 to 12 mm, and lengths range from 30 cm upward. We prefer 5 mm, 30–35 cm length instruments for our average patients. However, 45 cm or even longer instruments should be available and are typically used when mobilizing the splenic flexure. The type of grasper used will be dependent on the task. Surgeon preference is key with regard to the handle of the instruments. A ring handle offers a greater precision compared to the diamond or pincer grip. However, handles that allow for a greater form of a palm grip can be used for tasks involving power over precision (Fig. 2.4). Certain graspers may also have a locking mechanism, which is ideal when position of the grasper must be maintained for a prolonged period of time.

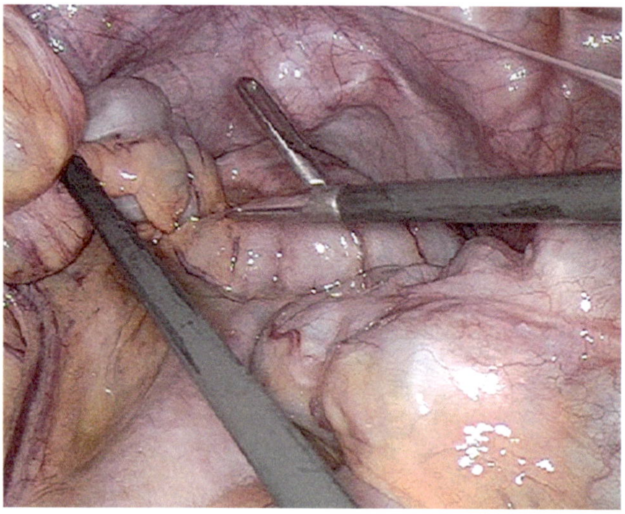

**Fig. 2.5** Fenestrated nontraumatic graspers, used for grasping bowel

Graspers used for bowel retraction should allow for a secure grip, without exerting excessive pressure. A variety of tips, including straight or flared, traumatic or atraumatic, single or dual, and fenestrated or solid, are available. To decrease traction injury, we prefer atraumatic fenestrated graspers (Fig. 2.5) with dull dual ends for most bowel retraction and bowel handling. Dual action is preferred, since single action type graspers with one movable jaw exert greater pressure on the tissue. Fenestrated tips exert less friction on grasped tissue, which also means they can be prone to slippage on the tissue. Care should be taken not to exert too much pressure, especially in directions perpendicular to the tip orientation. It is also pertinent to remember that the tip of the grasper, given its smaller surface area, exerts the greatest force. When retracting with the tip, avoid pushing blindly or excessively into the bowel wall to prevent inadvertent enterotomies.

Dissector graspers, such as Maryland graspers, and right angle graspers should be available for blunt dissection as needed but are generally not to be used for handling the bowel.

## Scissors

Laparoscopic scissors are also available as reusable, reposable (e.g., the tip is disposable while the shaft is reusable), or disposable. They can be used for sharp dissection and, with care, limited blunt dissection. In patients with prior abdominal surgery, scissors are invaluable with taking down adherent loops of bowel to the anterior abdominal wall. Monopolar cautery can be attached, allowing for use of energy during dissection for better hemostasis. Similar to graspers, these instruments are available in a variety of sizes and lengths.

## Laparoscopic Staplers

There are a variety of surgical stapling devices available on the market. Laparoscopic staplers can be used in lieu of energy devices or suturing for vessel ligation, as well as in the creation of anastomoses. Large prospective randomized trials have failed to demonstrate superiority of either stapled or hand-sewn anastomoses [8, 9]. The linear stapler (e.g., laparoscopic GIA) places 4 staggered rows of titanium staples and then divides the tissue between the staple lines. The device failure rate has been reported as 0.2–0.3 % [10, 11].

The appropriate stapler should be selected based upon the required function. Staplers are also classified into linear versus circular staplers, articulating versus straight, and cutting versus non-cutting. Staplers are also offered in a powered design (Video 2.1). Theoretically, powered staplers may optimize stapler deployment thereby achieving superior tissue apposition. However, to date no studies have validated their superiority. Cartridge length is variable for the staplers and is generally available in 30–60 mm lengths, and appropriate size should be selected to decrease the number of staple lines. However, shorter cartridges may be easier to deploy in the narrow pelvis.

Staples come in a variety of heights (2–5 mm) and are color-coded based upon the height. There is no uniform color-coded standard for labeling the stapling heights, and each manufacturer has their own color code. Height should be chosen based upon the tissue thickness. Failure to choose an appropriate height may result in incomplete tissue apposition or conversely inadequate compression of tissue (Fig. 2.6a) [12]. Ideal staple height selection to match the tissue thickness should result in formation of a "B" shape of the staples (Fig. 2.6b). The rectum, which is typically thicker than the colon, should be divided with at least a 4.0 mm staple, while the small bowel and colon can be stapled with ~3.5 mm staples. Staple line buttressing is also available with a variety of reinforcement material, though various studies have failed to show a significant difference in outcomes, and in our general practice, we do not use reinforcement [13].

Low anterior resection (LAR) can pose specific challenges to the surgeon, notably during division of the rectum. Division low in the pelvis can be challenging in terms of both articulation of the stapler and in the length of the staple line, especially in a narrow pelvis. A curved stapler has recently become available for bowel division, and one study has demonstrated feasibility and safety [14].

## Other Laparoscopic Instrumentation

Laparoscopic instruments that should also be available include needle driver for intracorporeal suturing, suction/irrigator device, and clip appliers for control of vessels. Clip appliers are indicated for ligation of appropriate size vessels or ducts. Clips vary in lengths (6–11 mm) and material (metallic or nonabsorbable plastic). They are available offered as disposable or reusable, and shaft diameters range from 5 to 11 mm.

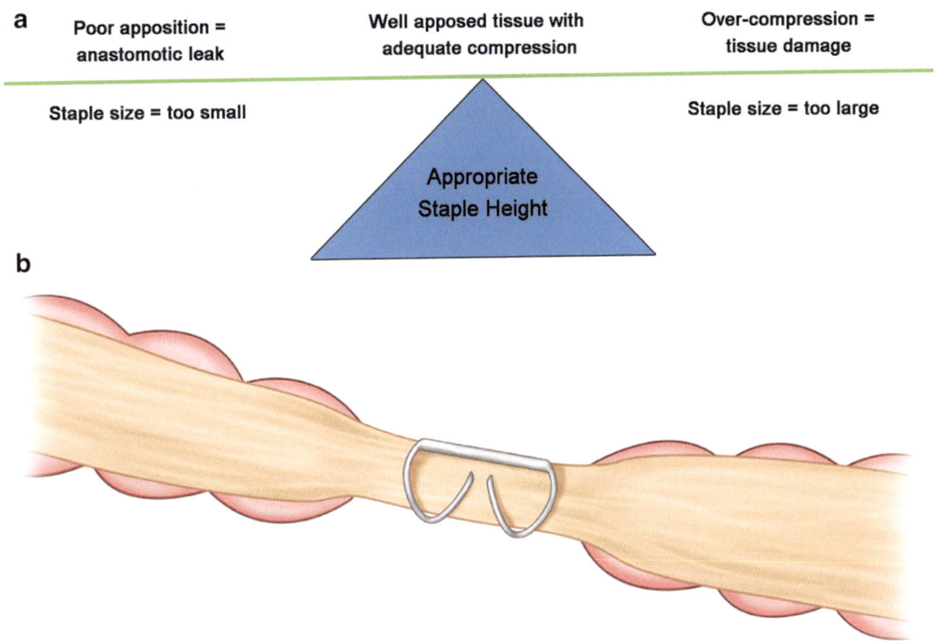


**Fig. 2.6** (**a**) Failure to choose an appropriate height may result in incomplete tissue apposition or conversely inadequate compression of tissue. (**b**) Ideal "B"-shaped staple configuration. *With Permission from Davis B, Rafferty JF. Technical Aspects. In: Steele SR, Maykel JA, Champagne BJ, Orangio GR, eds. Complexities in Colorectal Surgery: Decision-making and management. Springer, New York, 2014 © Springer in 2014*

## Energy Devices

Adequate hemostasis is key in any surgical procedure and is critical in laparoscopic surgery. The rapid control of vessels and hemorrhage will allow for maintenance of visualization and for the procedure to continue laparoscopically. However, hemostasis remains a challenge in laparoscopic surgery, given that traditional methods of controlling/dividing a vessel (i.e., suture ligation) is technically challenging in the laparoscopic setting; therefore, we have come to rely more heavily on surgical clips and staplers. However, these devices do have limitations in function. The surgical evolution of energy devices has become central in the laparoscopic era, for they allow for rapid control and division of named vessels. A general understanding of principles and knowledge of the advantages and complications of energy devices should be appreciated by all users.

### Monopolar Energy

Monopolar energy relies on electrical current flowing from the generator through the patient and return via a grounding pad. It can be used to facilitate dissection, achieve hemostasis, and ligate small vessels. Devices such as scissors, hook cautery, or graspers can be utilized, and the energy can be set as cutting or coagulation. Similar to monopolar "Bovie Electrocautery," advantages include speed, low voltage, and rapid hemostasis. It is important to recognize, however, that standard monopolar devices rely on heat and time to perform their duty. They also require the circuit to be intact. Inadvertent alternate site burns can occur if energy is allowed to complete the circuit outside of the designated grounding pad. Other disadvantages to standard monopolar energy include an increased lateral thermal spread when compared to the bipolar devices. This may be critical when dissecting in confined spaces adjacent to critical structures such as the pelvic plexus during the anterior portion of an LAR, where thermal damage to the nerves may have long-term consequences.

### Bipolar Energy

Traditional bipolar energy still relies on using electricity to perform its function. Unlike monopolar energy, bipolar energy requires no grounding pad, as the circuit is completed between the two instrument tips adjacent to one another. This results in a higher degree of current density at the tissue between the tips of the instrument. Advanced bipolar energy systems (i.e., LigaSure™, Covidien, CT, and Enseal™, Ethicon, Cincinnati, OH) add in the third component of vessel sealing (along with heat and time)—compression. This allows lower voltage to be used and, hence, lower heat to complete much larger tasks. Bipolar energy is used in a variety of vessel sealing devices and delivers a much smaller lateral thermal spread footprint. This energy, combined with the increased pressure delivered by the jaws of the instrument, allows for permanent sealing of up to 7 mm vessels (Video 2.2). The size of the vessel and thermal spread is variable depending on the instrument (Table 2.1). Many of these instruments are shaped in a blunt-tipped, versatile fashion. The advantage of bipolar devices is that these instruments can be used to grasp, dissect, and coagulate, thereby reducing the need to change instruments.

**Table 2.1** Bipolar energy devices [30]

| Device | Company | Thermal spread (mm) (reported) | Vessel seal (mm) |
|---|---|---|---|
| Enseal Trio® | Ethicon | 1 | 7 |
| Trissector PKS™ | Gyrus | 3.6 | 7 |
| LigaSure™ | Covidien | 0–4.5 | 7 |
| HALO PKS™ | Olympus | – | 7 |
| OMNI PKS™ | Olympus | – | 7 |

## Ultrasonic Energy

Devices such as Harmonic Scalpel® (Ethicon, Cincinnati, OH) and SonSurg® (Olympus, Southborough, MA) use ultrasonic technology. In essence, these devices convert electrical energy at the generator into mechanical motion at the jaw blade. Unlike monopolar and bipolar instruments, no energy flows through the patient. In fact, these instruments are more in line with surgical staplers than they are with the advanced bipolar devices. Yet, these devices can still reproducibly and reliably seal vessels ≤5 mm with minimal thermal damage, and newer models are FDA approved up to 7 mm vessels [15]. They only have one active blade that can be rotated. Depending on several factors such as the power setting at the generator, "max" or "min" activation at the device and degree of tissue tension applied by the user will all determine which end of the coagulation versus cut spectrum the device will function. These devices also have the advantage of serving multiple purposes (i.e., cut, coagulate, coapt, cavitate) and thereby eliminating the need to change instruments (Video 2.3).

## Hand-Assisted Devices

Although our practice does not include the use of hand-assisted devices, this option is available to aid in hand-assisted advanced laparoscopic operations. A variety of hand-assisted ports are available to provide a seal against the abdominal wall and allow for one of the surgeons' gloved hand to be inserted. Devices include Gelport (Applied Medical, Rancho Santa Margarita, CA), Dextrus (Ethicon Endosurgery, Cincinnati, OH) (Video 2.4), HandPort System (Smith & Nephew Inc., London, England), Dexterity Pneumo Sleeve device (Dexterity Inc., Roswell, GA), Omniport (Advance Surgical Concepts, Dublin, Ireland), and Intromit Device (Medtech Ltd, Dublin, Ireland).

## Positioning

Patient positioning should provide best possible access while maintaining patient safety (Fig. 2.7). Patient position should be discussed with the entire surgical team prior to the operation, and adequate personnel should be available for patient positioning. Optimal patient positioning involves adhering to basic principles, including avoiding those positions that may cause peripheral nerve injury and/or pressure ulcers. Peripheral nerve injuries have been reported as the second most common class of injury (16 %) by the Society of Anesthesiologists Closed Claims Project database [16]. Given that during laparoscopy the table incline is used to aid in retraction and dissection, the patient must be secured to the operating room table to avoid sliding.

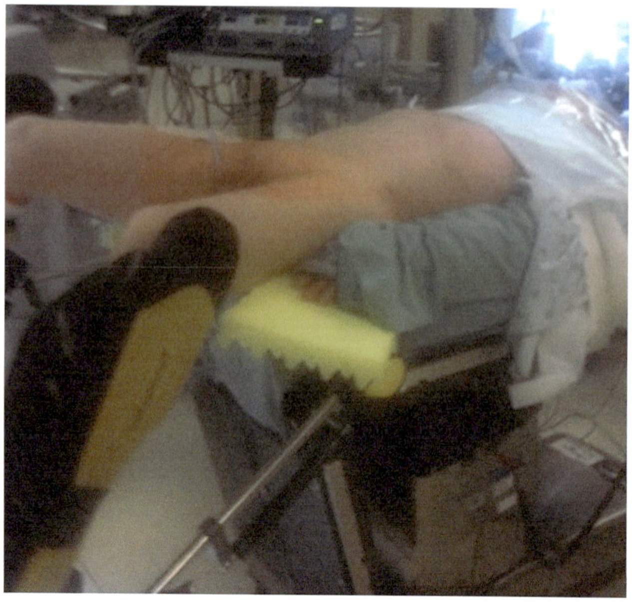

**Fig. 2.7** Patient positioning demonstrating appropriate padding of bony prominences and avoidance of nerve injuries

## Padding

At our institution we use a large high-density foam mat and a Velcro belt to prevent sliding. A beanbag, memory foam, and Z-flo (Sundance, White Plains, NY) can also be used to achieve the same results. Egg crate foam (Allen Medical Group, Acton, MA) can be used for padding and stabilization of the legs in stirrups.

Depending upon the specific procedure, patients are generally placed in a supine or modified lithotomy position for laparoscopic colorectal surgery. We prefer to have both arms tucked next to the patient's body, when feasible. If the arms are to be placed out on arm boards, care must be taken to avoid injury to the brachial plexus, and therefore they should not be abducted >90 degree. For supine procedures, the occiput, sacrum, and heels are at risk for pressure ulcers and should be padded, ideally with gel pads. Knees should maintain some degree of flexion to avoid hyperextension injuries. For modified lithotomy position, legs are placed into Yellow Fin® or Allen® stirrups with hips slightly flexed and abducted, feet flat within the stirrups, and pressure avoided along the lateral aspects of the legs. The ankle, knee, and contralateral shoulder should be aligned [16].

We prefer our patients to be placed supine with (at least) the left arm tucked to allow for both surgeon and assistant to stand on the left side of the patient for laparoscopic right colectomy. However, the patient can also be placed in modified lithotomy position, which will allow the operating surgeon to stand between the legs. For laparoscopic total abdominal colectomy, sigmoidectomy, low anterior resection, and abdominoperineal resection, we prefer our patients in the modified lithotomy position with both arms tucked. This will allow access to the perineum for rectal/vaginal exams, use of endoscopy, and the insertion of the circular stapler or access for hand-sewn anastomosis.

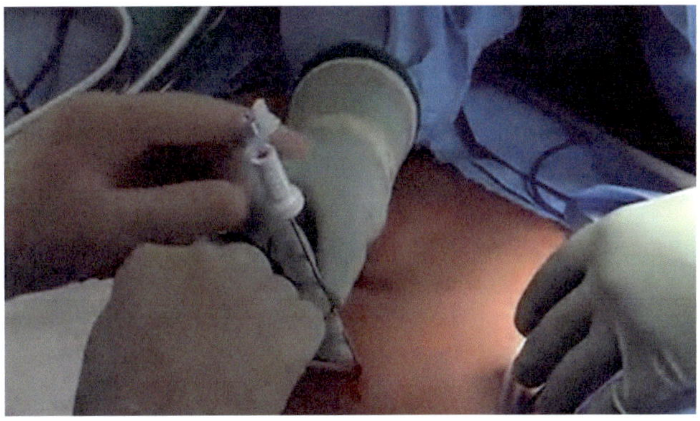

**Fig. 2.8** Veress needle placement at Plamar's point

## Gaining Access to the Peritoneal Space

### Laparoscopic Entry Techniques

The majority of major complications (>50 %) during laparoscopic surgery occur while gaining access to the abdomen [17–19]. There are multiple ways to gain access to the abdomen including Veress needle, direct trocar insertion, open "Hasson" technique and visual entry via optical needle or trocar technique. Each technique has potential complications and advantages. The decision of which method is most appropriate to gain entry should be dictated by patient's body habitus, history, and surgeon experience.

#### Veress Needle

The first report of Veress needle utilized for gaining pneumoperitoneum was described in 1947 by Raoul Palmer [20] and is the most commonly practiced method to access the abdomen [5, 17]. The disposable needle is a one-piece design with an external diameter of 2 mm, gauge of 14, and length of 70 and 120 mm. Reusable Veress needles are metal. Prior to entry to the abdomen, flush the needle to assure patency. The Veress needle has a blunt tip that will retract as it contacts resistance and spring forward when the needle is pulled away from the point of resistance. The use and exact location of Veress placement is surgeon dependent. In a patient without prior operation, we prefer placement 3 cm lateral to the umbilicus, which will be our preferred camera position. In patients with prior operation, we typically utilize Palmer's point (1–2 cm below the left costal border in the midclavicular line) (Fig. 2.8). The umbilicus is a less preferred option if the patient has had no prior operation. While the umbilicus is ideal in terms of cosmesis, its location is not ideal, as it is too close to the area of vessel division in many patients. The right upper quadrant is also an option; however, care must be taken to avoid injury to the liver.

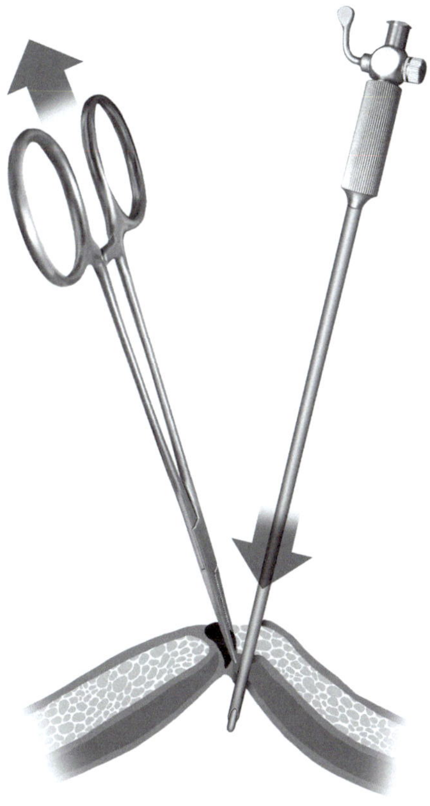

**Fig. 2.9** Proper placement technique of a Veress needle. *With Permission from Shin J, Lee SW. Laparoscopic Complications. In: Steele SR, Maykel JA, Champagne BJ, Orangio GR, eds. Complexities in Colorectal Surgery: Decision-making and management. Springer, New York, 2014 © Springer in 2014*

Once optimal position is determined based on patient history and surgeon preference, the needle is inserted. Grasping and elevating the anterior fascia with a tonsil clamp may decrease the risk of intra-abdominal injury (Fig. 2.9). As the needle traverses the anterior and then posterior fascia, there will be a sensation of resistance followed by a release at each layer of fascia, and then an absence of resistance as it enters the peritoneum. Once in the peritoneum, a click may be heard as the blunt tip of the needle inserts into the abdomen. Once entry is achieved, the needle should be aspirated to assure that no visceral or vascular injury has occurred. A drop test, which consists of observing the fluid enter the abdomen through the Veress rapidly, can help demonstrate accurate placement. It should be noted that the above maneuvers to ensure correct placement have not been proven to decrease complications, though remain, in general, good practice patterns to adhere to [21]. Once the above maneuvers are completed, pneumoperitoneum should then be attempted and initial pressure should be <10 mmg [5]. If high pressure is noted, the needle can be rotated to assure that the opening is not next to the abdominal wall. Maximal flow through a Veress needle (14 gauge) is 2.5 L/min regardless of flow settings. Avoid swaying the needle from side to side, given that this may enlarge a small visceral injury. However, if pressures continue to be high, attempt at repositioning should be made.

### Direct Trocar Insertion

Dingfelder first described direct trocar insertion in 1978 [22]. It involves the placement of the first trocar without prior pneumoperitoneum. This may allow an easier grasping and lifting of the abdomen and decrease complications related to Veress needle. Controversy continues to exist regarding the use of this technique [5, 17]. We do not practice, nor recommend, this technique.

### Hasson (Open) Technique

The open technique was introduced by Hasson in 1971 [23] and was designed to provide surgeons with a safe method of entry into the abdomen, thereby eliminating vascular and visceral injury [24]. It is mainly used in the high-risk population with prior abdominal surgeries, where blind entry into the abdominal is felt to be unsafe or is not feasible. It allows for direct visualization and division of abdominal wall layers. However, to date controversy exists regarding the best method to use for abdominal entry, and there is no definitive evidence that using an open technique will reduce intra-abdominal injury [17, 24, 25].

The open cannula system consists of an obturator, a plastic sheath, and a sleeve, with two rods that allow for fascial suture fixation. The two fascial sutures secure the cannula to the abdominal wall. However, this technique can be time-consuming, especially in the morbidly obese, and can cause difficulty in maintaining pneumoperitoneum due to gas leakage.

An incision is made at the selected entry site. In patients with previous abdominal surgery, this site should be away from preexisting abdominal scars or in the periumbilical skin incision. The abdominal wall is dissected with the aid of S-shaped retractors until the peritoneum is encountered. The peritoneum is then grasped and opened sharply. The surgeon's index finger is then placed intra-abdominally and adhesions are cleared. This is followed by trocar placement and securement to the fascia.

### Optical Trocar (Video 2.5)

This is a variation of the direct trocar technique with the exception that the trocar used is a clear visual trocar that allows for visualization during entry. The incision is usually made and two anterior fascial sutures are placed, the fascia is divided to the size of the trocar. These stay sutures will lift the abdominal wall against the advancing trocar. The entrance of the trocar can then be visualized via the 0-degree laparoscope, which is inserted simultaneously through the head of the trocar. Some surgeons have modified this technique to be used after achieving pneumoperitoneum with the Veress needle.

## Re-operative Surgery and Its Implications

As mentioned above, the decision for access to the abdomen should be made based upon patient history, body habitus, and surgeon experience. In patients who have had previous abdominal surgery, the initial access point and method should be considered carefully, taking into consideration prior incisions, prior areas of dissection, and expected pathology. Palmer's point entry and/or right upper quadrant access entry is often a safe option for previous midline laparotomy. An open technique or a visualized entrance should be considered if the Veress needle cannot be placed safely within the abdomen. After a failed attempt with the Veress needle, the area should be eventually carefully examined below the attempted insertion site to make sure that there is not any vascular or visceral injury.

## Trocar Positioning

As mentioned above, a wide variety of trocars are available. Once full pneumoperitoneum has been achieved, the Veress needle is removed. The first trocar is then placed. Some surgeons advocate that the initial insertion should occur while augmenting the pneumoperitoneum by lifting up the abdominal wall with a clamp at the fascia, a move we have found unnecessary. The trocar should be placed at 90-degree angle to the abdominal wall. However, care should be taken in the thin patient to avoid injury; aiming the trocars toward the pelvis to avoid injury may be necessary. There is typically moderate resistance; however, if excessive force is being used, the skin incision may be too small. Once within the abdomen, the valve should be opened to confirm intraperitoneal placement. The camera should be placed, and evaluation near the site should be made to ensure that no injury has occurred. All subsequent trocars should be placed under direct vision.

## Hand Assist

Hand-assisted laparoscopic surgery was introduced in the late 1990s, and it provided a means to overcome the limited tactile feedback and allow for gentle dissection of the tissue with the surgeon's hand [26]. Opponents feel its use can adversely affect the benefits of minimal invasive surgery given the need for a 7–8 cm incision [26]. However, in colorectal surgery, proponents note that the short-term outcomes have been found to be equivalent [27]. Long-term outcomes with regard to postoperative hernia rates favor a total laparoscopic approach. If a handport is to be used, we recommend using the extraction incision site (Pfannenstiel or minilaparotomy). Our preferred approach for extraction is a Pfannenstiel approach given its potential benefits for cosmesis and lower hernia rates [28]. Handports can also be placed at the site of planned ileostomy or colostomy. Despite the above considerations, the basic principles of laparoscopic surgery must be followed. Visualization is key to any surgical procedure, and therefore the port should be placed in a location that does not obscure laparoscopic view, and principles of triangulation will need to be maintained.

## Pearls and Pitfalls

### Avoiding Complications

Prior to starting any case, ensure:

1. The room step-up is sufficient for the anesthesiologist and surgeon.
2. Check all equipment.
3. Visualization is key in laparoscopic surgery; check the position of all monitors and place in optimal position.
4. Position cables in a manner to allow for maximal working space.

Trocars/instruments:

1. Minimally invasive surgery decreases tactile feedback and depth perception compared to open surgery [29]. Therefore, graspers should be used with caution given that it is difficult to judge how much force to apply.
2. Large "bites" of bowel, rather than small bites, should be taken during retraction to avoid tearing or perforating the bowel, as the larger surface area will spread out the applied force. This is especially true for the novice surgeon.
3. Monopolar devices can cause injury with the tip of the device and have a larger lateral thermal spread.
4. Inspect insulation of laparoscopic instruments. Failure of insulation can cause damage to the surrounding tissue.
5. Avoid tissue sticking when using monopolar devices by using Teflon-coated instruments.
6. When using bipolar devices, decrease tension during coagulation of the vessels to assure that the vessel is sealed and divided while still in the jaws [30].
7. For heavily calcified vessels, consider the use of clips or stapling devices.
8. Use the correct staple-height load for a laparoscopic stapler to decrease the risk of staple line failure.
9. Use appropriately sized cartridges for stapling devices. Using a longer load may lead to spillage of staples within the abdomen causing adhesions, while using too small of a staple load may lead to need for multiple staple lines. Similarly, ensure your staple height matches that of the tissue you are working on.
10. For pelvic procedures, consider the use of articulating staplers.
11. Avoid stapling of ischemic tissue.
12. Avoid creating a bridge of the tissue between two staple lines.

Positioning:

1. Ensure that the operating room table is in proper working condition and will allow for tilt. For cases in which perianal access is necessary, position the patient low on the table to allow for adequate access and visualization.
2. Assess joint mobility and motor deficit prior to the OR.
3. When placing a patient in modified lithotomy, be sure to avoid extreme flexion of the hip joints.
4. For lithotomy, flex both the hip and knees simultaneously.
5. Keep in mind that prolonged lithotomy may cause compression of the calves, and be aware of the risks of compartment syndrome after any procedure >5 h.

Abdominal access:

1. Obtain a full surgical history prior to beginning the case to aid in decisions of selecting the appropriate abdominal access site and technique.
2. Avoid multiple attempts with Veress needle and consider other options if unable to gain access easily.
3. Keep in mind the body habitus of the patient when inserting a Veress needle. For example, in a thin patient, the major vessels are approximately 1–2 cm below the umbilicus.
4. Avoid swaying the Veress needle once in the abdomen.
5. If pressures are high, reposition the Veress needle.
6. Avoid using previous scars to enter the abdomen blindly.

## Conclusion

Proper positioning, trocar placement, and instrumentation selection can either set you up for success right from the beginning or play a major role in your failure. Prepare well ahead of time, and have various selections available depending on your patient and your procedure. While standardization goes a long way in efficiency and avoiding errors, take the time up front to ensure things are exactly how you need them to be prior to embarking on the operation.

## References


1. Reynolds Jr W. The first laparoscopic cholecystectomy. JSLS. 2001;5(1):89–94. PubMed PMID: 11304004. Pubmed Central PMCID: 3015420.
2. Shukla PJ, Barreto G, Gupta P, Shrikhande SV. Laparoscopic surgery for colorectal cancers: current status. J Minim Access Surg. 2006;2(4):205–10. PubMed PMID: 21234147. Pubmed Central PMCID: 3016481.
3. Jayne DG, Thorpe HC, Copeland J, Quirke P, Brown JM, Guillou PJ. Five-year follow-up of the Medical Research Council CLASICC trial of laparoscopically assisted versus open surgery for colorectal cancer. Br J Surg. 2010;97(11):1638–45. PubMed PMID: 20629110.
4. Hatzinger M, Kwon ST, Langbein S, Kamp S, Hacker A, Alken P. Hans Christian Jacobaeus: inventor of human laparoscopy and thoracoscopy. J Endourol. 2006;20(11):848–50. PubMed PMID: 17144849.
5. Vilos GA, Ternamian A, Dempster J, Laberge PY. The Society of O, Gynaecologists of C. Laparoscopic entry: a review of techniques, technologies, and complications. J Obstet Gynaecol Can. 2007;29(5):433–65.
6. Passerotti CC, Begg N, Penna FJ, Passerotti AM, Leite KR, Antunes AA, et al. Safety profile of trocar and insufflation needle access systems in laparoscopic surgery. J Am Coll Surg. 2009;209(2):222–32. PubMed PMID: 19632599.
7. Theodoropoulou K, Lethaby DR, Bradpiece HA, Lo TL, Parihar A. Direct trocar insertion technique: an alternative for creation of pneumoperitoneum. JSLS. 2008;12(2):156–8. PubMed PMID: 18435888. Pubmed Central PMCID: 3016192.
8. Docherty JG, McGregor JR, Akyol AM, Murray GD, Galloway DJ. Comparison of manually constructed and stapled anastomoses in colorectal surgery. West of Scotland and Highland Anastomosis Study Group. Ann Surg. 1995;221(2):176–84. PubMed PMID: 7857145. Pubmed Central PMCID: 1234951.
9. Slieker JC, Daams F, Mulder IM, Jeekel J, Lange JF. Systematic review of the technique of colorectal anastomosis. JAMA Surg. 2013;148(2):190–201. PubMed PMID: 23426599.
10. Chan D, Bishoff JT, Ratner L, Kavoussi LR, Jarrett TW. Endovascular gastrointestinal stapler device malfunction during laparoscopic nephrectomy: early recognition and management. J Urol. 2000;164(2):319–21. PubMed PMID: 10893574.
11. Deng DY, Meng MV, Nguyen HT, Bellman GC, Stoller ML. Laparoscopic linear cutting stapler failure. Urology. 2002;60(3):415–9. discussion 9-20. PubMed PMID: 12350475.
12. Mery CM, Shafi BM, Binyamin G, Morton JM, Gertner M. Profiling surgical staplers: effect of staple height, buttress, and overlap on staple line failure. Surg Obes Relat Dis. 2008;4(3):416–22. PubMed PMID: 18226977.
13. Ho YH, Ashour MA. Techniques for colorectal anastomosis. World J Gastroenterol. 2010;16(13):1610–21. PubMed PMID: 20355239. Pubmed Central PMCID: 2848369.
14. Brescia A, Mari FS, Favi F, Milillo A, Nigri G, Dall'oglio A, et al. Laparoscopic lower anterior rectal resection using a curved stapler: original technique and preliminary experience. Am Surg. 2013;79(3):253–6. PubMed PMID: 23461949.
15. Phillips CK, Hruby GW, Durak E, Lehman DS, Humphrey PA, Mansukhani MM, et al. Tissue response to surgical energy devices. Urology. 2008;71(4):744–8. PubMed PMID: 18289646.
16. Knight DJ, Mahajan R. Patient positioning in anaesthesia. Continuing Education Anaesthesia. Critical Care & Pain. 2004;4(5): 160–3.
17. Jiang X, Anderson C, Schnatz PF. The safety of direct trocar versus Veress needle for laparoscopic entry: a meta-analysis of randomized clinical trials. J Laparoendosc Adv Surg Tech Part A. 2012; 22(4):362–70. PubMed PMID: 22423957.
18. Hashizume M, Sugimachi K. Needle and trocar injury during laparoscopic surgery in Japan. Surg Endosc. 1997;11(12):1198–201. PubMed PMID: 9373293.
19. Jansen FW, Kolkman W, Bakkum EA, de Kroon CD, Trimbos-Kemper TC, Trimbos JB. Complications of laparoscopy: an inquiry about closed- versus open-entry technique. Am J Obstet Gynecol. 2004;190(3):634–8. PubMed PMID: 15041992.
20. Palmer R. Safety in laparoscopy. J Reproduct Med. 1974;13(1):1–5. PubMed PMID: 4276707.
21. Teoh B, Sen R, Abbott J. An evaluation of four tests used to ascertain Veress needle placement at closed laparoscopy. J Minim Invasive Gynecol. 2005;12(2):153–8. PubMed PMID: 15904620.
22. Dingfelder JR. Direct laparoscope trocar insertion without prior pneumoperitoneum. J Reproduct Med. 1978;21(1):45–7. PubMed PMID: 151144.
23. Hasson HM. A modified instrument and method for laparoscopy. Am J Obstet Gynecol. 1971;110(6):886–7. PubMed PMID: 4254516.
24. Lal P, Vindal A, Sharma R, Chander J, Ramteke VK. Safety of open technique for first-trocar placement in laparoscopic surgery: a series of 6,000 cases. Surg Endosc. 2012;26(1):182–8. PubMed PMID: 21853393.
25. Merlin TL, Hiller JE, Maddern GJ, Jamieson GG, Brown AR, Kolbe A. Systematic review of the safety and effectiveness of methods used to establish pneumoperitoneum in laparoscopic surgery. Br J Surg. 2003;90(6):668–79. PubMed PMID: 12808613.
26. Litwin DE, Darzi A, Jakimowicz J, Kelly JJ, Arvidsson D, Hansen P, et al. Hand-assisted laparoscopic surgery (HALS) with the HandPort system: initial experience with 68 patients. Ann Surg. 2000;231(5):715–23. PubMed PMID: 10767793. Pubmed Central PMCID: 1421059.
27. HALS Study Group. Hand-assisted laparoscopic surgery vs standard laparoscopic surgery for colorectal disease: a prospective randomized trial. Surg Endosc. 2000;14(10):896–901. PubMed PMID: 11080399.
28. DeSouza A, Domajnko B, Park J, Marecik S, Prasad L, Abcarian H. Incisional hernia, midline versus low transverse incision: what is the ideal incision for specimen extraction and hand-assisted laparoscopy? Surg Endosc. 2011;25(4):1031–6. PubMed PMID: 20737171.
29. den Boer KT, Herder JL, Sjoerdsma W, Meijer DW, Gouma DJ, Stassen HG. Sensitivity of laparoscopic dissectors. What can you feel? Surg Endosc. 1999;13(9):869–73.
30. Smith R, Pasic R. The role of vessel sealing technologies in laparoscopic surgery. Surg Technol Int. 2008;17:208–12. PubMed PMID: 18802904.

# Surgical Anatomy

# 3

Todd D. Francone and Ron G. Landmann

**Key Points**

- A thorough understanding of the anatomy is imperative for proper exposure during minimally invasive operations. Every effort must be made to gain a clear understanding of the relationship and spacial arrangement of vital structures prior to proceeding with dissection.
- Excellent exposure, meticulous technique, and proper assistance cannot be overstated and are essential components to providing appropriate care to the patient, improving outcomes, and minimizing complications.
- Tension/counter-tension is an essential maneuver in developing and maintaining correct exposure of planes during any minimally invasive colon and rectal procedure.
- Retroperitoneal structures are always at risk during laparoscopic colectomy and must be identified and avoided throughout the dissection: right colectomy (duodenum), transverse colectomy (pancreas and mesenteric vessels), left colectomy (ureter/gonadal vessels, autonomic nerves), and pelvic dissection (ureter, hypogastric nerves).

## Introduction

Laparoscopic and robotic dissection of the abdominal colon and rectum have become increasingly utilized both for benign and malignant disease processes. Based on the underlying disease, and sequela of such processes, practicing and becoming facile with the various approaches will make exposure safer, quicker, and more reproducible.

A fundamental understanding of the surgical anatomy allows the surgeon to have the ability to proceed in a safe manner, perform an appropriate oncological resection, and allow for additional diagnostic and therapeutic maneuvering while maximizing quality of life and simultaneously reducing morbidity.

## Anatomy of Colonic Mesenteric Vasculature

### Ileocolic, Middle Colic, and Right Colic Arteries (Figs. 3.1, 3.2 and 3.3)

A clear understanding of colon mesenteric vascular anatomy is critical in performing laparoscopic colon resections. A thorough knowledge of vascular anatomy is especially important when performing resections for colon cancer where high ligation of mesenteric vessels is required.

Based on numerous anatomic, pathological, surgical, and radiologic studies, considerable variation exists in colonic vasculature (Fig. 3.3a–d). These variations need to be considered when approaching any dissection. One such example is that of the right colic artery (RCA) as a direct tributary of the superior mesenteric artery (SMA) – this occurs in only 11 % of cases. Depending on the study, the RCA is a derived from branches of the ileocolic (ICA) and middle colic arteries (MCA) in up to 80-100 % of patients. Other variations include single (95 %) and double (4 %) MCA's. When a double-MCA was found, the RCA was invariably absent. Rather than the typical SMA origin, the MCA itself can originate from either hepatic or distal splenic arteries.

***Pearl*: *When performing right colectomy, one can take advantage of the constancy of the ileocolic vessels. The ileocolic artery always courses toward the ileocecal junction (Fig. 3.1 and 3.2). By identifying the terminal ileum and the cecal junction and gently retracting the mesentery near the***

T.D. Francone, M.D., M.P.H. (✉)
Department of Colon and Rectal Surgery, Lahey Health and Medical Center, Lahey Hospital and Medical Center, Tufts University Medical Center,
41 Mall Road, Burlington, MA 01805, USA
e-mail: Todd.d.francone@lahey.org

R.G. Landmann, M.D., F.A.C.S., F.A.S.C.R.S.
Division of Colon and Rectal Surgery,
Mayo Clinic College of Medicine, Mayo Clinic,
4500 San Pablo Road, Jacksonville, FL 32224, USA
e-mail: landmann.ron@mayo.edu

H.M. Ross et al. (eds.), *Minimally Invasive Approaches to Colon and Rectal Disease: Technique and Best Practices*,
DOI 10.1007/978-1-4939-1581-1_3, 

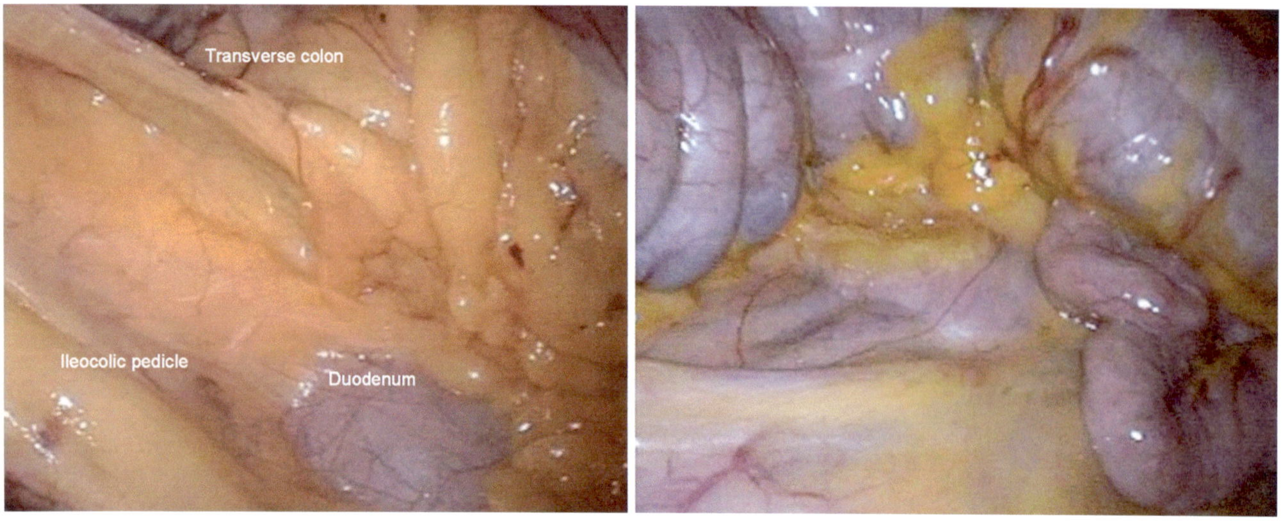


**Fig. 3.1** Demonstrates relationship of ileocolic pedicle, right colon, and transverse colon. Oftentimes, the duodenum can be seen in a relatively avascular plane toward the base of the mesentery and takeoff of the ileocolic pedicle

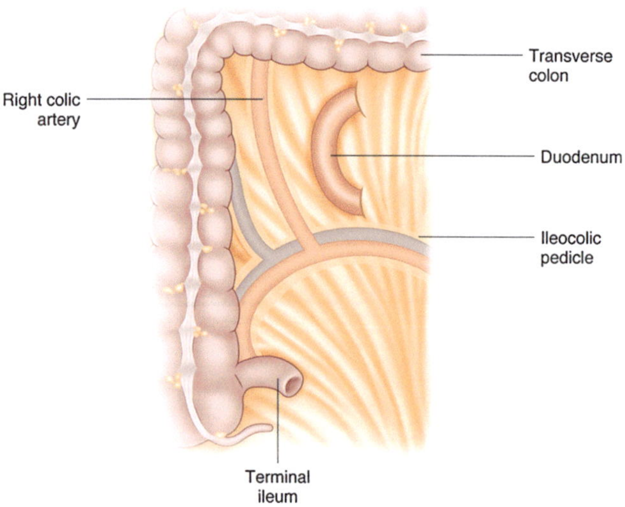


**Fig. 3.2** Relationship of the ileocolic pedicle to the duodenum and right colon

***ileocolic junction anteriorly and laterally, the ileocolic vessel will be tented or "bow stringed" for easy identification. The ileocolic artery is also the first and usually the only branch of the SMA located just below the duodenal sweep. Prior to ligating the ileocolic pedicle, the duodenal sweep located just above and near the origin of the duodenal sweep must be identified in order to avoid inadvertently injuring the SMA Ileocolic pedicle (Fig. 33.4).***

### Gastrocolic Trunk

An extreme caution should be exercised when dissecting the proximal transverse colon mesentery away from the duodenum and the head of the pancreas. Henle's gastrocolic

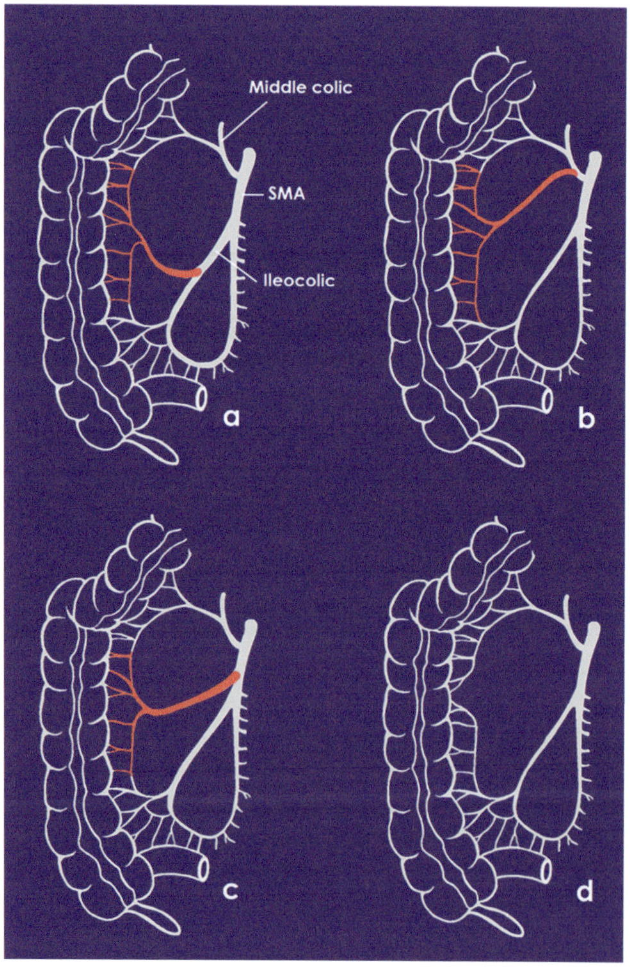


**Fig. 3.3 a–d** Variations in the blood supply to the right colon. *With permission from Yuko Tonohira*

trunk, a communicating vein between the gastroepiploic vein and the right branch of the middle colic vein or the main middle colic vein, courses behind the proximal transverse colon mesentery. Aggressive dissection in this area can tear the gastrocolic trunk, causing difficult to control hemorrhage.

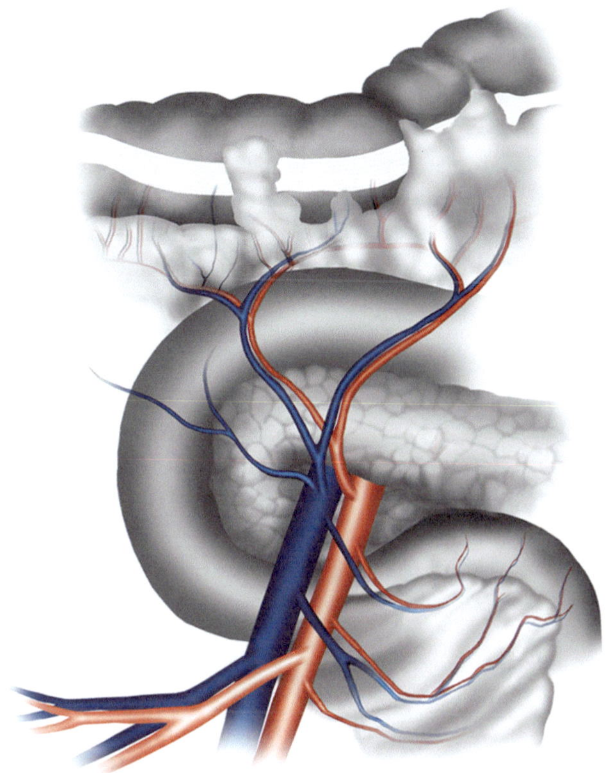

**Fig. 3.4** Superior mesenteric artery and its branches. *With permission from Yuko Tonohira*

## The Inferior Mesenteric Artery and Its Branches

The inferior mesenteric artery (IMA) is the last branch of the aorta prior to its bifurcation into the iliac vessels. The takeoff of the IMA occurs roughly at the level of L3 vertebrae, while the bifurcation resides roughly around L4 vertebrae of the anterior aorta and slightly to the left. The IMA and its branches are the vascular supply to the hindgut structures including the distal transverse, descending, and sigmoid colon, as well as the rectum. The left colic artery is the first branch off the IMA and is typically located 2 cm from the origin of the IMA from the aorta. The distal transverse colon and descending colon are vascularized via the ascending branch of the left colic artery. The bloody supply to the distal portion of the descending colon and proximal sigmoid colon is carried by the descending branch of the left colic artery. Distally, the IMA gives off various sigmoid branches. As the IMA courses over the left common iliac artery and vein, it gives rise to its terminal branch, the superior rectal artery (Figs. 3.5 and 3.6). As its name indicates, the superior rectal artery supplies the upper rectum in addition to the distal sigmoid colon. As the vessel courses into the pelvic cavity, it splits into two branches, which descend the lateral aspects of the rectum within the mesorectum and endopelvic fascia [1, 2].

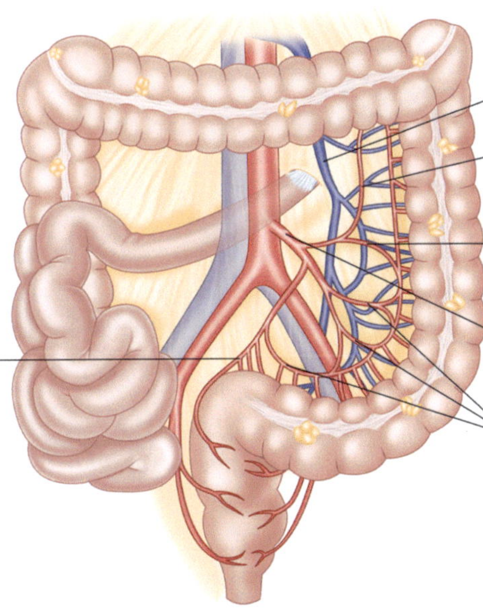


**Fig. 3.5** Blood supply to the left colon

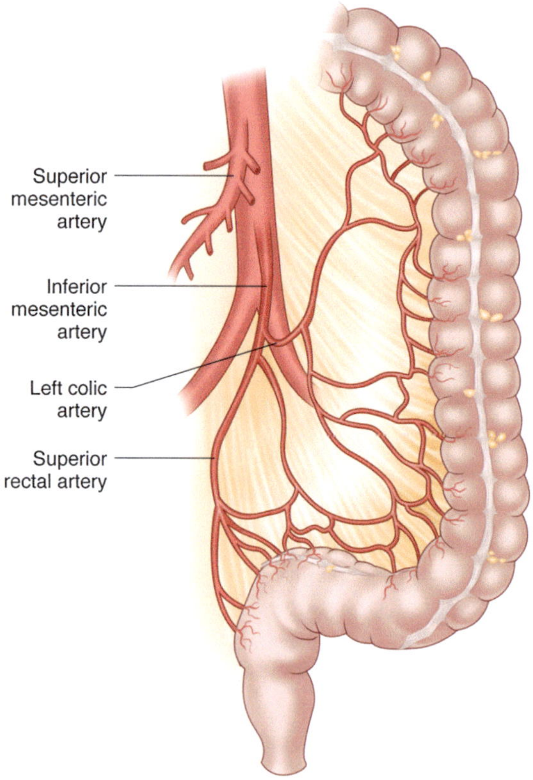


**Fig. 3.6** Mobilization of the IMA. Arrows point to the direction of mobilization toward the pedicle

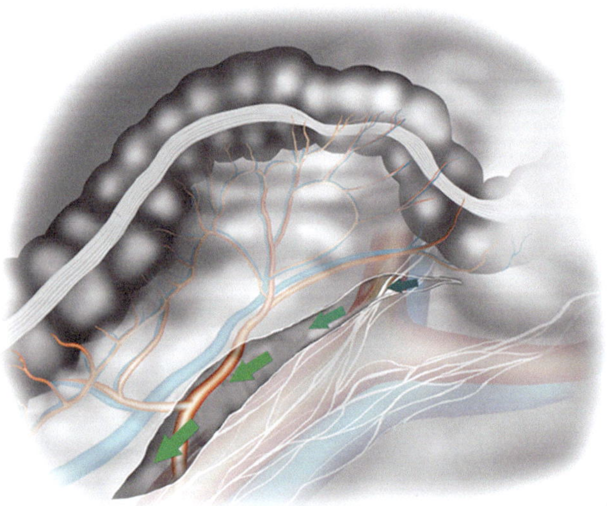

**Fig. 3.7** Mobilization of the IMA. Arrows point to the direction of mobilization toward the pedicle. With permission from Yuko Tonohira

***Pearls*:**

- ***There are no arterial branches coming off the IMA posteriorly. Dissection behind the IMA gives avascular access to the retroperitoneum. Dissection in this plane is best initiated at the level of the sacral promontory where there is the greatest separation between the retroperitoneal structures and the IMA (Fig.*** 3.7).
- ***In benign disease, the left colic artery can often be preserved by dividing the superior rectal artery (IMA as it crosses over the left common iliac artery), thereby maintaining collateral flow to the distal descending colon and proximal sigmoid colon. Typically, this is not a limiting factor in achieving adequate mobilization of the colon into the deep pelvis.***

### Splenic Flexure

The vascular anatomy distal to the middle colic artery and near the splenic flexure is variable. Connections between the left and the middle colic arteries are common. Most commonly (33 %), the ascending and descending branches of the left colic artery communicate through the marginal vessels. An additional third branch off the left colic communication with the middle colic (25 %) or the left colic artery as single arcade attached to the marginal vessels (25 %) is less frequent. In minority of cases (14.5 %), an accessory left colic artery arises from the superior mesenteric artery (Fig. 3.8).

## Embryologic Surgical Planes

During embryologic development, the colon starts off as a midline structure. As the embryo develops, the colon rotates laterally and fuses with the retroperitoneum. The white line of Toldt represents the lateral fusion line between the colon and the retroperitoneum (Fig. 3.9a, b). Regardless of type of dissection approach (medial to lateral vs. lateral to medial) one uses during a laparoscopic colectomy, the ultimate goal is to separate the colon and its mesentery away from the retroperitoneal structures and develop the colon as a midline structure. When performing the lateral-to-medial approach, the dissection must be started along or just medial to the white line of Toldt (Fig. 3.10a, b). Dissection in this area will allow an entry into the appropriate plane between the colon mesentery and the retroperitoneum. On the other hand, dissecting lateral to the white line will likely lead directly into the retroperitoneal space and will increase the likelihood of causing unwanted bleeding and injury to the retroperitoneal structures. When performing medial-to-lateral dissection, the mesenteric vessels are isolated and ligated before gaining an access into the retroperitoneum (Fig. 3.10a, b). Because there is no fusion plane between the colon mesentery and the retroperitoneum in the midline, closest to the named vessels, there is a tendency to veer off from the proper dissection plane (Fig. 3.11a). The surgeon has to make a conscious effort to stay within the appropriate surgical plane (Fig. 3.11b). The mantra "purple goes down" is useful to remind ourselves from getting too deep into the retroperitoneal space.

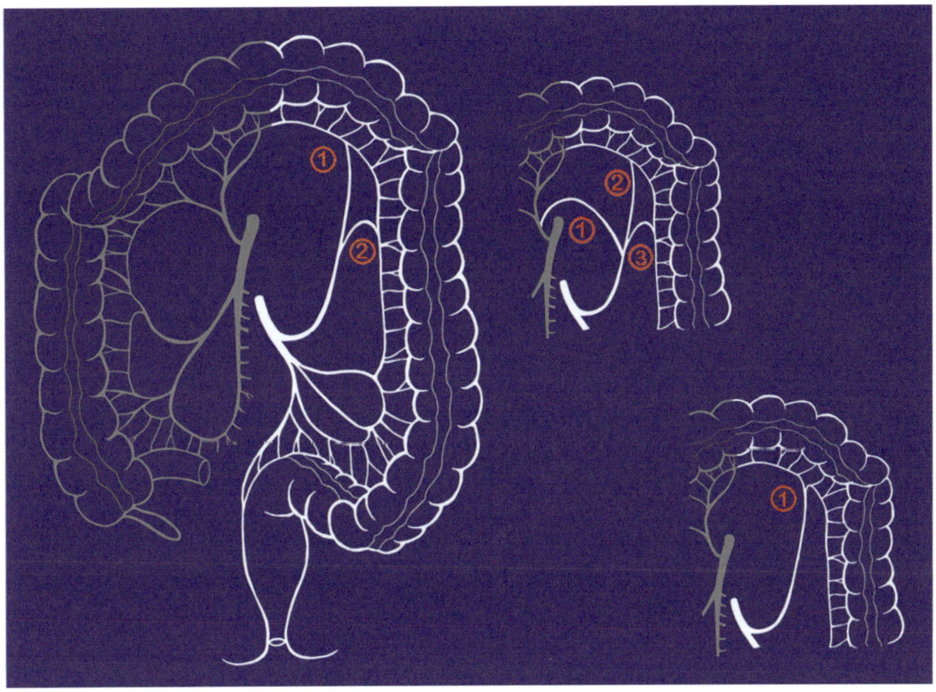


**Fig. 3.8** Variations in the blood supply to the left colon and splenic flexure (1, 2, 3 = Variations in left colic artery branches). *With permission from Yuko Tonohira*

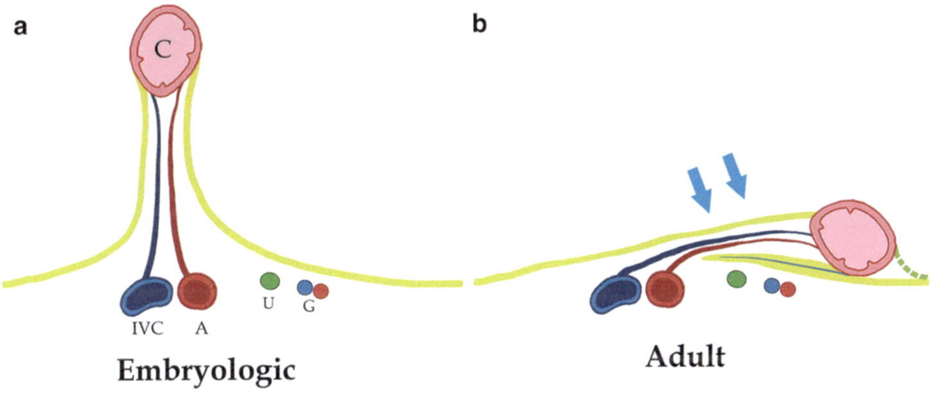


**Fig. 3.9** (**a**) Embryologic planes of the left colon (*C* colon, *U* ureters, *G* gonadal vessels, *IVC* inferior vena cava, *A* aorta). (**b**) In the adult, the colon has fused (*green arrows*) to the retroperitoneum. *With permission from Yuko Tonohira*

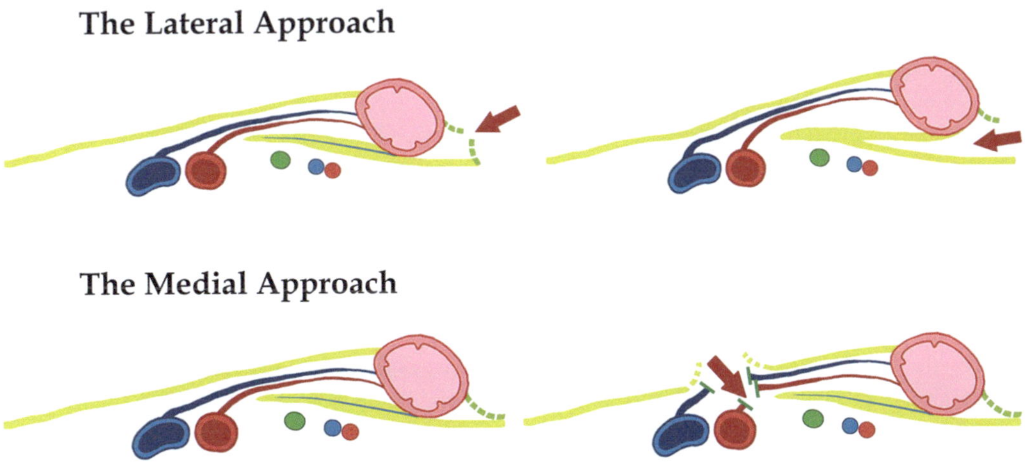


**Fig. 3.10** (**a**) Mobilization of the left colon through the white line of Toldt (*red arrow*); (**b**) continued dissection in the correct plane leaving the gonadal vessels and ureters in the retroperitoneum. *With permission from Yuko Tonohira*

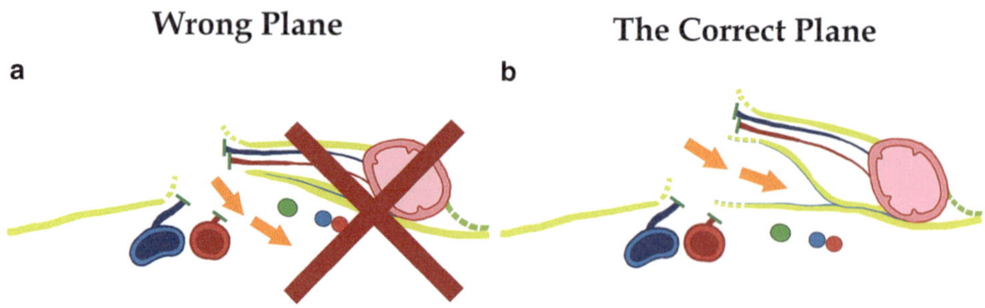


**Fig. 3.11** (**a**) Continuing mobilization in the posterior plane (*wrong plane*) will lead to elevation and possible damage to the ureter. (**b**) The correct plane is above the gonadals and ureter, leaving them in the retroperitoneum. *With permission from Yuko Tonohira*

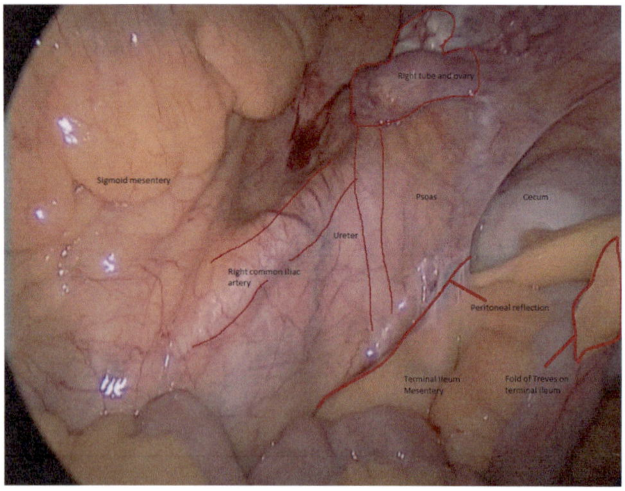


**Fig. 3.12** When mobilizing the terminal ileum mesentery, care must be taken to visualize the ureter which travels over the psoas and crosses the right external iliac artery

## The Ureter

The ureters lie under the parietal peritoneum and rest on the anterior surface of the psoas muscle (Fig. 3.12). The right and left ureters both follow a straight path from the renal pelvis to the pelvic, 4–5 cm laterally to the IVC and the aorta, respectively (Fig. 3.13). The ureters then cross over the iliac vessels to enter the pelvic brim. The right ureter classically traverses the external iliac artery (Figs. 3.16 and 3.17), whereas the left ureter lies slightly more medial and typically crosses the common iliac artery. The ureters then run posterior and inferior on the lateral pelvic sidewall. In males, the ureters continue to course medially and pass between the vas deferens (anterior) and the seminal vesicles (posterior). In females, the ureter descends posterior to the ovary and into the base of the broad ligament passing under the uterine artery. In males and females, the ureter enters the posterolateral surface of the bladder and travels at an oblique angle for approximately 2 cm until it forms the trigone [3].

In the course of performing laparoscopic right colectomy, the right ureter is typically not encountered when dissecting the right colon mesentery away from the retroperitoneal structures. Rather, the right ureter is typically visualized when the terminal ileum mesentery is sharply dissected away from the retroperitoneum over the pelvic brim (Fig. 3.19).

When performing a laparoscopic left colectomy or pelvic dissection, the ureters may be encountered in two locations: (1) where they cross over the common iliac vessels and (2) the lateral walls of the pouch of Douglas as they course beneath either the vas deferens or the uterine artery (Fig. 3.20). When dissecting behind the IMA into the retroperitoneal space, the left ureter is located medial to the gonadal vessels (Fig. 3.21). When developing the plane anteriorly, theoretically the ureters should not be seen at this level [4, 5].

***Pearls*:**

- ***Prior to dividing the IMA pedicle, the ureter must be visualized and dissected out of harm's way.***
- ***If the left ureter is not visualized and the psoas muscle appears bare, the plane of dissection is likely to be too deep. The left ureter and gonadal vessels may be adherent to the left colon mesentery in this case.***

## The Gonadal Vessels

The gonadal arteries typically arise from the anterior aorta just below the renal artery. Unlike the ureter, the gonadal vessels travel oblique toward the pelvic inlet. The gonadal arteries cross the abdominal ureters approximately halfway between the pelvic inlet and the renal pelvis. The ovarian vessels enter the broad ligament of the ovary at the pelvic brim. The testicular vessels cross the pelvic brim between the sacroiliac joint and the inguinal ligament to enter the deep inguinal ring. After traveling their respective courses, the right ovarian and testicular vein generally join the inferior cava while the left gonadal vein commonly joins the left renal vein [3].

**Fig. 3.13** Course of the ureters on the psoas

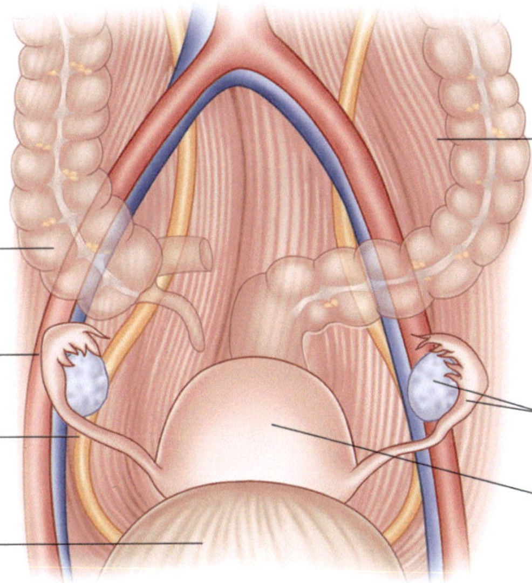


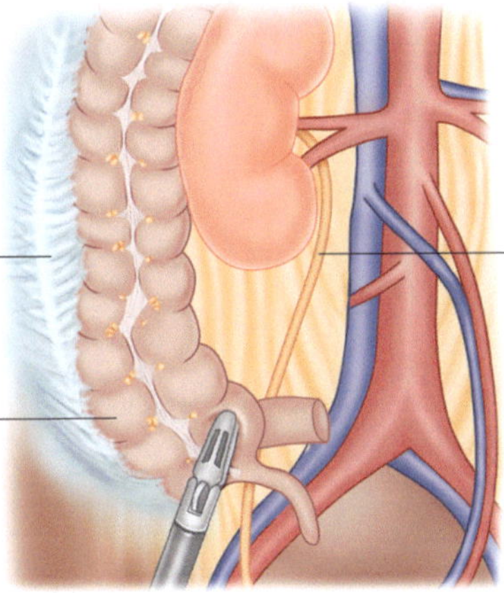


**Fig. 3.14** Entry into the presacral space. Notice the course of the ureter and the nerves at this level

## Anatomy of the Pelvis

Low anterior (rectal) resection requires an intimate knowledge of the pelvic anatomy. Appropriate understanding of the compartments and structures within these areas permits an easier, safer, more reproducible, and oncologically sound resection.

### Posterior and Lateral Compartments

The posterior compartment of the pelvis is comprised of the presacral fascia, rectum with its associated mesorectum, and surrounding fascia propria (Fig. 3.20). The presacral fascia overlies the concavity of the bony sacrum and coccyx (Figs. 3.18 and 3.23). It contains the middle sacral artery, the autonomic nerves, and the presacral veins known for causing perilous bleeding during a pelvic dissection [6, 7]. The rectum is enclosed by the fascia propria of the rectum, an investing extension of the endopelvic fascia. It encloses the mesorectum, fat, nerves, and the blood supply along the lateral extraperitoneal stalks of the rectum. The rectogenital septum marks the anterior border of the posterior pelvic compartment. The septum is clearly marked by the visceral pelvic fascia or Denonvilliers fascia that separates the extraperitoneal rectum anteriorly from the vagina (Figs. 3.24 and 3.25) or prostate and seminal vesicles [8]. Developing the plane anterior to the fascia propria or extramesorectal plane may lead to resection of Denonvilliers fascia and is associated with an increased risk of bladder and sexual dysfunction due to sacrifice of branches of the pelvic plexus of the hypogastric nerves.

***Pearls*:**

- ***Development of Denonvilliers fascia can be difficult and is often facilitated by developing the posterior and lateral planes initially and extending them circumferentially to the anterior plane.***
- ***If done correctly, the surgeon will notice an "open C"-type or "opening-zipper" configuration of this fascia that will demarcate the appropriate dissection plane (Figs. 3.26 and 3.27). In this instance, starting from a known to unknown dissection will help identify the appropriate dissection plane with loose alveolar tissue as the definitive marker.***

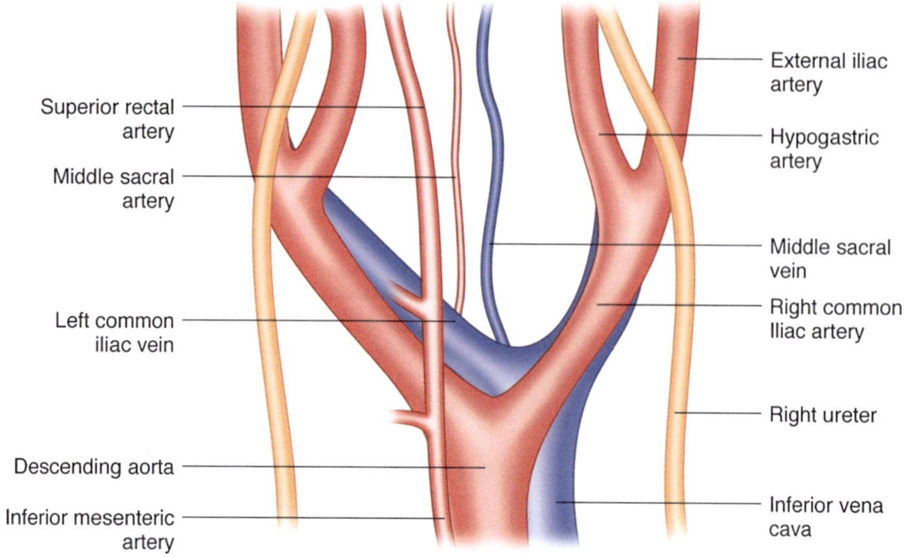


**Fig. 3.15** The right ureter will traverse the external iliac artery, while the left ureter will cross the travel slightly more medial crossing the left common iliac vessels

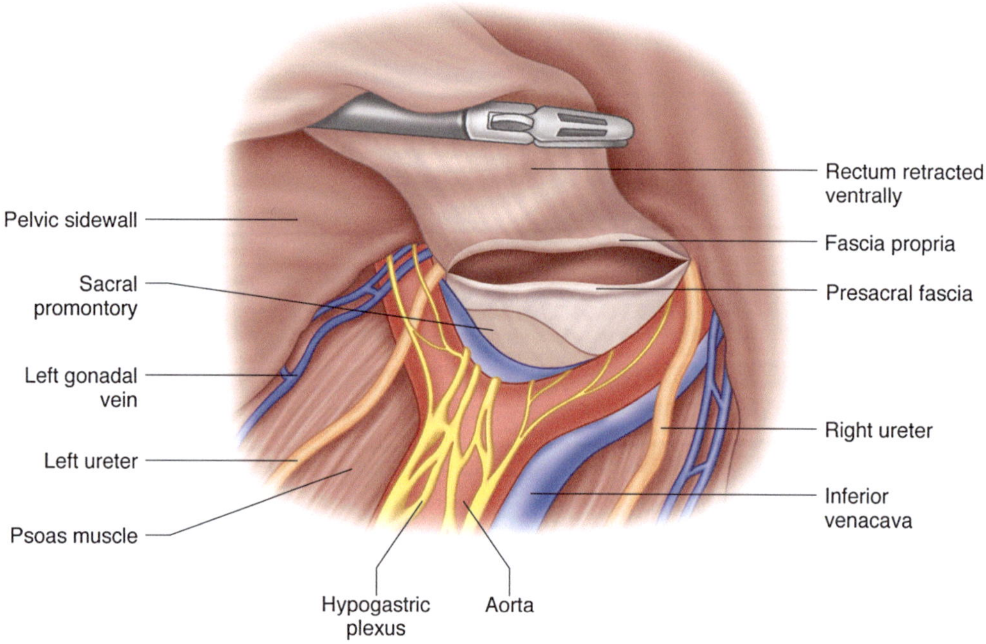


**Fig. 3.16** Entry into the presacral space. Notice the course of the ureter and the nerves at this level

## Innervation

The colon and rectum are innervated by the sympathetic and parasympathetic systems. The sympathetic supply of the left colon and the rectum arises from L1 to L3 and is distributed through the lumbar splanchnic nerves via the aortic and inferior mesenteric plexuses and the sacral splanchnic nerves through the superior and inferior hypogastric plexuses (Fig. 3.28). The preganglionic fibers synapse in the preaortic plexus, while postganglionic fibers travel along the IMA and superior rectal artery to the intestine. These nerves typically overlie the aorta, and care must be taken to identify and preserve these during dissection and ligation of

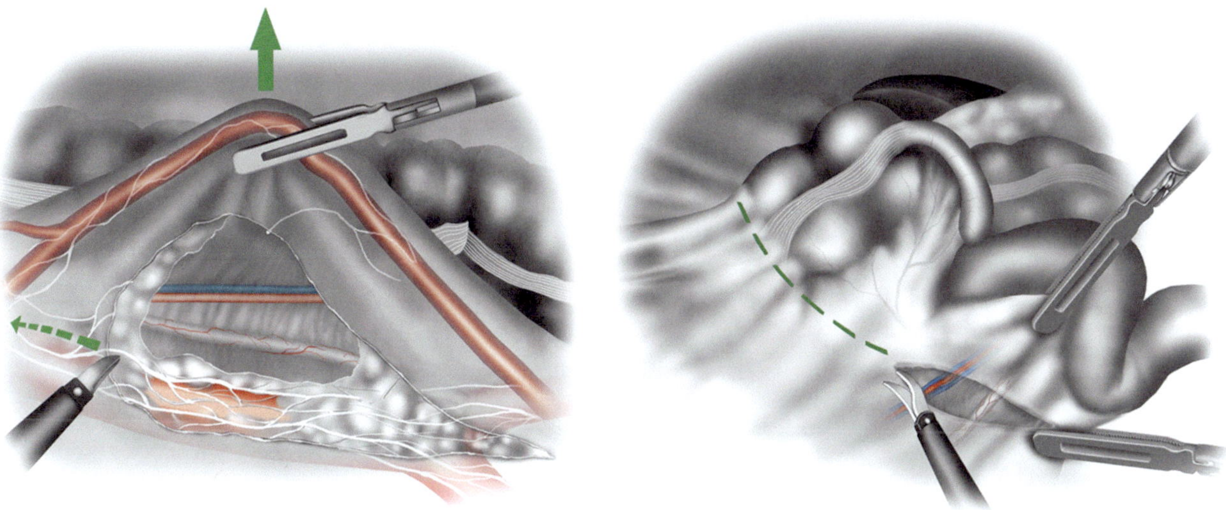

**Fig. 3.17** The right ureter will traverse the external iliac artery, while the left ureter will cross the travel slightly more medial crossing the left common iliac vessels

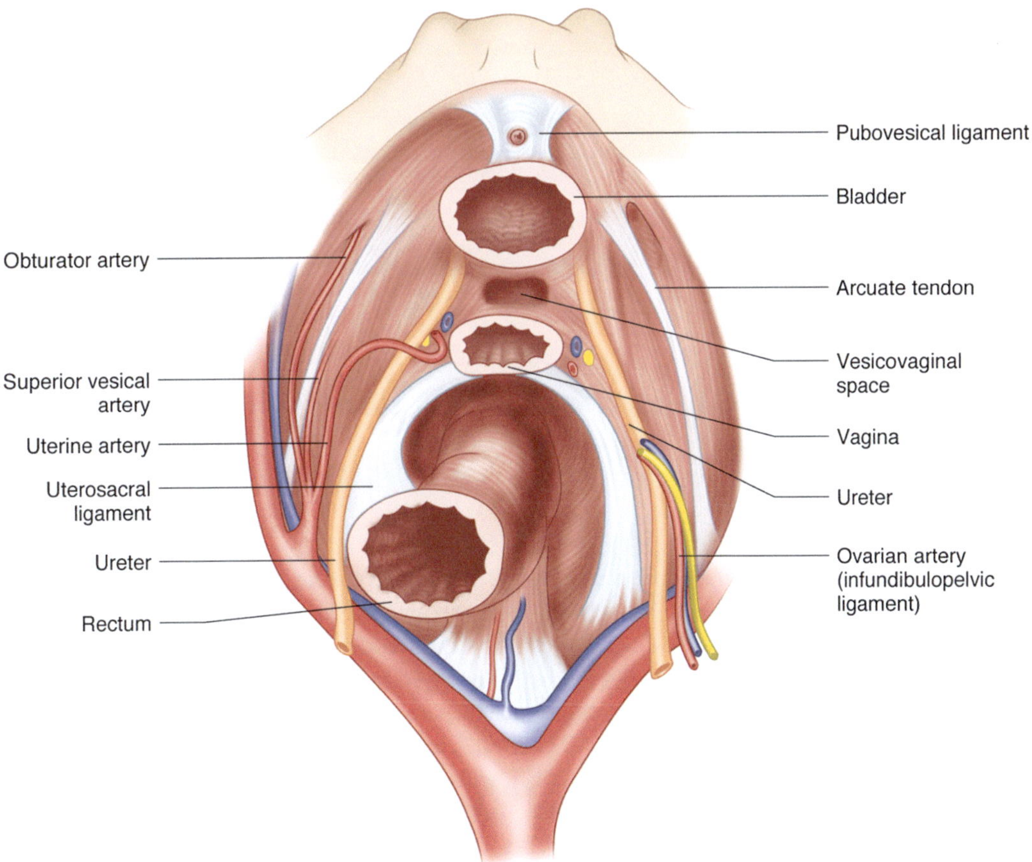


**Fig. 3.18** Course of the ureter as it enters the pelvic sidewall and travels under the uterine artery (vas deferens) and into the bladde

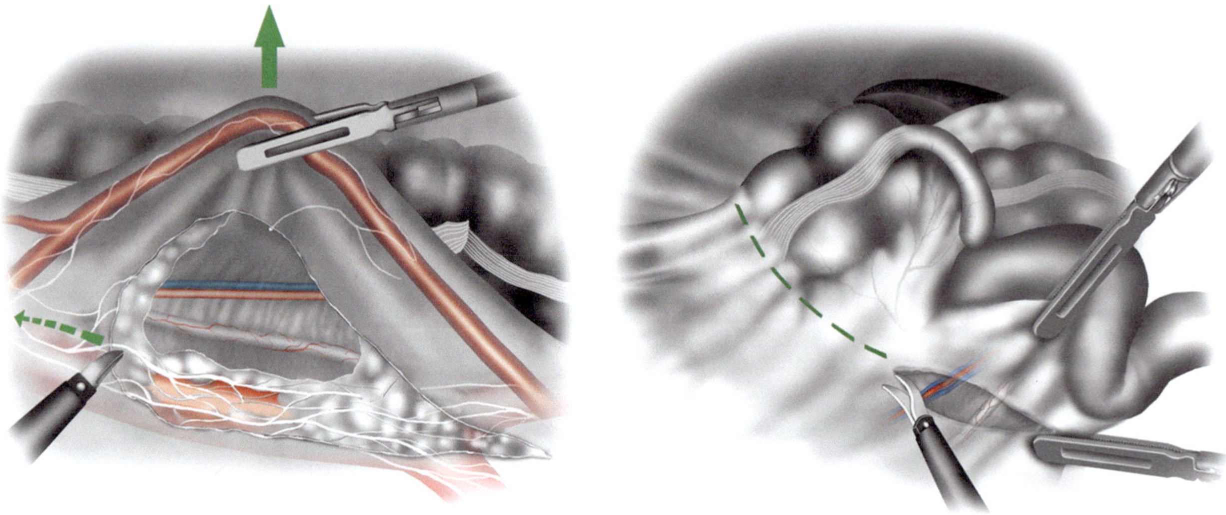

**Fig. 3.19** Mobilization of the left colon under the IMA (*green arrow* depicts elevation of the pedicle and *dashed arrow* depicts direction of dissection). Notice the relationship of the ureter to the gonadal vessels. *With permission from Yuko Tonohira*

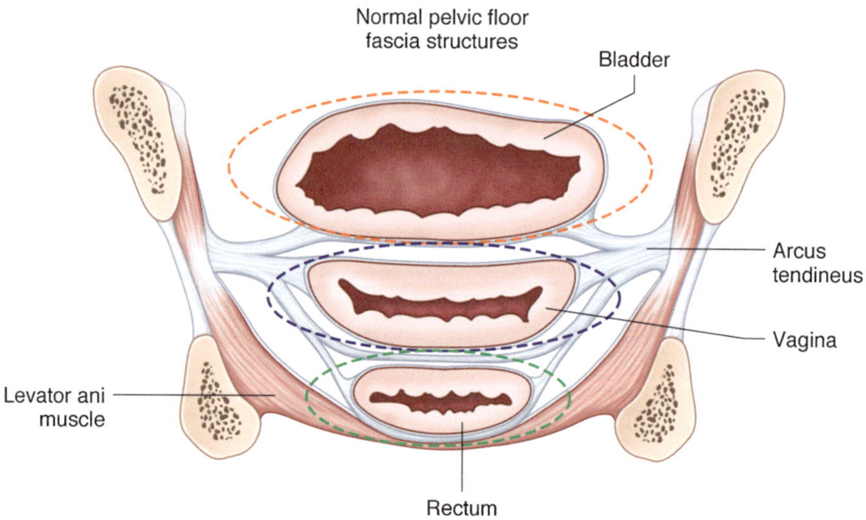


**Fig. 3.20** *Dashed green line* depicts the posterior rectum, while the *blue and orange lines* represent the middle and anterior compartments; the *middle compartment* is only present in females

the IMA off the aorta. The lower rectum is innervated by presacral nerves formed by the fusion of the lumbar splanchnic nerves and the aortic plexus. Subsequently, these nerves combine to form the hypogastric plexus located just below the sacral promontory (Figs. 3.29 and 3.30). The hypogastric plexus gives rise to two main hypogastric nerves which travel along the lateral sacrum and pelvic sidewalls into the pelvic plexus located in the lower rectum adjacent to what are typically conceived as the lateral stalks of the mesorectum [9, 10].

The parasympathetic innervation of the rectum and anal canal is comprised of sacral roots S2–4 and travels via the pelvic splanchnic nerves known as the latter (nervi) (Fig. 3.25). The nervi erigentes fuse with the sympathetic hypogastric nerves at the pelvic plexus. From here the pelvic plexus gives to the inferior mesenteric plexus and the periprostatic plexus. The inferior mesenteric plexus distributes both sympathetic and parasympathetic innervation to the lower rectum and anal canal. The periprostatic plexus supplies the prostate, seminal vesicles, vas deferens, urethra, ejaculatory ducts, and bulbourethral glands [10, 11].

Pelvic dissection poses a risk of injury to the pelvic nerves with increased risk of trauma at certain locations. High ligation of the IMA may lead to injury of the sympathetic preaortic nerves. Similarly, development of the avascular plane between the mesorectum and presacral fascia at the level of the sacral

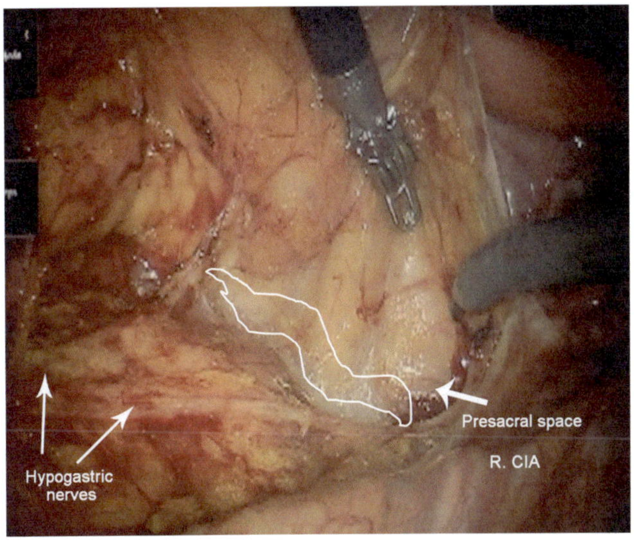


**Fig. 3.21** Pelvic anatomy highlighting the sacrum, hypogastric nerves, and avascular alveolar space between the fascia propria and presacral fascia

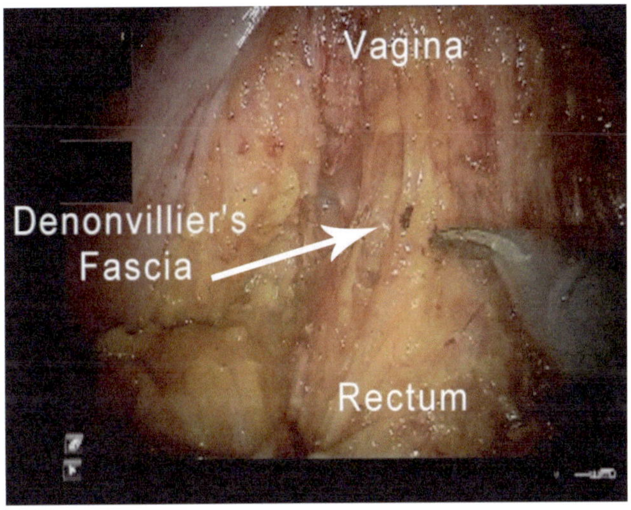


**Fig. 3.22** Denonvilliers fascia can often be a difficult plane to identify; careful tension/counter-tension between the rectum and the genitourinary structure will help develop the appropriate plane

promontory or the concavity of the sacrum exposes the superior hypogastric plexus and the hypogastric nerves to injury. Trauma at both levels results in sympathetic denervation with intact parasympathetic innervation leading to bladder dysfunction and retrograde ejaculation. As the dissection is extended caudally, the pelvic plexus may be damaged resulting in both sympathetic and parasympathetic denervation. Injury at this level can lead to rectal, urinary, and erectile dysfunction, vaginal dryness, and dyspareunia [12].

### Anterior and Middle Compartments

The anterior compartment is largely comprised of the bladder and the adjacent paravisceral fat pad. The nerve-vessel plate lies between the two structures. The middle compartment lies between the anterior and posterior compartment and exists only in females. It is outlined by the endopelvic fascia overlaying the uterus, vagina, and tuberosacral ligament (Fig. 3.22).

## Right Colectomy

With either approach, the patient is first placed in a Trendelenburg position with the operating table inclined toward the left. The omentum is retracted by lifting and placing this superiorly over the transverse colon and liver. The small bowel is then mobilized out of the pelvis and toward the left side of the abdomen. These steps will help isolate the terminal ileum, right colon, and mesentery from other vital structures (Figs. 3.1 and 3.2).

### Right Colectomy: Distinct Anatomy of Medial-to-Lateral Mobilization

***Pearl: The critical maneuver in performing a medial-to-lateral dissection for right colectomy is creation of a window around the origin of the ileocolic pedicle with appropriate tension near the bowel and then protection of the duodenum and other retroperitoneal structures during ligation and subsequent dissection.***

The right colon is supplied by the ileocolic artery branching off the superior mesenteric artery. Anatomically, it courses just infero-caudally to the third portion of the duodenum. This is best visualized by grasping either the cecum or mesentery close to the bowel wall anteriorly or ventrally. In thinner patients, identification of the duodenal sweep or C curve can be observed with superoanterior retraction of the transverse colon. In some patients, this must be preceded by division of congenital fusion attachments of the right colon mesentery to the proximal transverse colon mesentery. With anterolateral retraction of the ileocecal region, a tenting or bowstringing effect will be noted—with the mesenteric vasculature acting as the scaffold (Figs. 3.5 and 3.31). In general, when tracing named mesenteric vascular structures, such as the ileocolic vessels, to their origin, there will be a thinning out or paucity of adiposity in the mesenteric fat on both sides of the vessels. Careful dissection through the mesentery at this avascular point is critical. This is generally first performed by creating an opening in the peritoneum and mesentery inferiorly and then encircling the vessels superiorly. Some mobilization of the mesocolon from the retroperitoneal structures may be nec-

**Fig. 3.23** Schematic representation of the prostate, nerves, rectum, and pelvic structures

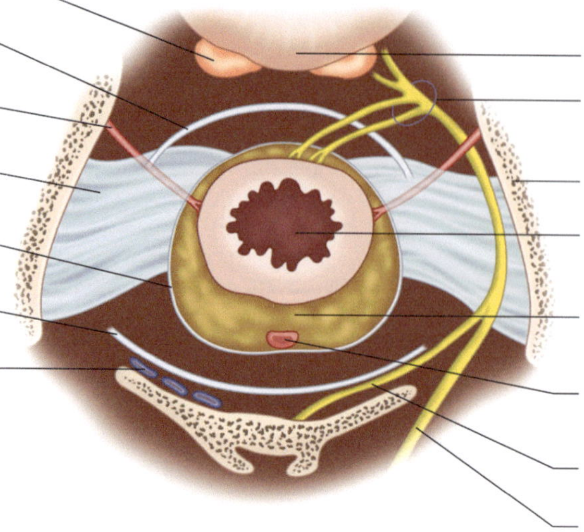


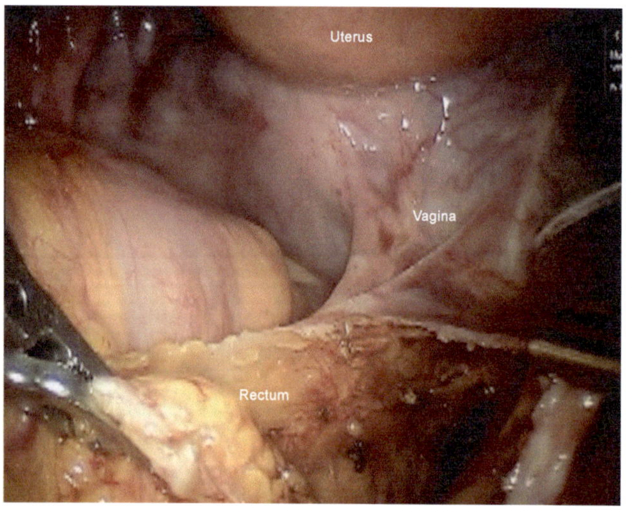


**Fig. 3.24** Reverse "C-shaped" plane during distal anterolateral dissection along the pelvic side

essary and can be performed with gentle blunt sweeping motions dorsally. When doing so, care must be taken to visualize the right ureter inferolaterally and, in particular, the duodenum posteriorly (Fig. 3.14a, b). Once these structures are well visualized and out of harm's way, a high or central ligation can be performed. This can be done in a variety of ways based on surgeon preference—endoscopic stapling devices, energy devices, or application of clips with intermediary division. At this point, the mesocolon can be safely grasped ventrally, and the retroperitoneal attachments can be safely dissected away from the right colon and its mesentery either sharply or with gentle brush movements. In this plane, one can see a thin white line of Toldt separating the retroperitoneal structures from the remainder of the mesocolon. Care must be taken to stay in the appropriate plane and not injure the duodenum or, more laterally, not mobilize the kidney (Fig. 3.32).

***Pearl***: ***(1) Identification of the duodenum is a helpful marker for confirming the correct plane of dissection and extent of dissection when performing the procedure for oncologic lymph node staging. (2) The critical maneuver in performing a medial-to-lateral dissection is to sustain proper tension and counter-tension. Only by doing so will the surgeon be able to identify and maintain the correct plane, allowing the procedure to continue along its natural progression.***

A key point in performing this maneuver is to gently push or sweep the peritoneal reflection line down rather than pull other structures down which generally causes more tearing and subsequent bleeding. Further distal dissection of the mesentery is performed to the level of the middle colic vessels. The middle colic vessel is the primary blood supply to the proximal two-thirds of the transverse colon and branches off the superior mesentery artery just inferior to and then overlies the pancreas. Care must be taken to use precise technique in this retroperitoneal space as the pancreaticoduodenal and gastroepiploic veins may cause significant hemorrhage if excess tension and shearing occur. Once the middle colic vessel is identified, the right branch of the middle colic vessel is then divided after isolation. This can be done with gentle anterosuperior retraction of the transverse colon and consequent identification of the takeoff of the right and left branches of the middle colic—a classic "Y" pattern may be seen (Fig. 3.33).

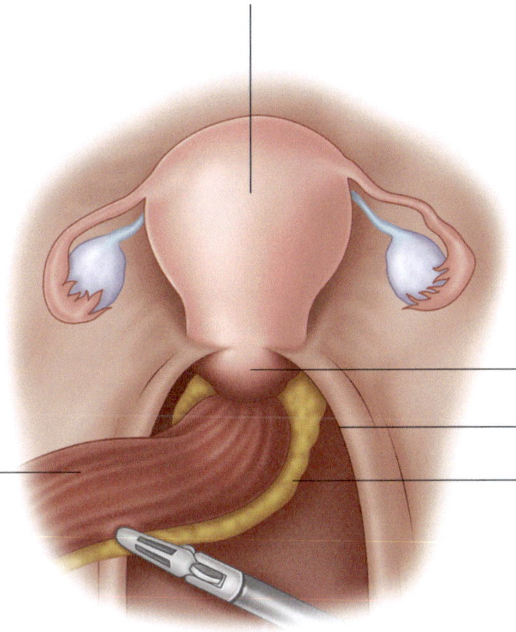


**Fig. 3.25** Entry into the presacral space involves retraction to the left to expose the right pelvic sidewall

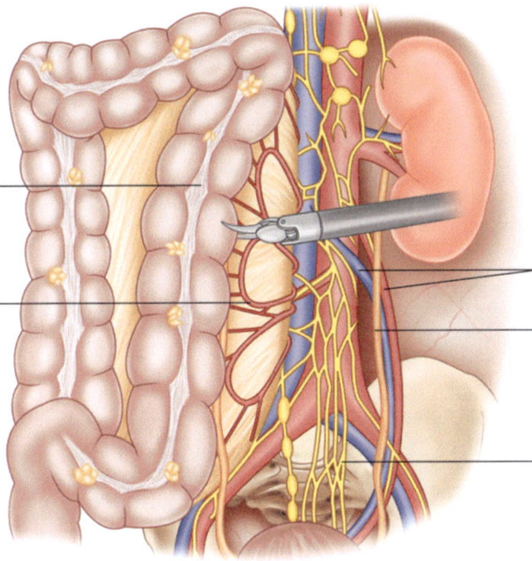


**Fig. 3.26** Medial mobilization of the left colon demonstrating the arterial blood supply, ureter, and nerves

In the vicinity of the hepatic flexure, the right colic vein, located lateral to the right branch of the middle colic artery, will be seen coursing from the pancreas to the hepatic flexure. This should also be carefully divided while preventing injury to the gastroepiploic vessels. Generally, after identifying the line of transection for the transverse colon, a window around the right branch of the middle colic artery (and right branch of middle colic vein) is created at the apex of the "Y" and is then divided in a left-to-right fashion. The dissection can then be extended inferiorly and proximally to mobilize the terminal ileal mesentery and also superiorly and distally to divide the mesentery to the level of the middle colic vessels. These latter vessels are preserved in anticipation of anastomosis of the small bowel to the transverse colon. At this point, the right colon will now only be held in place by lateral avascular attachments to the abdominal sidewall and then the hepatic flexure attachments and gastrocolic attachments of the omentum to the transverse colon. These can generally be easily divided by either a dissecting energy device (ultrasonic or bipolar type) or an energized, monopolar cautery/Metzenbaum scissors. Dissection proceeds proximally dividing the hepatic flexure (Figs. 3.34 and 3.35) and again carefully avoiding the gastroepiploic vein and then the lateral attachments to the ascending colon in a superior-to-inferior fashion into the pelvis while staying medial to the retroperitoneal structures, in particular Gerota's fascia. At the conclusion of the mobilization, one will have kept the retroperitoneal fascia intact and dissected to the point of visualization of the preserved right iliac vessels, right psoas muscle, and right ureter (Fig. 3.32a, b).

***Pearl*: *Maintenance of dissection in the appropriate plane and gentle dissection of the retroperitoneal reflection away from the target colon and mesentery allow for a safer and more appropriate complete and intact oncologic resection without invasion of the tissues*.**

Inferiorly, along the terminal ileal mesentery, there is a reflection noted at the attachment to the retroperitoneum (Fig. 3.36). This fold is medial to the ureter, overlies the right iliac vessels in the right pelvis, and is also superolateral to the sacral promontory. If entered appropriately with anterior retraction of the terminal ileum, this mobilization of the mesentery from the retroperitoneum can be performed sharply without any energy-type devices and then continued superiorly and separating the mesentery of the terminal ileum and right colon off the duodenum and pancreas as well.

***Pearls*:**

1. ***Leaving the lateral attachments to the abdominal sidewall (line of Toldt) and hepatic flexure until the very end of dissection allows for appropriate scaffolding of the tissue and aids in achieving counter-tension when necessary*.**
2. ***When completing the detachment of these lateral attachments, a visualization of a purple hue/discoloration will be noted due to the previously dissected planes held in place only by thin peritoneal tissue layers. This helps demarcate the appropriate dissection line*.**

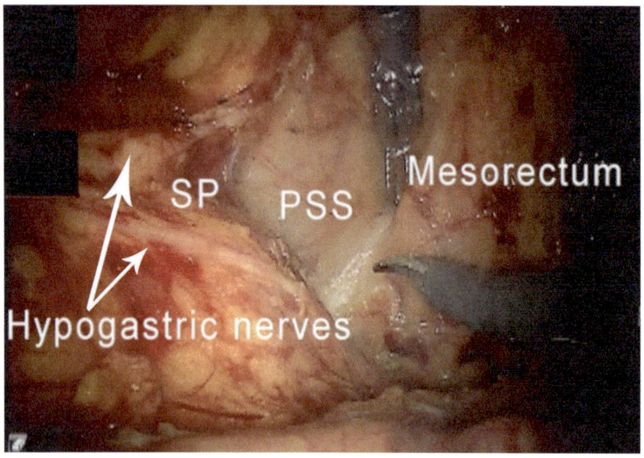


**Fig. 3.27** The hypogastric plexus located just below the *SP* sacral promontory; *PSS* presacral space

**Fig. 3.28** Cross-sectional view of the pelvis at the level of the sacral promontory

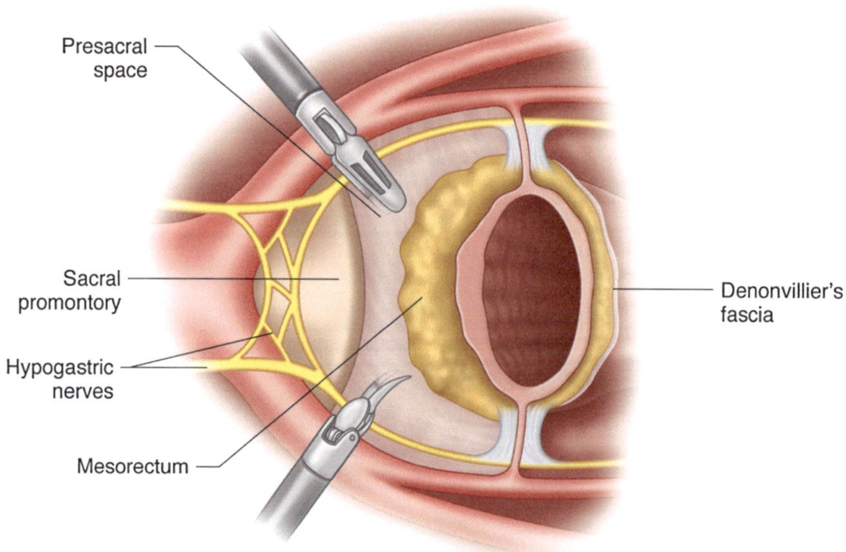

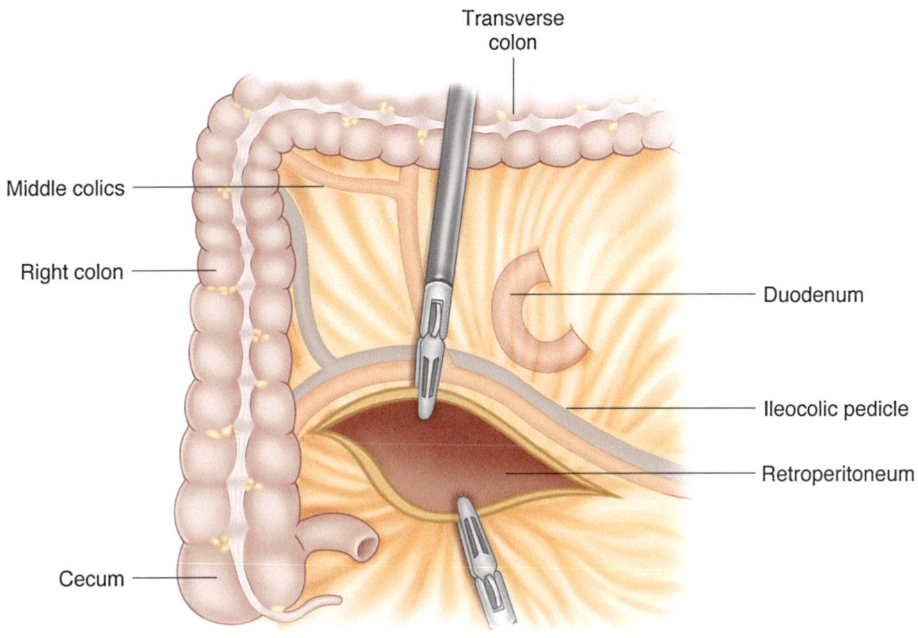


**Fig. 3.29** Dissection of the ileocolic pedicle from a medial approach

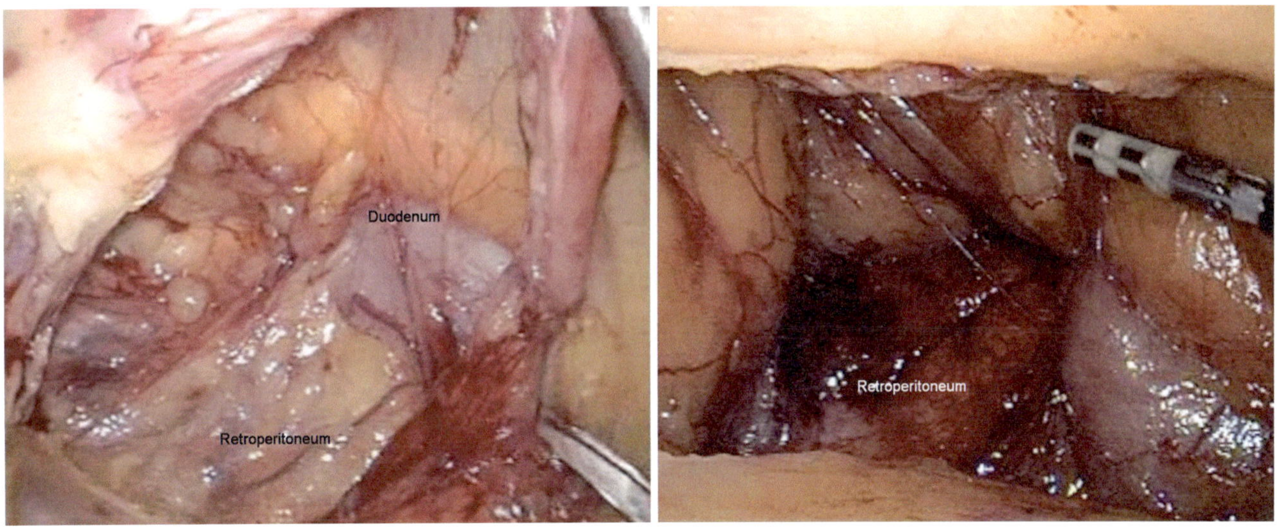


**Fig. 3.30** Medial-to-lateral mobilization highlighting the duodenum and white line of Toldt as the ascending colon and mesentery are ventrally retracted

## Right Colectomy: Distinct Anatomy of Lateral-to-Medial Mobilization

***Pearl**: Lateral-to-medial mobilization provides the surgeon the easiest transition to laparoscopic colectomy and also helps in teaching others. Care must be taken to first approach and identify the ureter and fold of the terminal ileal mesentery and its attachment to the retroperitoneum.*

This approach is generally the easier dissection to learn and perform. There are several critical anatomic landmarks that, once appreciated, can lead to a safer, more expedient and appropriate oncologic resection (sometimes termed total mesocolic excision—including the intact peritoneum encompassing the colon and mesenteric structures including high ligation of the pedicles). With the exclusion of a right colectomy for pathological enlargement of the appendix (i.e., mucocele, cystadenoma, cystadenocarcinoma, or carcinoid),

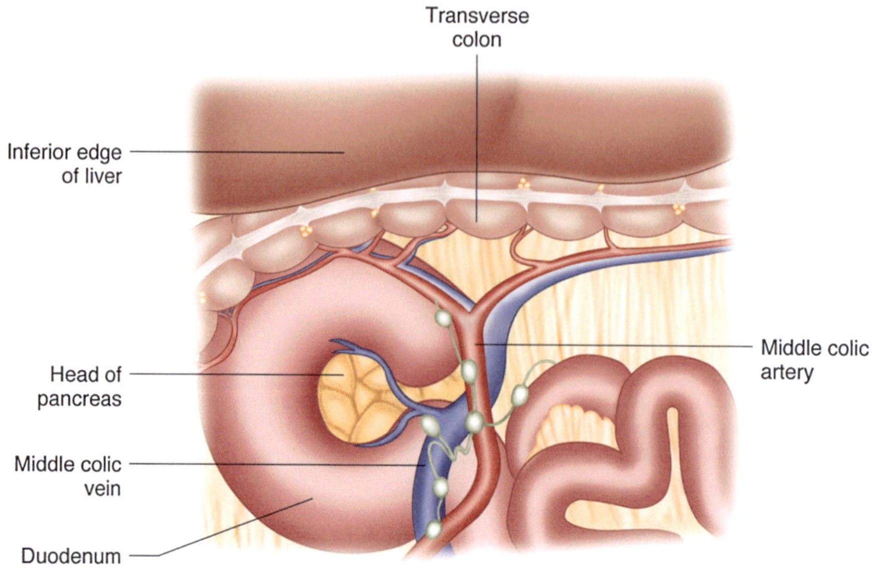


**Fig. 3.31** Depicts "Y" pattern of middle colic vessels

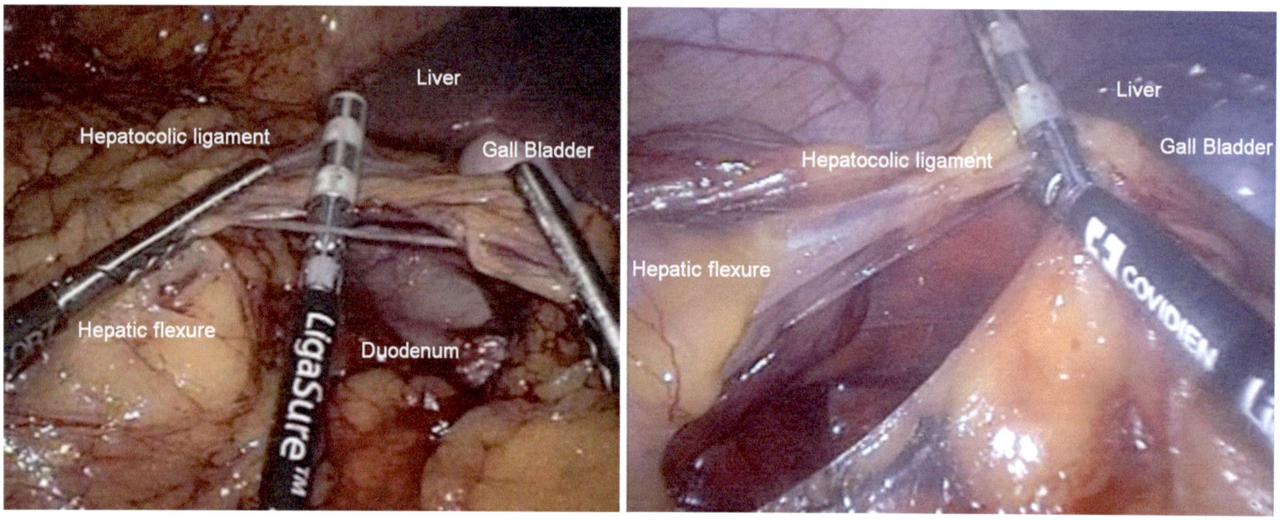


**Fig. 3.32** Hepatic flexure mobilization highlighting the liver, gallbladder, duodenum, and hepatocolic ligament (*HF* hepatic flexure, *GB* gallbladder)

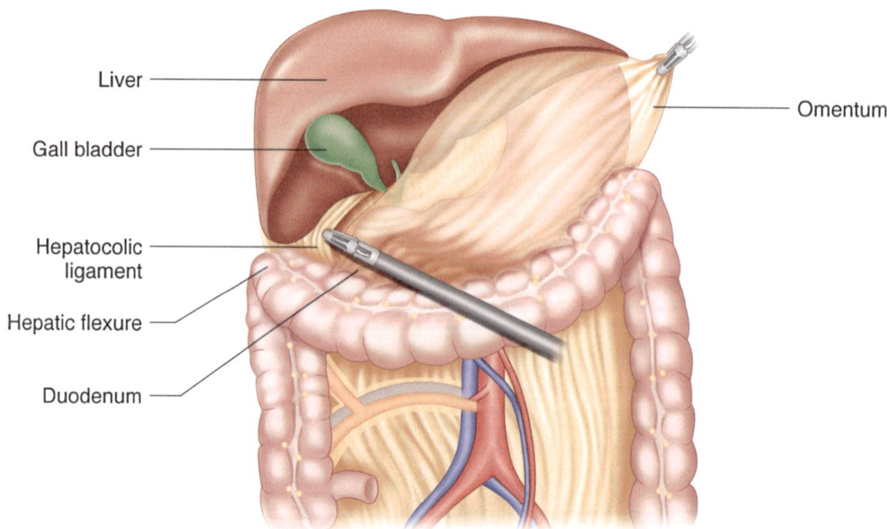


**Fig. 3.33** Mobilization of the hepatic flexure from the transverse colon

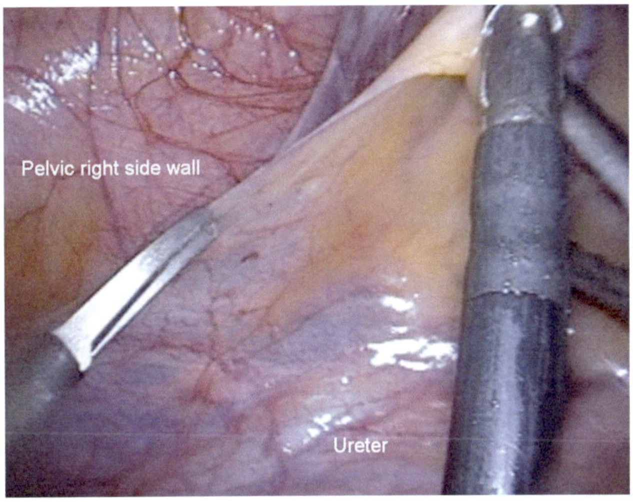


**Fig. 3.34** Visualization of the ureter while mobilizing the cecum and terminal ileum off the retroperitoneum. The ureter will course slightly more laterally on the right crossing over the right external iliac artery

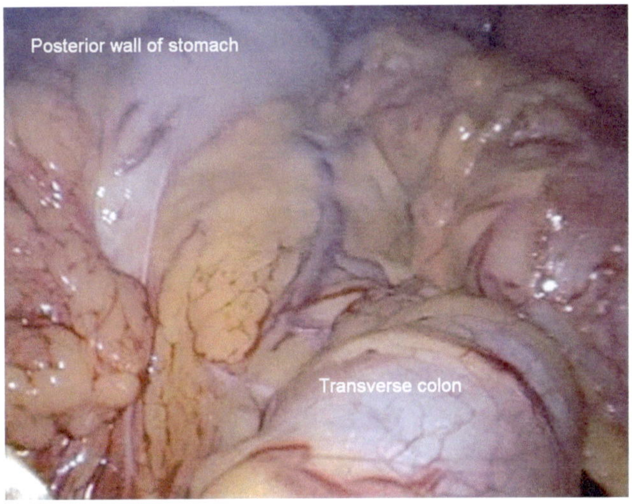


**Fig. 3.35** Laparoscopic view of the lesser sac from patient's right side

grasping this tubular structure can help significantly in retraction. Otherwise, either the terminal ileum or cecum can be gently and carefully grasped to mobilize the enteral structures anteriorly and toward the left upper quadrant. This will then clarify the lateral attachments of the colon and mesentery to the retroperitoneum. Along the colon, this will be the right lateral line of Toldt. Division of this will enter into a loose alveolar plane, and then dissection can proceed distally along the ascending colon to the hepatic flexure. In the vicinity of the ileocecal valve, however, care must be taken to identify and preserve the ureter as it crosses the right iliac artery bifurcation (Figs. 3.14a, b and 3.16). Care should be taken to stay within this appropriate plane and not too lateral—otherwise, entry into Gerota's fascia or mobilization of the kidney will ensue. Mobilization within the correct plane of the mesocolon from the retroperitoneum centrally (or medially) toward the takeoff base of the ileocolic pedicle will also expose the anterior surface of the duodenum and pancreas. The mesentery of the terminal ileum is then divided from the retroperitoneum to the level of the right iliac vessels as described above in the medial-to-lateral mobilization. At this point, as noted in the medial-to-lateral mobilization, the base of the ileocolic pedicle should now be easily visualized and divided as above.

## Right Colectomy: Common Steps

The gastrocolic attachments to the transverse colon need to be divided and then entry into the lesser sac is performed. The surgeon will first lift the omentum and retract this superiorly. Division can then be done sharply as the attachments are generally avascular or otherwise easily controlled with monopolar cautery or an energy device. For right colectomies, the distal extent of dissection is generally around the falciform ligament or in line with the middle colic vessels. It

**Fig. 3.36** Accessing the lesser sac through the omentum (gastrocolic ligament)

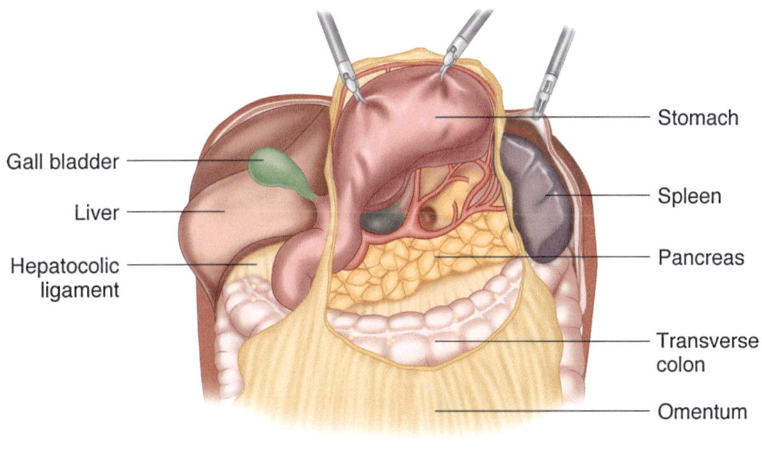

is sometimes best to start at this point and work retrograde toward the hepatic flexure. At a certain point, the omentum will then be fully mobilized. The lesser sac is entered and the proximal transverse mesocolon can then be sharply dissected from the other abdominal and retroperitoneal structures (Figs. 3.37 and 3.38). In particular, the posterior leaf of the omentum must be separated along its congenital attachments from the mesocolon. Care must be taken to completely and safely mobilize the mesocolon off of the duodenum and pancreas. As noted above, this area will have some vascular attachments that will need to be controlled. Another point of entry into the lesser sac will be the fusion or attachment of the gallbladder dome to the transverse colon or mesocolon. Similarly to above, entry at this level will also expose the lesser sac, and then one can proceed to mobilize the mesocolon off the duodenum. All that will remain at this point will be the hepatic flexure attachments, which should now be easily divided.

Once completely dissected, the right colon and mesentery should be able to be mobilized and expressed as a midline structure. Division of the intestines and subsequent anastomosis can now be performed either in a laparoscopic fashion intracorporeally or in an open fashion once extracorporealized through an extraction incision. Details of these techniques will be discussed in a later chapter.

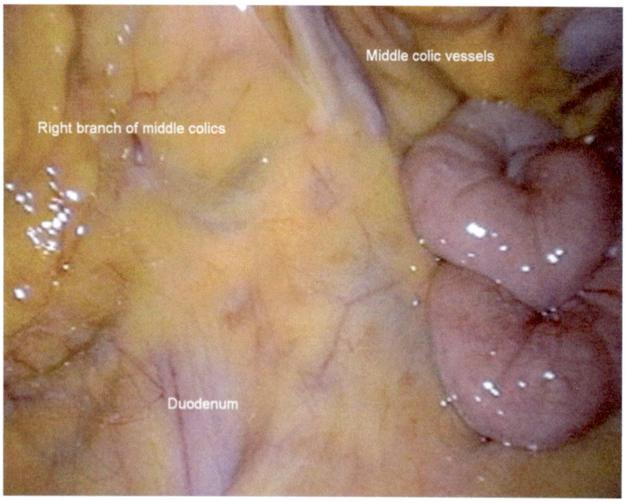


**Fig. 3.37** Transverse colon anatomy

## Transverse Colectomy and the Middle Colic Vessels

***Pearl*: *The critical maneuver in performing a transverse colectomy is identification of the middle colic artery and its distal right and left branches. In addition, care should be taken to prevent injury to the pancreas and right gastroepiploic vein. Ability to approach this from both sides of the patient will contribute to success.***

In cases requiring resection of the transverse colon, the middle colic vessel will need to be ligated and divided, sometimes in a high fashion (Figs. 3.39 and 3.40). This can proceed as a progression of the above steps. However, rather than isolating the right branch of the middle colic vessel, the entire middle colic vessel may be divided. This can be iso-

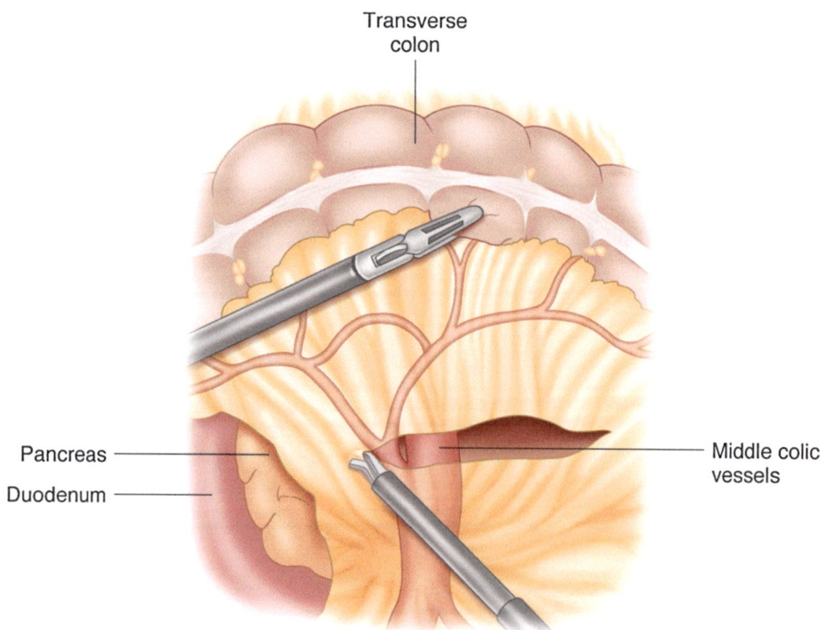


**Fig. 3.38** Middle colic vessels

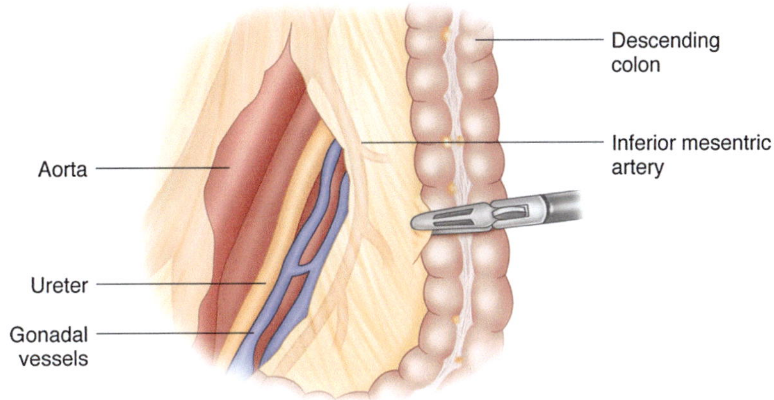


**Fig. 3.39** Dissection of the IMA via a medial-to-lateral approach

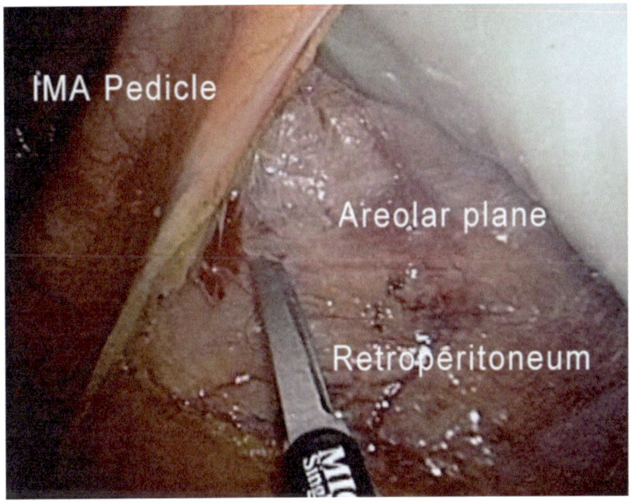


**Fig. 3.40** Laparoscopic hand-assist demonstrating the areolar plane between the colon mesentery and the retroperitoneum; *IMA* inferior mesenteric artery

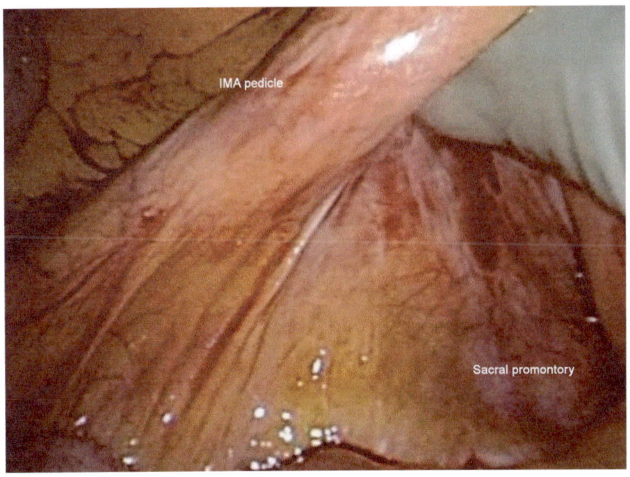


**Fig. 3.41** Anatomy of the left colon highlighting the IMA pedicle and sacral promontory

lated by gently retracting the mesentery of the transverse colon superiorly. The middle colic artery and its right and left branches will be identified. During dissection of the transverse colon mesentery off the pancreas and before division of the middle colic vein, the right gastroepiploic vein overlying the pancreas must be identified and preserved. In certain cases, the transverse mesentery may be divided as a proximal progression during total (procto)colectomy. This is generally done with the surgeon on the patient's right side after mobilization of the left colon. In this instance, after the splenic flexure is mobilized and divided, the transverse mesentery may then be serially ligated and divided in a retrograde fashion using an energy device. Alternately, a window can be created around the middle colic vessels and divided in an antegrade right-to-left fashion. This continues proximally to divide either the middle colic artery or both right and middle colic branches.

## Left Colectomy and Anterior Resection

***Pearl**: The critical maneuver in performing a medial-to-lateral dissection is to sustain proper tension and countertension. Only by doing so will the surgeon be able to identify and maintain the correct plane, allowing the procedure to continue along its natural progression.*

The patient is oriented in the Trendelenburg position with the left side tilted up, which assists in displacing the small intestine into the upper abdomen. This is an exceptional opportunity to appreciate the pelvic anatomy in its entirety before starting one's dissection. Take a moment to understand the multiple compartments of the pelvis including the relationship of pelvic vessels to the organs and the variations in pelvic anatomy between males and females.

Similar to a right colectomy, the initial dissection involves the development of the avascular plane between the

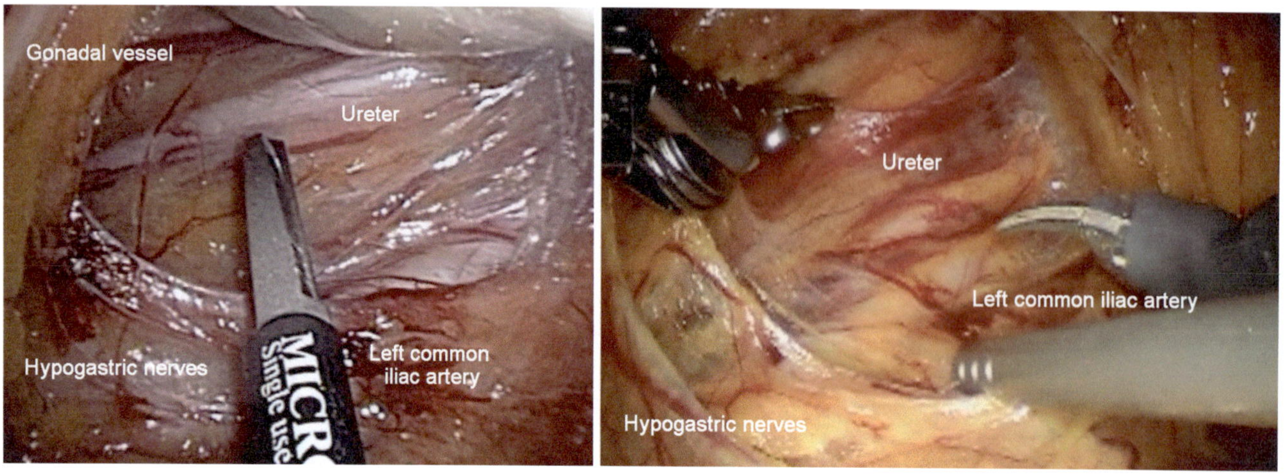


**Fig. 3.42** Medial-to-lateral mobilization of the left colon highlighting the IMA, ureter along the pelvic sidewall, and hypogastric nerve plexus overlying the aorta and iliac artery as the mesentery of the sigmoid colon is retracted anteriorly

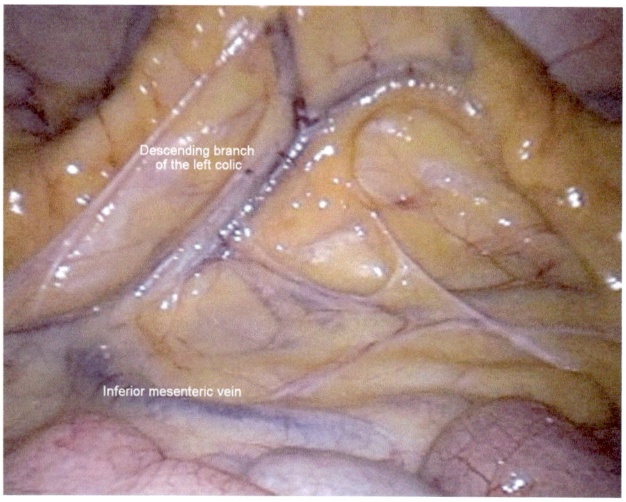


**Fig. 3.43** Left colic vessels (descending branch of left colic, *IMV* inferior mesenteric vein)

parietal peritoneum overlying the retroperitoneum and the mesentery of the left colon, along the left lateral line of Toldt. This may be achieved from a lateral-to-medial approach or vice versa. When performing a medial-to-lateral approach, the mesenteric fold containing the IMA can be found overlying the sacral promontory. Ventral retraction of the left colon mesentery will often outline the IMA pedicle entering into the pelvis to form the superior rectal artery, in a similar bowstring effect noted with the ileocolic pedicle. Scoring of the mesentery parallel to the posterior aspect of the IMA pedicle will often help enter into the avascular plane (Fig. 3.41). Gentle fenestration of the mesentery overlying the sacral promontory with an energy device (electrocautery or ultrasound) will create a ballooning pillow-type effect as the avascular plane expands and separates the mesentery away from the presacral fascia, aorta, iliac vessels, and autonomic nerves (Fig. 3.42). When performing a laparoscopic hand-assist approach, placing the thumb on the sacral promontory and pinching the mesentery of the left colon between the thumb and the index finger will aid in isolating the IMA pedicle and help initiate one's medial-to-lateral dissection (Fig. 3.43).

Paramount to any approach, retroperitoneal structures including the left gonadal vessels, left ureter, and the hypogastric nerve plexus must first be identified and preserved (Figs. 3.28 and 3.44). In cases where the ureter is not easily identified, commonly due to a surrounding fat pad, it would be prudent to alter the approach and mobilization to ensure visualization. In certain cases, the ureter may have been mobilized ventrally and placed on stretch with the mobilized left colon mesentery. Reorientation using a different approach may permit appropriate dissection away from the colon mesentery and avoid ureteral transection.

Once the ureter has been identified, the inferior mesenteric artery is often ligated and transected to facilitate the pelvic dissection. The medial-to-lateral mobilization is performed similar to that done on the right side. The retroperitoneal reflection is gently swept posterolaterally away from the colon and mesentery. The dissection proceeds cephalad to the level of the superior pole of the kidney. At this point, the IMV may be identified and mobilization of the splenic flexure may be performed (Figs. 3.6 and 3.45).

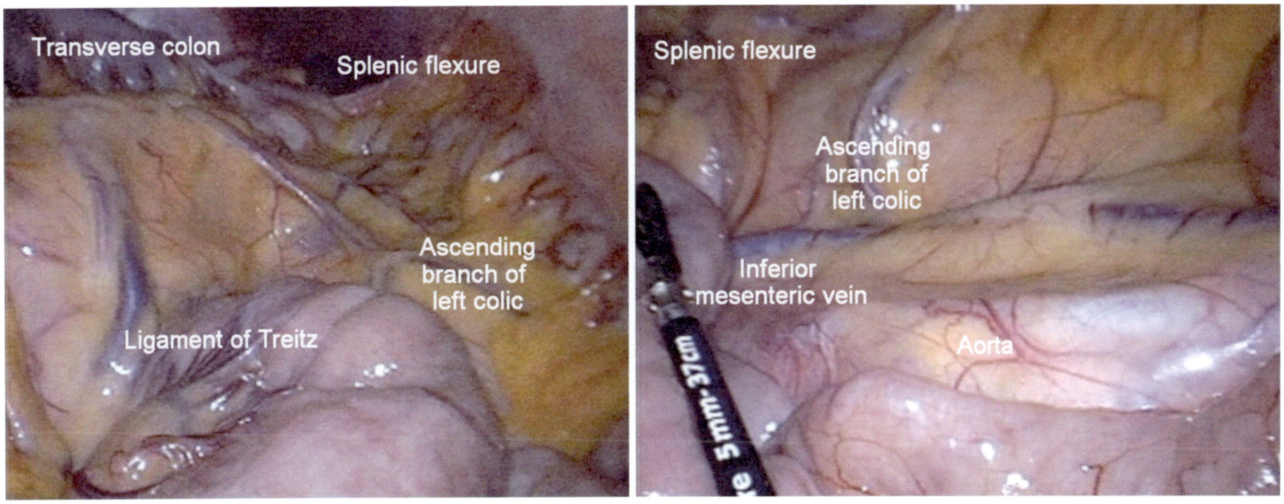


**Fig. 3.44** Left colon anatomy. *LBMC* left branch of middle colic, *ABLC* ascending branch of left colic, *SF* splenic flexure

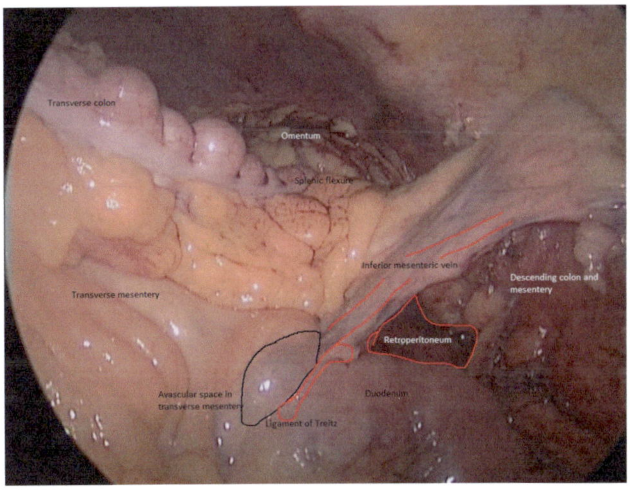


**Fig. 3.45** Ligation of the IMV transection is typically performed just caudal to the pancreas and ligament of Treitz, prior to its origin of insertion into the splenic vein. Dividing the IMV is a common technique in mobilizing the proximal colon during a low pelvic dissection

## Inferior Mesenteric Vein and Splenic Flexure Mobilization

***Pearl**: Careful technique should be used during the division of the IMV as the vessel can easily be sheared and retract if excess tension or inappropriate ligation is performed. Isolating the vessel by creating windows on either side should be performed prior to ligation such that an adequate pedicle may be grasped in case of sudden tear or dehiscence of a seal.*

The authors perform a proximal ligation of the IMV in almost all anterior or low anterior resections to aid in appropriate mobilization for tension-free colorectal or coloanal anastomoses. With the distal splenic flexure and proximal descending colon and mesentery retracted anteriorly, the inferior mesenteric vein (IMV) can be identified with avascular areas surrounding the vessel (Figs. 3.6 and 3.46). Often, the fourth part of the duodenum or proximal jejunum will have some attachments to the descending colon mesentery in this area that will need to be divided first. The IMV transection is performed just caudal to the pancreas and ligament of Treitz and prior to its origin of insertion into the splenic vein (Figs. 3.47 and 3.48). Ligation can generally be performed with an energy source such as ultrasonic shears or bipolar-type vessel sealing devices. Once this is performed, the mesentery of the splenic flexure can then be grasped superiorly and anteriorly, and the retroperitoneal reflection line of Toldt can then be gently swept posteriorly if not yet completed during the medial-to-lateral mobilization. This proceeds proximally and superiorly as high as possible toward the spleen. Careful technique should be used in IMV division as the vessel can easily be sheared and retract if excess tension or inappropriate ligation is performed.

***Pearl**: The complexity associated with mobilizing the splenic flexure may be conquered by a proper medial-to-lateral dissection to the level of the superior pole of the kidney. If done correctly, splenic flexure mobilization is reduced to simply dividing lateral attachments.*

Splenic flexure mobilization is generally performed using a combination of approaches. The patient is placed in

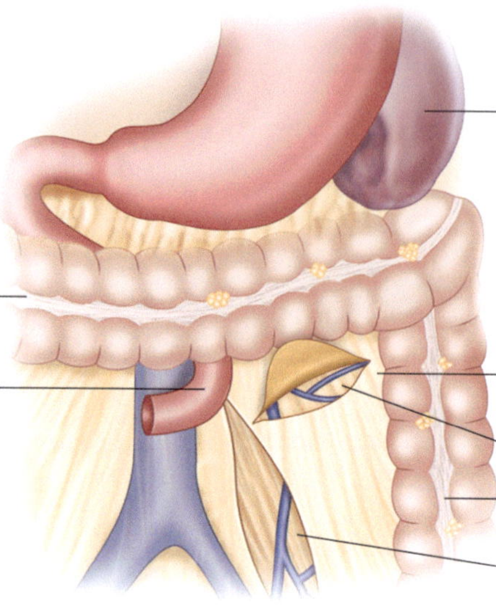


**Fig. 3.46** Ligation of the IMV involves access to the avascular space by the ligament of Treitz and an avascular window just lateral to its course

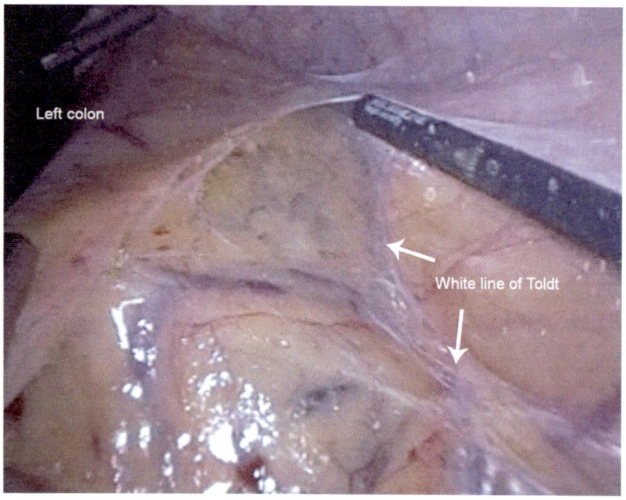


**Fig. 3.47** Lateral-to-medial mobilization of the left colon along the white line of Toldt

a reverse Trendelenburg position with the table inclined toward the right. Typically, if an adequate medial-to-lateral mobilization is performed of the left colon, then mobilization of the splenic flexure is reduced to division of the lateral attachments of the splenocolic ligaments. Laterally, the attachments to the sidewall and spleen are carefully divided while being mindful not to injure the splenic capsule (Figs. 3.49 and 3.50). Oftentimes, there will be close and dense adhesions of the colon to the spleen. The gastrocolic attachments of the omentum to the distal transverse colon are then also divided starting at the level of the falciform ligament. Congenital fusion attachments of the posterior leaf of the omentum to the mesocolon may need to be divided upon entry into the lesser sac. Similar attachments of the colonic mesentery to the stomach lead to inadvertent gastric injury. Dissection proceeds separating the attachments of the splenic flexure and its mesentery away from the spleen. At this point, an avascular plane is generally noted and dissection can safely proceed bluntly. The splenic flexure will then be held in place by thin mesenteric attachments that can be divided.

***Pearl*: *The avascular plane above the ligament of Treitz may offer an alternative pathway into the lesser sac and should be considered when the traditional approach through the omentum is not feasible due to poor exposure or pathology*.**

In some situations, the lesser sac may be dense with adhesions, and care must be taken not to proceed too posteriorly and into the pancreatic parenchyma. If the adhesions make dissection difficult, another approach to the splenic flexure may be afforded by an inferior-to-superior approach, starting at the ligament of Treitz. With the distal transverse colon mesentery retracted anteriorly, there is generally an avascular plane identified near and just above the ligament of Treitz along the transverse mesentery and above the duodenum. Entry into this window will lead into the lesser sac above the pancreas and behind the stomach (Figs. 3.51, 3.52, and 3.53). Dissection of the distal transverse colon mesentery and splenic flexure mesentery can then proceed in an antegrade distal fashion up to and including division of the IMV. Once mobilized, the transverse colon mesentery can be retracted anteriorly and dissected off the remaining retroperitoneal structures and then away from the

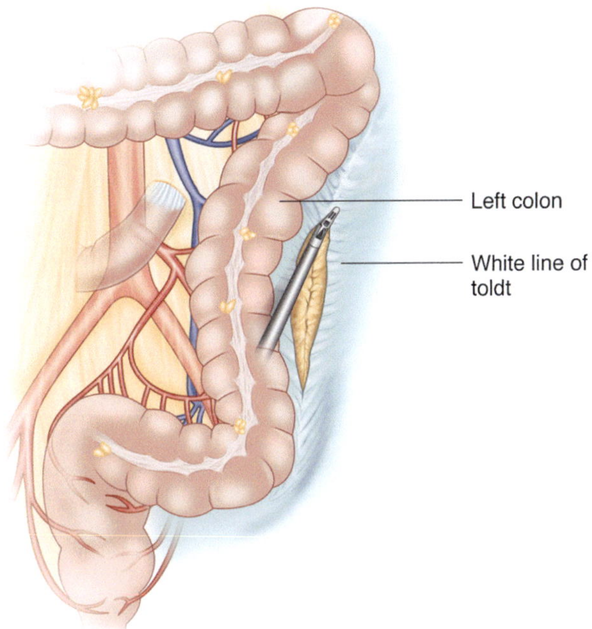


**Fig. 3.48** Mobilization of the left colon by taking down the lateral attachments

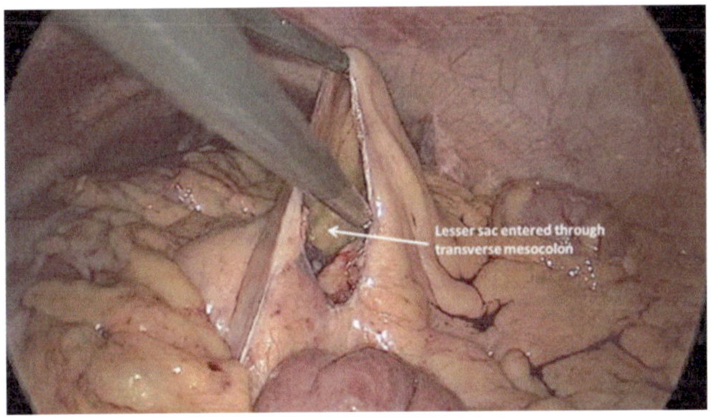


**Fig. 3.49** The avascular plane above the ligament of Treitz may offer an alternative pathway into the lesser sac

spleen. Care should be taken not to dissect the mesentery proximally and not to divide the left branch of the middle colic artery if the descending colon is to be utilized for anastomosis.

## Descending Colectomy

The descending colon and its mesentery are generally mobilized as continuations of sigmoid mobilization or splenic flexure mobilization. The key points during this mobilization are identification and preservation of the

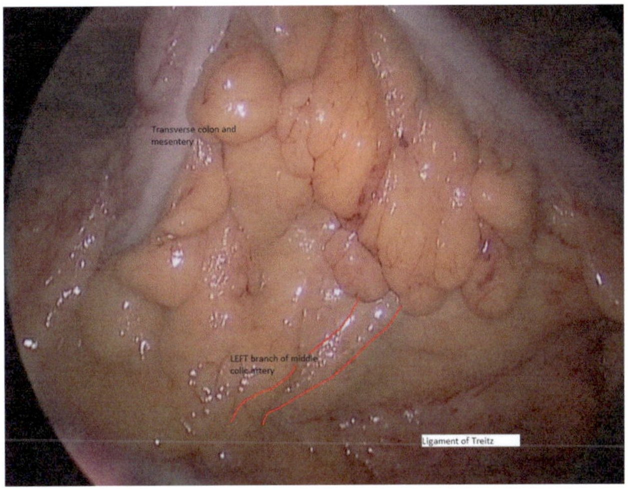


**Fig. 3.50** With the distal transverse colon mesentery retracted anteriorly, there is generally an avascular plane identified near and just above the ligament of Treitz along the transverse mesentery and above the duodenum. Entry into this window will lead into the lesser sac above the pancreas and behind the stomach

ureter and kidney during appropriate dissection of the avascular plane between the mesentery and retroperitoneum (Figs. 3.42–3.47 and 3.49).

## Low Anterior Resection

***Pearl**: Early development of the correct plane in the presacral space is critical in successfully performing a proper sharp total mesorectal excision. In an attempt to ensure proper oncologic resection, there may be a propensity to veer lateral from the proper plane. The loose areolar plane or "cotton candy" plane is often easily developed by staying close to the mesorectal fascia of the rectum. By doing so, one also minimizes the risk for injuring the hypogastric nerves and other retroperitoneal structures.*

When performing a pelvic dissection, the surgeon often initiates the dissection of the rectum posteriorly. The dissection plane is developed immediately posterior to the fascia propria of the rectum. This fascia is an extension of the pelvic fascia enveloping the rectum, fat, nerves, and blood and lymphatic vessels. There is a loose alveolar plane between this and the presacral fascia (Fig. 3.23). The dissection is carried down sharply to the levator ani and puborectalis sling posteriorly and laterally, taking care to avoid the pelvic nerves along the sidewalls whenever possible (Fig. 3.54).

When performing the posterior dissection, careful attention should be given to the presacral fascia. As described above, this is a thickened part of the parietal pelvic fascia that covers the sacrum, coccyx, nerves, middle sacral artery,

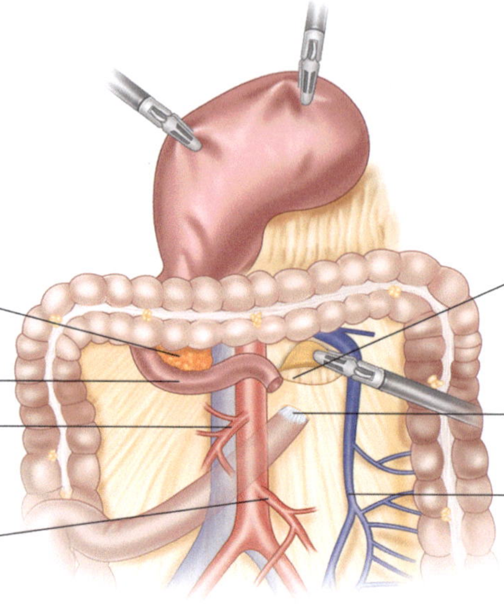


**Fig. 3.51** Accessing the lesser sac through the transverse colon mesentery

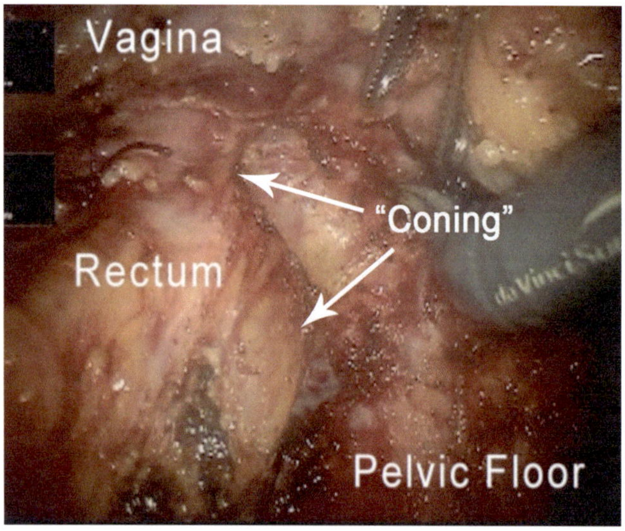


**Fig. 3.52** During a total mesorectal excision, the dissection may be extended to the level of the pelvic floor. At this point the mesorectum is thinned and the typical "coning" is seen

and presacral veins. Operating deep to the presacral fascia or tearing of the fascia due to retracting may cause excessive hemorrhage in an otherwise bloodless operation (Figs. 3.55 and 3.56).

The facial plane is then continued along the lateral aspects of the extraperitoneal rectum. The lateral ligaments or stalks are considered condensations of the pelvic fascia. They are comprised of connection tissue and nerves, but the middle rectal artery does not traverse them. Vessels may traverse the lateral stalks in 25 % of the time so care should be taken when dividing them [3, 13].

After developing the posterior and lateral planes, the anterior dissection is then performed. Continuation of the lateral and posterior dissection can often lead the surgeon in the right plane. Commonly, there is an "open C"-type or "opening-zipper" configuration of this fascia at this level that will demarcate the appropriate dissection plane (Fig. 3.26). In this instance, starting from a known to unknown dissection will help identify the appropriate dissection plane with loose alveolar tissue as the definitive marker. Here, too, there will be a loose alveolar space denoting the appropriate plane. The vagina, or prostate and seminal vesicles, will be visualized anteriorly as dissection proceeds caudally (Figs. 3.24 and 3.57).

As dissection continues distally, toward the level of the levator ani and puborectalis, there will be a paucity of mesorectal fat around the distal anorectal canal. This is typically the terminal limit of the abdominal dissection. In some advanced cases, an intersphincteric plane can also be developed, and careful dissection will reveal the space between the external sphincter and the anorectal tube.

## Uterine Retraction

It may be difficult at times to gain appropriate exposure to the anterior rectum and Denonvilliers fascia in a woman with a large uterus and poor suspension from the broad ligaments

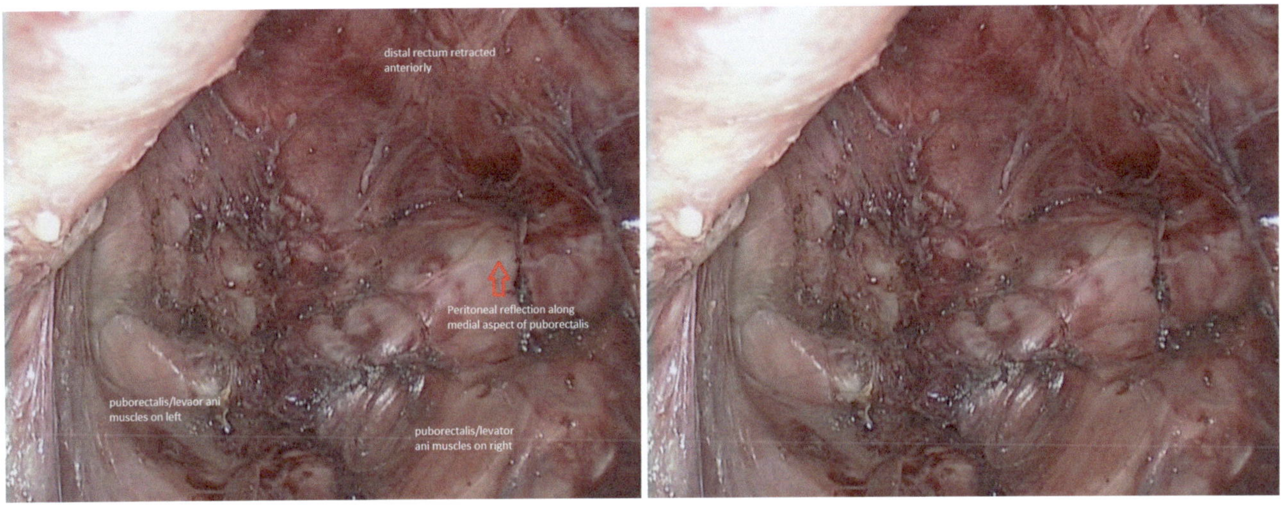


**Fig. 3.53** Posterior dissection. Note the fibers of the puborectalis and levator ani posterior bilateral with the distal rectal canal retracted anteriorly. Note the peritoneal reflection (*red arrow*) along the medial border of the puborectalis leading to the intersphincteric space

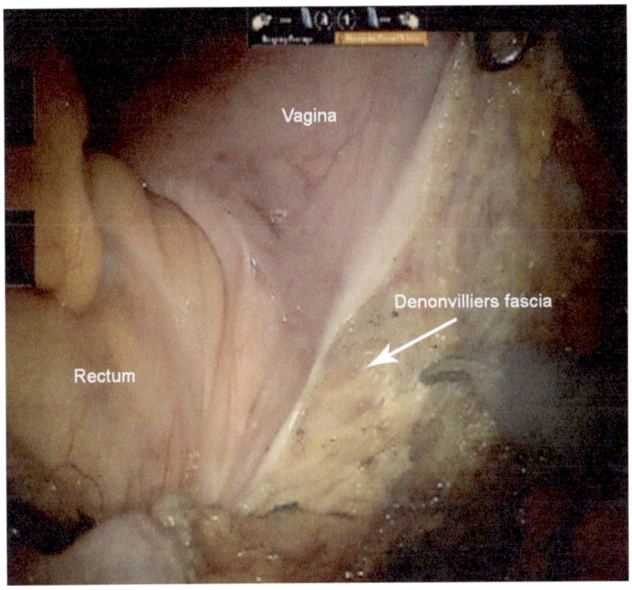


**Fig. 3.54** Anterior plane of dissection highlighting Denonvilliers fascia (DF)

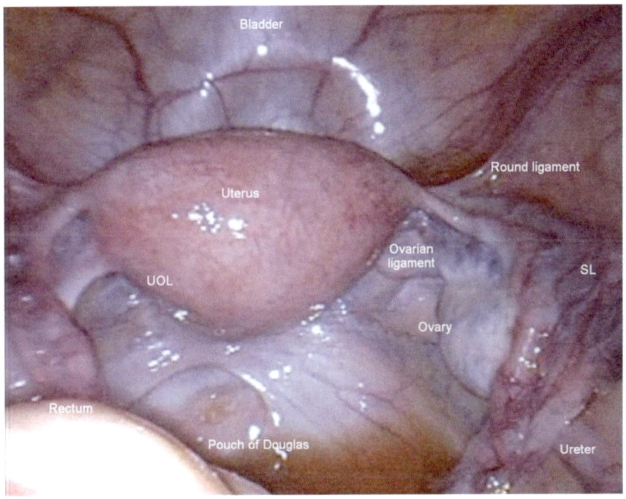


**Fig. 3.55** Uterine anatomy highlighting pouch of Douglas (*SL* suspensory ligament of the ovary, *UL* uterosacral ligament, *UOL* utero-ovarian ligament, *FT* fallopian tube, *OL* ovarian ligament)

(Fig. 3.58). In these cases, several options exist, with the authors generally preferring the last:

1. Endouterine manipulator—this is placed per vagina and held in place by an assistant or retractor.
2. Dynamic manual retraction via a grasper or fan retractor—this generally is performed by the assistant who is also manipulating the camera. This does provide for some limited dynamic control/retraction if needed.
3. Static retraction and suspension—performed by placing a transabdominal fixation stitch (i.e., 2-0 Prolene on a Keith needle) through the abdominal wall, then anterior to posterior through the broad ligament, around the fundus, and then again in a posterior-to-anterior fashion through the contralateral broad ligament and again out the abdominal wall. At this point, both ends of the suture are pulled taught and tied down while the uterus is being suspended ventrally. Rather than the broad ligament, some surgeons may prefer going directly through the uterine fundus, minimizing potential for uterine artery hemorrhage.

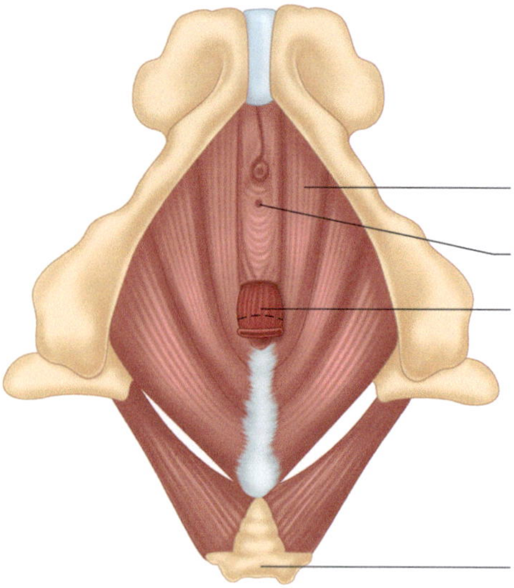


**Fig. 3.56** Anatomy of the pelvic floor demonstrating the perineal musculature

This last option provides significantly more retraction and exposure and frees up the assistant to utilize an additional laparoscopic grasper or retractor for additional dynamic retraction.

## Perineal Dissection

If an abdominoperineal resection is required, dissection must continue below the levator ani muscles. Following this, perineal dissection begins. The anal canal and lower rectum are dissected and removed through the ischiorectal fossa and urogenital diaphragm (Fig. 3.59). If the tumor is extensively invasive, removal of a female patient's vagina, vulva, and urethra may be required. The entire specimen may then be removed via an abdominal or perineal incision.

## Summary

A complete understanding of the normal anatomy as well as a generalized concept of some of the more commonly found variations is an absolute prerequisite to performing abdominopelvic surgery. While several factors such as obesity, previous surgery, or radiation therapy can alter traditional relationships, knowledge of tissue planes and where you are likely to encounter critical structures will serve you and your patients well in minimizing morbidity and maximizing outcomes.

## References

1. Milsom JW, Böhm B, Decanini C, Fazio VW. Laparoscopic oncologic proctosigmoidectomy with low colorectal anastomosis in a cadaver model. Surg Endosc. 1994;8(9):1117–23.
2. Bonnet S, Abid B, Wind P, Delmas V, Douard R. Anatomical basis of laparoscopic medial-to-lateral mobilization of the descending colon. Clin Anat. 2013;26(3):377–85.
3. Kadar N. Laparoscopic anatomy and dissection of the pelvis. Baillieres Clin Obstet Gynaecol. 1997;11(1):37–60.
4. Ostrzenski A, Radolinski B, Ostrzenska KM. A review of laparoscopic ureteral injury in pelvic surgery. Obstet Gynecol Surv. 2003;58(12):794–9.
5. Kutiyanawala, Scott, Jameson. Ureteric injuries during colorectal surgery: strategies for prevention. Colorectal Dis. 1999;1(6): 334–7.
6. Fritsch H, Lienemann A, Brenner E, Ludwikowski B. Clinical anatomy of the pelvic floor. Adv Anat Embryol Cell Biol. 2004;175:III–IX. 1–64.
7. Fritsch H, Hötzinger H. Tomographical anatomy of the pelvis, visceral pelvic connective tissue, and its compartments. Clin Anat. 1995;8(1):17–24.
8. Aigner F, Zbar AP, Ludwikowski B, Kreczy A, Kovacs P, Fritsch H. The rectogenital septum: morphology, function, and clinical relevance. Dis Colon Rectum. 2004;47(2):131–40.
9. Havenga K, Enker WE. Autonomic nerve preserving total mesorectal excision. Surg Clin North Am. 2002;82(5):1009–18.
10. Havenga K, DeRuiter MC, Enker WE, Welvaart K. Anatomical basis of autonomic nerve-preserving total mesorectal excision for rectal cancer. Br J Surg. 1996;83(3):384–8.
11. Havenga K, Grossmann I, DeRuiter M, Wiggers T. Definition of total mesorectal excision, including the perineal phase: technical considerations. Dig Dis. 2007;25(1):44–50.
12. Havenga K, Maas CP, DeRuiter MC, Welvaart K, Trimbos JB. Avoiding long-term disturbance to bladder and sexual function in pelvic surgery, particularly with rectal cancer. Semin Surg Oncol. 2000;18(3):235–43.
13. Boxall TA, Smart PJ, Griffiths JD. The blood-supply of the distal segment of the rectum in anterior resection. Br J Surg. 1963; 50:399–404.

# Part II

# Procedures

# 4 Right Colectomy: Straight Laparoscopic

Steven Robert Hunt

**Key Points**

- Gravity plays an important role in laparoscopic colon surgery, and patients should be prepared for extremes in positioning.
- Understanding the retroperitoneal anatomy of the right colon and its mesentery is important in performing a laparoscopic dissection.
- There are several different approaches to performing a laparoscopic right colectomy—each has advantages, and it is imperative to understand and be proficient at each approach.
- In the end, four steps must be accomplished: retroperitoneal mobilization, division of lateral and hepatic flexure attachments, ligation of the vascular pedicle, and resection/anastomosis.
- While laparoscopic colectomy has advantages over an open procedure, the safety of the patient should never be compromised, and conversion to an open procedure should not be considered a failure.

## Introduction

While a laparoscopic right hemicolectomy may be accomplished in a variety of approaches, in the end, the same maneuvers must be performed with each procedure. The order of these steps may vary with the approach, but each is necessary to satisfactorily complete the procedure. This chapter should allow the reader to personalize their approach to the laparoscopic right colectomy and also provide some insights that allow the surgeon to deal with challenging situations.

**Electronic supplementary material:** Supplementary material is available in the online version of this chapter at 10.1007/978-1-4939-1581-1_4. Videos can also be accessed at http://www.springerimages.com/videos/978-1-4939-1580-4.

S.R. Hunt, M.D. (✉)
Department of Surgery, Barnes-Jewish Hospital,
Box 8109, 660 South Euclid, St. Louis, MO 63110, USA
e-mail: hunts@wustl.edu

## Patient Preparation

Prior to beginning any colectomy, the operator must ensure that the lesion has been localized. The colonoscopy report should be reviewed, and the location of the lesion should be confirmed either by photographic visualization of the tumor within the cecum or by verifying that a tattoo has been placed at the site of the lesion. While the efficacy of bowel preparation is controversial, we use a mechanical bowel preparation with oral antibiotics. Ureteral stents are rarely needed for a laparoscopic right colectomy but can be considered for reoperative surgery or inflammatory conditions. All patients should receive DVT and intravenous antibiotic prophylaxis prior to the initiation of the procedure.

## Setup

Gravity plays an extremely important role in laparoscopic colon surgery, and an appropriate mechanical bed is a necessity for a laparoscopic colectomy. The patient should be secured to the bed either with a beanbag or a gel pad and taped across the chest to avoid sliding during the extremes of positioning. At our institution, all patients are placed in stirrups to allow the operator or assistant to stand between the patient's legs during portions of the procedure. If the patient is to be positioned in the lithotomy position, the hips should be flexed no more than 10 degrees to allow free movement of the instruments while operating in the upper abdomen (Fig. 4.1). For the majority of the procedure, the surgeon will stand on the patient's left side. The assistant generally stands between the patient's legs, and the camera operator stands on the patient's left side, cephalad to the surgeon. Occasionally, it is necessary for the surgeon to stand between the patient's legs in order to complete the right colon mobilization. The video monitor should be positioned off of the patient's right shoulder (Fig. 4.2).

The camera port should be placed in the center of the abdomen through a periumbilical incision centered between

H.M. Ross et al. (eds.), *Minimally Invasive Approaches to Colon and Rectal Disease: Technique and Best Practices*, DOI 10.1007/978-1-4939-1581-1_4, © Springer Science+Business Media New York 2015

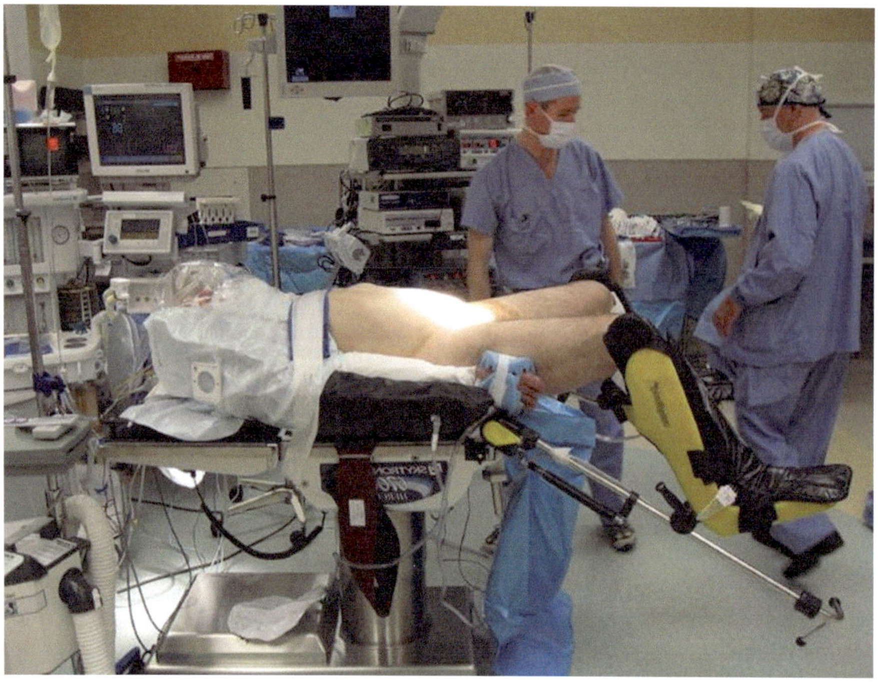

**Fig. 4.1** Positioning the patient in lithotomy position allows for a member of the surgical team to stand between the patient's legs. Hip flexion is minimal to avoid interference between the thighs and the instruments while working in the upper abdomen. This patient is secured to the table with a beanbag and tape to allow for extremes of table positioning

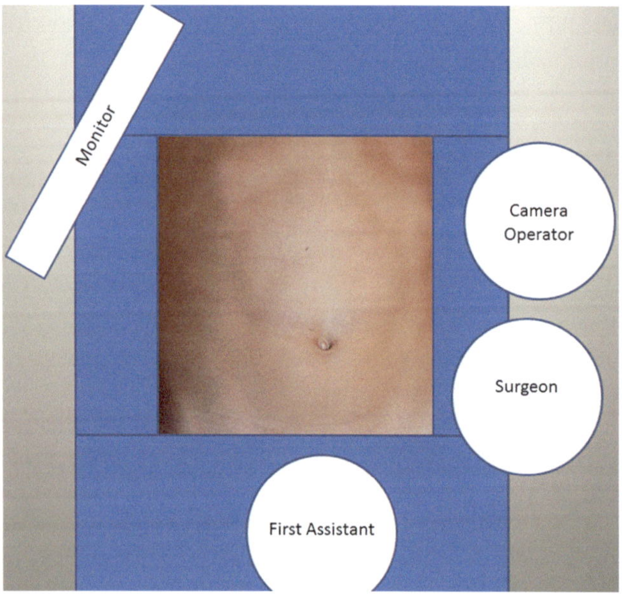


**Fig. 4.2** This schematic drawing depicts the positioning of the operating team and monitor during a laparoscopic colectomy. The first assistant can stand between the patient's legs

the patient's pubic synthesis and the xiphoid process at the top of the dome of the insufflated abdomen. Additionally, two or three other working ports are usually necessary to perform this operation. Generally, the umbilical camera incision can be extended and used as the extraction site. Two alternatives for placing the working ports are illustrated in Figs. 4.3 and 4.4.

## Clinical Anatomy

The right colon and its mesentery are intimately associated with the retroperitoneum in the right abdomen. It is suspended laterally by peritoneal attachments to the abdominal wall. The hepatic flexure has attachments to the posterior diaphragm and undersurface of the liver and gallbladder. Moving distally along the transverse colon, the colon fuses with the omentum and is attached to the greater curve of the stomach by the gastrocolic omentum. The superior aspect of the proximal transverse colon mesentery has avascular attachments to the posterior wall of the stomach. Proceeding distally along the transverse colon mesentery, the lesser sac forms the superior border. The blood supply to the right colon consists of the ileocolic vessels and, variably, the right colic or right braches of the middle colic vessels.

The retroperitoneal boundaries of the right colon and its mesentery form a triangle extending from the fourth portion of the duodenum inferolaterally to the cecum, up the right colic gutter, and then medially from the hepatic flexure to the middle colic vessels. The retroperitoneal attachments of the

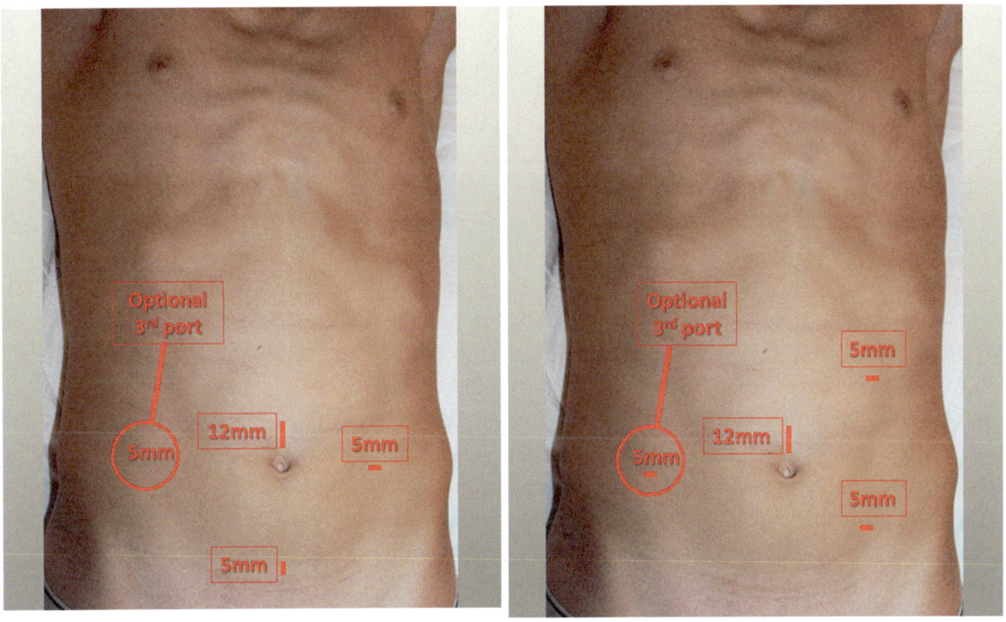


**Figs. 4.3 and 4.4** Two alternative port positions for a laparoscopic right colectomy. A third working port can be added in the right lower quadrant if needed

right colon are avascular. Within this retroperitoneal triangle posterior to the right colon, the right gonadal vessels are encountered first, moving from lateral to medial. The next vertically oriented structure is the right ureter, which crosses over the right common iliac vessels at the inferomedial border of this triangle. The vena cava is the next structure medial to the ureter running vertically in this plane. Proceeding cephalad in this plane, the second and third portions of the duodenum and head of the pancreas are encountered next. Just medial to the pancreatic head, the middle colic vessels are encountered. Lateral to these structures, the hepatic flexure lies over Gerota's fascia of the right kidney.

## Objectives of the Laparoscopic Procedure

Four objectives must be accomplished in order to complete a laparoscopic right colectomy: (1) the right colon and its mesentery must be mobilized off of the retroperitoneum and duodenum; (2) the vascular pedicles must be divided at the appropriate level for the disease process; (3) the lateral attachments, hepatic flexure, and omental attachments must all be divided; and (4) the specimen must be extracted and the anastomosis performed.

There are four commonly used approaches for a laparoscopic right colectomy—the medial, inferior, lateral, and superior approaches. Regardless of the method, the purpose is to mobilize the right colon completely from the retroperitoneum and the sweep of the duodenum. This accomplishes three purposes—it allows for safe ligation of the mesenteric vessels; it frees the colon so that it can be delivered out through the extraction site; and lastly, it allows for a tension-free ileocolic anastomosis.

## Medial Approach

The medial approach to the right colectomy involves an initial incision through the ileocolic mesentery underneath the ileocolic artery (Video 4.1). This vascular pedicle is identified by grasping the cecal mesentery and lifting it anteriorly down into the right lower quadrant. The vessels will form a bowstring in the mesentery. The peritoneum below the vessel is incised, and the retroperitoneal plane is identified. The initial retroperitoneal dissection is performed bluntly through this window. The duodenum is encountered early in the dissection and should be gently swept down from the mesentery. Once the duodenum has been identified and is safely dissected away from the pedicle, the ileocolic artery can be divided. Vascular ligation allows this window to be opened widely and greatly facilitates the remainder of the retroperitoneal dissection. Gentle blunt dissection should be carried out in this plane laterally beyond the colon and in a cephalad direction beyond the hepatic flexure. The entire sweep of the duodenum should be swept down in order to complete the mobilization.

## Inferior Approach

The inferior approach begins with a peritoneal incision underneath the terminal ileal mesentery extending from the distal mesentery up to the duodenum. As in the medial approach, the retroperitoneal dissection also proceeds superiorly and laterally. An advantage of this approach is that the window aperture is much wider than with the medial approach. The duodenum is again identified in the retroperitoneum and swept out of harm's way. This dissection should continue laterally beyond the colon and in a cephalad direction beyond the hepatic flexure, again including the entire sweep of the duodenum.

## Lateral Approach

The lateral approach is similar to the conventional open approach. An advantage of this approach is that it is more familiar for a traditional open surgeon and can ease the transition to performing laparoscopic colectomies. Additionally, this approach may be necessary when inflammation or adhesions preclude the medial or inferior approach. The disadvantage of this approach is that it can sometimes be difficult to perform the retroperitoneal dissection toward the operator and the camera. Again, the duodenum should be identified in the retroperitoneum and kept safe from harm.

## Superior Approach

The final approach is the superior-to-inferior approach. This approach is begun by incising the gastrocolic omentum and dissecting from medial to lateral in the plane cephalad to the mesentery of the proximal transverse colon. Dissection then proceeds inferiorly after the hepatic flexure attachments have been divided. The duodenum should be identified in the retroperitoneum as the hepatic flexure of the colon is mobilized and pulled down toward the patient's left hip. As with the lateral approach, it becomes more difficult as the dissection proceeds medially. The superior approach is invaluable in situations in which there is a large cecal mass or significant inflammation in the right lower quadrant or the ileocolic mesentery.

Every surgeon should be familiar with all of these approaches, as different patient habitus, anatomic variation, and disease presentation often necessitates some combination of these approaches in order to adequately mobilize the colon.

## The Procedure

For the purposes of this textbook, the operation will be described using the inferior approach. The other approaches will be referenced when appropriate.

After pneumoperitoneum has been established, the abdominal cavity should be visualized, and any abnormalities should be noted. If the resection is being performed for neoplastic disease, the liver should be closely inspected for metastatic disease. If a suspicious lesion is identified, it can usually be biopsied laparoscopically by passing a core needle biopsy device subcostally through a stab incision. If the resection is being performed for Crohn's disease, the small bowel should be visualized in its entirety.

The patient should then be placed in steep Trendelenburg and in the left lateral decubitus position. As described above, it is important to secure the patient to the table in order to avoid any mishaps. The omentum should be rolled over the top of the transverse colon and draped onto the stomach. This maneuver exposes the serosal surface of the transverse colon, keeps the omentum from displacing small bowel into your field of view, and allows access to the omental attachments of the transverse colon. Next, the small bowel is swept out of the pelvis into the left upper abdomen. The terminal ileum should then be placed alongside the ascending colon, exposing the inferomedial aspect of the terminal ileal mesentery. These steps are greatly aided by the gravity resulting from proper bed positioning.

## Mobilization of the Colon and Mesentery from the Retroperitoneum

The terminal ileal mesentery should be lifted off of the retroperitoneum, allowing visualization of along the base of the mesentery up to the fourth portion of the duodenum (Fig. 4.5). While it is not usually necessary to identify the right ureter during this procedure, it can often be seen at this

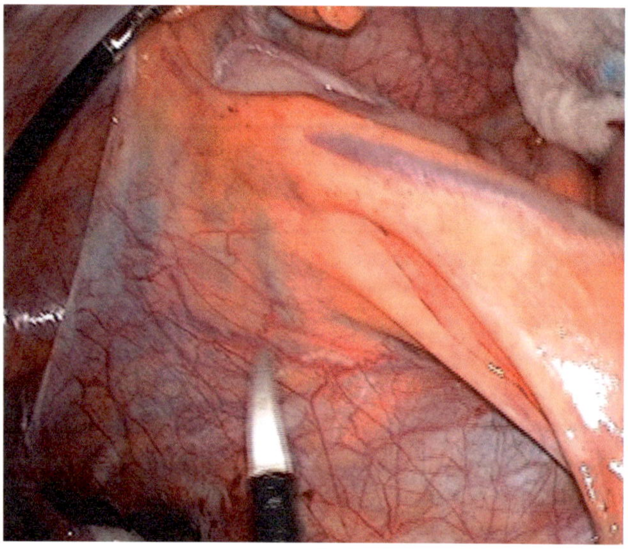

**Fig. 4.5** The inferior approach begins by elevating the terminal ileal mesentery off of the retroperitoneum. In this thin patient, the right ureter and inferior vena cava can be visualized through the peritoneum. Just offscreen to the right, behind that fold of mesentery, is the inferomedial aspect of the fourth portion of the duodenum

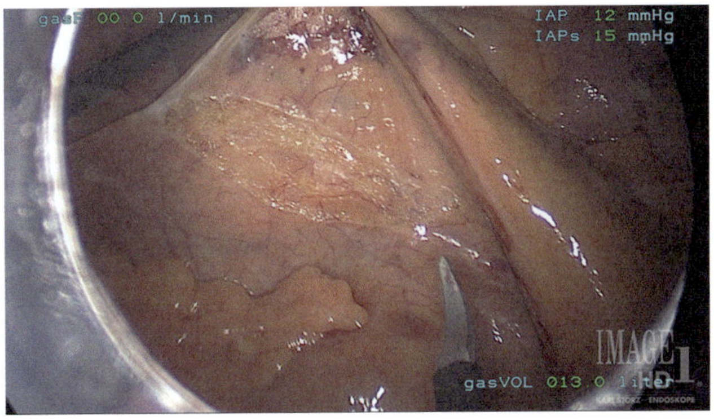


**Fig. 4.6** With the terminal ileal mesentery elevated, the peritoneum is excised in a line along the base of the mesentery up toward the duodenum—allowing access to the retroperitoneal space

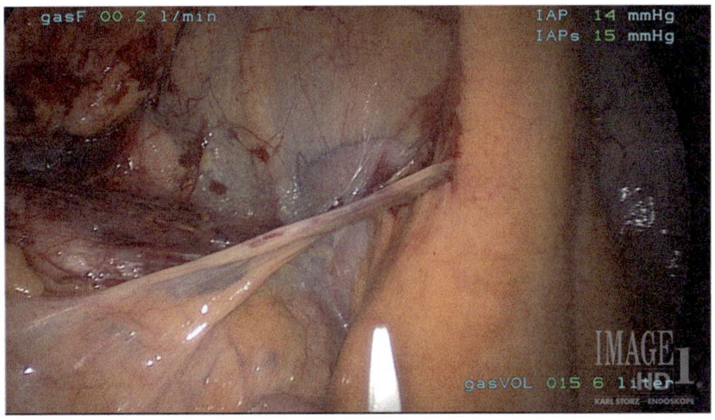


**Fig. 4.8** As the retroperitoneal dissection proceeds, the retroperitoneal duodenum is visualized (center). The areolar attachments of the duodenum to the right colon mesentery can then be bluntly dissected to separate the entire sweep of the duodenum from the mesentery

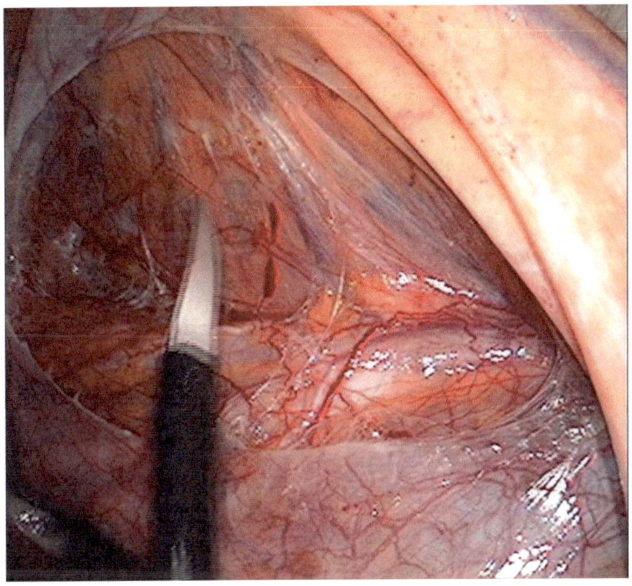

**Fig. 4.7** Once the peritoneum is incised, elevation of the mesentery and gentle blunt dissection in the retroperitoneum develops the avascular plane behind the ileocolic mesentery

point. A score should be made in the peritoneum along the base of the terminal ileal mesentery up to the duodenum (Fig. 4.6). The retroperitoneal fusion plane can then be accessed through this peritoneal entry point (Fig. 4.7). Often, the challenging part of this procedure is identifying the appropriate retroperitoneal plane. The simplest method by which this plane can be exposed is to place a blunt instrument behind the cecum and lift anteriorly and cephalad with modest force. This maneuver will usually reveal the appropriate areolar plane. Dissection should then be carried out bluntly in a lateral and cephalad direction. This is accomplished by elevating the mesentery upward with the left hand and using the right-handed instrument to develop the plane. It is not necessary to grasp tissue with the retracting instrument, and it may be kept closed during this portion of the procedure. If exposure is inadequate, a third 5 mm port may be added to allow the surgical assistant to facilitate exposure. Sweeping the right-handed instrument in the shape of a backwards "C" allows the dissection to progress in a cephalad direction. Occasionally, the dissection is better suited to using the right hand to lift the mesentery toward the anterior abdominal wall and developing the plane with the left-hand instrument. If the dissection becomes difficult, the surgeon should return back to a known plane, confirm the anatomy, and proceed with dissection from the known plane. The duodenum is identified during the cephalad portion of this dissection. Tension at the apex of the dissection is critical to progression, and the left hand should frequently be replaced to keep tension in this plane. The left hand can provide optimal tension by engaging the apex of the dissected plane and lifting anteriorly and toward the camera.

The duodenum will be found at the medial and superior aspect of this plane (Fig. 4.8). Once identified, it should be swept down and medially until the entire sweep of the duodenum and a portion of the pancreatic head have been freed from the mesentery. Once this is accomplished, dissection should be carried out laterally behind the hepatic flexure. Around the duodenum, it may be necessary to sharply divide some areolar tissue; however, energy should be used sparingly, if ever, in this avascular plane. If the duodenum is dissected posteriorly from the right colon mesentery, the right ureter is certain to be removed from harm's way.

If the duodenum cannot be easily identified using this inferior approach, the other approaches should be considered, as it is a necessity to free the duodenum from the colonic mesentery when mobilizing the right colon. Frequently, all four approaches are required before the duodenum can be safely identified and dissected away from the specimen.

## Identification and Division of the Vascular Pedicles

Once the retroperitoneal dissection has been accomplished, the vascular pedicles may be divided next. Alternatively, the right colon attachments can be divided at this point in the procedure, depending on the surgeon's preference. The ileocolic vessels are the most readily identified and should be the first vascular pedicle that is isolated and divided. This pedicle can be identified by grasping the cecum and pulling it down into the right lower quadrant and elevating it. This tension exposes a bowstring where the ileocolic pedicle exists. If an inferior approach has been used, there should be dark, purple windows on each side of the ileocolic vessels (Fig. 4.9). If there is uncertainty about its identity, the pedicle can be grasped and walked out to its distal extent to avoid confusion with the superior mesenteric artery. Once the ileocolic pedicle has been identified, the window should be opened on each side of the pedicle and the vessels ligated (Fig. 4.10). This author uses a vessel-sealing device, but clips and staplers offer equally effective means of vessel ligation. If the ileocolic pedicle is the only pedicle that needs to be divided for a specific disease, the operator may proceed to the next step. If the middle colic vessels are to be divided, it should take place at this point. The right branch of the middle colic artery can usually be identified by following the cut edge of the divided ileocolic pedicle onto the transverse colon mesentery (Video 4.2). The first fatty structure encountered will be the right branch of the middle colic artery. If this is to be divided intracorporeally, it should be isolated and divided in the same manner. Before applying an energy source to any middle colic vessels, the gastrocolic attachments to the superior transverse colon mesentery should be divided to avoid injury to the stomach.

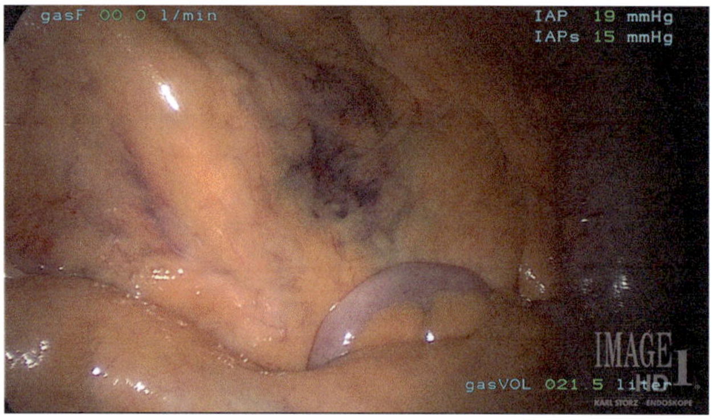


**Fig. 4.9** After the retroperitoneal dissection is completed, the ileocolic pedicle can be identified by pulling the cecum into the right lower quadrant and elevating it. The pedicle forms a bowstring, and the windows on each side of the vessels appear dark

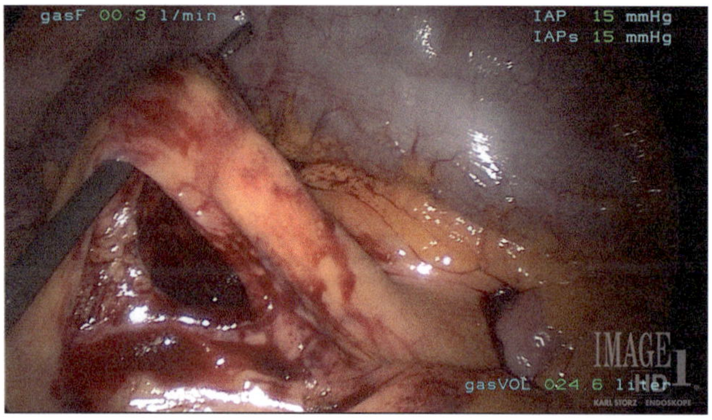


**Fig. 4.10** After the windows on each side of the ileocolic pedicle are opened, the vessels are easily identified, and the pedicle can be divided just distal to its origin

## Division of the Right Colon Attachments

The right colon attachments can then be divided. This is most easily accomplished with the patient in reverse Trendelenburg position. The simplest way to approach this is to start at the free edge of dissection just lateral and inferior to the cecum. The lateral attachments can then be lifted off of the retroperitoneum, as the posterior dissection should have already been performed lateral to the colon (Fig. 4.11). Division of these attachments should proceed in a cephalad direction. As this is an avascular plane, the division may be performed with scissors, cautery, or a vessel-sealing device. The surgeon should intermittently look both above and below the lateral attachments to confirm their location. A common mistake in dividing the lateral detachments is to continue dividing these attachments beyond the hepatic flexure lateral to the liver. The surgeon should take note of the location of the colon and divide only the colonic attachments. This will necessitate a deliberate medial turn at the hepatic flexure and to avoid going posterior to the kidney.

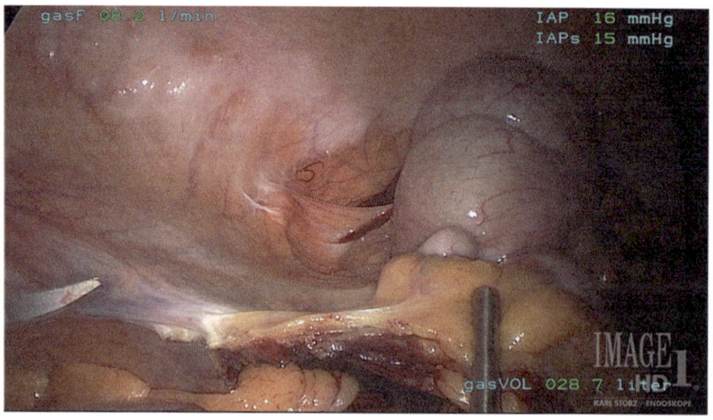


**Fig. 4.11** The lateral attachments of the right colon viewed from an inferior vantage point. The grasper is pulling the mesoappendix medially, and the retroperitoneal dissection is seen to extend laterally beyond the colon

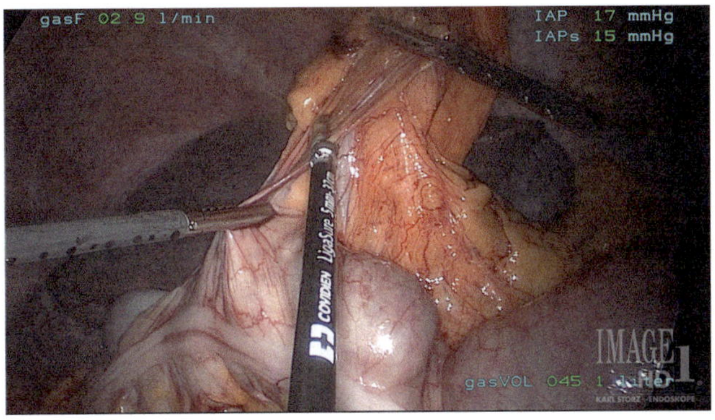


**Fig. 4.12** The superior approach is begun by incising the attachments between the omentum and the proximal transverse colon. This approach can be used in combination with other approaches to assist with mobilization of the hepatic flexure

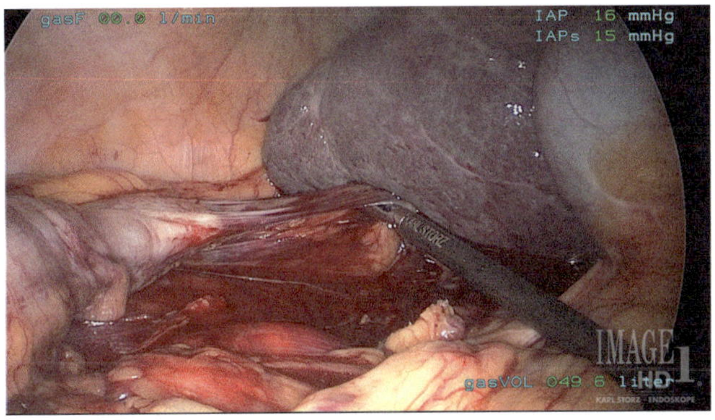


**Fig. 4.13** As the dissection proceeds proximally along the transverse colon in the fused gastrocolic plane, the remaining hepatic flexure attachments can be demonstrated by pulling downward and medially on the colon

Frequently, the most difficult part of a right colectomy is the final mobilization of the hepatic flexure. A helpful maneuver to better visualize the hepatic flexure attachments is to flatten out the colon just medial to the attachments and pull down toward the patient's left lower quadrant. If this still does not allow for continued mobilization of the hepatic flexure, a superior approach should be attempted.

The superior approach involves incising the gastrocolic omentum just cephalad to the proximal transverse colon (Fig. 4.12). Prior to beginning this dissection, the patient should be placed in reverse Trendelenburg position. A plane is usually easily identified just cephalad to the transverse colon mesentery. Dissection should be carried out bluntly in this plane laterally. As this dissection proceeds proximally along the transverse colon, the peritoneum of the gastrocolic attachments should be incised and the plane developed moving from medial to lateral toward the hepatic flexure. Eventually, the only remaining attachments will be the hepatic flexure attachments, and these can be visualized by grasping the colon proximal and distal to the flexure and pulling down toward the left lower quadrant (Fig. 4.13).

After the hepatic flexure attachments have been divided, the duodenum should be identified. There are often filmy attachments of areolar tissue that must be divided sharply before the right colon can be completely mobilized. Once the surgeon feels that the right colon has been mobilized adequately, this must be confirmed. Confirmation is best accomplished by grasping the hepatic flexure of the colon and dragging it down to the left lower quadrant well beyond the site of planned exteriorization. The operator should also assure that the colon has been mobilized sufficiently to lift it anteriorly up to and through the abdominal wall.

It is a grave mistake to attempt to exteriorize an incompletely mobilized colon. This can lead to excessive force in trying to deliver the colon through the extraction incision. Such force can cause avulsion of the middle colic vessels and rapid blood loss that can necessitate an emergent conversion to an open procedure.

## Extended Right Colectomy

If it is necessary to resect a significant portion of the transverse colon as part of the right hemicolectomy, the procedure need be modified only minimally. The retroperitoneal dissection is performed in exactly the same fashion as described above. This author prefers to divide the lateral attachments and mobilize the hepatic flexure prior to dividing the vessels when performing an extended right colectomy. After the hepatic flexure is mobilized, the omentocolic attachments across the transverse colon can then be divided. If the omentum is to be removed with the specimen, the gastrocolic omentum can be divided with a vessel-sealing device. Once the omental attachments are divided, the superior aspect of the transverse colon mesentery should be cleared down to the base of the mesentery by dividing the gastrocolic attachments to the posterior stomach. Only after these attachments are divided can high ligation of the middle colic vessels be accomplished safely.

## Exteriorization and Anastomosis

Once the colon is sufficiently mobilized, preparations should be made for exteriorization. Prior to desufflating the abdomen, the retroperitoneum and vascular pedicles should be inspected and hemostasis confirmed. If the camera port is in the center of the abdomen, the operator should note which incision would most easily allow for the specimen to be exteriorized with the least tension. Usually, this is a periumbilical incision. Infrequently, the incision is above or below the umbilicus. The fat fold at the cecum should be grasped and locked in a laparoscopic grasper. The periumbilical incision should then be extended to the appropriate size, usually around 3 cm. A self-expanding wound retractor facilitates extraction and may help to prevent wound infections [1]. The specimen can then be extracted by grasping it with a Babcock clamp after it is delivered up into this incision with the laparoscopic atraumatic grasper. The bowel should be maintained in an anatomic orientation during this portion of the procedure to prevent twisting prior to creating the anastomosis. The terminal ileum and colon can be divided, and the remaining mesentery to these points should also be ligated. After each portion of the bowel is divided, it should be held in place by an assistant or grasped with a Babcock clamp that is clipped to the drapes to avoid twisting the bowel. While some prefer to perform an intracorporeal anastomosis, we perform ours in an extracorporeal fashion. There is no proven advantage to the intracorporeal anastomosis, and the extraction incision does not need to be extended in order to perform the anastomosis extracorporeally. The anastomosis can be performed in a side-to-side, functional end-to-end fashion, or in an end-to-side fashion. We do not close our mesenteric defect, as this can be difficult to do through a small extraction incision. This has been shown to be a safe practice [2].

## Pearls and Pitfalls

When difficulty is encountered in a laparoscopic procedure, it can frequently be attributed to one of two simple things—lack of tension or a poor understanding of one's anatomic location. If a procedure is not proceeding according to plan, the surgeon must stop and ask oneself: (1) "Do I have enough tension?" and (2) "Do I know where I am?" If the answer to either question is negative, it should be corrected immediately. If the anatomy still cannot be determined after simple maneuvers, serious consideration should be given to converting to an open procedure.

In some cases, the anatomy may be obvious, but the procedure still is not progressing because of patient or disease factors. As long as there is no overt danger of proceeding laparoscopically, there are two options short of conversion to an open procedure. Extra 5 mm ports can be placed to aid exposure. Another option is to use a hand-assisted device. When adding a hand port, be cautious to place it in a position where it will be possible to extract the specimen without undue tension—usually in the periumbilical position. Such positioning of the hand port will necessitate moving the camera port to another location, such as the epigastrium.

Conversion to open is *not* a failure, and it is often the better part of valor. Any perception by the surgeon that proceeding laparoscopically would be unsafe or unsound oncologically demands conversion to an open procedure. It is preferential to convert before anything untoward occurs, rather than after. Litigation for laparoscopic mishaps is unfortunately common, but litigation for conversion should be nonexistent.

## Conclusion

The straight laparoscopic approach to a right colectomy or ileocolic resection is a safe, reproducible, and reliable technique that provides all the advantages of minimally invasive surgery. While the inferior approach is preferred in most cases by this author, surgeons should be aware of all methods available to effectively accomplish the retroperitoneal mobilization, division of lateral and hepatic flexure attachments, ligation of the vascular pedicle, and resection/anastomosis.

## References

1. Reid K, Pockney P, Draganic B, Smith SR. Barrier wound protection decreases surgical site infection in open elective colorectal surgery: a randomized clinical trial. Dis Colon Rectum. 2010;53(10):1374–80.
2. Causey MW, Oguntoye M, Steele SR. Incidence of complications following colectomy with mesenteric closure versus no mesenteric closure: does it really matter? J Surg Res. 2011;171(2):571–5.

# Right Colectomy: Hand-Assist

5

Kirk A. Ludwig and Timothy Ridolfi

**Key Points**

- Hand-assisted laparoscopic right colectomy, as described here, is a top-down approach.
- The anatomy is viewed from a laparoscope placed near the falciform ligament in a subxiphoid position.
- The operation is performed with a hand port placed in the midline and then only two additional 5 mm ports.
- This is a single-surgeon approach with no need for a trained assistant.
- Unlike other laparoscopic right colectomy techniques, the dissection starts and stays in a single plane throughout the operation, which minimizes operative time and makes for a smooth, clean, bloodless, and anatomic dissection.
- This approach gives the surgeon an excellent view of the middle colic vessels allowing for proximal ligation deep in the transverse colon mesentery.
- Since, at present, the ileocolic anastomosis that follows a right colectomy is most commonly performed extracorporeally, using the extraction site for a hand port makes intuitive sense.

## Introduction

Since the introduction of laparoscopic cholecystectomy in the late 1980s, laparoscopic techniques have been rapidly and successfully applied to multiple abdominal operations, including colon and rectal resections. However, in large part due to the degree of difficulty, oncologic concerns, and the difficulty in demonstrating dramatic advantages compared to the open approach, laparoscopic colon surgery was slow to evolve. In the early years, laparoscopic colectomy was targeted towards benign conditions such as Crohn disease and diverticulitis. As experience was gained, the technique was applied to not only all portions of the colon and rectum but to malignant disease as well. Initial concerns regarding oncologic outcomes, such as locoregional clearance of tumor, recurrence rates, and long-term survival, have largely been answered by four prospective, randomized, controlled trials demonstrating the equivalency of laparoscopic and open procedures [1–4]. In addition, minimally invasive colon surgery has been associated with a number of short-term benefits, including faster recovery, less pain, shorter hospitalization, and improved cosmetic outcome [5].

Technical difficulty with laparoscopic colorectal surgery is still an issue, which probably explains why the majority of colorectal surgery is still performed using open techniques [6]. There are a variety of techniques for performing a laparoscopic right colectomy: there is the (open) standard lateral to medial approach, there is the medial to lateral laparoscopic approach wherein the ileocolic artery is grasped and taken near its origin as the initial maneuver, and there is the bottom-up or retroperitoneal approach wherein the operation starts by incising the peritoneum at the base of the small bowel mesentery from the right lower quadrant up the duodenum and then the ileal and right colon mesentery are lifted off of the retroperitoneum to the hepatic flexure, while the lateral attachments are left in place to fix the colon in position. It is valuable for the laparoscopic surgeon to be facile with each, since in different situations, they can each be

**Electronic supplementary material:** Supplementary material is available in the online version of this chapter at 10.1007/978-1-4939-1581-1_5. Videos can also be accessed at http://www.springerimages.com/videos/978-1-4939-1580-4.

K.A. Ludwig, M.D. (✉) • T. Ridolfi, M.D.
Division of Colorectal Surgery, Department of Surgery, Medical College of Wisconsin, 9200 W. Wisconsin Ave., Milwaukee, WI 53226, USA
e-mail: kludwig@mcw.edu; tridolfi@mcw.edu

H.M. Ross et al. (eds.), *Minimally Invasive Approaches to Colon and Rectal Disease: Technique and Best Practices*, DOI 10.1007/978-1-4939-1581-1_5, © Springer Science+Business Media New York 2015

applied to advantage. However, the approach illustrated here is the hand-assisted laparoscopic right colectomy. What follows are the concepts underlying this operative approach and a description of the technique.

## Background

The concept of using the hand to facilitate a laparoscopic colon operation is based on a number of factors. The first and most basic concept is that as long as an incision will be made at some point in the case, for extraction and the anastomosis, why not make it at the beginning of the case and use the incision to facilitate the conduct of the operation? While there is legitimate argument over whether the hand-assisted laparoscopic colectomy is associated with the same short-term patient-related benefits as the standard laparoscopic operations, data from the literature suggests that it does [7–9]. Some find troubling the fact that a "large" incision has to be made on the abdominal wall for placement of the hand-assist device. For the average surgeon, the incision size will be about 7 cm. This compares favorably to the average extraction incision size in the COST trial, 6 cm, and the CLASICC trial, 7 cm [10, 11]. Some argue that the hand-assisted technique is not as "gentle" as the standard laparoscopic approach. While there is probably more abdominal wall "trauma" associated with this approach due to the stretching of the wound with the hand placed through it, one could reasonably argue that in terms of what happens inside the abdomen, there is no more gentle instrument than the hand: surely less "traumatic" than the 5 and 10 mm graspers that apply significant force, over small surface areas, especially on fragile tissues. Who would ever grasp the small bowel or the colon with clamps during open surgery?

Second, for surgeons who do not perform a high volume of colon surgery, it can be difficult to learn and utilize laparoscopic colon surgery techniques. In addition, with laparoscopic colectomy, operative times tend to be long, and there is a fairly high conversion rate, which can be frustrating. In the COST trial [10] and the CLASSIC trial [11], the average operative time for laparoscopic colectomy was almost an hour more than for the open colectomy. In the COLOR trial the open operations were 30 min faster than the laparoscopic procedures. In each of these trials, the conversion rate was greater than 20 %. While these conversion rates are quite a bit higher than rates reported in more recent series [6], there are still situations that can make laparoscopic colon surgery long, difficult, and frustrating. The hand-assisted technique may help reduce operative times significantly, and in the authors' experience, conversion to open operation rarely occurs. A surgeon with a good grasp of the pertinent anatomy and just a modicum of laparoscopic skill can learn and use this technique.

Third, there are simply a number of practical issues related to laparoscopic colon surgeries that a hand-assisted technique can help overcome. For example, the increasing number of obese patients is a problem. Over 60 % of adults in the United States today are considered either overweight or obese [12]. Unfortunately, due to the difficulty of performing standard laparoscopic colon surgery on these patients, the very patients who might benefit the most from a minimally invasive operation may simply be excluded due to their size. Difficulty will vary from patient to patient and will vary by patient gender. For example, women tend to carry much of their excess weight within the abdominal wall. While a laparoscopic colon resection in an obese female may seem a daunting task, in reality, the thicker the pannus, the more likely that the amount of intra-abdominal fat will be such that laparoscopic operation will be possible. With an obese woman, the most difficult part of the operation may not be the intra-abdominal dissection, but the exteriorization of the specimen and elevation of the bowel ends for the construction of an anastomosis. In the obese male, the situation is often exactly the opposite: the abdominal wall may be quite thin while the omentum and the mesentery may be extraordinarily thick, and the colon may be engulfed in its fatty appendages. Moving the heavy omentum and thick and heavy mesentery and bowel around with small-diameter laparoscopic instruments can be very difficult. The weight of the tissue increases the likelihood of tearing tissue and creating a tough situation with bleeding to contend with. This type of obese patient, that is, the one with most of the excess weight inside, as is most often the case in males, is generally not a good candidate for standard laparoscopic colon surgery. But they can often be managed well using a hand-assisted technique.

Fourth, when performing a standard laparoscopic colon operation with a large organ like the colon, where exposure is so important, it really helps to work with the same team on a regular basis, and this can be difficult to coordinate for the average surgeon. Many of the standard laparoscopic approaches to colon surgery require an assistant to help with exposure. This assistant must be trained, as this person has to provide the all-important exposure. Many surgeons do not have ready access to a trained assistant for a routine colectomy. The technique illustrated does not require a second surgeon to assist. The camera can be held by a nurse or surgical assistant. Many of the troubles with exposure can be overcome with this technique, and this technique makes laparoscopic colon surgery doable in obese patients. Five millimeter graspers do not work very well to lift and expose anatomy in obese patients, but the hand does this job very well.

Fifth, there are a number of anatomic issues that can challenge the surgeon when performing a laparoscopic right colectomy, and the hand-assisted approach can help overcome these difficulties. For example, the hand-assisted technique overcomes the difficulty in doing a laparoscopic right colectomy in a patient who has had a cholecystectomy with adhesions that fix the hepatic flexure into the gallbladder fossa or approaching the mesenteric vessels in the patient who has the omentum stuck down onto the right colon or the ventral surface of the right colon mesentery. Especially when operating for cancer, if the omentum is adherent to the right colon, it should be left in place, and this makes exposure of the vessels problematic. Patients who have had an appendectomy will also frequently have omental adhesions in the right lower quadrant that can make the standard laparoscopic approaches more difficult. The hand-assisted technique that is illustrated minimizes these difficulties significantly. Another problem for the standard laparoscopic approaches to the right colon is a bulky tumor. Laparoscopic instruments are just not very good at moving bulk around in the abdomen, while the hand works quite well.

Finally, the hand-assisted right colectomy technique makes proper management of the middle colic vessels fairly easy. Anyone who has performed any significant number of laparoscopic colon resections would agree that the middle colic vessels and the transverse colon mesentery are the hardest part of the colon anatomy to manage properly. The reasons are that the vascular anatomy in this area is quite variable, the arteries are surrounded by large veins that can bleed easily, the mesentery in this area is short, exposure is difficult, and bleeding in this area takes the surgeon right down onto the pancreas and the superior mesenteric artery. This can just simply be a difficult area to manage well using standard laparoscopic right colectomy approaches. Using the technique illustrated, the surgeon gains a very good view of the middle colic vessels. This is a particular concern with regard to resecting cancers up at the hepatic flexure or the proximal transverse colon. The primary advantage here is that the vessels are seen from above and are approached from the side, moving from the patient's left to right. The middle colic vessels can be hard to manage head on using laparoscopy. From the side, they are very straightforward. Ileocecal resections are frequently performed for ileocecal Crohn disease, but this is a different operation. With an ileocecal resection, there is no particular need to take the middle colic vessels. The hepatic flexure is mobilized simply to allow mobility for extraction of the ileum and right colon so that a safe extracorporeal anastomosis can be conducted in the ascending colon, not the transverse colon. When the issue is cancer, much concern about taking the vessels near their origin will be shown.

The vast majority of right colectomies are performed to manage neoplastic disease, either invasive cancer or large polyps that cannot be managed using a colonoscope. As a general rule, since the likelihood that a polyp will harbor a cancer increases with the size of the polyp, when the indication for colectomy is a large adenoma, a formal resection should be performed. Another, not infrequent, indication for laparoscopic segmental colon resection is in the management of a malignant polyp that has been removed colonoscopically. If the polypectomy fails to meet one or more of the accepted criteria for a curative polypectomy, a formal resection is indicated. In these situations, the operation is conducted to remove the area of bowel involved so as to ensure that there is no cancer left within the bowel wall itself and to do a regional lymphadenectomy to remove potentially involved nodes. Again, a formal resection is recommended. Other much less common indications for a laparoscopic right colectomy might include management of right colonic bleeding from a vascular malformation or inflammatory disease due to right colon diverticulitis.

The formal right colectomy for neoplasia involves the usual maneuvers that define an oncologic colon resection: (1) proximal lymphovascular pedicle ligation and complete lymphadenectomy, (2) wide en bloc resection of tumor-bearing bowel segment with adjacent soft tissue and mesentery, and (3) minimizing the possibility of tumor contamination to the abdominal cavity, the wounds, or the bowel above or below the tumor.

The formal oncologic right colectomy, then, involves proximal ligation of the ileocolic pedicle and the right branch of the middle colic artery for cecal tumors or the entire middle colic pedicle for tumors in the ascending colon up to the proximal transverse colon. The ileum is divided about 15–20 cm from the ileocecal valve which corresponds to a point on the small bowel at which the superior mesenteric artery ends. The transverse colon is divided at its midpoint.

## Operation (Video 5.1)

### Patient Positioning

For the hand-assisted right colectomy illustrated, the patient is placed on the operating table in the supine position. Intermittent compression devices are placed, a general anesthetic is administered, and a urinary catheter and an orogastric tube are inserted. Both arms are tucked alongside the body. The arms are held in position by a folded drawsheet that the patient lays on. The ends of the drawsheet are brought up alongside the body, the arms are placed next to the body, the drawsheet is pulled around the arms, and it is placed under the patient. In addition, the patient is secured to the bed with multiple pieces of three inch tape. One or more pieces are placed across the lower extremities and a piece is used across the chest. Foam pads can be placed beneath the tape. These maneuvers are used to keep the patient on the operative table during the extremes of bed tilt that are often required to obtain exposure (Fig. 5.1). Having both arms tucked is more secure for the patient, and it also provides the surgeon and the assistant with maximal mobility around the

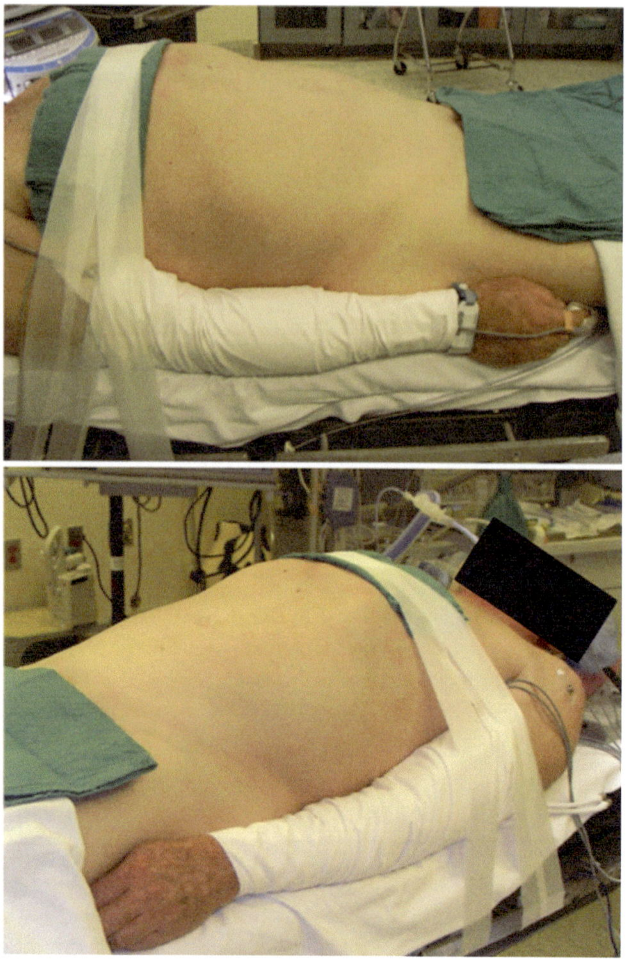

Fig. 5.1 The patient is positioned on the operating table in the supine position with both arms tucked at the side. Tape is used around the chest and the legs to ensure that the patient stays on the table in the extremes of bed tilt

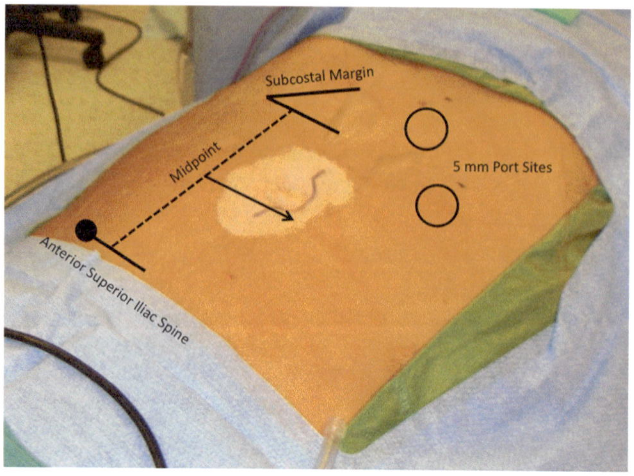


Fig. 5.2 The midpoint of the hand-assist incision is at the midpoint of a line drawn from the anterior superior iliac spine to the costal margin. For most patients, the incision will be centered on the umbilicus. For obese patients, it may be well above the umbilicus

operative table. The operative field should be lengthened by pushing the IV poles up towards the patient's head and asking the anesthesia personnel to push the table away from their equipment. Again, this simply gives the operative team more room to maneuver around the table. The field is prepped from the nipples to the mid-thigh level and the towels are placed wide on the abdomen. We prefer to have the towels held in position with an Ioban™ sheet. This is used to keep the towels in place, since when they are placed so widely on the abdomen, they can easily fall down the sides of the patient, exposing the un-prepped table. In addition, the Ioban™ sheet keeps instruments, cords, and cables from falling down alongside the patient outside the sterile field.

The exact routing of the camera cord, the fiberoptic light cord, and the insufflation tube will vary based on the arrangement of the operating room. The energy sources are brought onto the field at the patient's right shoulder. Typically, no suction is set up for this operation, as it is rarely used. If need be, it is brought on to the field at the foot of the bed. One or two video monitors will be placed along the right side of the patient, and the entire team focuses on these monitors. Additional monitors are really not needed for the illustrated procedure.

## Port Placement

For the hand-assisted laparoscopic right colectomy, the ports and the hand-assist device are placed as follows. The hand-assist device is placed in the midline. One should center this midline wound based upon palpable skeletal landmarks. The center of the hand port incision should be at the midpoint of a line drawn from the costal margin to the anterior superior iliac spine (Fig. 5.2). This will center the hand properly on the anatomy, independent of the location of the umbilicus, the location of which will vary based on the body habitus of the patient. In obese patients, the entire hand port incision may be well above the umbilicus, while in average weight patients, the incision is generally centered on the umbilicus. The midline wound is optimal, based upon surgeon ergonomics, consideration of extracorporeal anastomosis, and maintenance of videoscopic perspective of the relevant anatomy for right colectomy. Generally speaking, the size of the incision for the device will be the size of the surgeon's glove in centimeters. However, in practicality, one can usually cheat this size by a centimeter or so.

The authors use the GelPort™ device. It is easy to use and it provides the advantage of being able to place ports, instruments, or staplers right through the device even with the hand in place. Also, the surgeon's hand can be brought in and out of the abdomen without losing pneumoperitoneum. This feature helps for teaching purposes, as it is easy to go from the surgeon's to the assistant's hand in the abdomen.

Pneumoperitoneum is then established through a 5 or 12 mm port placed through the hand-assist device. The laparoscope is passed into the abdomen through this port. Two 5 mm ports are then placed in the left upper abdomen: one in the subxiphoid region and one in the left upper quadrant. The subxiphoid port will be for the 5 mm 30 degree laparoscope, and the left upper quadrant port will be for a 5 mm sealing/cutting device.

The position of the subxiphoid port will vary, some depending on the patient and what is being done. It will usually be placed at least a few centimeters to the left of midline. The further over to the left on the transverse colon one plans to go, the further to the left one should place this port. Generally, the port will be placed just to the left of the falciform ligament. At times, the falciform ligament is very large and long, it gets in the way, and it will need to be removed. This is easy to do working through the left upper quadrant ports, with or without the use of the hand in the hand port. The left upper quadrant port should not be placed too high on the costal margin; otherwise, getting to the right lower quadrant can be difficult. Also, it should not be placed too low, since the hand and the energy source will get in each other's way during dissection in the right lower quadrant. Placement in the midclavicular line, about halfway between the costal margin and the upper aspect of the hand-assist incision, will be about right.

In the patient who has had previous abdominal surgery, the hand-assist incision can be used initially to lyse adhesions. If there are more adhesions than can be reached by operating through the incision, the GelPort™ can be placed, the additional ports can be placed, and adhesiolysis can be carried out with or without the hand being placed through the device. If adhesions in the left abdomen interfere with placing the left upper quadrant ports, one can simply place 5 mm ports and instruments through the GelPort™, and it can be used as a working port for this activity.

Using this hand-assisted right colectomy approach, 5 mm ports can be used exclusively. If a stapling device is needed, it is inserted through a 12 mm port placed directly through the GelPort™ hand-assist device (Applied Medical, Rancho Santa Margarita, CA). A 5 mm, 30 degree laparoscope is used since this provides maximum flexibility as the scope can be moved to any port and the 30 degree angle allows the surgeon the best view in tight spaces.

There are a number of 5 mm energy sources that seal and cut well. With these tools, the surgeon has a 5 mm instrument that can be used to dissect bloodlessly and take any of the named mesenteric vessels.

## Operative Technique

It is important again to note that this is a single-surgeon operation. There is no need for a trained assistant to help with

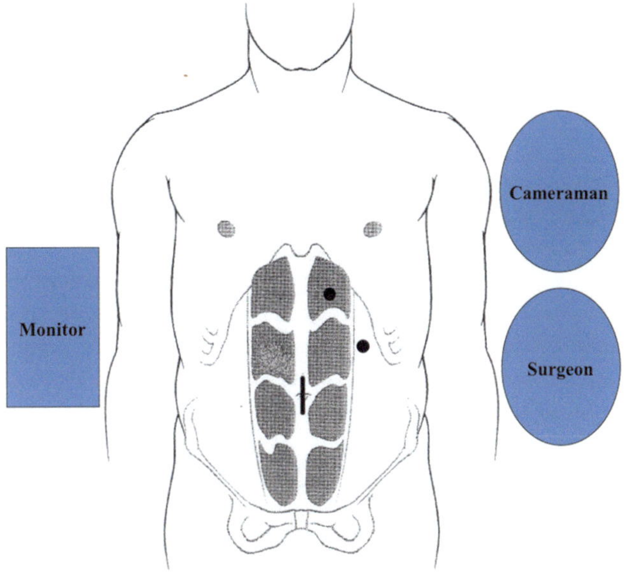


**Fig. 5.3** The position of the surgeon, camera holder, and monitor at the operating table

exposure. With the ports and the hand-assist device in position, the camera holder will be positioned at the patient's left shoulder and the surgeon will be on the patient's left side (Fig. 5.3). Both focus their attention on the monitor at the patient's right. The patient is placed in strong reverse Trendelenburg position and is tilted to the left. This brings the hepatic flexure down. The abdomen is explored with the laparoscope and the surgeon's hand.

An important aspect of hand-assisted laparoscopic surgery that is not often discussed is the use of the hand itself. The surgeon should keep in mind a couple of important points. First of all, the surgeon and the camera holder should work to keep the hand out of view of the laparoscope. The amount of the hand inside should be minimized: the hand is almost never put in to a point proximal to the wrist. At almost all points in the case, the scope should see not much more than a finger or two. The hand should be, for the most part, kept outside the field of vision. There should be parts of the case where it may not even appear that the hand is inside the abdomen.

Secondly, the hand should not be used as a substitute for a large laparoscopic clamp. The hand is a much more versatile instrument. There are but a very few points in the operation where the hand is actually used to "grasp" tissue. Rather the hand is used to expose anatomy. In this regard, the hand can take the place of multiple instruments. Often the third, fourth, and fifth digits are pushing back towards the palm to move tissue out of the field, usually out of view of the laparoscope, the index finger is being used to expose the anatomic feature that is being addressed with the cutting and sealing device, and the thumb is being used to counter the index finger so as to provide the classic "traction and countertraction."

The index finger and the cutting and sealing device are at the point of action and the laparoscope will follow them. Much of the cutting done with the cutting and sealing device will use the index finger as a "backstop" to protect the surrounding tissue. The finger then is used as a gentle guide for cutting, not as an anvil.

The surgical dissection described is unique and proceeds in a counterclockwise, top-down fashion beginning at the gastrocolic ligament. As opposed to other techniques described for laparoscopic right colectomy, this operative approach has the dissection and mobilization of all the important anatomy starting and ending in a single plane. There is no need to change orientations or connect tissue planes as one mobilizes certain parts of the right colon anatomy. The right colon, in essence, is lifted off the retroperitoneum and swept up and out of the right abdomen, moving from the right upper quadrant to the right lower quadrant. The surgical dissection described is unique and proceeds in a counterclockwise, top-down fashion beginning at the gastrocolic ligament. The procedure can be viewed in five steps as follows:

### Step 1: Hepatic Flexure Takedown

The surgeon uses his/her left hand to grasp the greater omentum along the greater curve of the stomach, and he/she makes a defect in it, just off of the gastroepiploic vessels. This puts the surgeon into the lesser sac, and the smooth, shiny ventral surface of the transverse mesocolon can be seen. Whether moving from left to right or right to left, it does not matter, as this space is developed by taking the greater omentum off the stomach. As one moves to the right, the anterior surface of the duodenum is exposed and the hepatic flexure comes into view. The hepatic flexure is taken down and Gerota's fascia comes into view. Alternatively, if the lesser sac cannot be well developed as an initial maneuver, the dissection can be started up at the hepatic flexure, and as soon as the proper plane is recognized on Gerota's fascia and the duodenum, the dissection can come from right to left back into the lesser sac, which will be very important later in the operation for managing the middle colic vessels.

### Step 2: Retroperitoneal Dissection and Takedown of Lateral Attachments

The surgeon then mobilizes the right colon mesentery up off of the retroperitoneum. Lifting the colon and ileum up off of the retroperitoneum is accomplished by gentle lifting off the bowel and mesentery and pushing back towards the retroperitoneum, just inside the white line, with the cutting and sealing device. As one starts to lift the bowel off of the retroperitoneum, oftentimes the bowel will be lying on the back of the hand, and the palm will be facing the smooth surface of the retroperitoneum. The temptation during this part of the operation is to go directly to the lateral attachments. One should fight this temptation. It is much easier to mobilize medially first, leaving the lateral attachments for later. These lateral attachments act as natural retractors fixing the bowel in place and providing a natural point of countertraction that makes lifting the colon off the retroperitoneal structures easier. The filmy attachments between the third part of the duodenum and the ileal and right colon mesentery should be completely divided. This will expose the duodenum completely, essentially over to the ligament of Treitz. This extensive mobilization will help later when taking the mesentery, and it will make extraction easy, even in the obese patient. After the right colon and ileal mesentery are lifted completely, the lateral attachments are easily seen and then divided from the right upper quadrant down to the right lower quadrant.

### Step 3: Mobilization of the Ileal Mesentery

With the right colon and ileal mesentery now completely freed from the retroperitoneum and with the right colon and ileum now folded over into the left lower abdomen, the surgeon puts the back of his/her hand on the iliac vessels and the ileal mesentery is now draped over the surgeon's hand, and the peritoneum at the base of the mesentery is incised from the right lower quadrant back up to the duodenum. This is the embryologic fusion plane for the small bowel mesentery. Once this is incised, the entire right retroperitoneum is bare. The duodenum, the head of the pancreas, and Gerota's fascia are all in plain sight. The ureter and gonadal vessels can be seen beneath Toldt's fascia, which is covering the right retroperitoneum. With mobilization complete, it is now time to take the mesentery and vessels. It is tempting at this point to simply stop, extract, and take the vessels extracorporeally. One should fight this temptation for two reasons. First, in a patient of any size, taking the ileocolic artery and the middle colic artery near their origins off of the superior mesenteric artery can be done much better inside than outside. It is very hard (if not impossible for the middle colic artery) to do a proper high ligation of the vessels when a bulky specimen is being pulled up through a 6 or 7 cm incision. Second, in a large patient with a thick abdominal wall, it will be the vessels that tether the bowel down and make extraction difficult. The goal should be to get the bowel completely mobilized and the vessels taken inside so that when it comes to extraction, the bowel comes up easily and there is no tension. The larger the patient, the more important it is to do a complete mobilization and the more important it is to divide the vessels on the inside. Especially with large patients, do not be tempted to do a minimal mobilization, and then think that the vessels can be taken after extraction. One should always try to mobilize a bit more than one thinks will be needed, and one should plan to take the vessels intracorporeally. This makes things easy during, and after, extraction of the specimen. Hand-assisted techniques really shine for obese patients, and it is actually easier to get things done inside rather than after extraction through the hand-assist device.

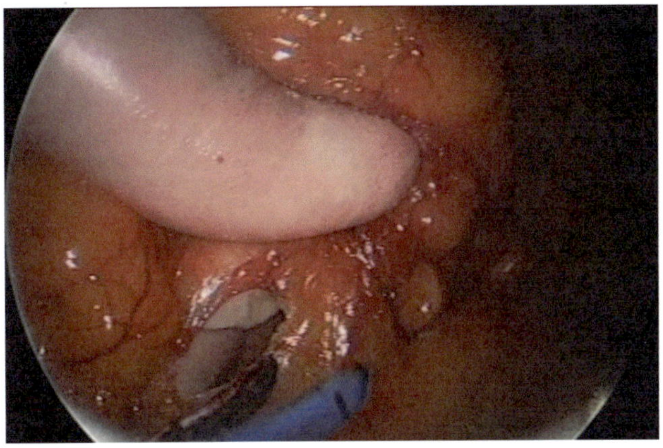

**Fig. 5.4** The surgeon is elevating the transverse colon, and a defect is made in the transverse mesocolon to the left of the middle colic vessels, which are here being taken with the LigaSure device

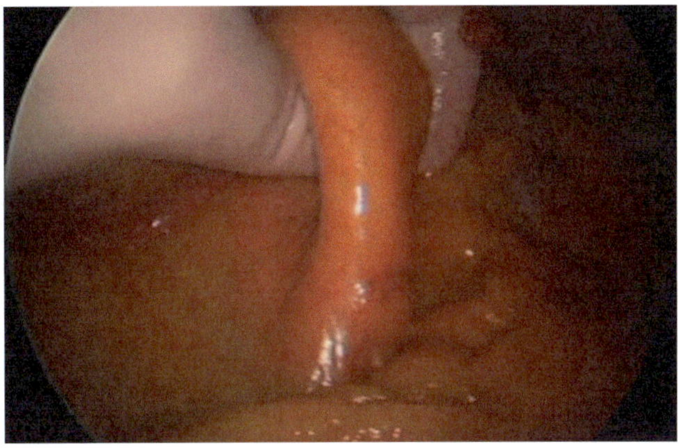

**Fig. 5.5** Before the ileocolic pedicle is taken, the right colon is put back in its normal anatomic position and the ileocolic pedicle is firmly identified. Here it is elevated by the surgeon off of the small bowel mesentery

## Step 4: Vessel and Mesentery Division

The vessels and the mesentery are taken as follows: the surgeon will grasp the transverse colon in his/her palm and then work his/her middle finger down to the base of the dorsal surface of the transverse mesocolon to the left of the middle colic vessels. A window is then developed in this area (Fig. 5.4). This is the same window, i.e., to the left of the middle colic vessels, which one might create to do a retrocolic gastrojejunostomy. The surgeon then moves across the base of the transverse mesocolon from left to right taking the right branch of the middle colic vessel or the entire middle colic vessel trunk (depending on the situation) just over the pancreas. These vessels are well seen from above and from the side as they come up out the retroperitoneum. One should move slowly through this area as bleeding here can be difficult to control. It is very important, before taking the middle colic vessels, that the mesentery is cleared right down to its base of any omental or gastric attachments. The lesser sac should be very well developed. This makes taking the vessels near their origin feasible, and it facilitates control of bleeding, should this be encountered. A short stump of vessel should be left in case there is bleeding in this area. This stump allows the surgeon room to control any bleeding with either a clip, a stapler passed through a 12 mm port passed through the hand-assist device, an ENDOLOOP™ (Ethicon, Cincinnati, OH) passed through the left upper quadrant port or the GelPort™, or a stitch placed intracorporeally using the hand and a laparoscopic needle holder placed through the left upper quadrant port. The surgeon should remember that the middle colic stump is sitting just deep to the GelPort™, and control of bleeding may be most easily managed by simply removing the cap of the GelPort™ and using a stick tie passed straight down on the mesentery. Once the middle colic vessels are taken, there is usually a free space in the mesentery, and the surgeon can sense the decrease in tension on the mesentery as the middle colic vessels are released. The surgeon then takes a sharp left turn and the ileocolic pedicle is encountered (Fig. 5.5). In about 90 % of patients, the right colic artery is a branch of the ileocolic artery or the middle colic artery, so one should not routinely expect to find a right colic artery between the middle colic and ileocolic vessels. If there is a right colic off of the superior mesenteric artery, it is taken and the surgeon moves on to the ileocolic. The ileocolic should always be confirmed to be the ileocolic, and not the superior mesenteric artery. This can be easily accomplished by putting the hepatic flexure back in its place in the right upper quadrant and then grasping the cecum and pulling it down and to the right. This will "tent" the ileocolic artery for anatomic confirmation. One can take the ileocolic vessels from their ventral surface with the hepatic flexure returned to the right upper quadrant, but it is better not to. Exposure is actually better, and problems are easier to manage with the hepatic flexure pushed back down into the left abdomen as it is after the mobilization. So if there is a problem with the ileocolic pedicle, the hepatic flexure is not falling down into the field, interfering with exposure. Just as with the middle colic vessels, a short stump of the ileocolic vessel approximately 2 cm long should be left. This gives the surgeon room to maneuver should there be bleeding. If there is bleeding, it can be managed as described above for the middle colic artery. While the named mesenteric vessels are routinely taken with the cutting/sealing energy source, if the surgeon can feel with his/her fingers that they are highly calcified, they should be taken with a vascular load of the laparoscopic stapler passed through a 12 mm port inserted through the GelPort™ device alongside the surgeon's hand. Once the ileocolic artery is divided, the mesenteric window between the ileocolic and the superior mesenteric vessels is incised out to the marginal vessel along the ileum.

### Step 5: Bowel Extraction and Anastomosis

Now that the bowel is completely mobilized and the major vessels have been taken, pneumoperitoneum is evacuated through the 5 mm ports, they are removed, and the bowel is extracted through the hand-assist device. The marginal vessels along the ileum and the transverse colon are divided, the bowel is divided, and a hand-sewn or stapled ileocolic anastomosis is fashioned. The bowel is dropped back into the abdomen, the hand-assist device is removed, and the incision at the umbilicus is closed with a running absorbable suture, and each of the wounds is closed with a subcuticular stitch and tissue adhesive. The mesenteric defect is generally not closed, but the surgeon should try to make sure that the anastomosis sits comfortably in the right upper quadrant and that the small bowel is returned to its proper anatomic position with no twist.

## Postoperative Care

Standardized postoperative care includes early and frequent ambulation starting on the day of surgery, minimizing the use of narcotics and making use of oral and intravenous NSAIDs, and early resumption of oral intake. Discharge comes when the patient can tolerate a diet and there has been resumption of bowel function. This usually occurs on day two to four depending on the patient's age, home situation, motivation, and/or anxiety level.

## Pearls and Pitfalls

1. Generally, the operation starts by entering the lesser sac along the greater curvature of the stomach. The lesser sac is best entered as proximal on the stomach as possible. If the lesser sac cannot easily be entered, just move over to the hepatic flexure and start the operation at the hepatic flexure, and at some point later, once the duodenum has been exposed, the dissection can move into the lesser sac so that the middle colic vessels can be exposed better in the transverse mesocolon.
2. The anterior surface of the duodenum is the most important landmark for the dissection. If there is any trouble at all in defining the plane behind the right colon, simply go back to the duodenum and reorient.
3. Try to resist the temptation to simply take down the lateral attachments to the right colon from the start. They are actually helpful in providing countertraction as the right colon and its mesentery are lifted up off of the retroperitoneum.
4. Take the vessels on the inside. They are better visualized, they can be taken closer to their origin, and bleeding from a pedicle is actually easier to manage inside.
5. If the vessels seem as if they would be better taken with a laparoscopic stapler, put a 12 mm port through the GelPort and pass the stapler through this port.
6. When operating on an obese patient, you may find that taking the marginal vessel along the ileum and then dividing the ileum intracorporeally may be quite helpful. It simply makes extraction easier, since there is less bulk coming through the hand-assist port.
7. If the ileum is divided intracorporeally, you must pay special attention to the orientation of the ileum as it is extracted so that there is no twist. Just follow the cut edge of the ileal mesentery right down to the base of the mesentery to avoid a twist.
8. Finally, consider that the more obese the patient, the more important it can be to develop the defect in the distal transverse colon mesentery and to take the entire middle colic pedicle. These maneuvers give the transverse colon significant mobility for extraction and anastomosis.

## Summary

In conclusion, the authors' experience and the surgical literature confirm that hand-assisted laparoscopic colon surgery is a sound technique. Using the hand can help shorten the learning curve for those surgeons trying to adopt laparoscopy for the treatment of colon pathology, shorten operative time, make marginal laparoscopic cases feasible, reduce the need for a fully trained operative team, and, especially for the surgeon just starting in laparoscopic colon surgery, significantly reduce the stress level in the operating room. It is very comforting having a hand in the abdomen. All these advantages are gained without any apparent price being paid in terms of the rapid return of bowel function and the reduced length of stay seen with standard laparoscopic resection.

## References

1. Fleshman J, Sargent DJ, Green E, Anvari M, Stryker SJ, Beart Jr RW, et al. Laparoscopic colectomy for cancer is not inferior to open surgery based on 5-year data from the COST Study Group trial. Ann Surg. 2007;246(4):655–62. discussion 662-4.
2. Colon Cancer Laparoscopic or Open Resection Study Group, Buunen M, Veldkamp R, Hop WC, Kuhry E, Jeekel J, et al. Survival after laparoscopic surgery versus open surgery for colon cancer: long-term outcome of a randomised clinical trial. Lancet Oncol. 2009;10(1):44–52.
3. Jayne DG, Guillou PJ, Thorpe H, Quirke P, Copeland J, Smith AM, et al. Randomized trial of laparoscopic-assisted resection of colorectal carcinoma: 3-year results of the UK MRC CLASICC Trial Group. J Clin Oncol. 2007;25(21):3061–8.
4. Lacy AM, Delgado S, Castells A, Prins HA, Arroyo V, Ibarzabal A, et al. The long-term results of a randomized clinical trial of laparoscopy-assisted versus open surgery for colon cancer. Ann Surg. 2008;248(1):1–7.

5. Aly EH. Laparoscopic colorectal surgery: summary of the current evidence. Ann R Coll Surg Engl. 2009;91(7):541–4.
6. Kang CY, Halabi WJ, Luo R, Pigazzi A, Nguyen NT, Stamos MJ. Laparoscopic colorectal surgery: a better look into the latest trends. Arch Surg. 2012;147(8):724–31.
7. Chang YJ, Marcello PW, Rusin LC, Roberts PL, Schoetz DJ. Hand-assisted laparoscopic sigmoid colectomy: helping hand or hindrance? Surg Endosc. 2005;19(5):656–61.
8. HALS Study Group. Hand-assisted laparoscopic surgery vs standard laparoscopic surgery for colorectal disease: a prospective randomized trial. Surg Endosc. 2000;14(10):896–901.
9. Marcello PW, Fleshman JW, Milsom JW, Read TE, Arnell TD, Birnbaum EH, et al. Hand-assisted laparoscopic vs. laparoscopic colorectal surgery: a multicenter, prospective, randomized trial. Dis Colon Rectum. 2008;51(6):818–26.
10. Clinical Outcomes of Surgical Therapy Study Group. A comparison of laparoscopically assisted and open colectomy for colon cancer. N Engl J Med. 2004;350(20):2050–9.
11. Guillou PJ, Quirke P, Thorpe H, Walker J, Jayne DG, Smith AM, et al. Short-term endpoints of conventional versus laparoscopic-assisted surgery in patients with colorectal cancer (MRC CLASICC trial): multicentre, randomised controlled trial. Lancet. 2005;365(9472):1718–26.
12. Flegal KM, Carroll MD, Kit BK, Ogden CL. Prevalence of obesity and trends in the distribution of body mass index among US adults, 1999–2010. JAMA. 2012;307(5):491–7.

# Laparoscopic Sigmoidectomy/ Left Colectomy

# 6

Toyooki Sonoda

## Key Points

- While medial and lateral approaches are equally effective, the medial approach offers certain potential advantages such as early vascular ligation and intrinsic colonic retraction.
- Confirm and mark your lesions preoperatively either with India ink, clips, or another strategy. Using distance from the anal verge alone is fraught with error and will lead to longer operative times, adjustments in the operative plan, or worse, inappropriate surgery or missed lesions.
- Gravity is your friend—use it. By properly securing the patient to the table, you can use extremes of positioning to retract the small bowel and improve visualization.
- If available, a dedicated camera operator will allow your assistant to use two instruments.
- Do not be wed to one position. Move around the table to improve visualization and ergonomics.
- Never sacrifice operative principles for the number of trocars. Add more if you need them.
- A sigmoidectomy/left colectomy has specific steps that need to be accomplished; however, you may need to alter the order to successfully and safely complete the operation.

## Introduction

There are two general approaches to the mobilization of the sigmoid colon, one where the colon is mobilized from its lateral attachments first (the lateral approach) and one where the vascular pedicles are initially ligated, followed by colonic mobilization (the medial-to-lateral approach). Both accomplish the same dissection, and there is no known clinical advantage to either approach. The author prefers the medial approach for the following reasons:

- Abiding with the Turnbull no-touch technique for cancer, the vascular pedicles are ligated prior to any mobilization of the tumor-bearing segment of the bowel. This limits the liberation of tumor cells into the mesenteric circulation during mobilization.
- The lateral attachments of the colon may act as a natural retractor, fixing it in place while the medial dissection is performed. On the other hand, when the bowel is first mobilized laterally, it can lead to excessive floppiness of the bowel, making retraction difficult.

## Indications

The most common indications for a laparoscopic sigmoid colectomy include a malignant neoplasm, a benign polyp not amenable to colonoscopic removal, and diverticular disease. Other indications include but are not limited to chronic sigmoid volvulus and segmental Crohn's disease.

## Contraindications

There are both absolute and relative contraindications to the laparoscopic approach to colectomy. Absolute contraindications are:

- Hemodynamic instability
- Known history of extensive adhesions from prior surgery

Relative contraindications to laparoscopy will depend on surgeon experience and level of comfort. A minimally invasive approach can still be considered on a case-to-case basis. These include:

- Large tumor size (>8 cm)
- Invasion of other structures
- Bowel dilation from obstruction
- Emergency surgery

**Electronic supplementary material:** Supplementary material is available in the online version of this chapter at 10.1007/978-1-4939-1581-1_6. Videos can also be accessed at http://www.springerimages.com/videos/978-1-4939-1580-4.

T. Sonoda, M.D. (✉)
Section of Colon and Rectal Surgery, New York Presbyterian Hospital, Weill Medical College of Cornell University, 525 East 68th Street, New York, NY 10021, USA
e-mail: tos2003@med.cornell.edu

H.M. Ross et al. (eds.), *Minimally Invasive Approaches to Colon and Rectal Disease: Technique and Best Practices*,
DOI 10.1007/978-1-4939-1581-1_6, © Springer Science+Business Media New York 2015

The location of the sigmoid colon makes invasion of other organs possible, for example, colovesical and colovaginal fistulas. This is the case in both malignancy and inflammatory conditions, including diverticulitis and Crohn's disease. These complex fistulas can be treated laparoscopically in experienced hands, but a more robust en bloc resection will be required in malignancy as opposed to benign conditions, where the attached two organs need merely to be separated. These cases are also highly appropriate for hand-assisted laparoscopic surgery (HALS; see Chap. 7), where the area of fistulization is dealt with using open surgery techniques through either a small Pfannenstiel or low midline incision utilizing a hand port.

## Preoperative Planning

The patient's comorbidities and nutritional status are assessed to see whether a patient is an acceptable candidate for surgery. Every effort is made to maximize the patient's medical condition prior to surgery.

When patients are referred with neoplastic lesions in the sigmoid colon, the true location of the neoplasm must be confirmed. This is because the measured location of the tumor during colonoscopy may not be exact depending on whether the patient's buttocks are large or whether the measurement was taken during insertion or withdrawal of the colonoscope. For example, a lesion advertised to be at 20 cm may in fact be at 8 cm from the anal verge. This could have a major impact on the level of resection (and therefore technical difficulty), or for locally advanced tumors, this may even impact on the decision for neoadjuvant chemoradiation. A tumor large enough will be identified on CT scan, but in other cases the surgeon should perform a rigid or flexible proctosigmoidoscopy prior to any operation.

An endoscopic tattoo (i.e., using India ink) should be used to mark all neoplastic lesions, and this is especially important for lesions that may not be visible on the serosal surface. This allows for laparoscopic identification of the tumor-bearing segment and helps eliminate the possibilities of removing an incorrect segment of the intestine or resecting a tumor with inadequate lateral margins. The tattoo should be placed in multiple quadrants to assure that it is visible on the serosal surface and not hidden by the mesentery. The author favors a tattoo in three quadrants, distal to the tumor itself. Placing tattoos both proximally and distally may lead to confusion if only one area is visible.

The usefulness of routine ureteral stenting in laparoscopic sigmoidectomy can be debated. In straightforward cases, the left ureter can usually be identified during mobilization, and this practice is probably unnecessary. However, selective preoperative ureteral stenting should be considered in complex cases where retroperitoneal or pelvic adhesions could exist (i.e., in locally advanced tumors, in re-operative pelvic surgery, or in diverticulitis/Crohn's disease with abscess). Surgeons early in their laparoscopic learning curve may also benefit from the use of lighted ureteral stents during sigmoid colectomy.

## Surgery

Patients should receive appropriate intravenous antibiotics within 1 h of skin incision. For a lengthy operation, antibiotics should be re-dosed intraoperatively based on their pharmacokinetics. Prophylaxis against deep vein thrombosis should be given preoperatively; this includes both sequential compression stockings and subcutaneous heparin.

## Positioning

The laparoscopic sigmoid colectomy is performed with extreme positioning such as steep Trendelenburg and side-to-side "air-planing." To avoid slippage of the patient during these maneuvers, the patient needs to be secured to the operating table. The author places a gel pad underneath the patient for this reason, but a beanbag can also be used. Both arms are tucked at the sides, with adequate padding to avoid pressure points. In larger patients, the arms are placed in padded sleds or toboggans, which may additionally help with patient slippage. The patient's legs are placed in a modified lithotomy position in padded stirrups, and adequate access to the anal orifice is confirmed. It is common for the patients' hips to slide upward on the operating table during steep Trendelenburg positioning, so generous access to the anus at the time of setup is recommended. Hip flexion while in stirrups must be kept to a minimum (i.e., hips as straight as possible), so that the laparoscopic instruments are not obstructed by the patient's thighs during the splenic flexure dissection. A heating blanket is placed on the chest to prevent hypothermia.

## Technique (Videos 6.1 and 6.2)

### Port Placement

The camera port is placed in an infraumbilical position. The author favors the blunt Hasson technique for initial entrance, with a 10-mm or 12-mm port placed for the camera. The subsequent port placement is illustrated in Fig. 6.1. A suprapubic port is optional and can be helpful for lateral sigmoid colon mobilization.

The laparoscopic sigmoid colectomy is facilitated by a dedicated cameraperson (2nd assistant), as this allows the assistant to help with two instruments. This is important for

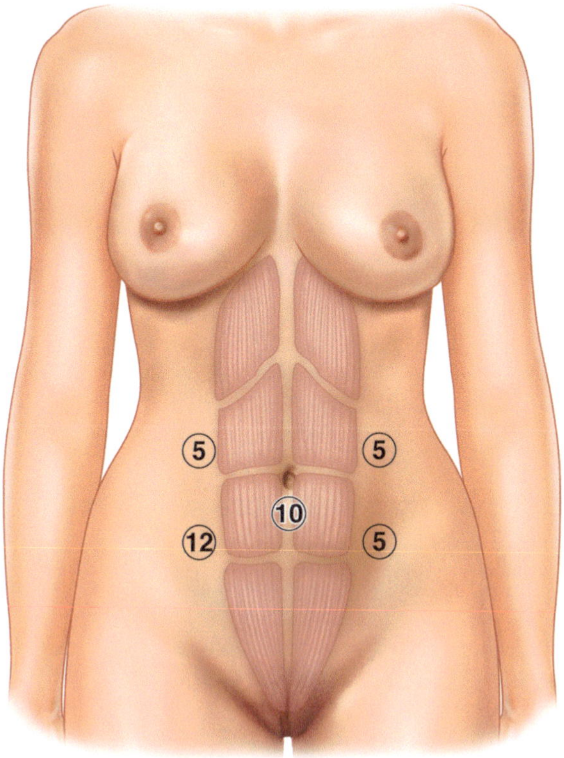


**Fig. 6.1** The port placement for a medial-to-lateral laparoscopic sigmoidectomy/left colectomy. Optional port$^{5\text{-mm}}$

adequate retraction of a floppy sigmoid colon and during splenic flexure mobilization. At the start of the operation, the surgeon stands at the right side of the patient and uses the two right-sided ports for dissection, and the camera assistant stands to the left of the surgeon. The assistant is positioned on the left side of the patient, using the two left-sided ports to retract the sigmoid colon. Two monitors are helpful at this point, placed on both sides of the patient near the knees, as the assistant and surgeon should view separate monitors (Fig. 6.2).

For splenic flexure mobilization, a monitor is moved to the patient's left shoulder. The surgeon moves in between the legs and uses the two left-sided ports for dissection. The assistant moves to the patient's right side, using the two right-sided ports to assist (Fig. 6.3).

It is important to remember that different port placements are used by different surgeons, and what is described above is only one option of many. A minimally invasive sigmoid colectomy by two operators using 2 or 3 working ports has been described, and port placement should eventually be tailored by each surgeon to meet one's needs. However, one should never limit the number of ports to the point that basic surgical principles such as tissue triangulation are sacrificed. An additional 5-mm trocar presents minimal morbidity to patients and could be of tremendous benefit during a difficult laparoscopic colectomy. The port placement described above remains the most common configuration used by the author.

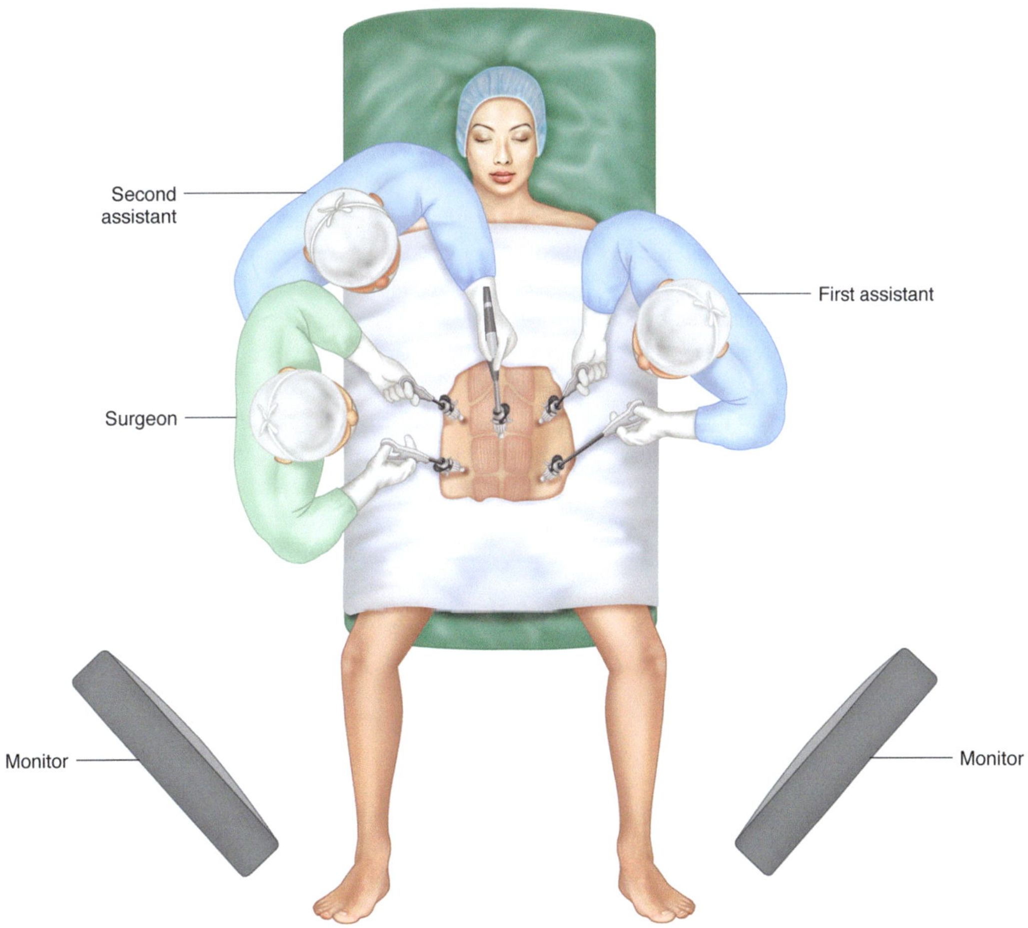


**Fig. 6.2** Position of the monitors and surgical team for vascular ligation, medial and lateral bowel mobilization, and anastomosis

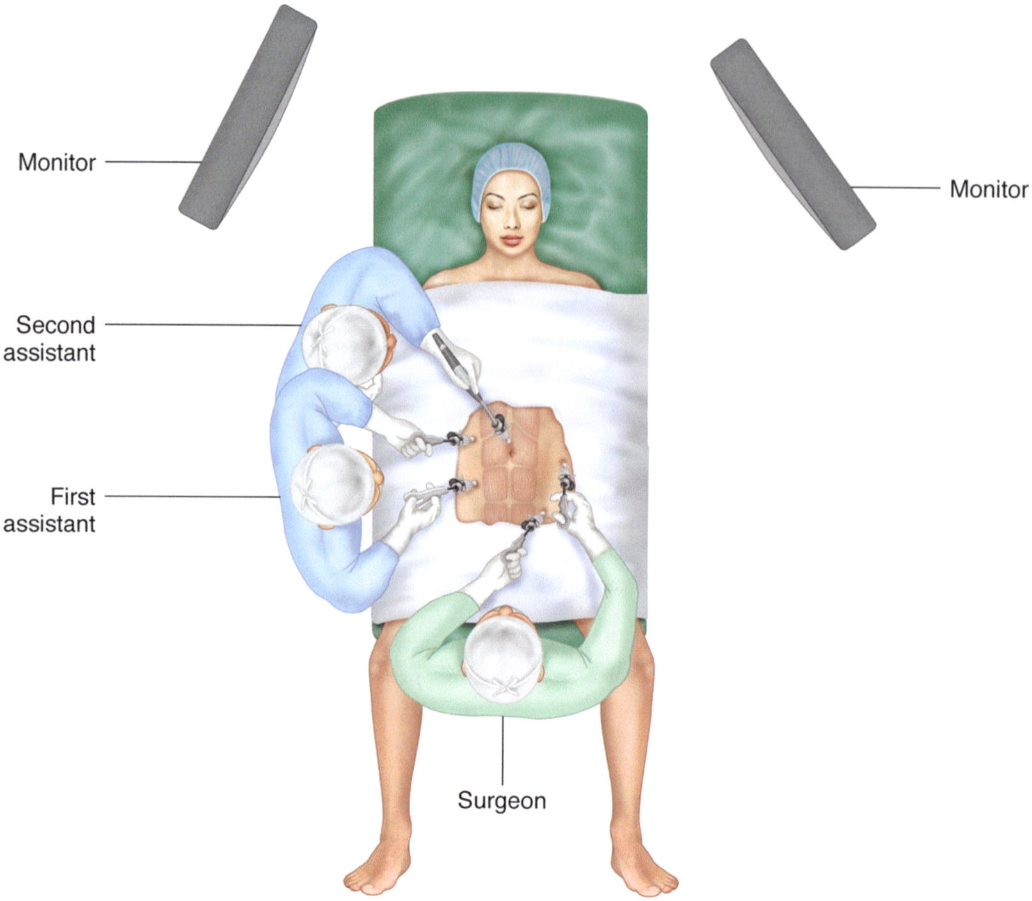


**Fig. 6.3** Ports on the patient's left abdomen should be in the same position as Fig. 6.1. It's a little off in this illustration

## Operative Steps

The following are the general operative steps in a medial-to-lateral laparoscopic sigmoid colectomy:

- Isolation and division of the inferior mesenteric artery
- Isolation and division of the inferior mesenteric vein, ligated together or separately from the artery
- Separation of the sigmoid colon and mesentery from the retroperitoneal fascia in a medial-to-lateral direction
- Dissection of the lateral attachments of the sigmoid and descending colon
- Splenic flexure mobilization (when necessary)
- Division of the bowel proximally and distally
- Anastomosis

## Vascular Isolation and Division

It is common for the distal small bowel loops to drape into the pelvis and obstruct the exposure of the sigmoid mesentery, and retraction of these loops out of the pelvis can at times be difficult. Gravity is used to help with this cause, and thus, positioning of the patient is very important. Initially, the patient is placed in a steep Trendelenburg position and tilted (airplaned) with the left side up. The omentum is lifted over the transverse colon, and the small bowel loops are swept into the right upper quadrant away from the mesosigmoid. It is important that the sacral promontory is visualized and can be palpated with a laparoscopic instrument at this point. The terminal ileum not uncommonly is adhered to the right pelvis, making superior retraction of the terminal ileum impossible. In this case, the ileum must be freed from the right pelvis as the initial step.

The sigmoid colon is then retracted by the assistant in two areas. The sigmoid mesentery is retracted in a ventral direction and toward the left. Especially in a redundant "pelvic" sigmoid colon, traction must also be in a superior direction (pulling the sigmoid colon out of the pelvis). The surgeon feels for the sacral promontory using a laparoscopic instrument as this should be the initial location where the peritoneum overlying the sigmoid mesentery is incised. Access to the proper avascular plane posterior to the inferior mesenteric vessels is easiest at the sacral promontory. While adequate

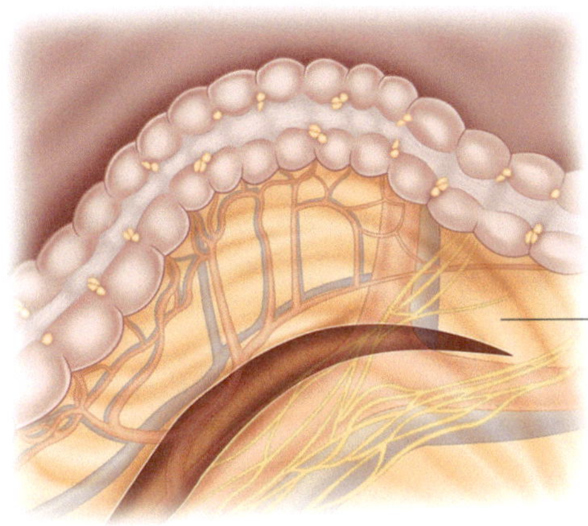


**Fig. 6.4** The peritoneal incision of the sigmoid mesentery commences at the sacral promontory. This is extended in a cephalad direction around the origin of the inferior mesenteric artery toward the inferior mesenteric vein

mesenteric traction is provided by the assistant, a wide mesenteric window is created around the origin of the inferior mesenteric artery (IMA) toward the inferior mesenteric vein (IMV) (Fig. 6.4). The right and left hypogastric nerves are adhered to the inferior mesenteric vessels and must be bluntly swept in a dorsal direction and preserved in order to avoid autonomic nerve injury that causes retrograde ejaculation. The dissection must stay anterior to the iliac vessels and these autonomic nerves and posterior to the inferior mesenteric vessels. Inability to find the correct avascular plane is usually due to inadequate ventral traction on the vessels. Creating a mesenteric window that is wide enough will allow for better traction on the vessels and avoiding "tunneling," which results in limited visualization.

The line of the fusion of the sigmoid mesentery and retroperitoneal fascia is identified underneath the inferior mesenteric vessels, and the retroperitoneal fascia is bluntly swept dorsally. It is with this step that the left ureter and left gonadal vein should be identified and preserved (Fig. 6.5). It is easy to dissect in a plane that is too deep, i.e., deep to the ureter and gonadal vessels. Only after identification of the left ureter should the IMA be divided. The origin of the IMA is cleaned off and skeletonized as the preaortic superior hypogastric plexus is further swept away from the origin of the IMA and preserved (both left and right branches). A mesenteric window is created lateral to the IMV, isolating the inferior mesenteric vessels. The IMA and IMV are then divided using a vessel-sealing energy device, clips, or a laparoscopic vascular stapler (Figs. 6.6 and 6.7). It is common practice to leave a 1–2 cm stump on the IMA so it can be grasped and sealed in the case it bleeds. Vascular calcification leads to failure of energy devices, and thus in cases of long-standing diabetes or cardiovascular disease, the use of a vascular stapler or clips is preferred. The IMV is usually not calcified and can be readily divided with an energy device.

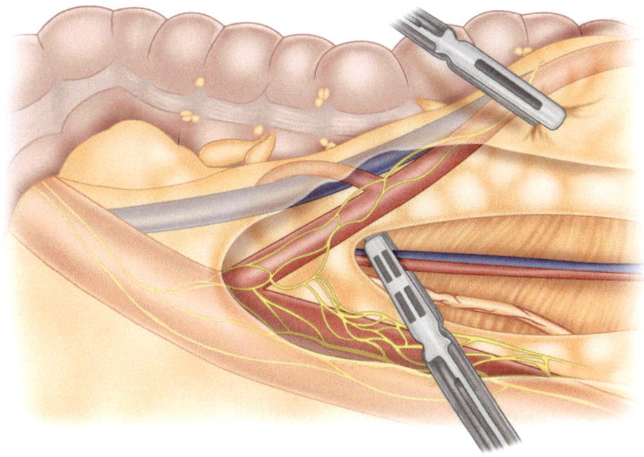

**Fig. 6.5** Dissection of the inferior mesenteric artery, with preservation of the hypogastric nerves and left ureter and gonadal vessels

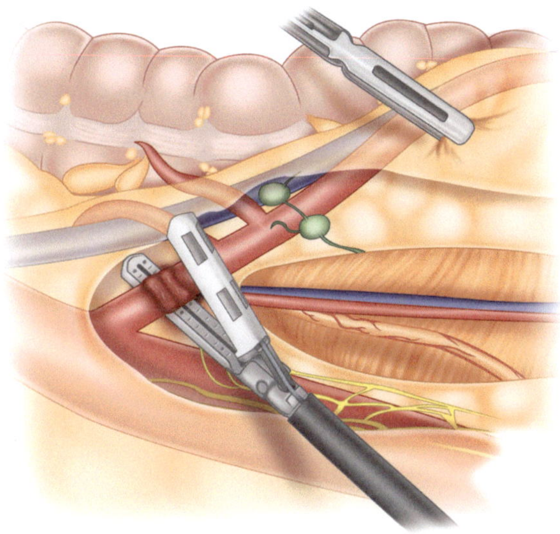

**Fig. 6.6** The division of the inferior mesenteric artery

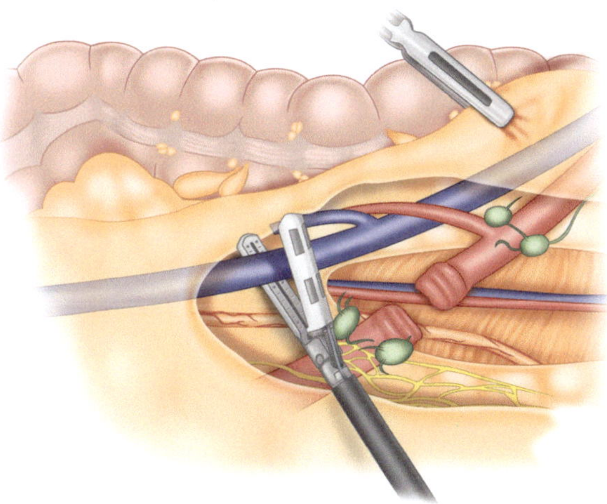

**Fig. 6.7** Division of the inferior mesenteric vein

Alternatively, the IMV can be isolated and divided independently of the IMA. In difficult cases, it is actually helpful to isolate and divide the IMV before the IMA. The IMV is identified adjacent to the ligament of Treitz in a location superior to the IMA, and in this location, it is isolated and divided. This provides an excellent entry point to the correct dissection plane between the left colon mesentery and retroperitoneal fascia and can aid in the mobilization of the splenic flexure.

## Pearls and Pitfalls

### Difficulty in Identifying the Left Ureter

The left ureter may be difficult to find when one is not dissecting in the correct plane. As mentioned previously, the tendency is to dissect deep to the retroperitoneal fascia, into the retroperitoneum itself, and keep the left ureter and gonadal vessels still attached to the sigmoid mesentery. An attempt should be made to reestablish the proper dissection plane anterior to the retroperitoneal fascia (Figs. 6.8 and 6.9). The retroperitoneal structures tend to stain purple in color, and the mantra of "purple goes down" should be remembered.

If this is not effective, a medial mesenteric dissection is started in an easier area, lateral to the inferior mesenteric vessels. Find the left colic vessel, make mesenteric windows isolating the vessel, and divide it close to its origin. The cut left colic vessel is lifted and the retroperitoneal fascia is identified and bluntly swept in a dorsal direction separating the retroperitoneum from the mesentery. Then, the cut medial edge of the mesenteric window attached to the inferior mesenteric vessels is lifted, and this plane is bluntly dissected toward the midline. When the inferior mesenteric vessels are freed from the retroperitoneal structures from a lateral direction, just to the left of the IMV should be the left ureter. Once the ureter is found in this location, it is traced more inferiorly.

If this step is not successful, a lateral mobilization of the sigmoid colon should be carried out in order to identify the left ureter more distally. In this location, the most reproducible location is as the ureter crosses the bifurcation of the common iliac artery. If the left ureter is not identified by any of the aforementioned methods, then the operation should be converted to open surgery. Even in this case, however, one should first mobilize the splenic flexure before the conversion so the open incision could be kept small in size.

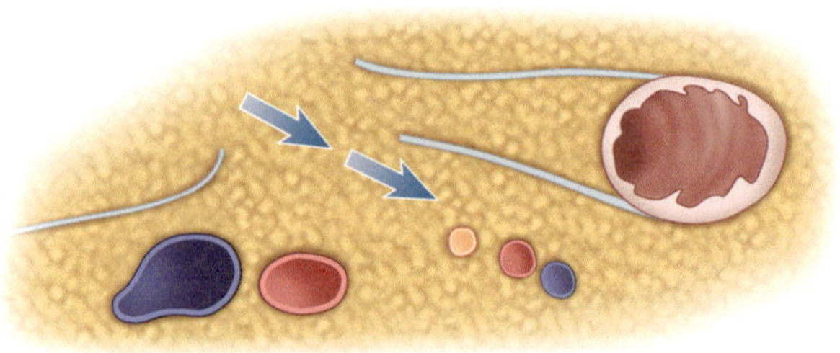

**Fig. 6.8** Congenital fusion of the sigmoid mesentery to the retroperitoneal fascia makes it easy to dissect in the wrong plane. The left ureter and gonadal vessels in this case will be anterior to the dissection

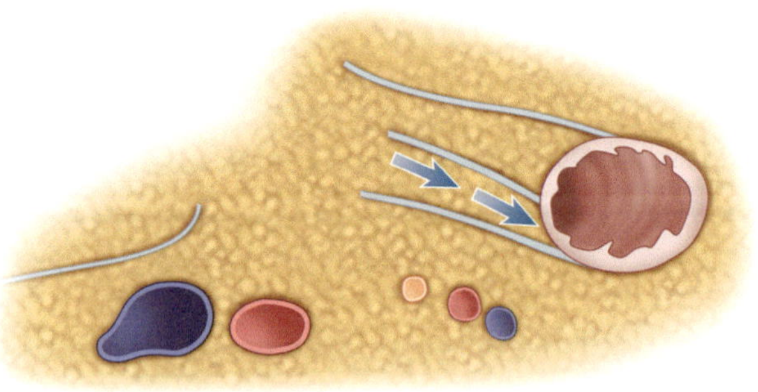

**Fig. 6.9** The proper dissection plane requires the conscious separation of the mesentery and retroperitoneal fascia

## Retromesenteric Dissection

The divided medial edge of the mesentery is grasped, exposing a wide mesenteric window. The retroperitoneum is further swept in a dorsal direction, separating it from the left colon mesentery in a medial-to-lateral direction (Fig. 6.10). Since the mesentery is congenitally adhered to the retroperitoneum, the tendency is to dissect in a plane that is too deep. Instead, it is important to repeatedly identify the true line

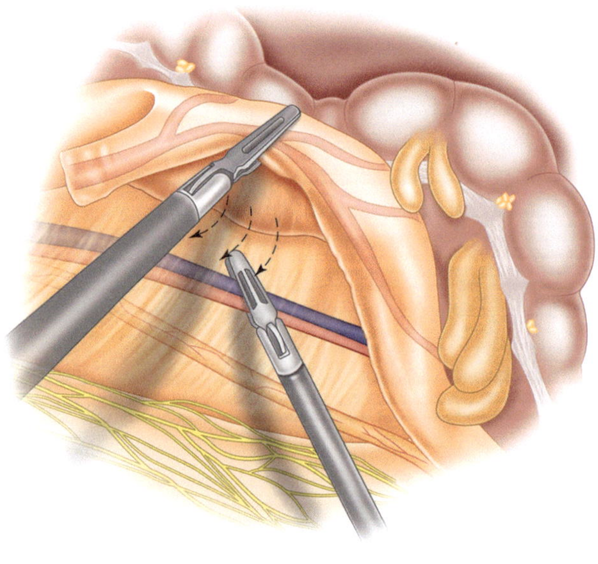

**Fig. 6.10** The dissection of the retromesenteric plane from a medial-to-lateral direction

of fusion between the mesentery and retroperitoneum. The retromesenteric plane is extended laterally to the abdominal wall, superiorly toward the upper half of the left kidney, and inferiorly past the left psoas muscle.

## Lateral Dissection

The sigmoid colon is retracted in a medial direction, and its lateral attachments are dissected from laterally. It is important to identify the left ureter and gonadal vessels again to avoid injury to them. After initial dissection, the prior dissection plane from the medial side should be encountered. If the medial dissection had been carried out lateral enough to the abdominal wall, what is left of the lateral attachment should be a thin peritoneal layer. This lateral mobilization is taken in a superior direction toward the splenic flexure (Fig. 6.11).

## Splenic Flexure Mobilization

Unless the sigmoid colon is redundant, splenic flexure mobilization will be necessary for many of the sigmoid and left colon resections. This step can be very tedious, especially in obese patients. One must understand the anatomic attachments of the splenic flexure, which include splenocolic, renocolic, and gastrocolic ligaments.

A systematic approach to splenic flexure takedown should be utilized. The splenic flexure takedown is greatly facilitated by a generous posterior retromesenteric dissection, and thus, the posterior renocolic attachments are first mobilized.

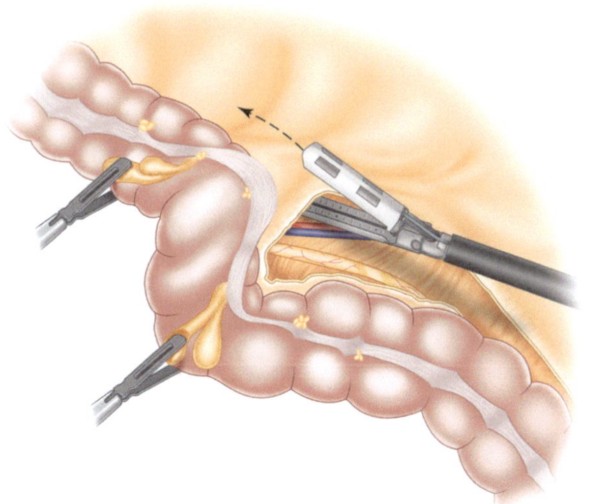

**Fig. 6.11** The lateral dissection of the sigmoid colon and descending colon is facilitated by a robust medial mobilization

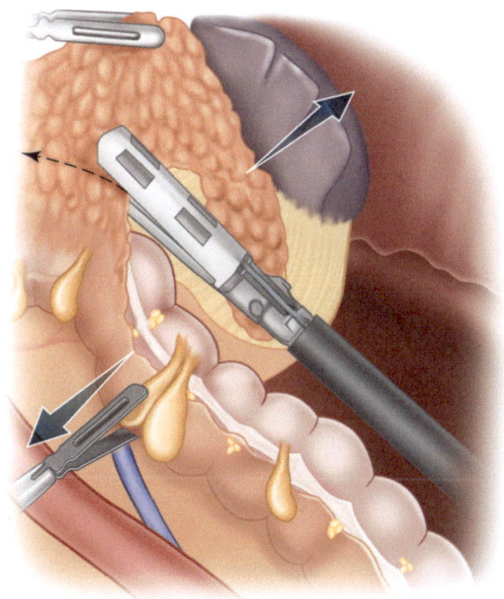

**Fig. 6.12** Splenic flexure: the splenic flexure is mobilized from the descending colon in a cephalad direction

Then, the prior lateral dissection along the white line of Toldt is further taken in a cephalad direction and around the splenic flexure from left to right (division of the splenocolic ligament) (Fig. 6.12). The assistant helps with retraction of the omentum and the surgeon retracts the descending colon in a caudal and medial direction. One must be careful not to use excessive traction in either medial or inferior direction since the splenic capsule could easily tear. The key to expeditious flexure takedown is to remain close to the colon as the omentum is dissected from the splenic flexure. It is helpful to look for the most distal point of omental attachment to the splenic flexure and begin separating the omentum from the colon and epiploic appendages here. Attention should be paid to the dorsal attachments of the flexure to the tail of the pancreas. The lesser sac is entered, and the omentum is dissected off of the distal transverse colon until the splenic flexure mobilization is complete. As soon as the lesser sac is entered, one should try to identify the stomach, because it can adhere close to the colon leading to inadvertent injury.

## Pearls and Pitfalls

### Difficult Splenic Flexure

This could be from obesity, complex omental adhesions, or close proximity of the splenic flexure to the spleen. One should first refer back to the general guidelines for splenic flexure takedown. Has an adequate posterior dissection been performed? Has the splenic flexure mobilization been performed close to the colon wall? Is the patient positioning

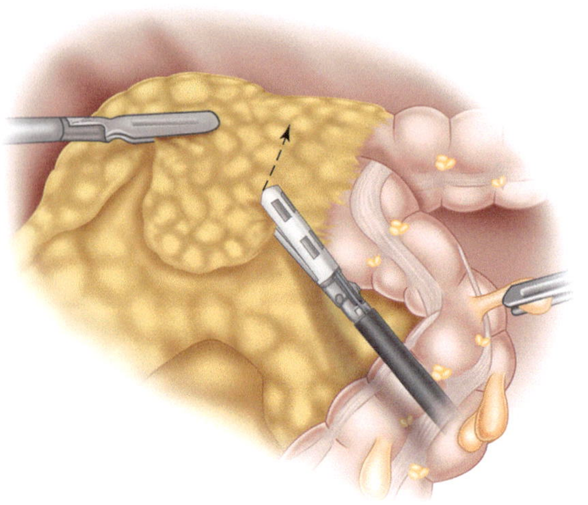

**Fig. 6.13** Splenic flexure: the splenic flexure is mobilized from the transverse colon side, taking down the omental attachments

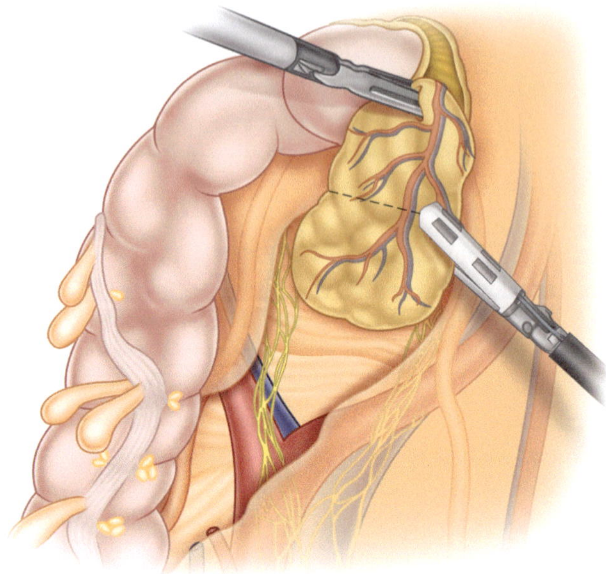

**Fig. 6.14** The mesorectum is cleared off

adequate, i.e., out of the steep Trendelenburg position? If the patient is large and the assistant's right lower quadrant port is useless due to lack of reach, consider placing an additional 5-mm right epigastric port.

The next step in a difficult splenic flexure mobilization is to start a medial dissection (i.e., from the transverse colon side) (Fig. 6.13). The omentum is dissected off of the distal transverse colon, again staying close to the colonic wall and entering the lesser sac. This dissection is extended to the left to the splenic flexure. Dissecting on both the right and left sides of the splenic flexure, the mobilization is completed.

## Bowel Division, Exteriorization, and Anastomosis

The site of distal transection is identified. The distal bowel division is performed intracorporeally. In cancer, the site of distal resection is 5–10 cm distal to the tumor, and in diverticulitis it is the top of the rectum. The mesentery is scored at this point close to the bowel wall. With care not to injure the bowel wall, the mesorectum is divided at this location including the superior hemorrhoidal vessels using a dissecting energy device (Fig. 6.14).

Using an endoscopic linear 60-mm stapler placed through the 12-mm right lower abdominal port, the bowel is divided (45-mm stapler for smaller patients) (Fig. 6.15). Attempt should be made to make a transection perpendicular to the bowel wall with one firing, but if two firings are necessary, the spike of the circular end-to-end stapler should be brought out at the confluence of the two firings. Next, the site of proximal transection is assessed intracorporeally; this location should allow for a tension-free anastomosis with good blood flow. The sigmoid mesentery located cephalad to the cut inferior mesenteric vessels is then dissected toward this point of proximal transection. This site should be identifiable when it is exteriorized, and it is helpful to mark an epiploic appendage in this area with cautery or clips. A laparoscopic grasper is then used to grasp the end of the colon to be exteriorized.

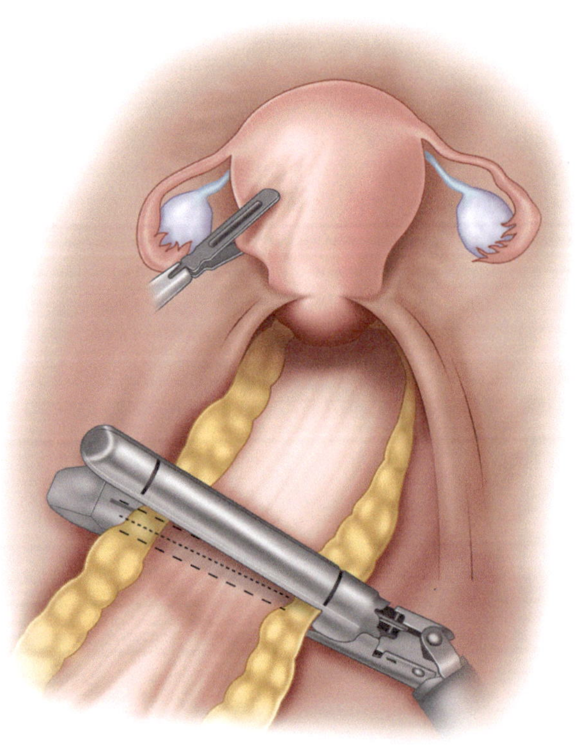

**Fig. 6.15** Distal bowel transection using an endoscopic 60-mm stapler

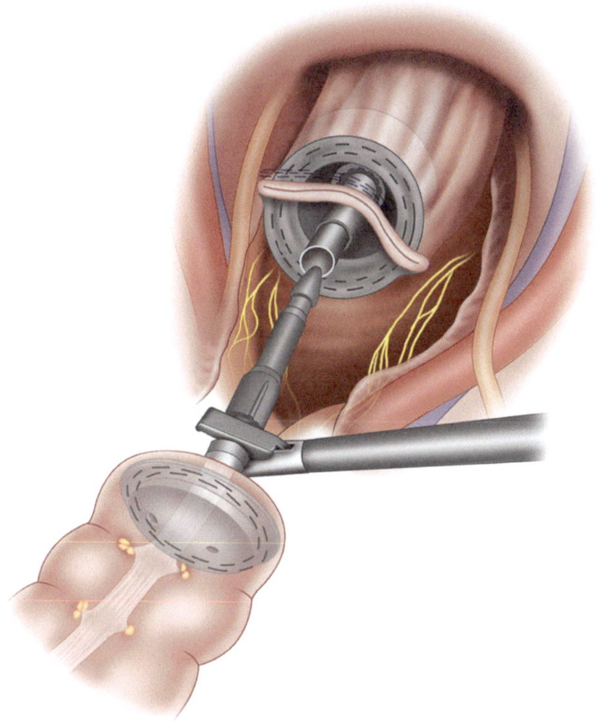

Fig. 6.16 Circular double-stapled end-to-end anastomosis

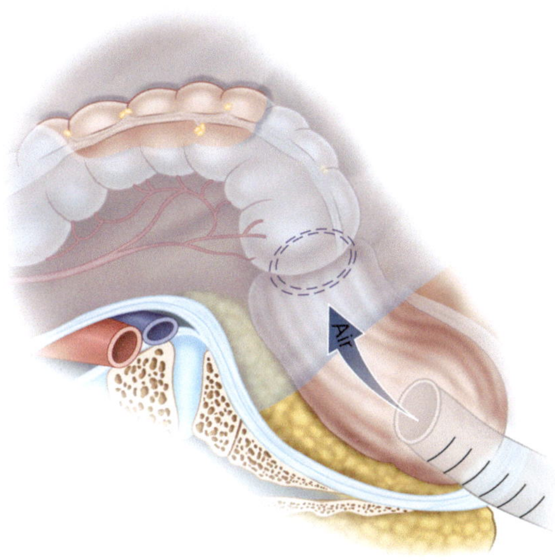


Fig. 6.17 The water level should be brought lower, to about mid rectum so that the anastomosis is underwater

A minilaparotomy is created for exteriorization. The reasonable sites are the umbilicus, left lower quadrant port site, and suprapubic position. The wound is enlarged to 3–5 cm or larger depending on the size of the pathology. A wound retractor is placed. The stapled end of the colon is found and the bowel is exteriorized, and the marked area of proximal transection is located. The marginal vessel is divided at this level, and the bowel is divided. Good blood flow from the marginal vessel and to the end of the colon must be confirmed. A purse-string suture is placed into the open mouth of the colon and tied around the anvil of a circular stapler. The author's preference is to use a 28-mm stapler in most cases unless the rectum is capacious. Especially in diverticulitis, the upper rectum is often contracted, and you may be unable to pass a circular stapler of larger diameter. In cases of extensive diverticulosis where the proximal bowel still contains multiple diverticula, one should consider bringing the anvil out from the antimesenteric colon more proximally and performing a side-to-end anastomosis.

The bowel is returned back inside the abdomen, and the minilaparotomy is closed with facial sutures. Under laparoscopic visualization, the circular stapling device is inserted into the rectum and through the end of the rectal stump. After confirmation that the mesentery is not twisted, a stapled end-to-end circular anastomosis is performed (Fig. 6.16).

The pelvis should then be filled with saline using a laparoscopic irrigation device, and a leak test performed. The bowel is occluded with a laparoscopic grasper proximal to the anastomosis, and the anastomosis is immersed in saline while the rectal lumen is insufflated with air or carbon dioxide (Fig. 6.17). Care is taken to be sure there is no migration of small bowel loops underneath the cut mesenteric edge.

Alternatively, an extracorporeal anastomosis can be performed. In this case, rather than perform an intracorporeal distal bowel division, a low midline or Pfannenstiel incision is created and the distal transection is performed using open techniques. It is still helpful at times to divide the mesorectum intracorporeally even in this case. After distal transection, the bowel is further exteriorized and the proximal division, anastomosis, and leak test are all performed through the small incision.

## Pearls and Pitfalls

### Positive Leak Test

One must first clearly identify the area of leak. This is best done with continuous $CO_2$ insufflation through a flexible sigmoidoscope. Carbon dioxide is absorbed from the lumen of the bowel much faster than air, limiting distension that can obscure the surgical field. If there is a single defect, the defect is small and can clearly be visualized laparoscopically, interrupted intracorporeal sutures can be used to close the defect. The subsequent leak test must be negative. For all other defects, the defective anastomosis should probably be resected and a new one created. This can still be accomplished laparoscopically if the rectum is cleaned off distal to the prior anastomosis and the rectum is divided using a laparoscopic linear stapler. The anastomosis is then exteriorized through the prior minilaparotomy wound and is resected, and a new anvil placed into the bowel. If this intracorporeal revision is technically challenging, it can be completed through a Pfannenstiel or a low midline incision.

According to one study of colorectal anastomoses, a positive leak test occurred in 7.9 % of tested anastomoses. Higher rates of clinical leak occurred in those with positive air leak tests compared with negative ones (7.7 % vs. 3.8 %). When a leak test was positive, the subsequent clinical leak rates were 0 % with reanastomosis versus 12 % with suture repair [1].

## Conclusion

A straight laparoscopic approach to the sigmoid and left colon can be successfully utilized as the surgical procedure of choice for a number of colorectal conditions. While this approach can be technically demanding and requires advanced laparoscopic skills, in most cases, your patient will reap the benefits from a minimally invasive approach. Undoubtedly, there are many technical approaches to this procedure, and while the basic steps remain the same, the approach for each surgeon should be individualized.

## Reference

1. Ricciardi R, Roberts PL, Marcello PW, Hall JF, Read TE, Schoetz DJ. Anastomotic leak testing after colorectal resection: what are the data? Arch Surg. 2009;144:407–11.

# 7 Hand-Assisted Left Colectomy

Steven Lee-Kong and Daniel L. Feingold

## Key Points

- The hand-assisted approach to colectomy is a versatile technique that facilitates dissection in difficult clinical circumstances.
- During standard "straight" laparoscopic colectomy, the surgeon must rely on the experience and skill set of the assistant. In hand-assisted surgery, the surgeon is able to perform much of the dissection and uses the assistant essentially as a camera holder.
- The surgeon can advance through the learning curve by dividing the operation into individual steps and focusing on what needs to be accomplished in each step; in this fashion, the operation becomes a standardized, reproducible method.
- Laparoscopic colectomy is a challenging operation; oncologic adequacy should not be compromised for the sake of performing a less invasive procedure.
- A major benefit of the hand-assisted approach to colectomy is that the surgeon can approach the dissection from all directions (medial, lateral, cephalad) and, in complex cases, can easily change from one approach to another in order to complete the dissection.

## Background

The most common indications for elective left colectomy include sigmoid adenocarcinoma, diverticular disease, and adenomatous polyps not amenable to endoscopic removal. Open colectomy has largely been supplanted by minimal access surgery; the benefits of laparoscopic-assisted colectomy over open surgery include accelerated postoperative recovery, earlier return to baseline level of functioning, decreased length of stay, decreased pain and narcotic use, and decreased operative blood loss [1–3]. The straight laparoscopic approach results in longer average operative times and can be particularly challenging in obese patients, re-operative patients, and patients with advanced disease. A variation of the standard laparoscopic approach, hand-assisted colectomy, shortens operative times, decreases conversion rates, and restores tactile feedback that aids in dissecting otherwise difficult anatomy without compromising the benefits of a minimally invasive approach [4]. Hand-assisted laparoscopy is a versatile approach to colectomy that allows for dissection of complicated anatomy, palpation to facilitate intraoperative tumor localization, and dissection through the hand-port access in open fashion or by using straight laparoscopy.

## Preoperative Planning

A relevant history and physical examination, assessment of prior abdominal surgery and the location of abdominal scars, and review of the available cross-sectional imaging and colonoscopy report are important as these can influence the operative plan. With the exception of patients with selected very large tumors, tumors requiring complex en bloc resection, and patients known to have severe adhesions, nearly all patients contemplating left colectomy are candidates for hand-assisted surgery.

**Pearls: Potential alterations in bowel function should be discussed preoperatively as patients can be frustrated by unexpected changes in bowel habits. The possible need for a defunctioning stoma should also be discussed in advance of left colectomy; however, diversion is rarely required. Ideally, a complete colon evaluation should be performed prior to colectomy to exclude synchronous pathology.**

**Electronic supplementary material:** Supplementary material is available in the online version of this chapter at 10.1007/978-1-4939-1581-1_7. Videos can also be accessed at http://www.springerimages.com/videos/978-1-4939-1580-4.

S. Lee-Kong, M.D. • D.L. Feingold, M.D. (✉)
Department of Surgery, New York Presbyterian Hospital, Columbia University, 161 Fort Washington Avenue, New York, NY 10032, USA
e-mail: sal116@cumc.columbia.edu; df347@cumc.columbia.edu

H.M. Ross et al. (eds.), *Minimally Invasive Approaches to Colon and Rectal Disease: Technique and Best Practices*, DOI 10.1007/978-1-4939-1581-1_7, © Springer Science+Business Media New York 2015

## Procedure

### Setup

Lower extremity sequential compression devices are placed and activated and general anesthesia is induced. The patient is placed in either modified lithotomy position with adjustable stirrups or in split-leg position with a bariatric-type table (Fig. 7.1). It is important to adequately pad patients to minimize the risk of neuropraxia or pressure-related skin breakdown. This positioning allows the surgeon to stand between the legs during mobilization of the splenic flexure and permits access to the anus for colonoscopy or insertion of the circular stapler. If stirrups are used, the thighs should be kept parallel to the floor, as greater than 10° of flexion of the hip can often limit the ability to access the upper abdomen through lower abdominal ports. The right arm is padded and tucked in neutral position to allow the surgeon and assistant to stand on the right side of the table. A strap is placed across the chest to secure the patient to the operating table to facilitate extreme positioning during portions of the operation that require gravity to aid exposure. A bladder catheter is placed and the abdomen is prepared and draped, per usual. Deep venous chemoprophylaxis should be administered prior to the procedure, and appropriate intravenous antibiotics should be given within 1 h of the skin incision. To further reduce surgical site infection, patients are oxygenated with 0.8 $FiO_2$ during the case. Core body temperature should be maintained according to individual institutional protocols.

The surgeon should confirm that all equipment is either in the room or is readily available (Table 7.1). A 30° angled laparoscope is used to look over the horizon of the operative field; this scope is more versatile than a standard 0° scope. Additional suggested equipment includes a colonoscope ($CO_2$ insufflation is preferred over ambient air) and lighted handheld deep pelvic retractors that facilitate pelvic dissection through the hand-port access. In general, disposable devices (hand port, energy device, and suction irrigator) are not opened until the surgeon enters the abdomen and confirms the feasibility of a hand-assisted approach.

### Procedure Steps

#### Hand-Assisted Left Colectomy (Videos 7.1, 7.2, and 7.3)

**Port Placement**

Hand-port placement: A Pfannenstiel incision placed two fingerbreadths above the symphysis pubis is used for the majority of patients. In patients with prior lower midline incisions and in patients considered at higher risk of conversion, a lower midline incision is typically used. When dissecting through the subcutaneous fat down to the fascia through a Pfannenstiel incision, avoid skiving towards the symphysis pubis as placing the port too close to the pubis may restrict access through the port and may cause the hand port not to sit well. Adequate flaps must be created between the anterior rectus sheath and the rectus muscle to ensure sufficient space for the operating surgeon's hand. Once the abdomen is

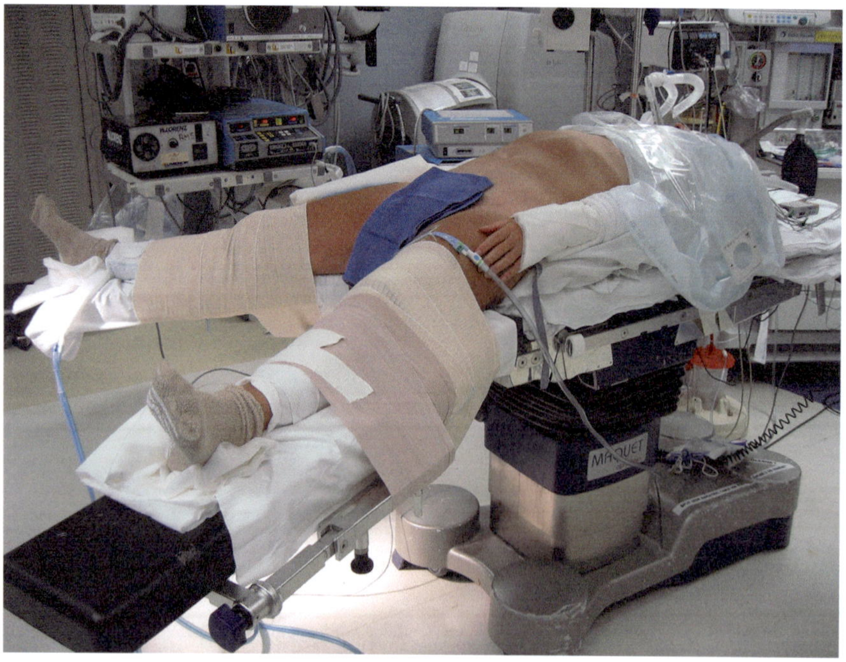


**Fig. 7.1** Positioning of the patient on a split-leg table

**Table 7.1** Equipment

| |
|---|
| • 5 mm 30° laparoscope |
| • Trocars (5 mm×4), hand-access port |
| • Laparoscopic blunt atraumatic graspers and scissors |
| • 5 mm blunt tip LigaSure™ (Covidien, Mansfield, MA) or other energy device, per surgeon preference |
| • Bowel stapler with appropriate loads |
| • End-to-end stapling device (appropriate sizes available) |
| • Colonoscope with carbon dioxide insufflation device |
| • Standard laparoscopic instrumentation (i.e., atraumatic graspers, Maryland dissector, etc.) |

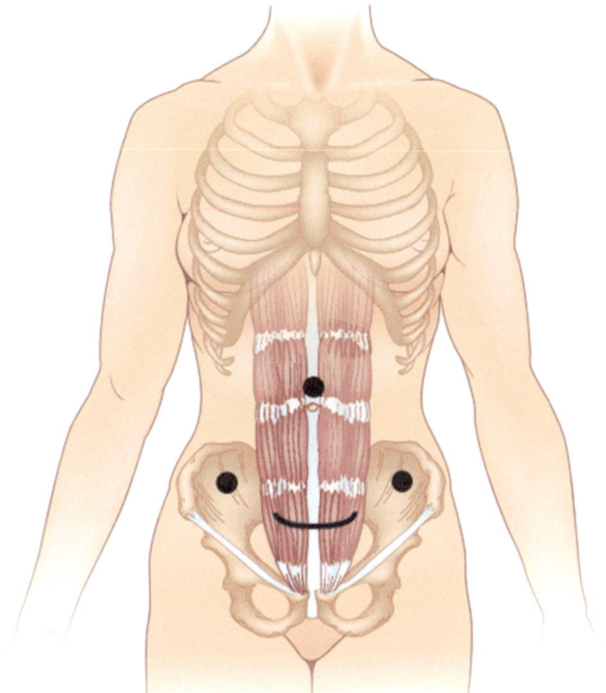

**Fig. 7.2** Hand-assisted device and port site placement for a left colectomy

entered, inspection of the field and palpation through the wound allows the surgeon to determine whether or not to proceed in hand-assisted fashion. If confirmed, a reusable 5 mm camera port is then placed near the umbilicus with the surgeon's hand within the abdomen protecting the viscera, and the abdomen is insufflated. Two additional 5 mm working ports are placed under direct laparoscopic visualization in the left lower quadrant and right lower quadrant lateral to the inferior epigastric vessels (Fig. 7.2). Once the ports are placed, and before the dissection is begun, the abdomen is surveyed and thoroughly explored for any abnormalities (metastases, adhesions, injury due to port placement, etc.).

In patients likely to have adhesions from prior surgery that might interfere with hand-assisted colectomy, it may be preferable to place upper quadrant ports to evaluate the adhesions and to potentially perform adhesiolysis to allow hand-port placement.

A laparotomy pad (with an attached radiopaque ring) is placed within the abdomen prior to securing the hand-port device. The pad facilitates exposure by keeping the small bowel out of the field, keeping the operative field dry, and allowing the surgeon to clean the scope without actually removing the scope from the abdomen. In order to reduce the risk of a retained foreign body, a hemostat is placed on the surgeon's surgical gown as a reminder that a laparotomy pad is within the abdomen. When the pad is removed and handed back to the scrub nurse, the hemostat is handed back as well.

### Left Colon Dissection

Mobilization of the splenic flexure: In the majority of cases, the splenic flexure will need to be mobilized to ensure a tension-free colorectal anastomosis. In order to decrease the risk of splenic injury, care should be taken to avoid undue traction on splenic attachments during the mobilization. Manipulation of the splenic flexure mesentery must also be done carefully, as injury to the marginal artery may compromise the vascular supply to the bowel being used for the anastomosis. There are several ways to approach taking down the splenic flexure (medial at the inferior mesenteric vein (IMV), lateral up the left paracolic gutter, entering the lesser sac at the midline). Typically, and especially in cases with an extreme splenic flexure, a combination of all three approaches is utilized to mobilize the flexure all the way to the ligament of Treitz.

#### Medial-to-Lateral Approach at the IMV

This is the preferred approach to the flexure because it allows relatively easy mobilization of the colon and mesocolon up off of the retroperitoneum, while the lateral-to-medial approach requires the surgeon to dissect in a plane while looking up over the horizon. Placing the patient in reverse Trendelenburg position with the table tilted right side down allows the small bowel to be placed in the right side of the abdomen and aids in exposing the anatomy. The assistant stands on the right side of the patient holding the camera and using a grasper through the right-sided port to retract the greater omentum and transverse colon cephalad over the liver exposing the paraduodenal fossa with the left colon mesentery and ligament of Treitz (Fig. 7.3). The surgeon, standing between the legs with the left hand in the abdomen and the energy device in the left-sided port, should appreciate the location of the aorta, the 4th portion of the duodenum, and the IMV. The intra-abdominal laparotomy pad helps to keep the small bowel out of the field of dissection. The peritoneum overlying the paraduodenal space is incised and a retromesenteric plane is developed in medial-to-lateral fashion (Fig. 7.4). This peritoneum should be taken sharply to avoid

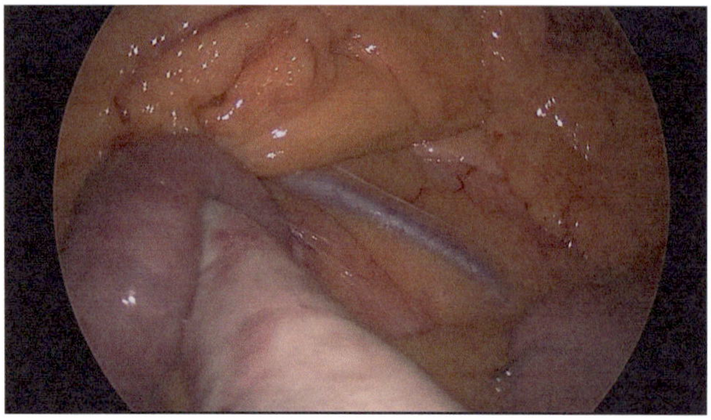

**Fig. 7.3** Paraduodenal fossa at the ligament of Treitz demonstrating the inferior mesenteric vein (IMV)

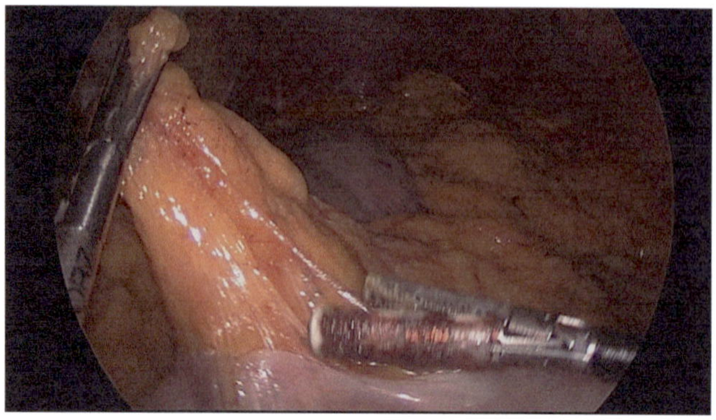

**Fig. 7.5** Entering the lesser sac near the midline

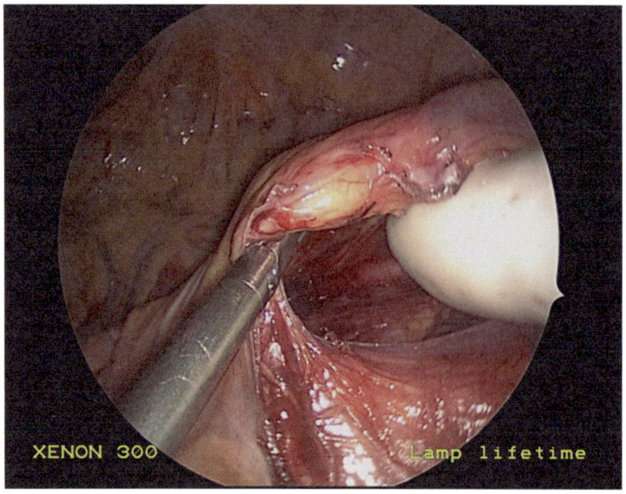


**Fig. 7.4** Medial-to-lateral dissection at the IMV in the avascular plane

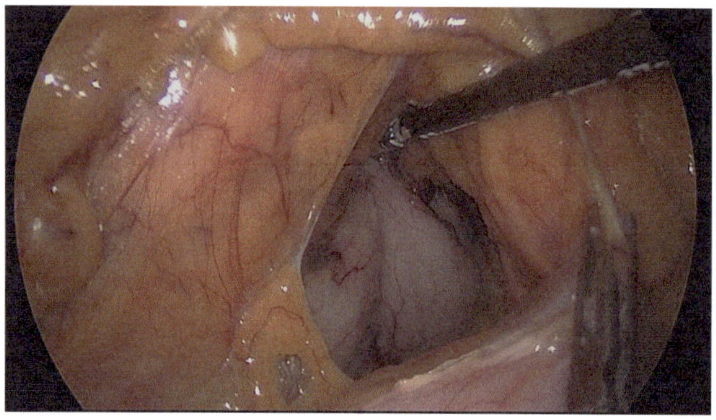

**Fig. 7.6** The lesser sac is entered—notice the back wall of the stomach

using energy so close to the duodenum. The retroperitoneum including the ureter, the gonadal bundle, and Gerota's fascia are pushed dorsally and the mesocolon is swept ventrally. If the correct plane is entered, this dissection is relatively avascular. This dissection is carried as far laterally to the abdominal wall as possible and cephalad to the inferior border of the pancreas. Care should be taken to avoid dissecting behind the pancreas or into the retroperitoneum as this can jeopardize the retroperitoneal structures. Once this dissection is completed, the IMV can be divided using the energy device.

The greater omentum is retracted anteriorly and cephalad by the assistant and the transverse colon is retracted caudally by the surgeon. This retraction facilitates exposure to enter the avascular plane that separates the greater omentum from the transverse colon and mesocolon (Fig. 7.5). This dissection, most easily started near the midline at the falciform ligament, enters the lesser sac and is carried laterally towards the splenic flexure (Fig. 7.6), fully releasing the omentum, which can now serve as an omental pedicle flap. During the dissection, the surgeon's left hand protects the colon and the stomach from collateral damage from the energy device. As the dissection progresses along the left transverse colon, it is important to use tissue triangulation to actually see the colon as it courses cephalad into the left upper quadrant at the splenic flexure; this helps prevent injury to the colon.

While the left colon is gently retracted by the assistant grasping an epiploica, the surgeon's left hand is placed into the retromesenteric space and is used to demonstrate the plane of dissection. Using the energy device through the left-sided port, the colon is released from its lateral attachments (commonly referred to as the white line of Toldt), and the retromesenteric dissection plane that had been mobilized previously in medial-to-lateral fashion is entered. The dissection is carried cephalad towards the splenic flexure (Fig. 7.7). The mesocolon is dissected free from the inferior border of the pancreas, completely releasing the splenic flexure. Once the left colon is mobilized, the surgeon performs a sweep with his hand to confirm the colon is completely mobilized from the retroperitoneum, the omentum, and the

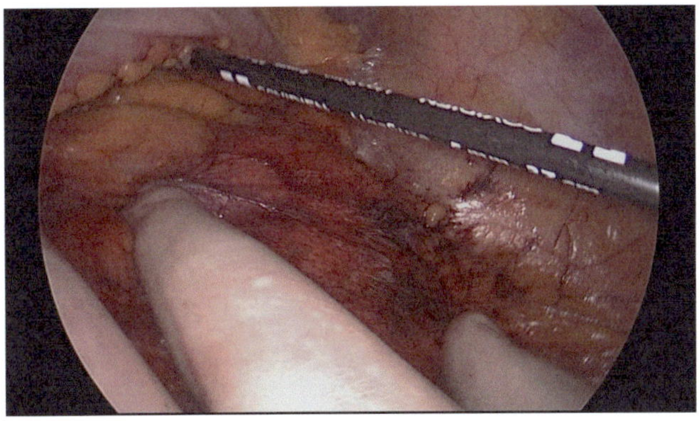

**Fig. 7.7** Taking down the remaining lateral colonic attachments while working cephalad towards the splenic flexure

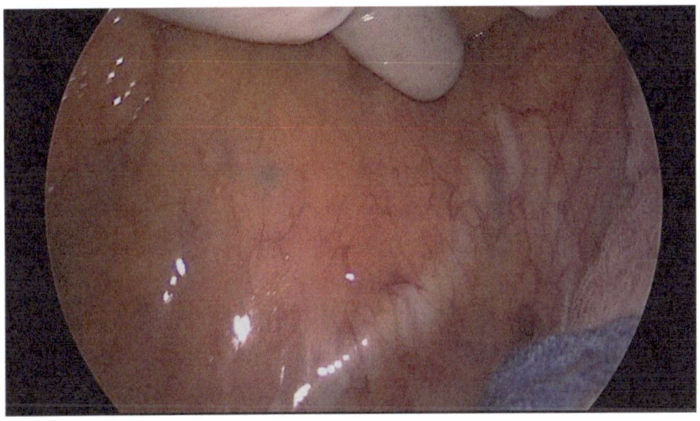

**Fig. 7.8** Exposure of the sigmoid mesocolon. The aortic bifurcation and common iliac vessels can be seen. In addition, the *right* ureter is often seen crossing over the iliac in this view

spleen, as persistent attachments can jeopardize reach to the pelvis and the ability to exteriorize the specimen.

### Sigmoid Colon Mobilization

This mobilization is typically performed using a medial-to-lateral approach. Occasionally, in cases with complicated anatomy like severe inflammation or significant redundancy of the colon, the lateral-to-medial approach may be technically easier.

### Medial-to-Lateral Dissection of the IMA

With the patient in steep Trendelenburg position, the assistant stands at the right shoulder holding the camera and the surgeon stands at the right hip with the right hand in the abdomen and the energy device in the right-sided port. The mesosigmoid is exposed by retracting the small bowel out of the pelvis and towards the right upper quadrant. The laparotomy pad again helps keep the small bowel out of the way. The surgeon should appreciate the aorta and the aortic bifurcation, the common iliac arteries, and the right ureter (Fig. 7.8). The sacral promontory is an important landmark as it is a midline structure and helps keep the surgeon oriented. Using the hand, the IMA pedicle is elevated and retracted towards the patient's left side (Fig. 7.9). The peritoneum just dorsal to the pedicle is scored with the energy device and the retromesenteric plane is entered. The window into the retromesenteric space is extended caudal past the sacral promontory to allow wide exposure of the retroperitoneum. This plane is developed bluntly by pushing the retroperitoneal structures (hypogastric nerves, left ureter (Fig. 7.10), left gonadal vessels) dorsally while dissecting laterally towards the left sidewall (Fig. 7.11). With the

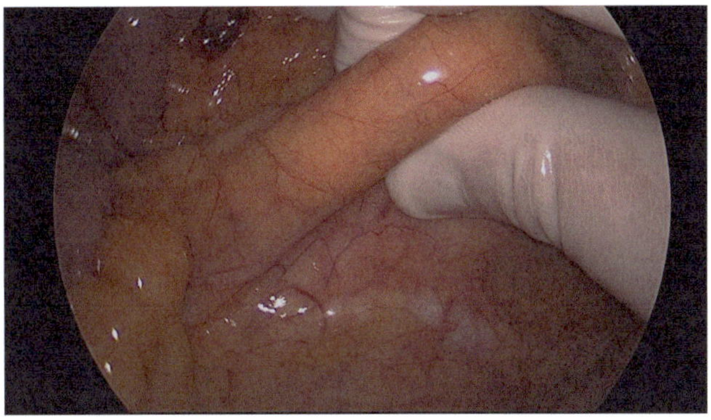

**Fig. 7.9** Grasping the inferior mesenteric artery pedicle

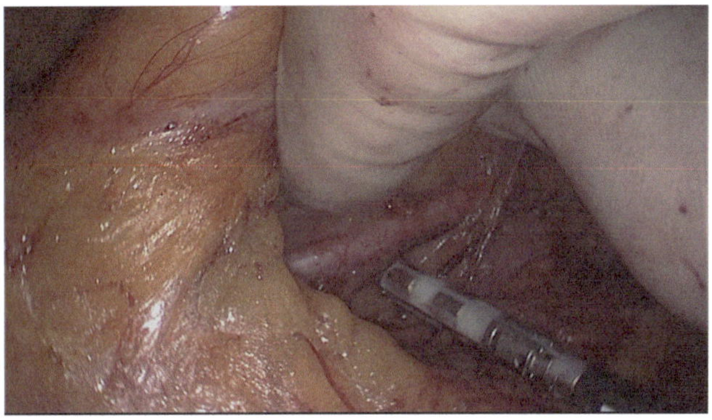

**Fig. 7.10** Identification of the left ureter

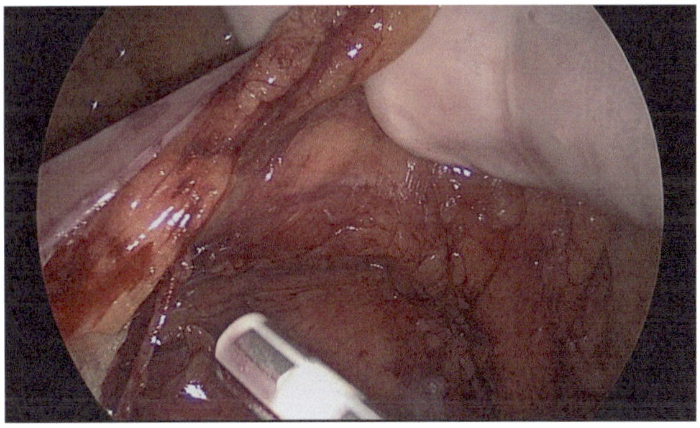

**Fig. 7.11** Developing the left retromesocolic plane

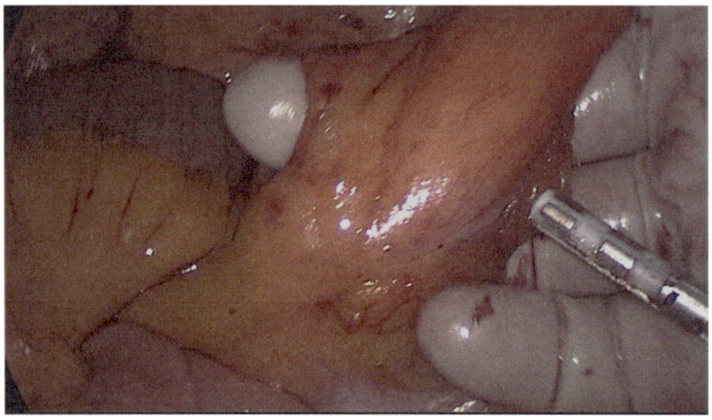

**Fig. 7.12** Isolation of the IMA pedicle

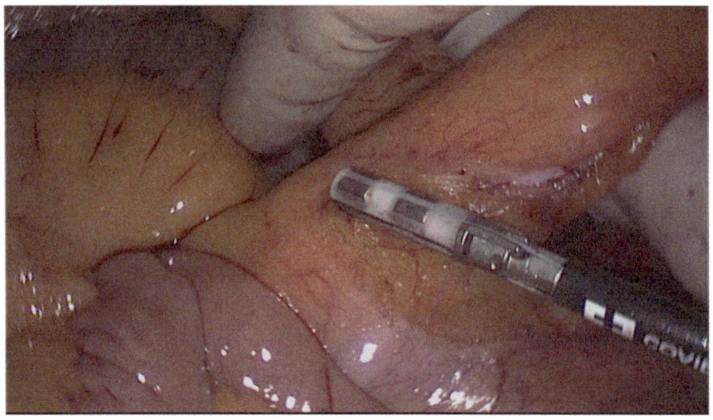

**Fig. 7.13** IMA division using an energy device

IMA elevated, the retromesenteric plane is developed cephalad as well, meeting the prior IMV dissection plane which was developed during splenic flexure mobilization. By supinating the hand underneath the mesosigmoid, a mesenteric window is identified on the left side of the IMA pedicle. This avascular mesentery is incised, isolating the IMA (Fig. 7.12). The IMA (proximal to the left colic artery takeoff) or the main sigmoidal artery (distal to the left colic artery takeoff) is divided with the energy device after confirming that the left ureter is protected (Fig. 7.13). The "stay-side" (proximal) stump of the pedicle is reinforced, as needed, with a preformed looped ligature.

An alternative to ligating the mesenteric pedicle as described is to perform a mid-mesenteric dissection whereby the superior hemorrhoidal artery is preserved and the actual sigmoid branches are sequentially ligated. This may be done for benign disease processes. This approach keeps the field of dissection off of the retroperitoneum and preserves the IMA blood supply to the proximal rectum, which is the distal side of the planned colorectal anastomosis. Patients with stricturing disease or who, for whatever reason, have not had neoplasia excluded preoperatively should undergo a cancer-type operation.

Once the pedicle is ligated, the retromesenteric plane is further developed as far laterally as possible and cephalad over Gerota's fascia. To mobilize the sigmoid colon from its lateral attachments at the pelvic inlet, it is helpful to retract the colon medially using a grasper in the right-sided port and to use the energy device placed through the hand-access port to take the lateral attachments down. Alternatively, the lateral attachments can be dissected out in open fashion through the hand-port site. In order to mobilize the proximal rectum, the presacral space is entered. This facilitates creating a colorectal anastomosis (as opposed to a colo-colonic anastomosis) and helps to straighten the rectum to allow passage of the EEA stapler.

#### Bowel Division and Anastomosis

The detachable cap of the hand port is removed leaving the self-retaining wound retractor/protector and the colon is exteriorized. Any residual mesentery not already taken laparoscopically is taken at this point in open fashion. Open staplers (as opposed to laparoscopic devices) are used to transect the proximal and distal colorectal margins; the specimen is delivered and oriented for the pathologist and is evaluated on a dirty back table to grossly evaluate the pathology and the margins.

Working through the hand port in open fashion, adequate blood supply to the end of the colon is confirmed and the anvil of an appropriately sized EEA stapler is seated and secured. Care should be taken to exclude any false diverticula from the anticipated site of the colorectal anastomosis as these can increase the risk of leak. The remaining part of the operation can be completed in open fashion or by resuming hand-assisted laparoscopy. The rectal staple line is leak tested; this allows for repair of a defect prior to creating the anastomosis. The colonic end is brought down to the pelvis and reach is assessed. Orientation of the colon is confirmed by verifying that neither the anti-mesenteric edge of the mobilized colon nor the cut edge of the mesentery is twisted. The anus is sequentially dilated and the EEA anastomosis is created in usual fashion. The anastomotic donuts are evaluated and the anastomosis is leak tested, per usual. We prefer leak testing with colonoscopic visualization to blindly insufflating the rectum.

Prior to closing, hemostasis is confirmed and the intra-abdominal laparotomy pad is removed. The surgeon also performs a manual and visual sweep to minimize the risk of undetected retained foreign bodies and confirms that the small bowel is not herniated underneath the mobilized colon. Finally, the omental pedicle is placed over the anastomosis and under the Pfannenstiel wound.

## Postoperative Care

Enteral nutrition is initiated with a clear liquid diet starting the day of operation and the diet is advanced as patients tolerate without waiting for flatus or a bowel movement. Nasogastric tubes are not utilized immediately postoperatively in elective colectomy cases. Progressive ambulation is encouraged beginning the day after the operation and incentive spirometry is uniformly implemented. Multi-pharmacy pain control relies on the combination of intravenous patient-controlled narcotic analgesia, intravenous ketorolac, and oral acetaminophen. Intravenous narcotics are replaced with enteral formulations once patients tolerate a diet. Deep vein thrombosis chemoprophylaxis is initiated prior to incision with subcutaneous unfractionated heparin or enoxaparin and continues through the hospitalization together with sequential compression devices. Urine catheters are typically removed within 24–48 h. Postoperative laboratory blood tests are minimized and are typically drawn on the first postoperative day only or not at all.

## Complications

As in any surgical procedure, complications from hand-assisted colectomy invariably occur. Intraoperative complications may include excessive bleeding, bowel injury (due to port placement, tissue handling, or delayed thermal injury), and ureteral injury. The incidence of technical complications can be reduced by verifying the operative anatomy rather than relying on pattern recognition, by minimizing the laparoscopic use of monopolar energy, and by being mindful of potential injuries that can occur "off screen".

Early postoperative complications may include infection, Pfannenstiel wound hematoma and other wound complications, prolonged ileus or early postoperative bowel obstruction, thromboembolic events, cardiac complications, as well as the dreaded anastomotic dehiscence. The risk of many of these complications can be reduced by adhering to sound perioperative principles like appropriate use of perioperative antibiotics and DVT prophylaxis, early ambulation and pulmonary toilet, timely removal of bladder catheters, and creating tension-free anastomoses with healthy bowel and adequate blood supply (Table 7.2).

**Table 7.2** Complications

| |
|---|
| *Intraoperative* |
| • Vascular injury |
| • Enterotomy |
| • Ureteral injury |
| *Postoperative* |
| • Early |
| – Urinary tract infection |
| – Respiratory infection |
| – Surgical site infection |
| – Anastomotic dehiscence |
| – Hemorrhage |
| • Late |
| – Anastomotic stricture |

## Pearls and Pitfalls

- Ureteral stenting may facilitate dissection in selected complicated cases such as morbidly obese patients, irradiated patients, patients undergoing reoperation, and patients whose preoperative imaging suggests abnormal anatomy.
- One should have a low threshold for utilizing a lower midline incision over a Pfannenstiel incision for hand access, particularly for patients in whom you anticipate a higher chance of conversion (extensive prior intra-abdominal surgery, large tumors, fistulizing disease, etc.).
- Surgeons unfamiliar with hand-assisted surgery can have difficulty "keeping the hand out of the way" and can feel that the hand actually interferes with performing the operation. Cupping the hand like a "C" and extending the fingers so that the knuckles do not buckle improve visualization and access to the field. As surgeons progress along the learning curve, they learn how to use the hand more effectively and transition from using the hand only as a grasping-type retractor to utilizing the hand and individual fingers for blunt dissection, maintaining exposure, palpation of the anatomy, and keeping other structures out of harm's way.
- Ureter identification is not always straightforward. If the retromesenteric dissection is too deep (posterior), the left ureter may actually be above the plane of dissection (on the ceiling of the space). If the patient's body habitus and camera port placement do not allow identification of the ureter looking through the retromesenteric window under the IMA pedicle, the surgeon can incise the mesentery cephalad to the IMA (described above) and find the ureter through that window. In cases where the medial-to-lateral approach does not expose the left ureter, alternating to the lateral-to-medial dissection may help identify the ureter.
- Cases with confounding anatomy and cases that are not progressing over time should be converted to an open approach. Conversion should not be viewed as a failure; rather, it may be safer than persisting laparoscopically and it is a powerful teaching tool that allows the surgeon to understand complex anatomy and master a challenging learning curve.
- A potential catastrophic complication of creating a colorectal anastomosis using a circular stapler is passing the stapler through the vagina instead of the anorectum. This can be prevented by performing a confirmatory vaginal exam and pulling the posterior vaginal wall away prior to firing the stapler.
- Splenic bleeding from a capsular tear can usually be managed with a combination of electrocautery, absorbable hemostatic agents, and manual compression using the laparotomy pad.

- The actual order in which the individual operative steps are performed is not usually important. Part of the sophistication of the hand-assisted technique is that if the dissection does not progress due to the anatomy (tumor, inflammation, abdominal fat, etc.), you can switch to a different approach (lateral-to-medial dissection, straight laparoscopy, open dissection though the hand-port access, etc.). Oftentimes, complicated cases can be successfully completed by alternating between these approaches rather than by dogmatically sticking to one particular technique.
- Extreme splenic flexures (due to the cephalad location of the flexure and/or difficult colonic attachments) can be challenging. Placing the patient in steeper reverse Trendelenburg position with the right side of the table down can facilitate the dissection by bringing the operative field closer to the surgeon. Using longer (bariatric-type) laparoscopic instruments can also be helpful in this situation. Placing an additional 5 mm port in the right upper quadrant can help with retraction and exposure. Approaching the flexure by alternating between the left paracolic gutter, the medial-to-lateral plane, and the lesser sac helps release the splenic flexure by creating a knuckle that accentuates whatever attachments remain of the flexure.
- Prior to creating the anastomosis, adequate reach of the colon should be confirmed. In general, the end of the colon should stay, by itself, resting in the pelvis while the patient is in steep Trendelenburg position. In cases where there is insufficient reach, after confirming that all left upper quadrant attachments have been released, sacrificing the left colic artery and/or taking the IMV (if not already done) may be required. Incising the medial aspect of the colon mesentery permits straightening of the colon and helps with reach; when performing this maneuver, care should be taken to preserve the blood supply through the marginal artery. On occasion, ligating the left branch of the middle colic artery to further release the transverse colon mesentery may be needed to afford reach.
- If a leak is demonstrated while testing the rectal staple line prior to creating the anastomosis, suture repair can be performed through the hand-port access. A leak demonstrated after firing the circular stapler may be addressed by suture repair, creating a new anastomosis or, in certain circumstances, proximal diversion.
- On occasion, an anastomotic donut may be thin, incomplete, or missing. These situations, typically, do not require a specific remedy as long as the endoscopic exam is normal and the leak test is negative.
- In cases with a difficult retroperitoneal dissection, the integrity of the ureters can be evaluated, to some degree, by administering intravenous indigo carmine.
- The descending colon mesentery may restrict the reach of the end of the colon to the pelvis. Rather than sacrificing the mesentery (and potentially compromising blood flow to the anastomosis), consider configuring the anastomosis in a side-to-end fashion (Baker anastomosis) that might permit tension-free reach while preserving the mesentery.
- When securing the anvil of the circular stapler with the purse-string suture, the colon may not cinch down tightly onto the anvil leaving a gap between the colon and the device. An alternative to tying the purse string tighter (this often results in breaking the suture) is to place a 4-point "U" stitch using a braided suture through the colon around the anvil. This suture can be tied down tightly and pulls the colon snug onto the anvil.

## Conclusion

Hand-assisted left colectomy has the advantages of shorter operative times and decreased conversion rates compared with the "straight" laparoscopic approach; otherwise, the two techniques have equivalent clinical outcomes. This versatile technique restores tactile feedback to the surgeon and facilitates dissection in cases of complicated anatomy. In colectomy cases where difficulties are encountered using straight laparoscopy, conversion to a hand-assisted procedure can potentially avoid the need for conversion to an open approach.

## References


1. Clinical Outcomes of Surgical Therapy Study Group. A comparison of laparoscopically assisted and open colectomy for colon cancer. N Engl J Med. 2004;350:2050–9.
2. Guillou PJ, Quirke P, Thorpe H, Walker J, Jayne DG, Smith AM, et al. Short-term endpoints of conventional versus laparoscopic-assisted surgery in patients with colorectal cancer (MRC CLASICC trial): multicenter, randomized controlled trial. Lancet. 2005;365:1718–26.
3. Jayne DG, Thorpe HC, Copeland J, Quirke P, Borwn JM, Guillou PJ. Five-year follow-up of the Medical Research Council CLASICC trial of laparoscopically assisted versus open surgery for colorectal cancer. Br J Surg. 2010;97:1638–45.
4. Marcello PW, Fleshman JW, Milsom JW, Read TE, Arnell TD, Birnbaum EH, Feingold DF, Lee SW, Mutch MG, Sonoda T, Yan Y, Whelan RL. Hand-assisted laparoscopic vs. laparoscopic colorectal surgery: a multicenter, prospective, randomized trial. Dis Colon Rectum. 2008;51(6):818–26.

# 8 Total Abdominal Colectomy: Straight Laparoscopic Approach

Amanda V. Hayman and Eric J. Dozois

**Key Points**

- A clear understanding of the embryonic planes when mobilizing the colon will significantly reduce the risk of bleeding and inadvertent injury to retroperitoneal structures.
- Appropriate port placement allows and greatly facilitates the ability to perform optimal traction and countertraction necessary for a straight laparoscopic approach to colonic dissection.
- Multiple strategies are available, and should be employed, to prevent rectal stump dehiscence in patients undergoing subtotal colectomy for fulminant colitis.
- Exposing the lesser sac completely greatly facilitates ligation of the transverse colon mesentery.
- When extracting the entire colon through a small incision, removing the right colon first may prevent an inadvertent perforation of the thin-walled cecum.

## Background

Total abdominal colectomy (TAC) is performed for a variety of conditions. The main surgical indications are fulminant or toxic colitis resulting from infection (i.e., *Clostridium difficile*) or, more commonly, refractory ulcerative colitis, diffuse colonic Crohn's disease, slow transit constipation, familial adenomatous polyposis, and Lynch syndrome. In some settings, such as fulminant colitis, an end ileostomy and Hartmann's rectal stump are performed as an immediate anastomosis has a high risk of failure. In most other circumstances, an ileorectal anastomosis can be performed safely in order to restore intestinal continuity.

Several studies have demonstrated that a minimally invasive approach to TAC is feasible, safe, and associated with significant short-term benefits [1, 2]. A number of minimally invasive techniques to colectomy exist including: hand-assisted laparoscopy, straight laparoscopy, laparoscopic-assisted laparoscopy, and single-port laparoscopy [3–5]. As more experience has been gained in minimally invasive approaches, straight laparoscopy—in which all dissection, vessel ligation, and the manufacturing of the anastomosis are performed intracorporeally—has become increasingly popular among surgeons. Although a straight laparoscopic approach to TAC is associated with a longer operative times [6], it avoids the larger incision associated with a hand-assisted approach, which increases the risk of skin and soft tissue infections and hernias. Moreover, if extraction of the colon can be done through a stoma site, or a natural orifice (rectal stump or vagina), instead of a formal abdominal wall incision, even further benefits may be seen [7].

In this chapter, we will outline the technical steps we use when performing a straight laparoscopic TAC followed either by an ileorectostomy or by an end ileostomy and Hartmann's rectal pouch.

## Preoperative Planning and Decision Making

When deciding to use a straight laparoscopic approach to TAC, appropriate timing for surgery and proper patient selection are imperative to optimizing surgical outcomes. Patients that need an emergency colectomy who are critically ill are typically not suited for a straight laparoscopic approach. Patients with severe colitis that have a dilated toxic megacolon will be a high risk for intra-abdominal bowel perforation using a straight laparoscopic approach as this technique requires significant manipulation of the colon with bowel graspers. In these patients we perform an open procedure, which is fast and safe in terms of bowel manipulation.

---

**Electronic supplementary material:** Supplementary material is available in the online version of this chapter at 10.1007/978-1-4939-1581-1_8. Videos can also be accessed at http://www.springerimages.com/videos/978-1-4939-1580-4.

A.V. Hayman, M.D., M.P.H. • E.J. Dozois, M.D. (✉)
Division of Colon & Rectal Surgery, Department of Surgery, Mayo Clinic, 200 1st Street SW, Gonda 9-S, Rochester, MN 55905, USA
e-mail: dozois.eric@mayo.edu

H.M. Ross et al. (eds.), *Minimally Invasive Approaches to Colon and Rectal Disease: Technique and Best Practices*, DOI 10.1007/978-1-4939-1581-1_8, © Springer Science+Business Media New York 2015

Many hospitalized patients with inflammatory bowel disease (IBD) that surgeons are asked to see for colectomy are nutritionally deplete, anemic, and on high-dose corticosteroids and/or immunomodulators. These patients will benefit from some medical optimizing if they do not need immediate surgery. Moreover, these patients may also have a superimposed *Clostridium difficile* or cytomegalovirus infection in addition to their underlying IBD, and a short course of antibiotic or antiviral therapy may assist in avoiding an emergency colectomy. Patients with a history of corticosteroid use will need a steroid prep at the time of surgery, followed by a postoperative taper.

Whenever possible, patients should meet with an enterostomal therapist preoperatively to have all potential stomal sites identified and marked and be educated about living with a stoma. Some surgeons recommend mechanical bowel preparation in patients undergoing laparoscopic colectomy, not because they believe it reduces infection, but because a large stool load in the colon makes laparoscopic manipulation of the colon difficult. We have not found that to be true for most patients and only perform mechanical bowel preparation in patients undergoing TAC for slow transit constipation. However, we do perform 2 tap water enemas in the morning of surgery in all patients to clear the lower colon and rectum, which facilitates stapling of the ileorectal anastomosis. Ultimately, the decision of whether or not to use mechanical bowel preparation should be individualized based on the operating surgeon's best judgment.

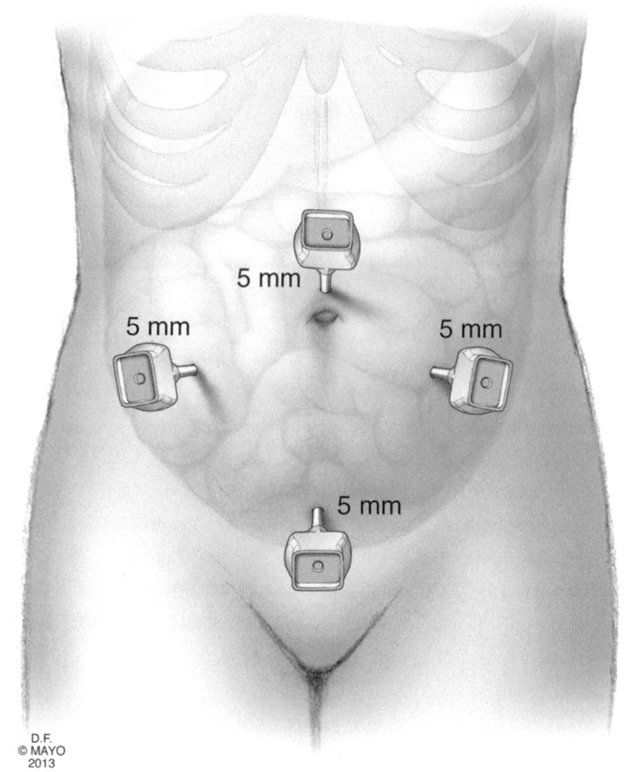


**Fig. 8.1** "Asymmetric baseball diamond" laparoscopic port positioning for total abdominal colectomy (*With permission from Mayo Clinic*)

## Operation

### Setup

Intravenous antibiotics and 5,000 units of heparin are given within 60 min of incision. Once the patient has undergone general anesthesia, a urinary catheter and orogastric tube are placed. Even if planning only an end ileostomy with Hartmann's stump, we prefer lithotomy position so that the operating surgeon can stand between the legs for certain parts of the procedure and also have access to the anus and rectum. Proctoscopy during the operation can be useful to assess adequate closure of a difficult rectal stump, to evacuate all stool and mucus, and in some cases, to leave a draining rectal tube. When a rectal drainage tube is indicated, we use a large urinary catheter with a 30 cc balloon. The catheter is passed into the mid-rectum and the balloon is inflated above the level of the pelvic floor to keep it in place. This obviates the need for perineal sutures to secure a tube, which is extremely uncomfortable for patients. Both arms are tucked and well padded with gel or foam mats to avoid extremity nerve compression injury. Chest straps are routinely utilized to accommodate the steep medial-lateral and caudad-cephalad bed tilts required for the procedure.

### Accessing the Abdomen and Port Placement

Either an OPTIVIEW® (Ethicon, Cincinnati, OH), Hasson, or Veress technique can be used to secure safe access to the abdomen. For most cases, we access the abdomen using a 5 mm OPTIVIEW port, placed just above the umbilicus. A 0° scope is used for the OPTIVIEW access step, and then a 30° scope is used for the rest of the operation. Our preference is to utilize all 5 mm ports, whenever possible, as these port sites do not require fascial closure and have a smaller risk for postoperative hernia. Three other 5 mm ports are then placed under direct vision in a slightly asymmetric "baseball diamond" pattern, one suprapubic, another in the right lower quadrant (if appropriately positioned a hand's breadth away, the ileostomy site can be used), and the last in the left lower quadrant slightly more cephalad than the right lower quadrant port (Fig. 8.1). When intracorporeal stapling is required, one port (usually the right lower quadrant port) will be upsized later to a 12 mm port to accommodate the stapler. Some port site modifications may be necessary based on patient anatomy. For example, in patients with a low hypogastrium, the camera port may need to be shifted superiorly from the umbilicus. In obese patients, the left lateral port may need to be medialized in order to reach the hepatic flexure, and the suprapubic port placed more superior to reach the splenic flexure. In addition, we always have a set of extra-long bowel graspers that come in handy when operating on tall patients or those with high splenic and hepatic flexures.

## Operative Steps (Video 8.1)

### Right Colon

The right or left colon can be approached first. We prefer to start with the right side and use a modified medial-to-lateral approach to the colonic mobilization. The patient is placed in steep Trendelenburg with the right-sided tilt. The small intestine is swept out of the pelvis and placed into the left upper quadrant. The ileum, or a leaf of ileal mesentery near the cecum, is grasped and retracted up and slightly left which exposes the areolar plane between the distal ileal mesentery and the retroperitoneum. Using hot scissors, the peritoneum overlying this indentation just anterior to the iliac artery is incised and carried proximally and medially exposing the retroperitoneum. This dissection can be carried as far as the ligament of Treitz, if needed. This exposes the plane between Toldt and Gerota's fascia and, when in this avascular plane, blunt dissection is performed in a medial-to-lateral fashion across to the underside of the ascending colon mesentery and superiorly to the inferior border of the duodenum (Fig. 8.2). It is critical during this dissection to stay cleanly between Toldt and Gerota's fascia as this avoids unnecessary bleeding and decreases the risk of injury to retroperitoneal structures. If significant bleeding is encountered, the surgeon is likely not in the correct plane. The ureter and gonadal vessels should be clearly visible at this point. The dissection is then continued inferiorly and laterally toward the cecum. The appendix is grasped and the peritoneum incised laterally to separate the cecal attachments from the pelvic sidewall (Fig. 8.3). Care must be taken to stay just next to the bowel to avoid injury to retroperitoneal structures. The final step in fully mobilizing the right colon is to grasp the colon and to pull it medially so that the lateral line of Toldt is placed under tension and can be easily incised. Very little dissection is required at this point to join the previous medial dissection plane. Once complete, this mobilization provides excellent visualization of the right colon mesenteric vessels (Fig. 8.4). The vessels to the right colon are taken by opening a plane between the ileocolic and right colic arteries (Fig. 8.5). The vessels can either be taken close to the colon or more proximally close to the superior mesenteric artery and vein. High ligation of these vessels is done in IBD patients who have dysplasia in the right colon and in patients with known malignancy (Fig. 8.6). In benign cases, the vessels are taken where easy and convenient.

### Transverse Colon and Hepatic Flexure

The patient is then placed level (side-to-side) and in a slight reverse Trendelenburg position. The omentum is addressed first. In most cases it is preserved and taken off the transverse colon and hepatic and splenic flexure regions by pulling

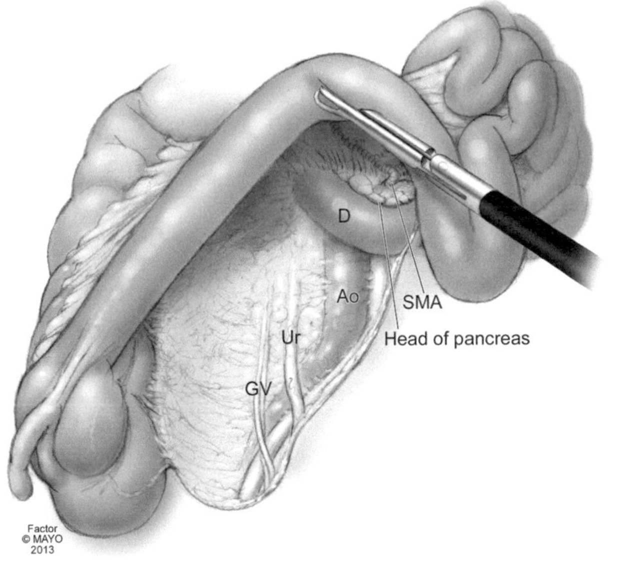


**Fig. 8.2** Retroperitoneal exposure during medial-to-lateral dissection of the right colon (*D* duodenum, *Ao* aorta, *SMA* superior mesenteric artery, *Ur* ureter, *GV* gonadal vessels) (*With permission from Mayo Clinic*)

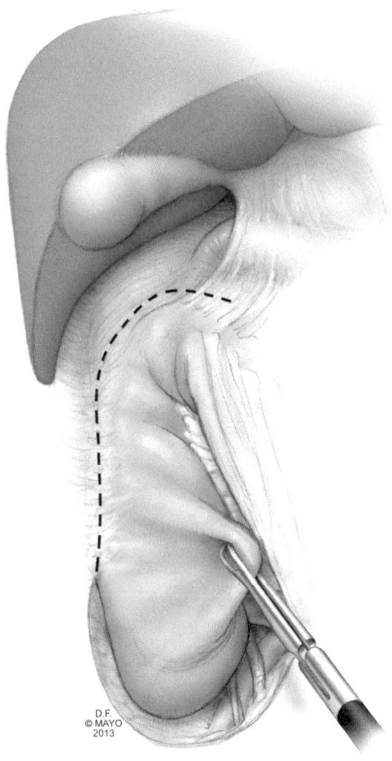


**Fig. 8.3** Dissection plane for separating the lateral attachments of right colon from the sidewall (*With permission from Mayo Clinic*)

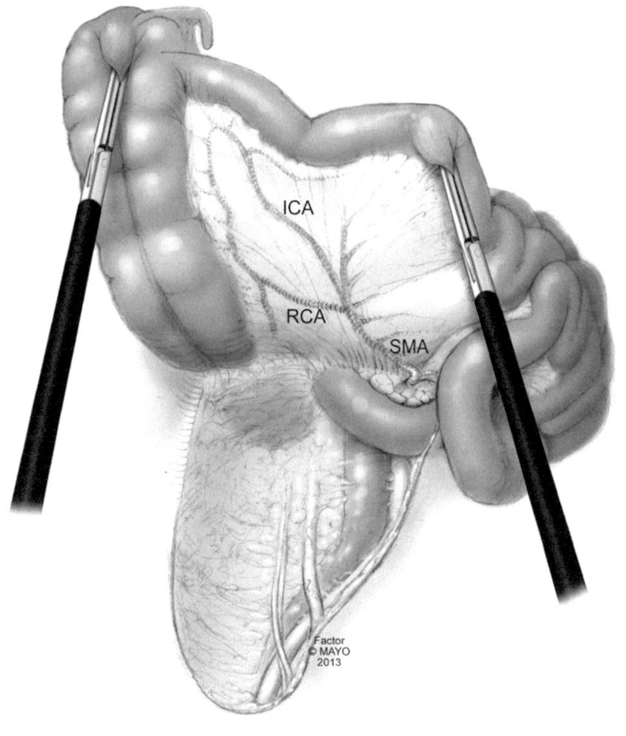


**Fig. 8.4** Posterior view of right colon after complete mobilization (*RCA* right colic artery, *ICA* ileocolic artery, *SMA* superior mesenteric artery) (*With permission from Mayo Clinic*)

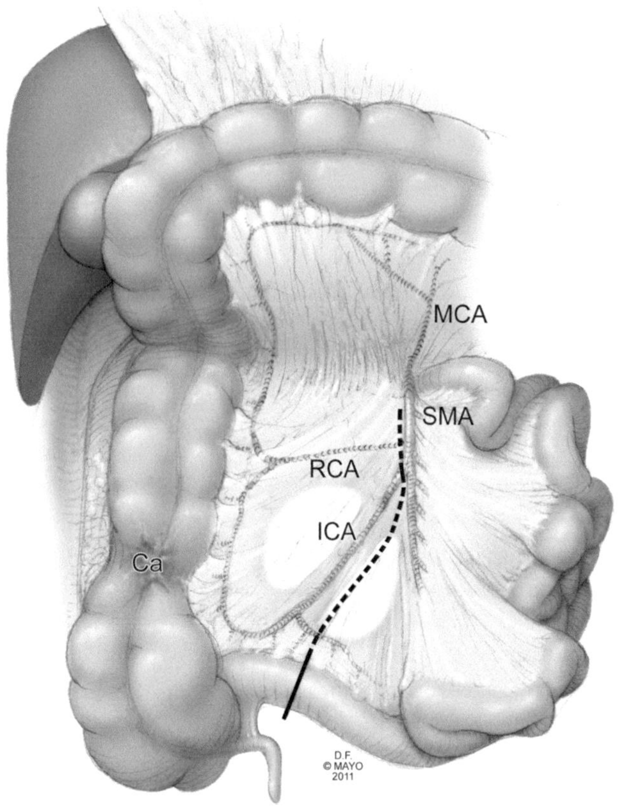


**Fig. 8.6** Plane for high ligation of mesentery near the SMA (*MCA* middle colic artery, *RCA* right colic artery, *ICA* ileocolic artery, *SMA* superior mesenteric artery, *Ca* cancer) (*With permission from Mayo Clinic*)

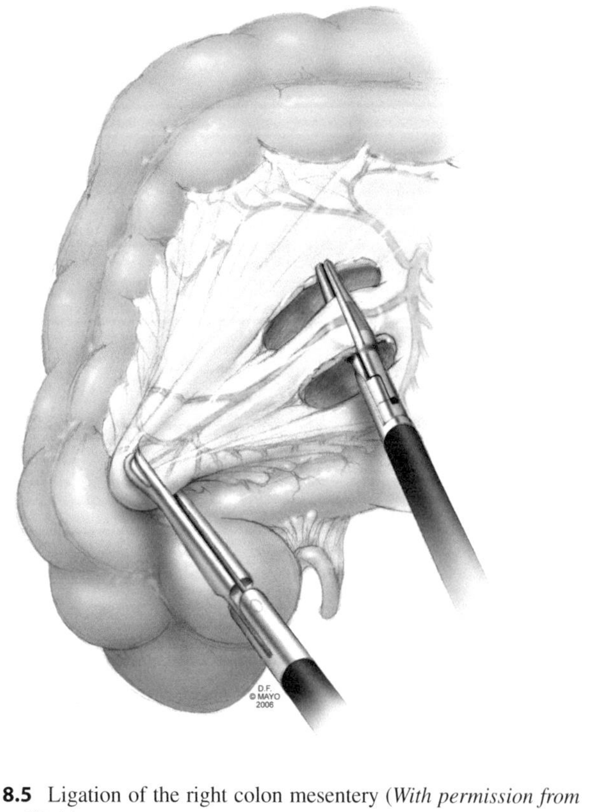


**Fig. 8.5** Ligation of the right colon mesentery (*With permission from Mayo Clinic*)

downward to the transverse colon and upward to the omentum. Caution must be taken when taking the omentum off the splenic flexure as it is sometimes adherent to the splenic capsule, and too much tension may result in splenic capsule avulsion and significant bleeding (Fig. 8.7). The hepatic flexure can be mobilized from the left by taking down the hepatocolic ligaments, exposing the plane between Gerota's fascia, identified by its pale white appearance and the transverse mesocolon (Fig. 8.8). Downward traction of the colon at the hepatic flexure toward the pelvis greatly facilitates this portion of the dissection as this motion puts the hepatocolic ligaments under maximal tension. Ultimately, the avascular plane around the flexure is fully developed bluntly all the way to the right abdominal side wall, forming a tunnel, and the transverse mesocolon is separated from the gastrocolic, duodenal, and pancreatic attachments (Fig. 8.9). This plane ultimately joins the dissection done when mobilizing the right colon earlier. At this point, the right and left branches of the middle colic are easily exposed and can be taken (Fig. 8.10). Once the left branch of the middle colic artery is taken, we address the sigmoid and left colon.

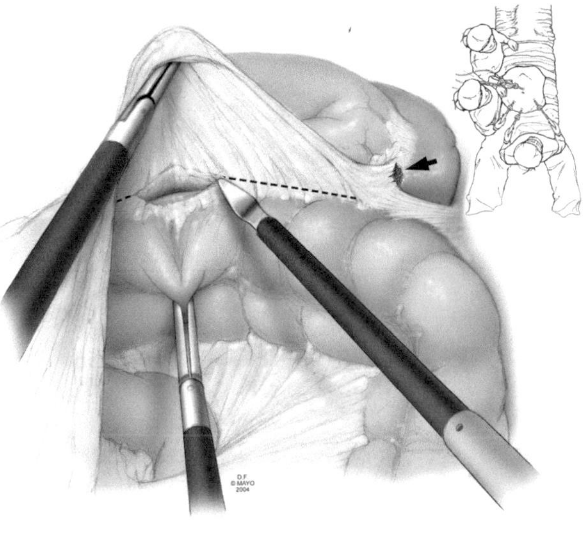


**Fig. 8.7** Separation of the omentum from the distal transverse colon mesentery during splenic flexure mobilization (*With permission from Mayo Clinic*)

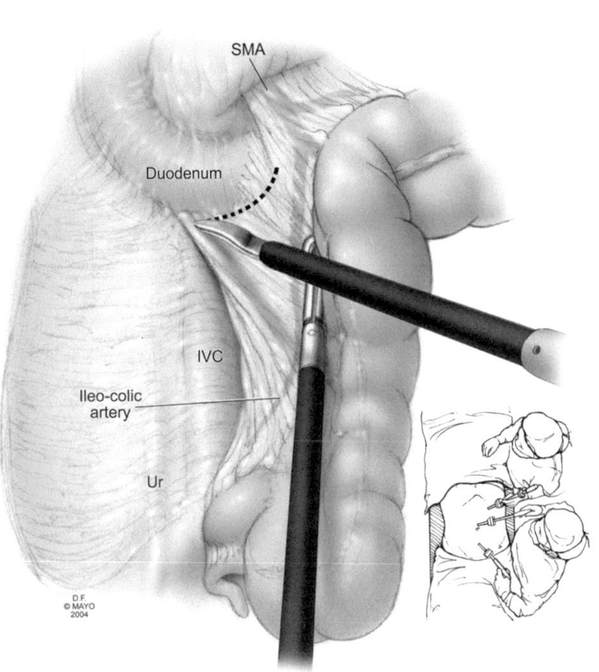


**Fig. 8.9** Exposure of right retroperitoneal structures with downward traction of hepatic flexure after completion of mobilization (*SMA* superior mesenteric artery, *Ur* ureter, *IVC* inferior vena cava) (*With permission from Mayo Clinic*)

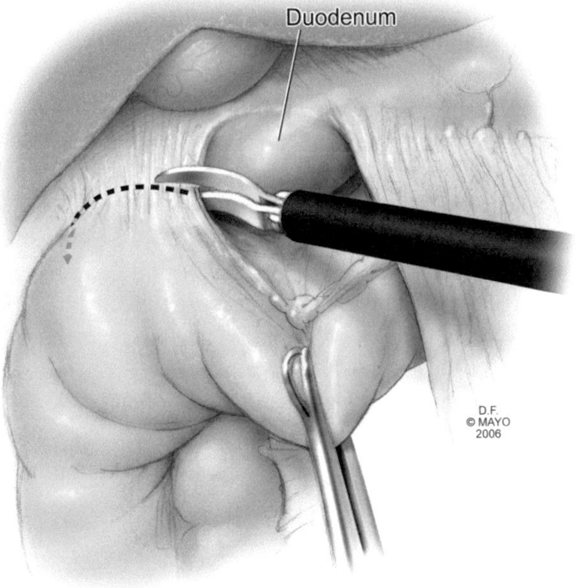


**Fig. 8.8** Excision of the hepatocolic ligament during mobilization of the proximal transverse colon at the hepatic flexure, exposing the duodenum below (*With permission from Mayo Clinic*)

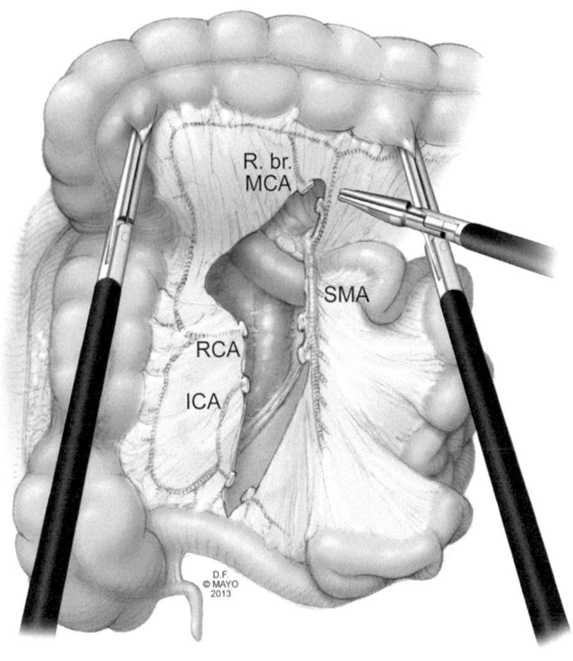


**Fig. 8.10** Ligation of major colic arteries and mesentery of right colon (R. br. *MCA* right branch of middle colic artery, *RCA* right colic artery, *ICA* ileocolic artery, *SMA* superior mesenteric artery) (*With permission from Mayo Clinic*)

## Sigmoid Colon, Left Colon, and Splenic Flexure

For this portion of the operation, the patient is placed in steep Trendelenburg with the patient's left side tilted maximally up. The small bowel is placed in the right upper quadrant, exposing the left colon mesentery. The left colon is grasped and pulled medially, putting the lateral line of Toldt under maximal tension (Fig. 8.11). The sigmoid and left colon are then fully mobilized to the midline of the abdomen in a lateral-to-medial fashion. Again, it is critical during this point of the dissection to stay cleanly between Toldt and Gerota's fascia. This exposes the retroperitoneal structures (gonadal vessels and ureter) and avoids injury (Fig. 8.12).

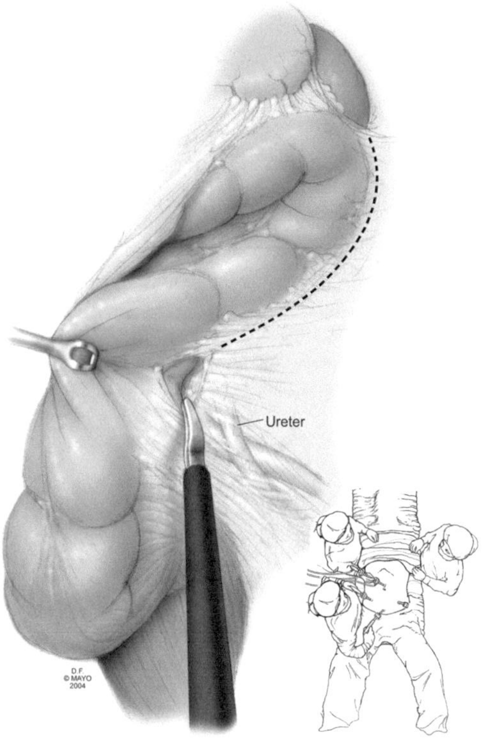


**Fig. 8.11** Dissection plane for separating the lateral attachments of left colon from the sidewall (Ur: ureter) (*Inset*: position of surgeon and assistants around patient) (*With permission from Mayo Clinic*)

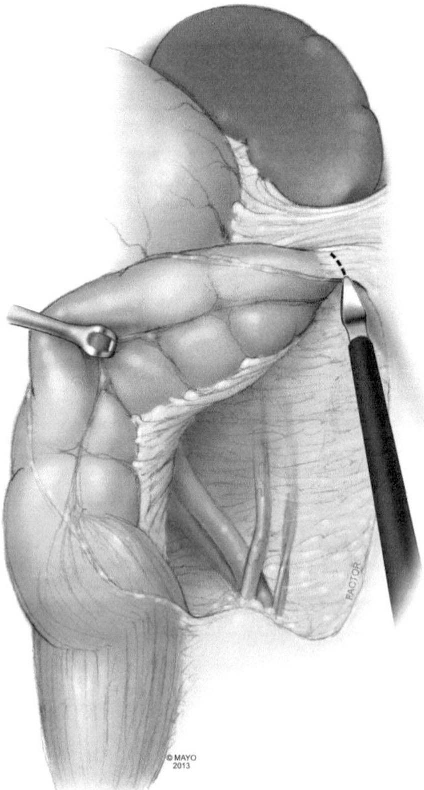

**Fig. 8.12** Exposure of retroperitoneal structures during lateral mobilization of left colon

The mobilization is then carried proximally to the splenic flexure. The splenic flexure is taken down enough to visualize the mesentery for a safe, tension-free vessel ligation. The splenocolic, phrenocolic, and pancreaticocolic ligaments are identified and incised for full splenic flexure mobilization as needed to ensure safe vessel ligation (Fig. 8.13a, b).

Once full mobilization of the left colon and splenic flexure is completed, the decision of where to transect the colon must be made. If there is concern for a high-risk rectal stump, as in the case of a patient with fulminant colitis, we transect the sigmoid at a point that leaves enough length so it can be brought up to the suprafascial position at the suprapubic port site or lower part of the incision if one is made (Fig. 8.14). If the stump is low risk for leak, or if ileorectostomy is going to be performed, transection should be at the top of the rectum. In either case, we typically preserve the superior rectal artery to the rectal stump.

For patients who will get an ileostomy and who have a high-risk distal bowel stump, the mid-sigmoid is transected with the Endo GIA stapler (60 mm load) after upsizing the right lower quadrant 5 mm port to a 12 mm port (Fig. 8.15a, b). Alternatively, the rectum can be transected transabdominally if a Pfannenstiel extraction port is planned. The sigmoid colon is then grasped and retracted medially and anteriorly up toward the abdominal wall, and a vessel-sealant device is then used to ligate all remaining mesentery until the site of the planned colon transection is reached proximally (Fig. 8.16).

For patients undergoing ileorectostomy, a window in the mesentery at the level of the distal sigmoid is created by taking the marginal artery. The mesentery is then taken from this point inferiorly to the top of the rectum, staying close the colon (Fig. 8.17). This preserves the superior rectal artery blood supply to the rectal stump and significantly decreases the risk of sympathetic nerve injury. Once the top of the rectum is adequately cleared of mesentery, the right lower quadrant port can be upsized and the 60 mm Endo GIA stapler is used to transect the rectum with a single firing (Fig. 8.18). The sigmoid colon is then grasped and retracted medially and superiorly, and all the remaining mesentery proximally from this point up to the transected mesentery in the transverse colon done earlier is taken (Fig. 8.19).

## Specimen Extraction

Before closing the abdomen and making the ileostomy or ileorectostomy, the entire abdomen should be inspected for inadvertent injuries to the small bowel and for bleeding (especially near the spleen). Options for specimen extraction fall into two main groups: through a natural orifice route or through a traditional abdominal incision. Traditional abdominal incisions can be low midline, periumbilical, Pfannenstiel, or off midline. Our preferred approach in patients who require an ileostomy is to use the stoma site to extract the entire colon, avoiding a formal

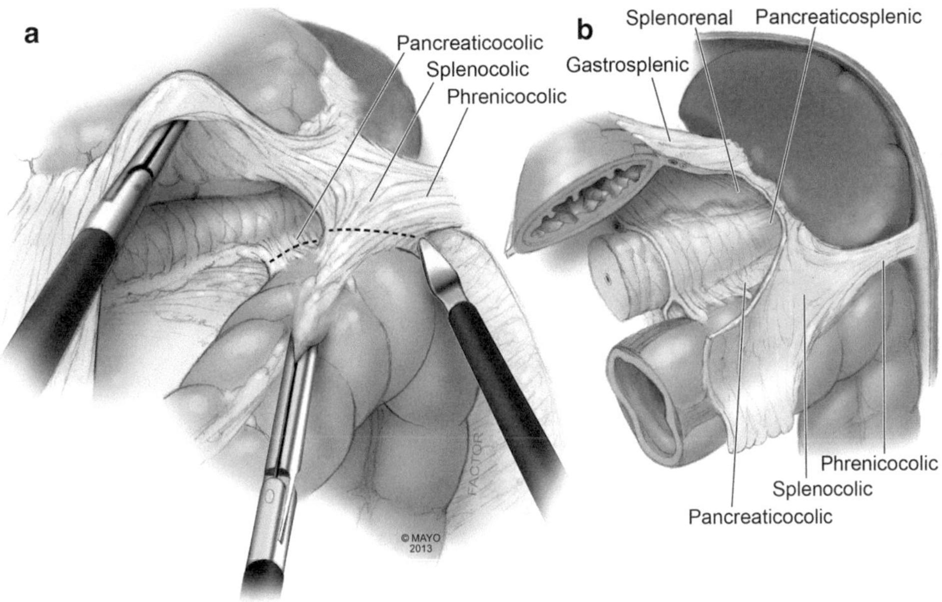


**Fig. 8.13** (**a**) Exposure of splenocolic ligament; (**b**) Splenic flexure recess with associated ligaments (*With permission from Mayo Clinic*)

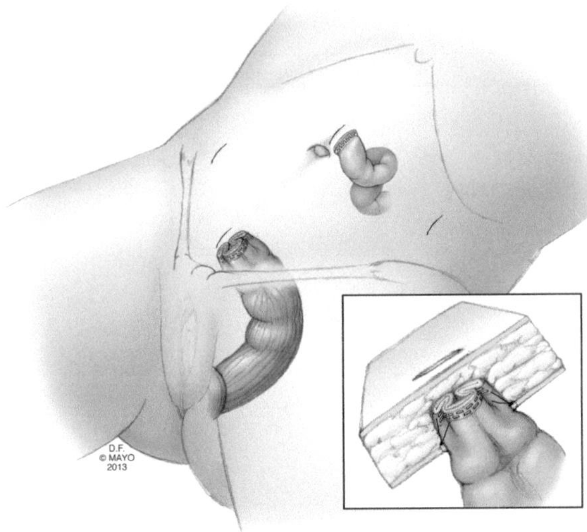

**Fig. 8.14** Creation of a suprafascial sigmoid mucous fistula (*With permission from Mayo Clinic*)

abdominal wall incision (Fig. 8.20). The other option for extraction is to use a natural orifice. We have successfully used the transvaginal route in our Lynch patients undergoing transvaginal hysterectomy at the time of TAC [7]. The gynecologic surgeon performs the transvaginal hysterectomy and leaves the vaginal cuff open. We then place a wound protector through the cuff and bring out the colon and the terminal ileum (Fig. 8.21). The ileum is transected and the EEA anvil is placed into the lumen, secured with a purse-string suture or device, and then placed back into the abdominal cavity. The vaginal cuff is closed transvaginally, pneumoperitoneum is restored, and the EEA stapler is docked to the anvil using laparoscopic techniques. Alternatively, the ileum can be brought out through one of the port sites for anvil placement (Fig. 8.22).

If using a Pfannenstiel, the suprapubic port's skin incision is extended bilaterally, and the anterior fascia incised. The rectus muscle is swept down bluntly, with care taken to avoid any muscle trauma and subsequent bleeding. The peritoneum is incised and a wound retractor placed transabdominally. This approach also allows the passage of a small transverse stapler, such as the TA30 or 45 to transect the rectum or mid-sigmoid in lieu of the Endo GIA. As the cecum is the widest portion of the colon and has the thinnest wall, it is best to extract the right colon first when removing the whole colon to prevent inadvertent colonic rupture when extracting through very small incisions. One must confirm that the small bowel has been gathered in the left upper quadrant and that the colon will not get caught on the small bowel mesentery upon extraction.

## End Ileostomy

If creating an end ileostomy, the ostomy site is grasped with a Kocher and a circular quarter-sized incision is made. A cylinder of subcutaneous tissue is also excised, and a cruciate incision made in the anterior fascia above the rectus abdominis. Via a muscle-spreading technique, the peritoneum is then exposed and incised so that two fingers can easily pass. This technique is slightly more challenging than when

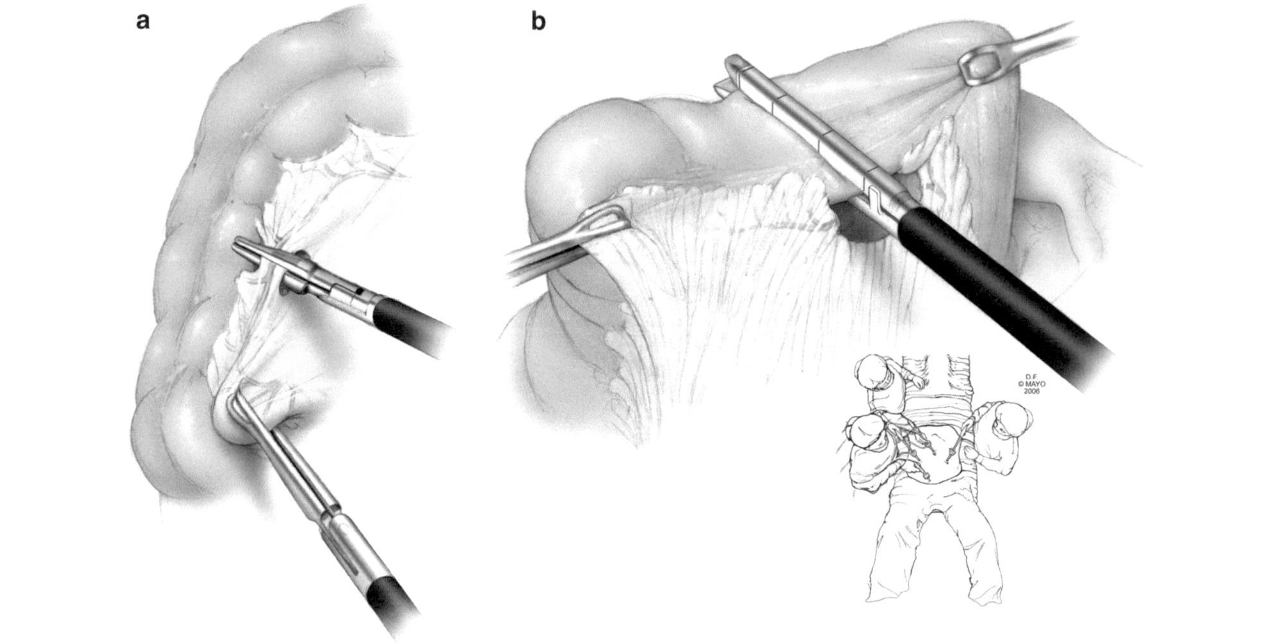


**Fig. 8.15** (**a**) Ligation of marginal artery in sigmoid colon mesentery; (**b**) Intracorporeal transection of sigmoid colon with laparoscopic stapler to create a rectal stump (inset: position of surgeon and assistants around patient) (*With permission from Mayo Clinic*)

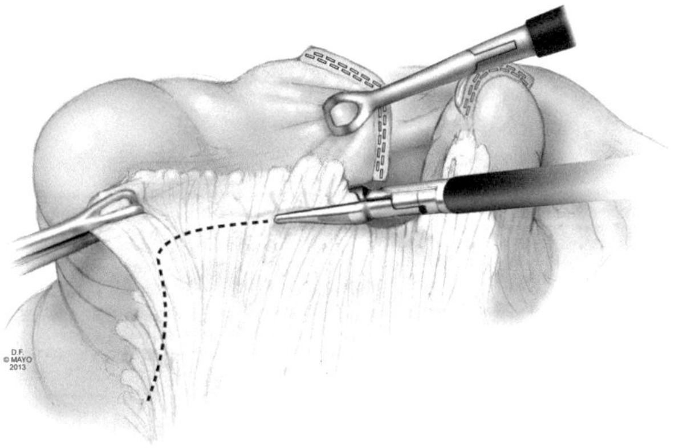

**Fig. 8.16** Ligation of proximal sigmoid mesentery with vessel sealer after transection (*With permission from Mayo Clinic*)

approached open, as minimal counter tension can be applied intra-abdominally. If using a Pfannenstiel, the laparoscopy camera cable can be disconnected and used as a "flashlight" to identify the ileal stump (if not already grasped with a locking bowel grasper) to be delivered to the ileostomy site. It is of paramount importance at this point to make sure that the ileum and ileal mesentery are not twisted or rotated. When in proper orientation for a right-sided end ileostomy, the cut edge of the ileal mesentery should be seen going directly to the head of the pancreas and splayed out flat. Moreover, all of the small bowel should be placed in the left side of the abdomen and pulled out from under the ileal mesentery if

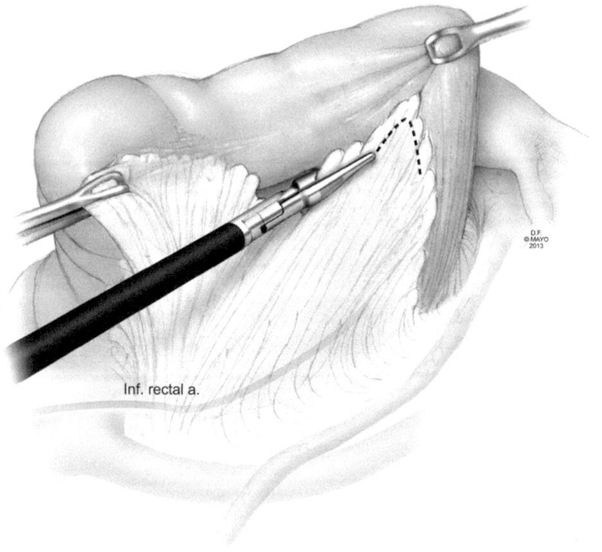


**Fig. 8.17** Ligation of sigmoid mesentery prior to transection (inf. rectal a.: inferior rectal artery) (*With permission from Mayo Clinic*)

loops are seen in the right upper quadrant to prevent internal herniation. A Brooke ileostomy is then made after closing all port sites (Fig. 8.23).

### Ileorectostomy

If performing an ileorectal anastomosis (end-to-end), the ileal stump is delivered through the extraction site, and a run-

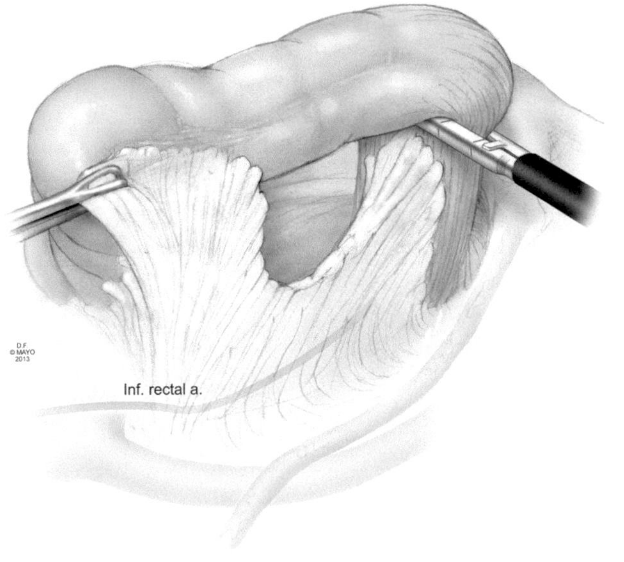


**Fig. 8.18** Open transection of sigmoid colon to create rectal stump (inf. rectal a.: inferior rectal artery) (*With permission from Mayo Clinic*)

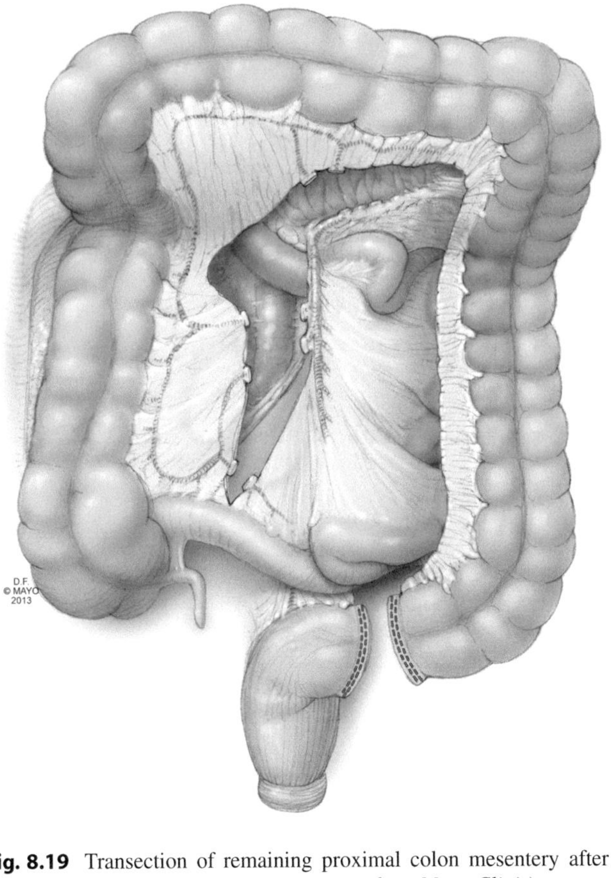

**Fig. 8.19** Transection of remaining proximal colon mesentery after sigmoid colon transection (*With permission from Mayo Clinic*)

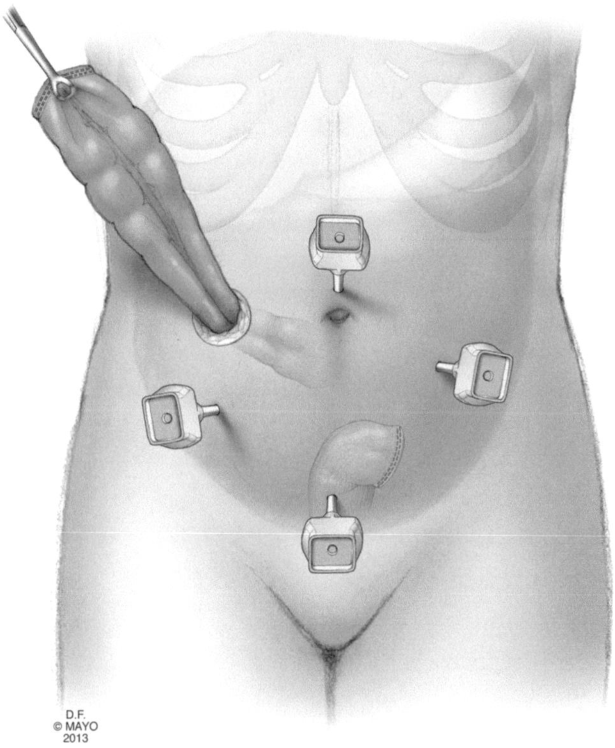

**Fig. 8.20** Specimen extraction via planned ileostomy site (*With permission from Mayo Clinic*)

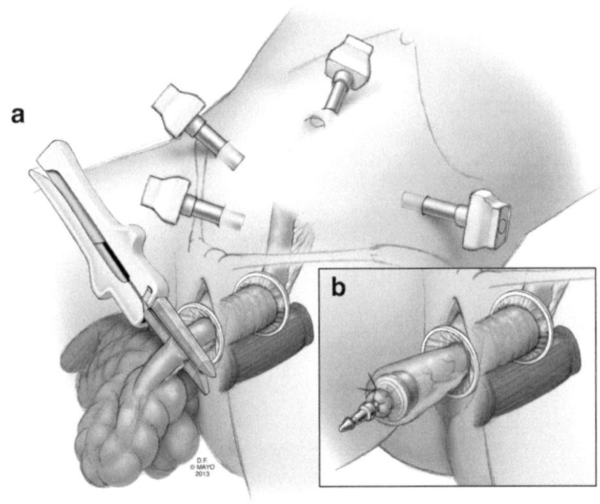


**Fig. 8.21** (**a**) Transvaginal extraction of specimen and transection of the ileum with a GIA stapler; (**b**) Transvaginal insertion of anvil into the ileum for planned ileorectal anastomosis with an EEA stapler (*With permission from Mayo Clinic*)

ning purse string is created with 2.0 PDS suture. The anvil from the 28 mm EEA is inserted intraluminally and secured with the purse-string suture. The EEA stapler is carefully maneuvered transanally to the end of the rectal stump after using rectal sizers to dilate the sphincter. The pin is advanced through the rectal stump, usually just superior to the rectal staple line, and the anvil secured with a click, after ensuring the colon mesentery is not twisted. Generally, the splayed taeniae will be positioned anteriorly. The stapler is closed completely and fired. If desired, interrupted sutures can be placed at the crossing staple lines to better secure the "dog-eared" areas (Fig. 8.24a, b). An alternative anastomotic approach is the side (the ileum) to end (the rectum) ileorectal anastomosis. The end of the ileum is stapled and oversewn with interrupted 3.0 Lambert silk sutures. An enterotomy to place the anvil must be made on the antimesenteric side of the ileum 3–4 cm proximal to the transected end of the ileum to avoid an ischemic segment between the circular staple line and the transected end of the ileum. A purse-string stitch is used to secure the anvil. Finally, a proctoscope is introduced into the distal rectum to insufflate the anastomosis under a water bath after occlusion of the ileum above the anastomosis. In the event of a "positive leak test," we generally revise the anastomosis instead of suture repairing it, but ultimately this decision is made on a case-by-case basis. If technically satisfied with the operation, and if there is no tension and an excellent blood supply, we do not perform a defunctioning loop ileostomy. In very rare cases where patient factors and tissue quality are not ideal, a diverting loop ileostomy is done.

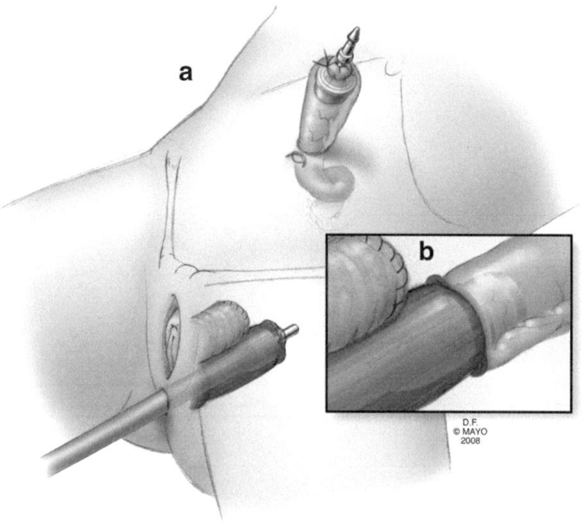


**Fig. 8.22** (**a**) Insertion of anvil into the ileum via laparoscopic port site extraction after intracorporeal transection and transvaginal extraction in setting of shortened mesentery; (**b**) Creation of ileorectal anastomosis using an EEA stapler after vaginotomy repair (*With permission from Mayo Clinic*)

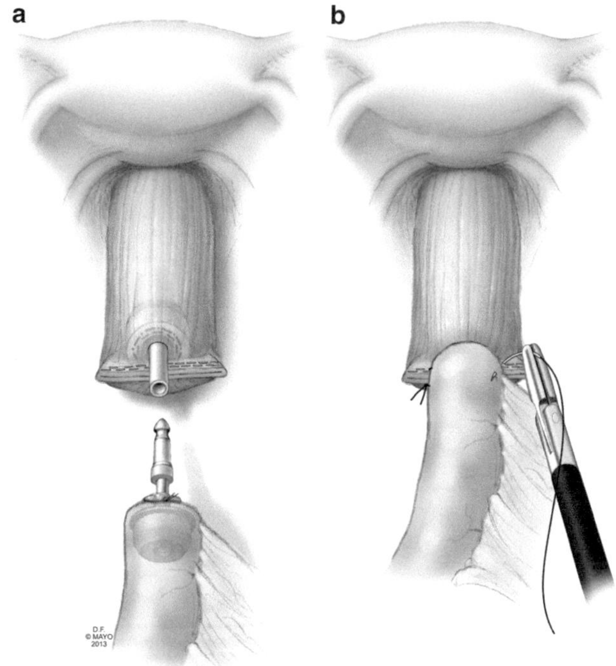


**Fig. 8.24** (**a**) Creation of ileorectal anastomosis using an EEA stapler; (**b**) Sutures used to secure lateral "dog ears" on rectal side of ileorectal anastomosis (*With permission from Mayo Clinic*)

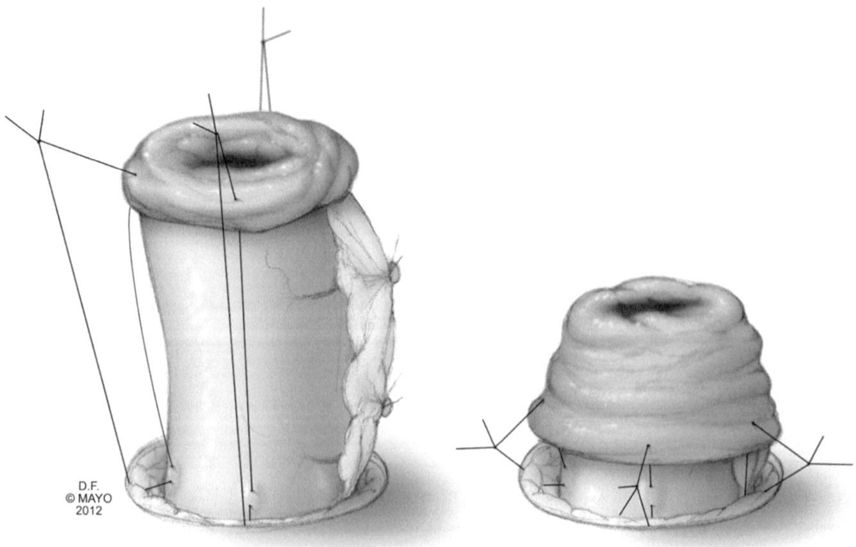


**Fig. 8.23** Creation of a Brooke ileostomy (*With permission from Mayo Clinic*)

## Postoperative Care

At our institution, almost all patients are enrolled in an enhanced recovery pathway that has been reported previously [8]. Key components of the pathway include:

- Absence of mechanical bowel preparation
- Preoperative intrathecal injection (when appropriate)
- Intraoperative fluid restriction
- General diet (apart from fresh fruits and vegetables) starting the night of surgery
- Routine pre- and postoperative oral NSAIDs and acetaminophen administration
- Avoidance of intravenous opioids
- Early ambulation
- Removal of urinary catheter on the first postoperative day
- Cessation of intravenous fluids on the first postoperative day

We check electrolytes and a complete blood count on the first postoperative day and then only when indicated afterward. For patients who have an ileostomy, postoperative stoma teaching is essential. Patients with stomas are not discharged until the stoma output is between 500 and 1,500 ml per day. In the ileorectostomy patients, a bowel movement prior to discharge is required.

## Complications

### Intraoperative

First and foremost, conversion to an open procedure should never be viewed as a failure, but instead, as the appropriate measure to take to avoid major complications. In some cases, we have converted from straight to hand-assisted laparoscopy if for technical reasons a hand inside will make the operation safe and still provide the benefits of minimally invasive surgery. Intraoperative complications during straight TAC are similar to that of minimally invasive colectomy and include: trochar or cautery injury to hollow or solid organs or vessels, inadvertent ligation of the ureter, vascular pedicle bleeding, and delayed thermal injury to the small bowel from cautery. Thermal injuries when noticed are treated with intracorporeal Lembert sutures of the bowel to seal the site of injury.

Care must be used when using vessel-sealant devices in patients with severe atherosclerotic diseases, as these devices will not be as effective or reliable when sealing large calcified vessels. When mobilizing the splenic flexure, injudicious retraction can lead to splenic capsular bleeding and, occasionally, the need for emergent splenectomy [9].

Another important safety issue is to ensure that the patient is properly secured to the table. Given the extreme changes in table angulation during this case, it is important to confirm that the patient is both properly padded and secured, using chest and/or shoulder straps. One tip is to have the anesthetist simulate extreme Trendelenburg and lateral positions prior to prepping and draping to confirm no excessive patient movement.

Delay in diagnosis of an intraoperative injury usually results in greater morbidity for the patient than when recognized at the time of operation. It is essential to be prepared for the unexpected and to be vigilant about exploring the abdomen at the end of the procedure to search out potential problems. We have found that most intraoperative injuries can be avoided by ensuring that the surgeon stays in the correct plane of dissection at all times, avoids excessive and blind retraction, and always visualizes the critical anatomy.

### Postoperative

Ileorectostomy is notorious for an increased risk of postoperative complications when compared to other anastomoses, both for anastomotic leaks [10, 11] and postoperative bowel obstructions [12]. Reasons are manifold but likely include difficulty with size mismatch, ischemia, or excessive mobility of the small intestine mesentery leading to volvulus.

For all straight laparoscopic TAC cases, there are risks of an unrecognized enterotomy, small bowel thermal injury (leading to a delayed enterotomy), and ureterotomy. Postoperative bleeding can result from poorly sealed or tied mesenteric vessels, from splenic capsular bleeding, or from the abdominal wall where ports have been placed. Ports placed through the inferior epigastric vessels that bleed in the postoperative period can lead to life-threatening bleeding when the tamponade effect of the trocar is gone. Other postoperative complications specific to a subtotal colectomy also include mesenteric or portal vein thrombosis [13] or, most frequently, early small bowel obstruction from adhesions, mesenteric volvulus, or at the site of the ileostomy (either from edema or too small of a fascial aperture). Postoperative bowel obstruction requiring reoperation has been reported in up to 8 % of patients [14]. In cases of fulminant colitis (i.e., ulcerative colitis or *Clostridium difficile*), rupture of a high-risk rectal stump can occur, resulting in abdominal sepsis. If a high-risk sigmoid stump was tacked in the suprafascial position, it may later rupture, resulting in a wound infection. The wound can be opened, and controlled mucus fistula can be managed with a stoma appliance. As mentioned previously, one may consider leaving a urinary catheter with inflated balloon or red rubber catheter in the rectum for a day or so to promote drainage of bloody stool and mucus and release of air in order to decrease subsequent risk of "stump blow out." Meticulous technique is essential as postoperative bleeding or anastomotic leaks can result in pelvic hematomas or subsequent abscesses, which may compromise future surgery.

## Outcomes

Studies conflict over the absolute benefits of laparoscopy versus open approach to TAC in regard to postoperative complications [15–18]. One of the purported, but not proven, benefits of laparoscopic TAC is the prevention of adhesions, which is especially relevant if a future ileoanal pouch is planned [17, 19]. Multiple studies have shown that laparoscopic TAC is safe and feasible in experienced hands and results in shorter lengths of stay and a decrease in wound infections compared to open approaches [17].

## Pearls and Pitfalls

Perhaps the most important consideration for surgeons to recognize is that a laparoscopic TAC is a technically challenging procedure, necessitating the ligation of multiple vessels and working in multiple quadrants of the abdomen. Moreover, straight laparoscopy requires advanced knowledge of embryologic planes and regional anatomy to avoid collateral damage. An experienced laparoscopic camera operator and frequent table adjustments are required to maximize visualization. Surgeons at the beginning of their learning curve may want to consider getting more experience with straight laparoscopic segmental colectomy and hand-assisted TAC early in their career prior to undertaking a straight laparoscopic approach to the entire colon when independent operating experience is limited. Having a senior colleague that can mentor can greatly facilitate the learning curve.

For the most challenging cases (obese, adhesions from prior surgery), adding more ports can greatly facilitate successful completion of the operation [7]. Traction and countertraction are critical to make the straight laparoscopic approach successful, and one should not hesitate adding ports to facilitate this. Patient selection (less obese patients, no previous surgery) and staying consistent with a standardized technical approach will improve efficiency as the surgeon's experience grows.

## Conclusion

A straight laparoscopic approach to TAC with either end ileostomy or restorative ileorectal anastomosis can be utilized as the surgical procedure of choice for a number of colorectal conditions. This approach is highly technical and requires advanced laparoscopic skills. In most cases, the operation is associated with shorter length of stay and fewer wound complications and may prove to decrease adhesion burden, giving the patient a greater chance to benefit from laparoscopic procedures in the future. There are many technical approaches to straight laparoscopic TAC, and the best approach for each surgeon is individualized. This chapter serves as a guide to what we believe to be a safe, efficient, and effective approach. For the surgeon early in the learning curve for advanced laparoscopy, we hope that the systematic approach we have outlined here will facilitate further learning leading to confidence in performing a straight laparoscopic TAC.

## References

1. Holubar SD, Larson DW, Dozois EJ, Pattana-Arun J, Pemberton JH, Cima RR. Minimally invasive subtotal colectomy and ileal pouch-anal anastomosis for fulminant ulcerative colitis: a reasonable approach? Dis Colon Rectum. 2009;52(2):187–92.
2. Fichera A, Zoccali M, Gullo R. Single incision ("scarless") laparoscopic total abdominal colectomy with end ileostomy for ulcerative colitis. J Gastrointest Surg. 2011;15(7):1247–51 [Comparative Study].
3. Paranjape C, Ojo OJ, Carne D, Guyton D. Single-incision laparoscopic total colectomy. JSLS. 2012;16(1):27–32 [Case Reports Review].
4. Cahill RA, Lindsey I, Jones O, Guy R, Mortensen N, Cunningham C. Single-port laparoscopic total colectomy for medically uncontrolled colitis. Dis Colon Rectum. 2010;53(8):1143–7 [Comparative Study Research Support, Non-U.S. Gov't].
5. Ozturk E, Kiran RP, Remzi F, Geisler D, Fazio V. Hand-assisted laparoscopic surgery may be a useful tool for surgeons early in the learning curve performing total abdominal colectomy. Colorectal Dis. 2010;12(3):199–205 [Comparative Study].
6. Boushey RP, Marcello PW, Martel G, Rusin LC, Roberts PL, Schoetz Jr DJ. Laparoscopic total colectomy: an evolutionary experience. Dis Colon Rectum. 2007;50(10):1512–9.
7. Dozois EJ, Larson DW, Dowdy SC, Poola VP, Holubar SD, Cima RR. Transvaginal colonic extraction following combined hysterectomy and laparoscopic total colectomy: a natural orifice approach. Tech Coloproctol. 2008;12(3):251–4 [Case Reports].
8. Lovely JK, Maxson PM, Jacob AK, Cima RR, Horlocker TT, Hebl JR, et al. Case-matched series of enhanced versus standard recovery pathway in minimally invasive colorectal surgery. Br J Surg. 2012;99(1):120–6.
9. Merchea A, Dozois EJ, Wang JK, Larson DW. Anatomic mechanisms for splenic injury during colorectal surgery. Clin Anat. 2012;25(2):212–7.
10. Hyman N, Manchester TL, Osler T, Burns B, Cataldo PA. Anastomotic leaks after intestinal anastomosis: it's later than you think. Ann Surg. 2007;245(2):254–8.
11. Alves A, Panis Y, Trancart D, Regimbeau JM, Pocard M, Valleur P. Factors associated with clinically significant anastomotic leakage after large bowel resection: multivariate analysis of 707 patients. World J Surg. 2002;26(4):499–502.
12. Pemberton JH, Rath DM, Ilstrup DM. Evaluation and surgical treatment of severe chronic constipation. Ann Surg. 1991; 214(4):403–11. [Research Support, U.S. Gov't, P.H.S.]; discussion 11–3.
13. Broucek JR, Francescatti AB, Swanson GR, Keshavarzian A, Brand MI, Saclarides TJ. Unusual thrombotic complications. Am Surg. 2012;78(6):728–9 [Case Reports].
14. Alves A, Panis Y, Bouhnik Y, Maylin V, Lavergne-Slove A, Valleur P. Subtotal colectomy for severe acute colitis: a 20-year experience of a tertiary care center with an aggressive and early surgical policy. J Am Coll Surg. 2003;197(3):379–85.

15. Parnaby C, Ramsay G, Macleod C, Hope N, Jansen J, McAdam T. Complications after laparoscopic and open subtotal colectomy for inflammatory colitis: a case-matched comparison. Colorectal Dis. 2013;15(11):1399–405.
16. Frid NL, Bulut O, Pachler J. Acceptable short-term outcome of laparoscopic subtotal colectomy for inflammatory bowel disease. Dan Med J. 2013;60(6):A4645.
17. Tilney HS, Lovegrove RE, Purkayastha S, Heriot AG, Darzi AW, Tekkis PP. Laparoscopic vs open subtotal colectomy for benign and malignant disease. Colorectal Dis. 2006;8(5):441–50 [Meta-Analysis].
18. Seshadri PA, Poulin EC, Schlachta CM, Cadeddu MO, Mamazza J. Does a laparoscopic approach to total abdominal colectomy and proctocolectomy offer advantages? Surg Endosc. 2001;15(8):837–42 [Comparative Study].
19. Fowkes L, Krishna K, Menon A, Greenslade GL, Dixon AR. Laparoscopic emergency and elective surgery for ulcerative colitis. Colorectal Dis. 2008;10(4):373–8.

# Total Abdominal Colectomy: Hand-Assisted Approach

9

Kiyokazu Nakajima, Tsunekazu Mizushima, and Riichiro Nezu

## Key Points

- Don't make the minilaparotomy wound too small.
- Select a hand-access device and energy device carefully to suit your needs.
- Don't do everything under HALS. Use straight laparoscopic as well as both "open" and "HALS" techniques effectively.
- Consider "lateral-to-medial" rather than "medial-to-lateral" approach for inflammatory conditions. The mesentery can bleed easily.
- Don't use your hand randomly. The "palm-up" and "palm-down" are different techniques. Be comfortable with both and use them effectively.
- Communicate with your surgical crew consciously. You are the only person with tactile feedback, so ensure they are aware of what you are doing and your next steps.

## Introduction

Total abdominal colectomy (TAC) is one of the most complex and extensive operations. It requires a full mobilization of the entire abdominal colon, division of the mesentery with safe ligature of all major colonic vessels, colonic resection, and anastomosis (or ileostomy) while exposing all necessary anatomical structures effectively in each of the abdominal quadrant [1, 2]. These steps become further technically challenging when using laparoscopy, since TAC is mostly indicated for patients with inflammatory conditions such as ulcerative colitis (UC) and Crohn's disease, where anatomy is often distorted with adhesions, abscesses, and fistulae [2, 3].

Hand-assisted laparoscopic surgery (HALS) has been proposed as a practical alternative to both open and straight laparoscopic surgery. With HALS, surgeons regain their tactile sensation and gentle handling of the bowel, which may enhance efficacy and safety of complex colorectal operations such as laparoscopic TAC and total proctocolectomy [1, 2, 4]. In this chapter we describe our recent technique of HALS TAC and discuss its potential advantages over straight laparoscopic TAC.

## Indications

The indications for HALS TAC are basically similar to open or laparoscopic TAC, such as UC and Crohn's extensive colitis. In fulminant UC, TAC with end ileostomy is indicated as first-stage operation. In Crohn's colitis, ileorectal anastomosis can be considered when the perianal disease is absent or well controlled with local therapy [2]. HALS can be considered even in "semi-emergent" settings in patients with inflammatory bowel disease when the hemodynamic status remains stable. However, open TAC should be selected when safe pneumoperitoneum is not physiologically achievable. Currently the authors do not use HALS for cases with megacolon, since laparoscopic exposure is not optimal due to distended colonic segments.

Other indications involve slow transit constipation resistant to medical treatment, familial adenomatous polyposis with rectal sparing, and hereditary non-polyposis colorectal cancer. TAC is not usually indicated for colorectal cancers, expect for limited cases with synchronous multiple lesions located in two or more separated colonic segments.

---

**Electronic supplementary material:** Supplementary material is available in the online version of this chapter at 10.1007/978-1-4939-1581-1_9. Videos can also be accessed at http://www.springerimages.com/videos/978-1-4939-1580-4.

K. Nakajima, M.D., F.A.C.S. (✉) • T. Mizushima, M.D.
Department of Gastroenterological Surgery, Osaka University Graduate School of Medicine, 2-2, E-2, Yamadaoka, Suita, Osaka 565-0871, Japan
e-mail: knakajima@gesurg.med.osaka-u.ac.jp

R. Nezu, M.D., Ph.D.
Department of Surgery, Nishinomiya Municipal Central Hospital, 8-24, Hayashida-cho, Nishinomiya, Hyogo, Japan

H.M. Ross et al. (eds.), *Minimally Invasive Approaches to Colon and Rectal Disease: Technique and Best Practices*, DOI 10.1007/978-1-4939-1581-1_9, © Springer Science+Business Media New York 2015

## Patient Positioning

Under general anesthesia, the patient is placed in the modified lithotomy position with the legs positioned in padded stirrups. The trunk should remain fixed adequately on an operating table even in a steep Trendelenburg position. The operating surgeon stands between the patient's legs. The assisting surgeon(s) stands on the both sides of the patient. The surgeon first stands on the patient's right side and then moves to the left side, as the procedure proceeds from the left colon to the right colon (Fig. 9.1).

## Hand-Access Device Placement

A 7–8 cm minilaparotomy is made. We exclusively use muscle-splitting Pfannenstiel incision for UC cases, though we prefer a lower midline incision for Crohn's patients to keep the lateral abdomen free of incisions for possible future ostomy [1, 2]. Too small of a wound may complicate free and deep insertion of the device, therefore, interfering with the HALS procedure. After confirming the adequacy of wound size by inserting surgeon's hand into the abdomen, a hand-access device is assembled to the wound. Our favorite device is GelPort laparoscopic system (Applied Medical, Rancho Santa Margarita, CA), which provides stable wound retraction during open procedure and enables unlimited hand exchanges into every abdominal quadrant without significant gas leakage during laparoscopic procedure [5, 6].

## Surgical Ports and Energy Devices

Two standard trocars are used: one in the periumbilical region for laparoscopy and the other in the left mid-abdomen for the energy device, respectively (Fig. 9.2). We currently prefer bipolar vessel-sealing device (LigaSure™, Covidien, Mansfield, MA) for colonic mobilization, takedown of the omentum, and mesenteric division. We do not find that the LigaSure™ device gets too hot, even after repeated activations, and thus enables safe use of surgeon's hand simultaneously [6]. We do not use monopolar electrocautery or ultrasonically driven scalpel since these devices may make hand assist difficult with an inability to take large vessels (monopolar) and increased heat production. We also do not routinely use any laparoscopic clips. However, device and instrumentation selection is up to the individual surgeon, and preferences differ pending experience and comfort level.

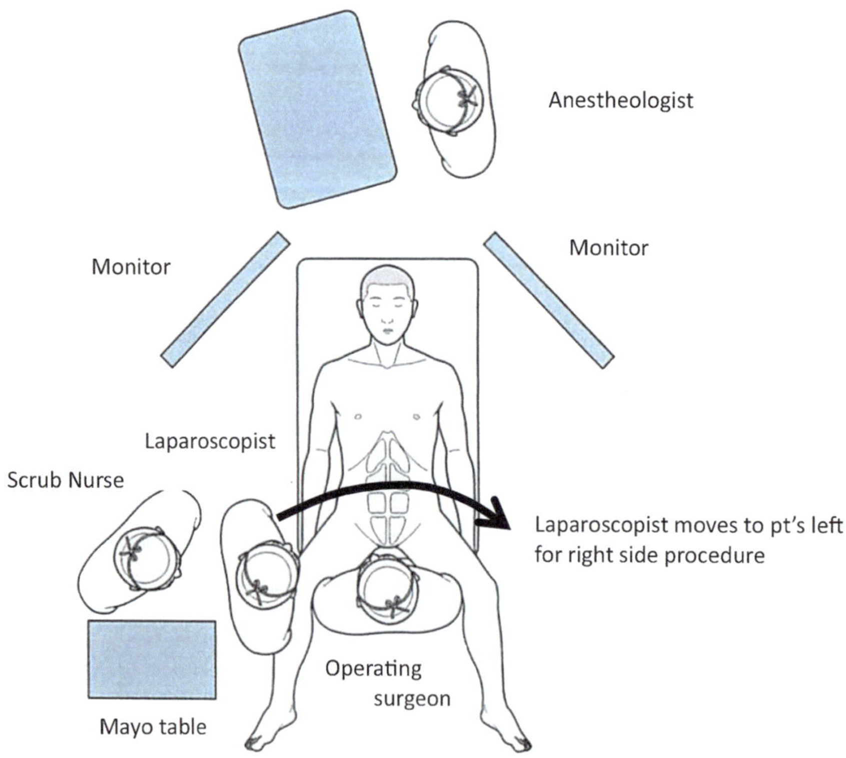


**Fig. 9.1** Patient positioning and OR setup. The operating surgeon stands between patient's legs. The surgeon stands on patient's right side for left colon procedure and then moves to left side for right colon procedure

## The "Palm-Down" and "Palm-Up" Techniques

HALS requires logical and systemic use of surgeon's hand. A random use of hand may interfere with the procedure, rather than assist the procedure. The authors have systematized and categorized the use of hand into two simple techniques: "palm-down" and "palm-up" techniques.

Most of HALS procedures can be performed using "palm-down" technique (Video 9.1). This technique facilitates free and delicate use of the 2nd/3rd fingers. This is best suited for extending an avascular plane under continuous traction, e.g., colonic mobilization (Fig. 9.3a). A blunt dissection using 2nd finger is possible, as needed.

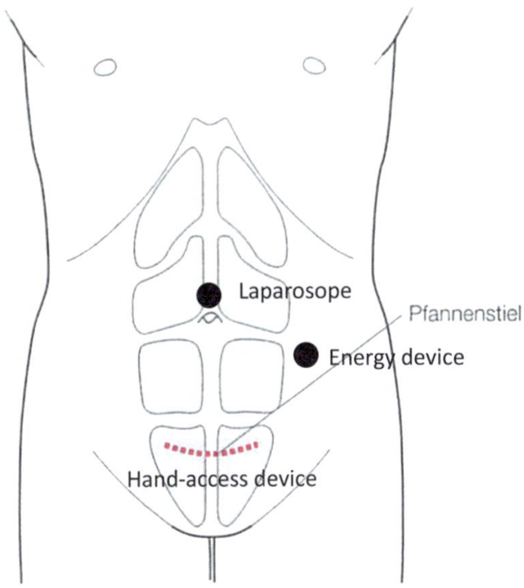


**Fig. 9.2** The sites for hand-access device, laparoscope, and energy device

In "palm-up" position, on the contrary, the surgeon can more positively use his/her 1st finger (Video 9.2). This technique is effective for palpation and for dividing structures containing vessels. In mesenteric division, for example, a fine palpation and rapid division is possible by pinching the mesentery with 1st and 2nd fingers (Fig. 9.3b). Additionally, a wider displacement/retraction is possible with intentional use of dorsal surface of the hand. This is extremely useful in dividing the mesentery while keeping small-bowel loops out from the operative field.

## Technical Aspects Step-by-Step

Our technical principles of TAC are similar either in open, straight laparoscopic or HALS approach, which involve entire colonic mobilization followed by the mesenteric division, both in an inferior-to-superior fashion initially, followed by counterclockwise approach. Since the high ligation of major colonic arteries is often unnecessary (except in the rare situation of multiple synchronous cancers), the authors exclusively use a "lateral-to-medial" approach for colonic mobilization. A "medial-to-lateral" approach can still be used; however, it is not as straightforward as in usual cancer cases due to inflamed mesentery and fragile peri-colonic tissue. The key is to maximally utilize the minilaparotomy to facilitate "open" procedures, i.e., procedures achievable under direct vision, such as small-bowel exploration, partial colonic mobilization, and anastomosis.

### Step 1. Partial Colonic Mobilization Under Direct Vision (Fig. 9.4)

The procedure begins under direct vision with the hand-access device left uncapped (opened). First, the small bowel

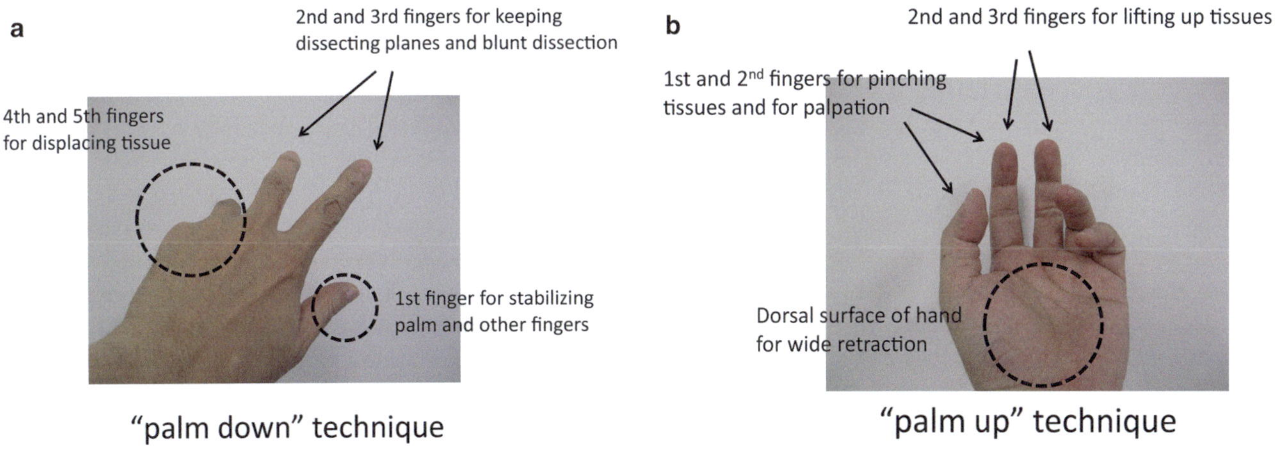


**Fig. 9.3** Schematic representations of (**a**) "palm-down" and (**b**) "palm-up" techniques

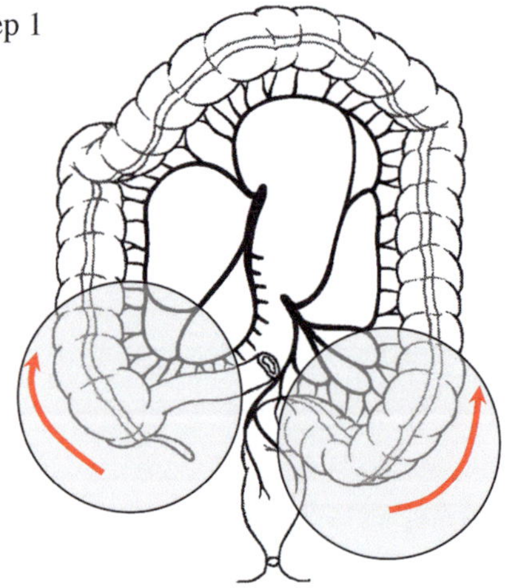


**Fig. 9.4** Step 1 (partial colonic mobilization under direct vision)

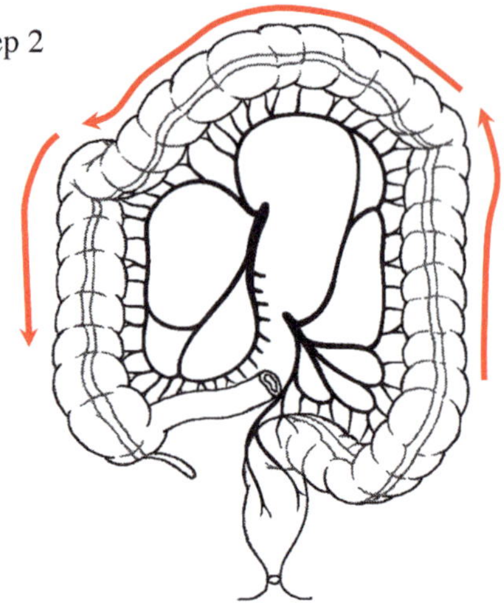


**Fig. 9.6** Step 2 (completion of colonic mobilization under HALS)

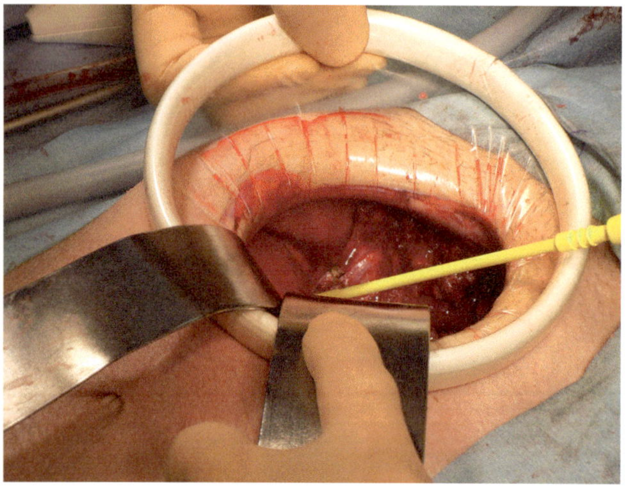

**Fig. 9.5** Mobilizing the sigmoid-descending colon junction under direct vision

is identified and exteriorized to evaluate any "extracolonic" pathologies. This step is extremely important in Crohn's patients, since additional strictureplasty and/or small-bowel resection can be immediately performed under direct vision when a significant lesion is identified during the exploration. This exploration is also important in UC patients to exclude any possibility of "Crohn's disease mimicking UC."

While the hand-access device is kept uncapped, the descending colon and its junction to the sigmoid colon is exposed and partially mobilized (Fig. 9.5). The left ureter can be identified as it crosses over the iliac bifurcation in thin patients (Video 9.3). The dissection can be extended towards the splenic flexure as long as the exposure is adequate and constant. The ileocecal mobilization is then performed on the right side as well (Fig. 9.4). The key is to use long retracting devices for effective displacement of the small-bowel loops.

## Step 2. Completion of Colonic Mobilization Under HALS (Fig. 9.6)

The hand-access device is then sealed, and a pneumoperitoneum is established. HALS begins with the insertion of surgeon's nondominant hand into the abdominal cavity. The colonic mobilization under HALS is initiated from the left side by extending the dissecting plane made at Step 1 (Fig. 9.7). The descending colon is medially retracted using "palm-down" technique. The 2nd and 3rd fingers are used to maintain the dissecting plane onto the lateral attachment. After mobilizing the descending colon, the splenic flexure is cupped with the palm and gently retracted caudally (Fig. 9.8). The splenocolic ligament is thus stretched and effectively taken down with LigaSure™ device. Care is taken to avoid too much traction at this stage to avoid an inadvertent tearing of the splenic capsule.

The omentum is then freed from the transverse colon at its attachment, from the left side to the right side, by inserting the hand between the omentum and transverse mesocolon using "palm-down" technique. During the omental dissection, each finger can be used for effective retraction: stretching the omentum with 2nd and 3rd fingers, while displacing the transverse colon with 4th finger (Fig. 9.9). Alternatively, the lesser sac is first opened at the mid-transverse colon, and the window is then extended to the left side to meet the initial dissecting plane over the splenic flexure.

As the omentum takedown proceeds beyond the mid-transverse colon, the dissection gradually becomes challenging due to mismatch of the working axis of LigaSure™ device and the direction of dissection. This can be solved simply by moving the dissecting area into the effective working area of LigaSure™ device. This so-called "move-the-ground" technique is also useful when the operative field is too close to the laparoscope (Fig. 9.10). The overview can be

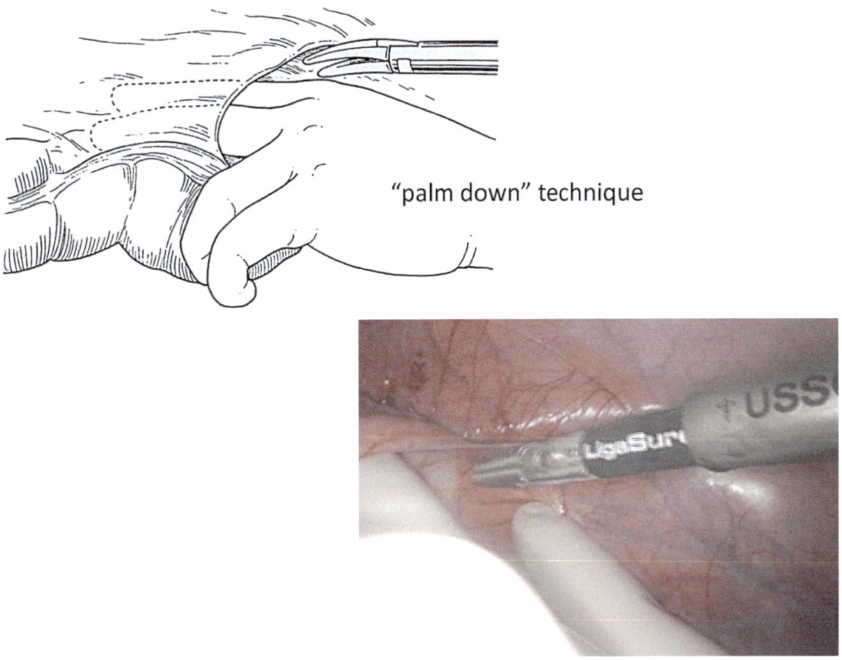


**Fig. 9.7** Mobilizing the descending colon using "lateral-to-medial" approach

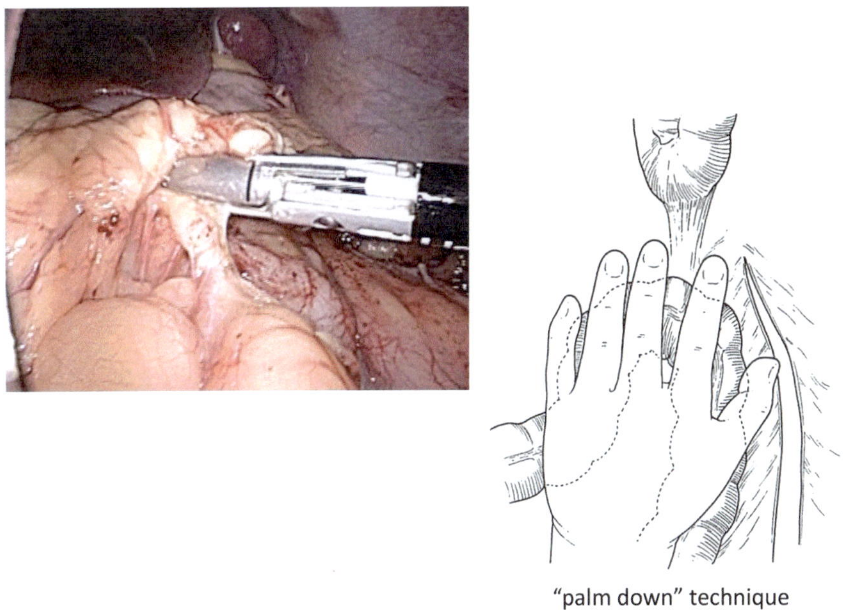


**Fig. 9.8** Taking down the splenic flexure by cupping both the descending and transverse colon in the palm and gently retracting them caudally

obtained by pushing the operative field, not by pulling back the laparoscope (Video 9.4). In order to accomplish this effectively, you must ensure you have adequate mobilization to avoid tearing of the often-fragile tissues.

The transverse colon is mobilized from the duodenum with blunt dissection using the 2nd finger and tip of LigaSure™ device. The hepatic flexure is then mobilized by dissecting the hepato-colonic ligament. The dissection is extended caudal and lateral to the ascending colon, till it meets with the plane made previously at Step 1. The colonic mobilization is completed when the cecum is freed and secured in the surgeon's palm.

## Step 3. Mesenteric Division Under HALS (Fig. 9.11)

The mesenteric division is performed again in a counter-clockwise fashion (from the left side to the right side). Using the "palm-up" technique, the fingers are inserted onto the

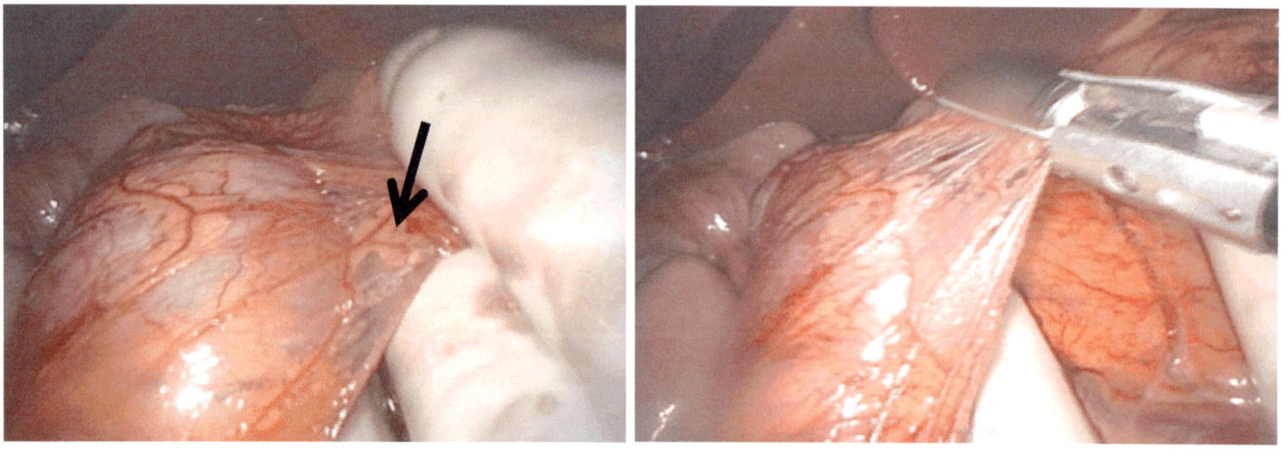

**Fig. 9.9** Taking down the omentum from the transverse colon, using 2nd and 3rd fingers to pinch the omentum and 4th finger to displace the transverse colon

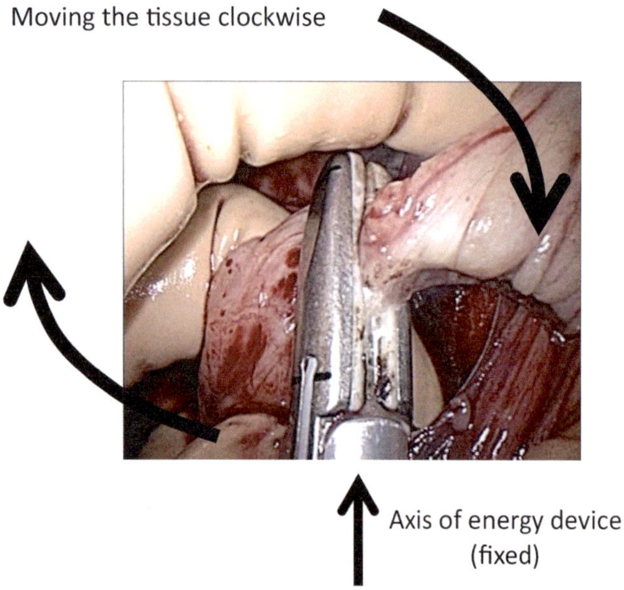


**Fig. 9.10** The concept of "move-the-ground" technique

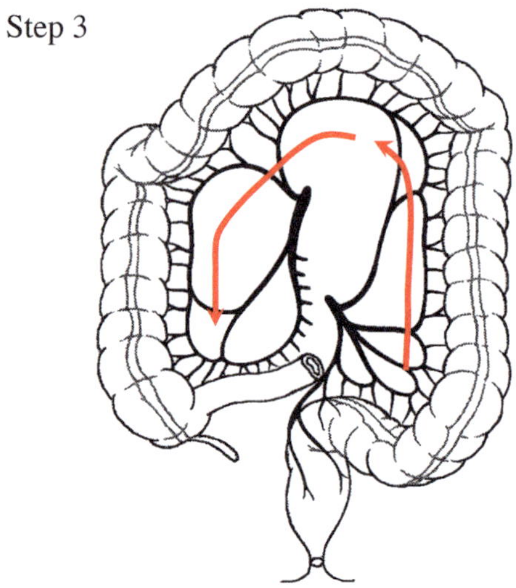


**Fig. 9.11** Step 3 (mesenteric division under HALS)

colonic mesentery behind the descending colon (Fig. 9.12). The mesentery is thus stretched laterally and is easily divided with LigaSure™ device just proximal to the marginal vessels. All major colonic arteries should be positively palpated with 1st and 2nd fingers and then sealed with LigaSure™ device.

As the division reaches to the transverse mesocolon, the small-bowel loops escape from the mesenteric window and might compromise surgical exposure. This can be prevented by "palm-up" technique: the mesentery is pushed up with 2nd and 3rd fingers, while the small bowel is pushed down with the dorsal surface of the hand (Fig. 9.13). Again, the use of "move-the-ground" technique should be considered when the directions of LigaSure™ device and dissecting line are not matched. The entire abdominal colon is freed in the peritoneal cavity when division of the right mesocolon is completed. If the small bowel continues to be a hindrance to clear visualization, changing the position of the patient during this step is often helpful.

## Step 4. Resection, Specimen Extraction, and/or Anastomosis

The hand-access device is opened, and the abdominal colon is exteriorized. Additional mobilization/division can be performed under direct vision when necessitated. The distal colon is then staple transected at the level of the sacral promontory (Fig. 9.14). Brooke end ileostomy or ileorectal anastomosis is completed in a usual fashion.

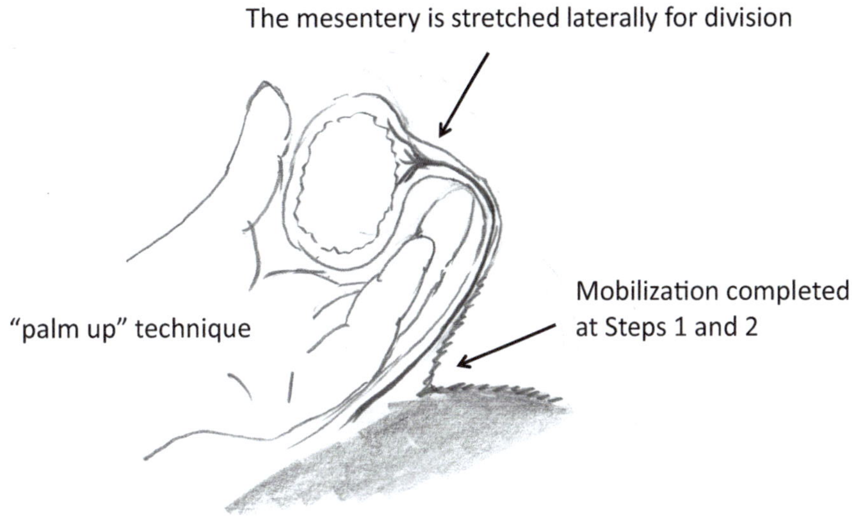


**Fig. 9.12** The mesenteric division using "palm-up" technique. The 2nd to 4th fingers are inserted underneath the mobilized colon, to stretch the mesocolon laterally

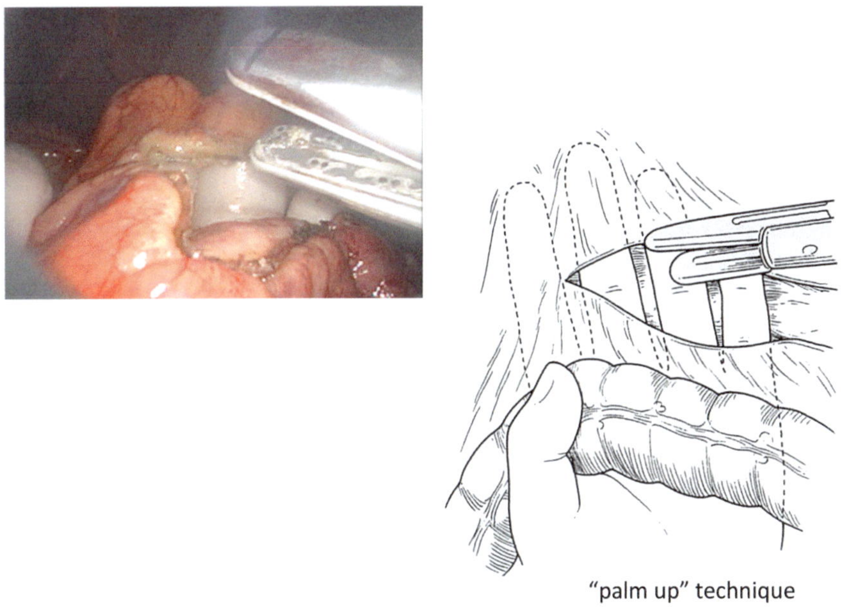


**Fig. 9.13** Dividing transverse mesocolon using "palm-up" technique. The small-bowel loops are displaced from the operative filed using the dorsal surface of the hand

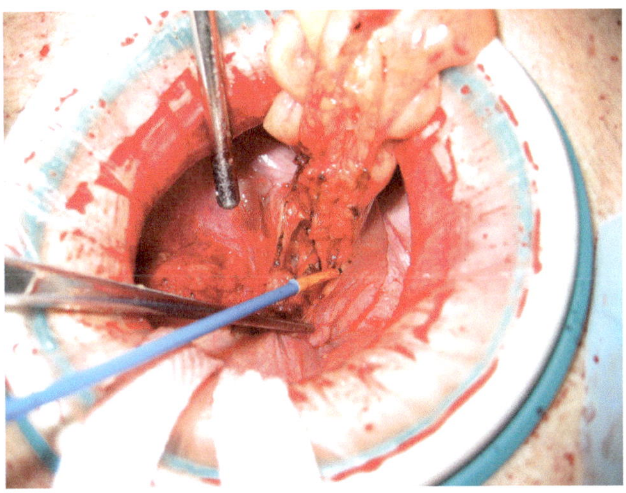

**Fig. 9.14** The remainder of mesenteric division is completed under direct vision

## Special Considerations

Theoretically HALS is suitable for operations that require minilaparotomy for completion [1, 2]. The recovery of tactile sense further contributes to better exposure, easier identification of anatomy, and rapid control of bleeding. HALS thus has been increasingly accepted as practical alternative to straight laparoscopy for complex and extensive colorectal operations such as TAC. Several previous studies including ours have suggested that HALS reduces operative times of TAC, while retaining acceptable morbidity rates and recovery benefits of minimally invasive surgery [1, 2, 4, 7].

HALS is virtually a "solo surgery," since regained tactile feedback can only be enjoyed by the operating surgeon, whereas the other members have to assist him/her only through conventional laparoscopic visual cues [2].

To make HALS procedure most effective and safe, the operating surgeon should deliver his/her sense of palpation verbally to other surgical crew, making timely orientation and understanding possible. The authors believe HALS is not a simple "bridge" for novice, but should be performed by experienced surgeon, since abundant experience and profound understanding with both open and laparoscopic surgery is necessary to give adequate feedback for coordinate performance of the surgical members during the procedure.

## Summary

HALS provides many things to surgeons, e.g., tactile sensation, gentle tissue handling, blunt dissection, and rapid hemostasis. Though these are the "lost items" in the straight laparoscopic era, they are very helpful in performing complex and extensive colorectal procedures such as TAC.

## References

1. Nakajima K, Lee SW, Cocilovo C, Foglia C, Sonoda T, Milsom JW. Laparoscopic total colectomy: hand-assisted vs standard technique. Surg Endosc. 2004;18:582–6.
2. Nakajima K, Nezu R, Hirota M, Nishida T. The role of hand-assisted laparoscopic surgery in subtotal/total colectomy for Crohn's colitis. Surg Endosc. 2010;24:2713–7.
3. Fichera A, McCormack R, Rubin MA, Hurst RD, Michelassi F. Long-term outcome of surgically treated Crohn's colitis: a prospective study. Dis Colon Rectum. 2005;48:963–9.
4. Marcello PW, Fleshman JW, Milsom JW, Read TE, Arnell TD, Birnbaum EH, Feingold DL, Lee SW, Mutch MG, Sonoda T, Yan Y, Whelan RL. Hand-assisted laparoscopic vs. laparoscopic colorectal surgery: a multicenter, prospective, randomized trial. Dis Colon Rectum. 2008;51:818–26.
5. Nakajima K, Lee SW, Cocilovo C, Foglia C, Sonoda T, Milsom JW. Hand-assisted laparoscopic colorectal surgery using GelPort. Surg Endosc. 2004;18:102–5.
6. Nakajima K, Nezu R, Ito T, Nishida T. Hand-assisted laparoscopic restorative proctocolectomy for ulcerative colitis: optimization of instrumentation towards standardization. Surg Today. 2010;40:840–4.
7. Wilhelm TJ, Refeidi A, Palma P, Neufang T, Post S. Hand-assisted laparoscopic sigmoid resection for diverticular disease: 100 consecutive cases. Surg Endosc. 2006;20:477–81.

# 10 Operative Details of Laparoscopic Rectal Resection for Cancer

Martin R. Weiser

**Key Points**

- Preoperative considerations in the setting of rectal cancer are extensive. Meticulous evaluation of the patient before surgery will help identify potentially difficult aspects of the operation.
- Proper radiographic imaging can demonstrate the local extent of the tumor, facilitating a detailed operative plan.
- The single most important factor in optimizing outcomes is complete excision of the tumor with negative macroscopic and microscopic margins.
- Total mesorectal excision (TME) for malignancy involves sharp dissection in relatively avascular planes under direct visualization.

## Introduction

Surgical therapy for rectal cancer encompasses several different operations, ranging from local excision or TEM/TAMIS to total mesorectal excision (TME) and abdominal perineal resection. In properly selected patients, each can provide standard of care for oncologic resection of rectal cancer. A laparoscopic approach to rectal lesions, which is the focus of this chapter, offers an oncologically sound solution to a complex problem, with the added benefits witnessed in other minimally invasive procedures. When performed by experienced surgeons facile in the laparoscopic TME technique, the potential morbidity associated with radical surgery (including major medical complications, impaired sexual and urinary function, wound problems, and the need for a permanent stoma) is in large part reduced compared to an open approach. With the proper selection of appropriate candidates, laparoscopic proctectomy stands as a useful and valuable tool in the surgeon's armamentarium.

## Indications

Benign, premalignant, and cancerous lesions of the rectum involving the various layers of the rectal wall may be removed via a laparoscopic approach. This technique depends in part upon accurate preoperative staging to avoid inadequate resection of more advanced lesions (i.e., T4). Endorectal ultrasound has reported rates of up to 90 % accuracy for determining tumor depth of penetration, along with sensitivity rates of 60–70 % and specificity rates of 70–80 % for nodal metastases. Similarly, MRI is associated with accuracy rates of up to 85 % for primary rectal wall involvement, nodal sensitivity rates of 60–70 %, and specificity rates of 70–80 % [1]. In general, radical resection offers lower recurrence rates when compared to local excision [2]. This is especially true for T2 tumors, where local recurrence has been cited to be as high as 47 % after standard transanal excision. Similarly, lesions possessing poor prognostic risk factors, such as lymphovascular invasion (LVI), poor differentiation, tumor budding, and mucinous or signet cell adenocarcinoma, should typically be resected with a standard TME [3].

## Patient Preparation

Patients receive a full bowel preparation to allow for intraoperative endoscopy. Low molecular weight heparin is given in the preoperative area, and antibiotics are administered within an hour of incision. In the operating room, each calf is wrapped in pneumatic compression stocking and then placed in modified lithotomy position, with legs in padded adjustable stirrups. The legs are positioned in a 20- to 25-degree

**Electronic supplementary material:** Supplementary material is available in the online version of this chapter at 10.1007/978-1-4939-1581-1_10. Videos can also be accessed at http://www.springerimages.com/videos/978-1-4939-1580-4.

M.R. Weiser, M.D. (✉)
Department of Surgery, Memorial Sloan Kettering Cancer Center, 1275 York Avenue, New York, NY 10065, USA
e-mail: weiser1@mskcc.org

H.M. Ross et al. (eds.), *Minimally Invasive Approaches to Colon and Rectal Disease: Technique and Best Practices*, DOI 10.1007/978-1-4939-1581-1_10, © Springer Science+Business Media New York 2015

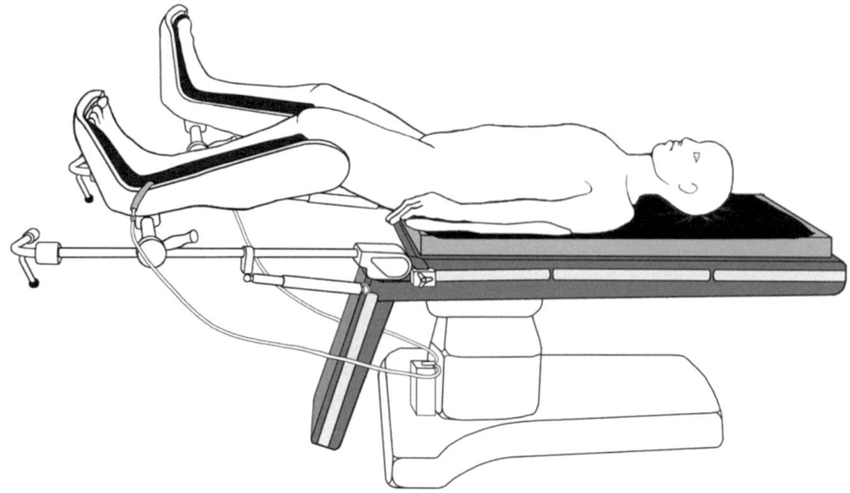

**Fig. 10.1** Patient positioning. *With permission from Nakajima K, Milsom JW, Böhm B. Patient Preparation and Operating Room Setup. In: Milsom JW, Böhm B, Nakajima K, eds. Laparoscopic Colorectal Surgery, 2nd ed. Springer, New York 2006*

abducted position, with the thighs only minimally elevated above the level of the abdomen; higher elevation may cause the surgeon's hands to collide with the thigh when mobilizing the splenic flexure (Fig. 10.1). The patient is positioned with the pelvis just above the break at the lower end of the operating table. This facilitates free access to the perineum for intraoperative endoscopy, pelvic manipulation, perineal resection, or transanal anastomosis. A beanbag or other securing device is used to help maintain position during table rotation and tilt. The hands and arms are padded and tucked at the patient's sides. After the induction of general anesthesia, an indwelling ureteral catheter and orogastric tube are inserted to decompress the bladder and reduce gastric distension.

## Operative Technique (Video 10.1)

The author routinely utilizes the five following ports: one for the laparoscope, two for the operating surgeon, and two for the assistant. A 10-mm infraumbilical port is initially placed using an open technique. A balloon port—which creates an airtight seal—is preferred, as this port is mostly used for the camera. Five-millimeter ports are then placed in the right upper, left upper, and left lower quadrants, under direct laparoscopic vision. A 12-mm port is placed in the right lower quadrant and ultimately utilized for endoscopic stapling. A fascial suture (#0 Vicryl) is placed at the 12-mm stapling port site, using a suture passing technique for fascial closure at the end of the case. All ports are placed at least 8 cm apart on each side to prevent the instrument shafts from crossing each other. I generally use three monitors; however, two monitors are sufficient. One monitor is placed at the patient's left leg and can swing to the left shoulder during splenic flexure mobilization; the other monitor is placed on the right and can be maneuvered between the patient's legs for pelvic dissection (Fig. 10.2).

## Surgeon, Assistant, and Nurse Positioning

Depending on the operative step, all team members will stand in varying positions. It is important to adapt the position based on the patient's body habitus and the particular step of the operation, to maximize ergonomics. For dissection of the mesocolon and mobilization of the splenic flexure, the surgeon and second assistant (camera person) stand on the patient's right side, and the first assistant stands on the patient's left. The nurse is positioned at the patient's left leg. For mesocolon dissection, the surgeon views the monitor positioned near the patient's leg. For splenic flexure mobilization, the second assistant moves between the patient's legs; all team members look at the left-sided monitor, which is repositioned to the patient's left shoulder. For pelvic dissection, the surgeon and second assistant stand on the patient's right side, and the first assistant stands on the left side. All team members view the monitor between the patient's legs.

## Dissection of the Mesocolon and Vascular Pedicle

Following initial inspection of the peritoneal cavity, including liver, omentum, and pelvis, the patient is positioned in Trendelenburg for dissection of the mesocolon and vascular pedicle. The omentum is placed superiorly above the colon and onto the liver. The patient is tilted right-side down; this allows placement of the small intestine in the right upper quadrant, out of the area of dissection. Using 5-mm bowel

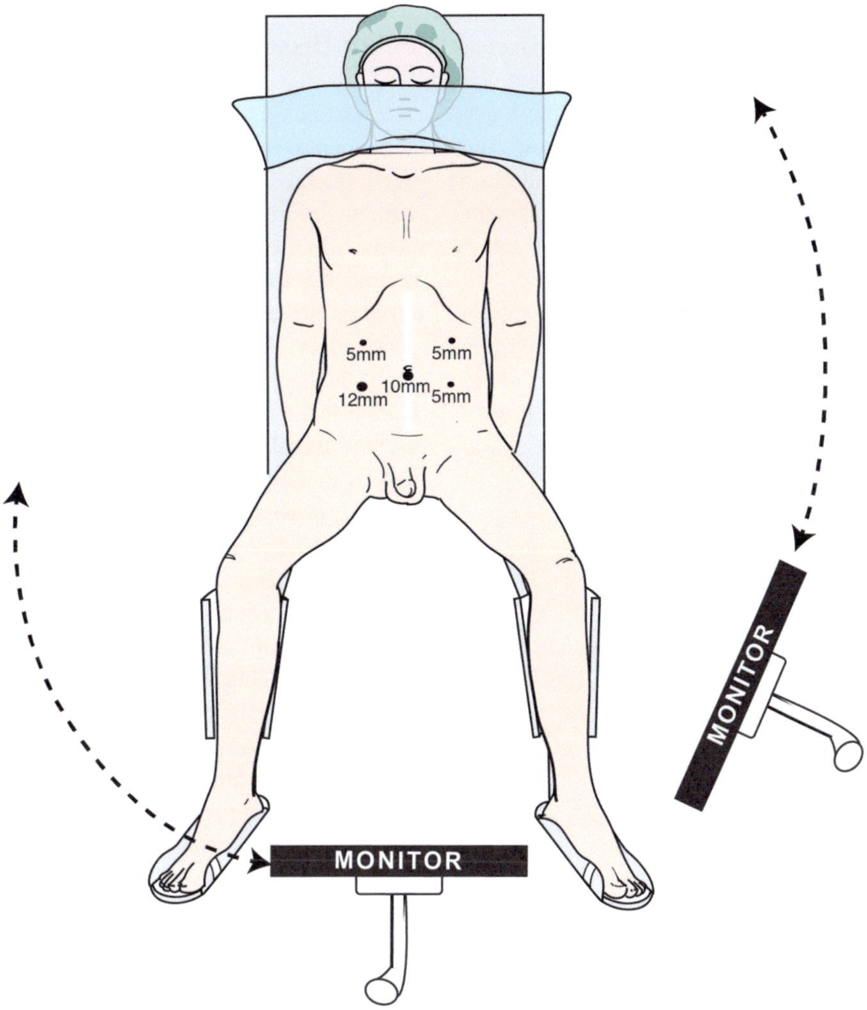


**Fig. 10.2** One monitor is placed at the patient's left leg and can swing to the left shoulder during splenic flexure mobilization; the other monitor is placed on the right and can be maneuvered between the patient's legs for pelvic dissection. *With permission from Memorial Sloan Kettering Cancer Center*

graspers through the left-sided cannulas, the assistant holds the sigmoid ventrally under traction and to the left. In a medial to lateral fashion, the inferior mesenteric artery (IMA) is identified and the retroperitoneum is incised, starting at the sacral promontory to the right of (i.e., under) the vessel. Dissection is continued in a cephalad direction to the base of the IMA. Using gentle blunt dissection, the mesentery is dissected off the retroperitoneum. Dissection proceeds adjacent to and just below the IMA, which is swept ventrally, to ensure that the preaortic hypogastric sympathetic nerves are preserved and swept dorsally. Dissection beneath the mesentery is continued laterally, until the left ureter and gonadal vessels are identified and swept posteriorly. Once the origin of the IMA is identified, the peritoneum is incised anteriorly over the pedicle and away from the left colic artery. A peritoneal window is made just lateral to the inferior mesenteric vein (IMV). This permits ligation of the IMA and IMV pedicle, generally distal to the left colic artery (Fig. 10.3). We employ a bipolar device for vascular ligation, but occasionally use endoscopic staplers or clips. Care is taken to revisualize the left ureter before ligation and division of the IMA and IMV.

## Splenic Flexure and Left Colon Mobilization

The second phase of the procedure is left colon mobilization. Through the peritoneal window, the left mesocolon is bluntly dissected from the underlying retroperitoneal structures, including the gonadal vessels, ureter, Gerota's fascia, and pancreas (Fig. 10.4). If splenic flexure mobilization is necessary, the submesenteric dissection is continued until the spleen is visible and the lesser sac is entered. This can also be performed in a medial to lateral fashion by dissection just under the IMV adjacent to the ligament of Treitz and the pancreas. The IMV is divided adjacent to the pancreas, before it joins the splenic vein to form the portal vein. This enables full mobilization of the left colon and mesentery. The greater omentum is then freed from the transverse colon edge toward the midline, as far as necessary, to allow the descending colon to reach to the pelvis. The left colon is then mobilized by sharply dividing the lateral peritoneal attachments along the white line of Toldt (Fig. 10.5).

After the mobilization of the left colon, the sigmoid mesocolon is divided to the appropriate area of the colon; this will become the proximal resection line. The colon is transected at this level with an endoscopic stapler (Fig. 10.6).

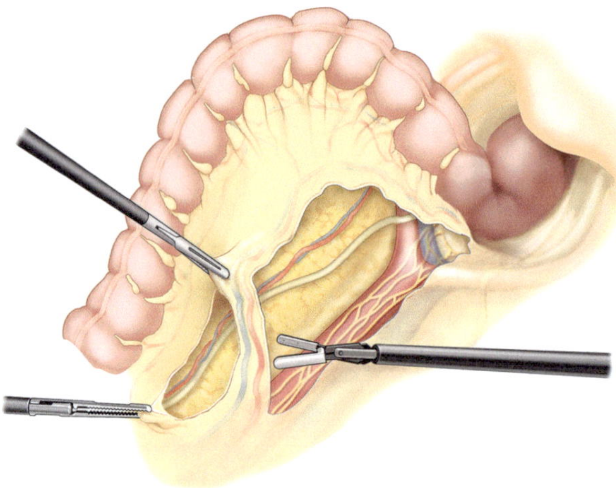

**Fig. 10.3** A peritoneal window is made just lateral to the inferior mesenteric vein (IMV), permitting ligation of the IMA and IMV pedicle. *With permission from Memorial Sloan Kettering Cancer Center*

## Pelvic Dissection

The next phase of the operation is mesocolic dissection. The surgeon moves back to the right side of the table. The goal is to completely remove the rectum with an intact mesorectum, without injuring the pelvic autonomic nerves. The peritoneum is incised along both sides of the rectum down to and around the anterior peritoneal reflection. The dissection is initiated posterior to the rectum, at the level of the sacral promontory. The plane between the parietal and visceral layers of the endopelvic fascia is dissected sharply with cautery. Care is taken to immediately identify the hypogastric nerves as they travel anterolaterally across the aortic bifurcation, approximately 2 cm medial to the ureters bilaterally. Dissection along the visceral peritoneum (fascia propria of the rectum) will maintain the plane of dissection above the hypogastric nerves and avoid injury to these structures.

Dissection continues posterolaterally until the junction of the mesorectum and pelvic autonomic nerve plexus is encountered. This area is referred to as the lateral rectal stalks, and care is taken to maintain sharp dissection along the mesorectum to avoid parasympathetic nerve injury (Fig. 10.7). The area of dissection may contain small blood vessels emanating from the pelvic sidewall, which can generally be well controlled with cautery or—rarely—bipolar. The surgeon must be wary of straying into the pelvic sidewall, as this can result in substantial bleeding and nerve injury. The area of dissection is enhanced using the laparoscope, because of the magnification it provides. Inferior to the level of S3, the rectosacral ligament (Waldeyer's fascia) is divided sharply with cautery or bipolar. Blunt dissection

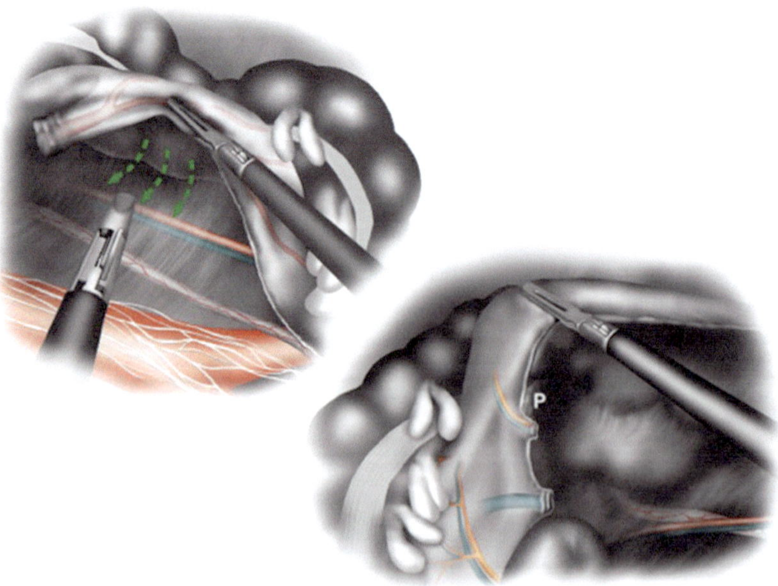


**Fig. 10.4** Medial dissection. (*Top*): an avascular plane exits between Toldt's fascia and the mesocolon, which is briefly dissected medial to lateral after IMA and IMV ligation. (*Bottom*): medial to lateral dissection beneath the left mesocolon provides excellent views of the distal pancreas (P), the base of the left transverse mesocolon and retroperitoneum. *With permission from: Leroy J, Henri M, Rubino F, Marescaux J. Sigmoidectomy. In: Milsom JW, Böhm B, Nakajima K, eds. Laparoscopic Colorectal Surgery, 2nd ed. Springer, New York 2006*

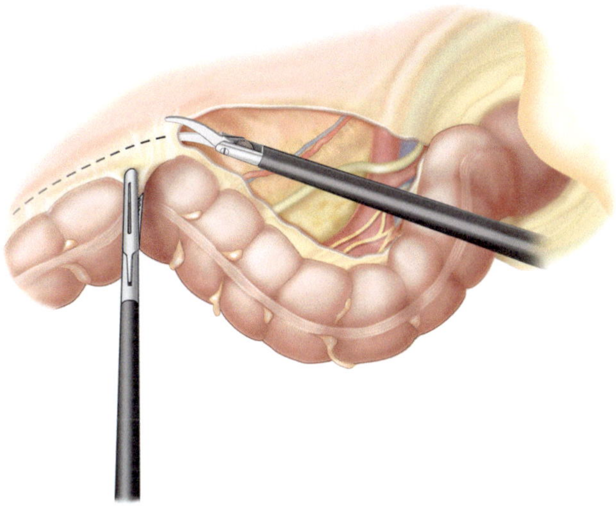

**Fig. 10.5** Mobilization of the left colon is achieved by sharply dividing the lateral peritoneal attachments along the white line of Toldt. *With permission from Memorial Sloan Kettering Cancer Center*

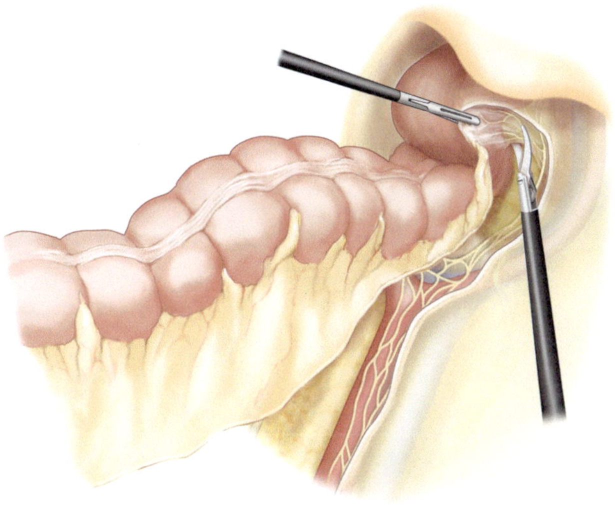

**Fig. 10.7** Dissection posterolaterally to the junction of the mesorectum and pelvic autonomic nerve plexus. This area is referred to as the lateral rectal stalks, and care is taken to maintain sharp dissection along the mesorectum to avoid parasympathetic nerve injury. *With permission from Memorial Sloan Kettering Cancer Center*

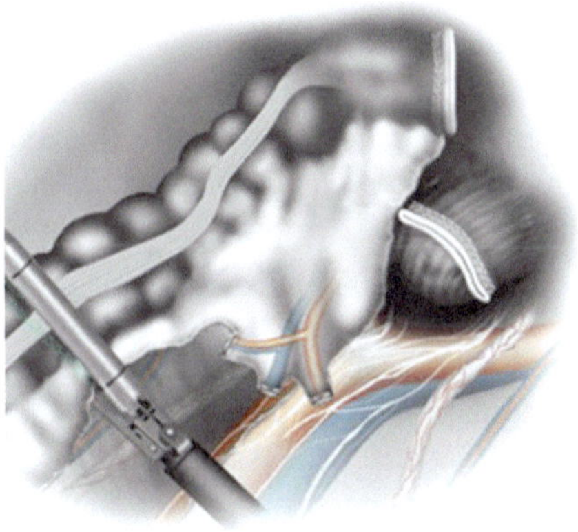

**Fig. 10.6** Division of the sigmoid. (*Top*): proximal bowel division is performed after dividing the mesocolon up to the chosen site. (*Bottom*): specimen extraction at the suprapubic site involves double protection: (1) wound protector. *With permission from: Leroy J, Henri M, Rubino F, Marescaux J. Sigmoidectomy. In: Milsom JW, Böhm B, Nakajima K, eds. Laparoscopic Colorectal Surgery, 2nd ed. Springer, New York 2006*

should be avoided to prevent tearing into the mesorectum or presacral fascia and injuring the presacral venous plexus. The angle of dissection follows the curves of the sacrum, proceeding in an anterior direction to the pelvic floor.

Anterior dissection of the peritoneum in the pouch of Douglas is usually performed last. For anterior tumors in male patients, dissection is anterior to Denonvilliers' fascia, exposing the seminal vesicles bilaterally (Fig. 10.8). In female patients, dissection occurs in the rectovaginal septum. Anterior elevation of the vagina, by an assistant holding a sponge stick in the vaginal vault, helps provide appropriate tissue tension for dissection.

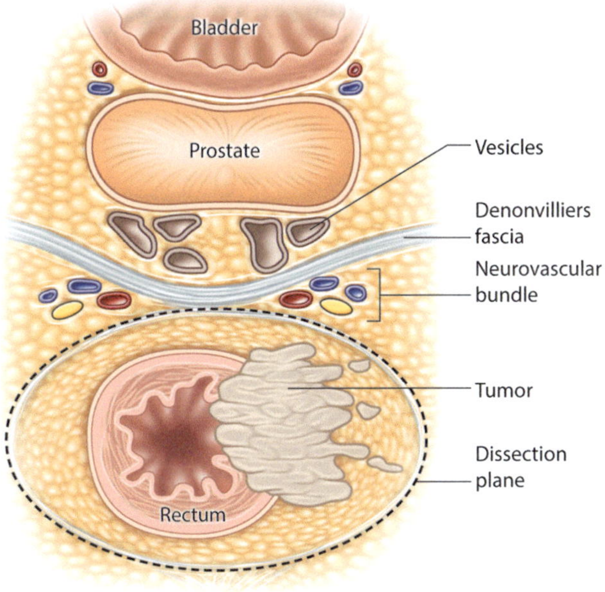


**Fig. 10.8** Denonvilliers' fascia

The precise point of distal resection is determined by sigmoidoscopy, which is performed at the time of resection. The proximal bowel is closed with a laparoscopic bowel clamp, and a flexible sigmoidoscope/proctoscope locates the

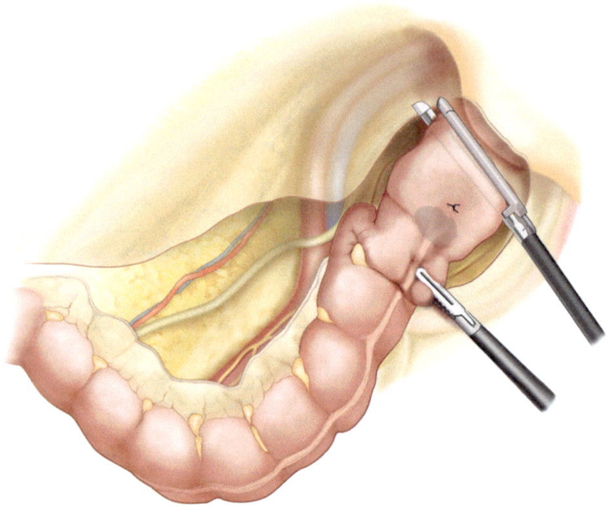

**Fig. 10.9** Before stapling, the rectum is occluded below the level of the tumor, and the distal rectum is irrigated with saline. *With permission from Memorial Sloan Kettering Cancer Center*

lesion. By transillumination or palpation of the sigmoidoscope with a laparoscopic instrument, the lower edge of the tumor in the rectum is identified.

## Division of the Rectum (Video 10.2)

The rectum is then divided at least 2 cm below the mid- and distal lesions and 5 cm below upper rectal lesions. If the pelvis is wide, an endoscopic stapler can be used under laparoscopic guidance to divide the rectum. Before stapling, the rectum is occluded below the level of the tumor, and the distal rectum is irrigated with saline (Fig. 10.9). A laparoscopic stapler is then deployed below the clamp on the bowel. After enlarging the port site and placing a wound protector, the specimen is usually removed at the umbilicus.

In the case of a narrow pelvis in which the endoscopic stapler cannot be properly positioned, a low transverse incision with a wound protector is usually employed. The rectum is occluded, irrigated, stapled, and divided using an open technique.

## Colorectal/Coloanal Anastomosis

The final stage of the operation is the creation of an end-to-end anastomosis with a circular stapler. If a low transverse incision is utilized, the anastomosis can be performed using an open technique. If the distal rectum was successfully stapled laparoscopically, the anastomosis is performed laparoscopically. The mobilized descending colon is delivered through either the enlarged umbilical port site or the low transverse incision (Fig. 10.10a). The anvil of the circular stapler is then placed into the descending colon lumen, and a purse-string is tied around the center rod in the usual manner (Fig. 10.10b). The proximal bowel is then returned to the peritoneal cavity, and the abdominal wall is closed by occluding the wound protector. Pneumoperitoneum is reestablished; the shaft of the stapler is brought to the stapled end of the rectum, and the pin is advanced through the rectal wall. The groove in the center rod is held with an endoscopic clamp through the right lower quadrant cannula and by locking the center rod into the center post of the circular stapler (Fig. 10.11). This locking action requires that the axes of the center rod and the center post be in a perfect line. Because the center rod protruding from the proximal colon is grasped with an instrument from the right lower quadrant, its tip will be slightly directed to the right side of the pelvis. Thus, the circular stapler head should be directed slightly to the left side. After deploying the stapler, it is removed, and the tissue rings are inspected. The anastomosis is tested for leaks by filling the pelvis with saline, occluding the left colon, and insufflating air into the rectum via a proctoscope (Fig. 10.12). The anastomosis is visualized for completeness and hemostasis.

When performing ultralow coloanal anastomosis with intersphincteric dissection, the specimen is removed via the perineum. The descending colon is then divided at the level of the anal canal in preparation for a hand-sewn reconstruction. Full thickness colon is secured to the mucosa of the anal canal, with the incorporation of muscle with interrupted suture in a single layer technique.

A loop ileostomy is placed in patients with coloanal anastomosis who have received preoperative chemoradiation. This can be performed with laparoscopic assistance. It is placed in the right lower quadrant, at a site ideally marked by an enterostomal nurse preoperatively. A flat drain is passed through the 5-mm right upper quadrant cannula and guided into the pelvis with a bowel grasper.

## Pearls and Pitfalls

- When starting the dissection at the sacral promontory, ensure that you have all of the redundant sigmoid colon out of the pelvis. This will help you identify the IMA and avoid getting in the wrong plane.
- When performing a medial approach to the left colon, avoid tunneling after scoring the mesentery underneath the IMA. Keep a broad plane of dissection as you work toward the base of the IMA to allow for maximal visualization and safe dissection.
- Dissection, aside from dealing with the major vascular pedicles, should be relatively avascular. If you encounter moderate-significant bleeding, you are likely in the wrong plane and need to stop and reassess.
- Applying perineal pressure will push the pelvic floor superiorly and can aid in dissection.

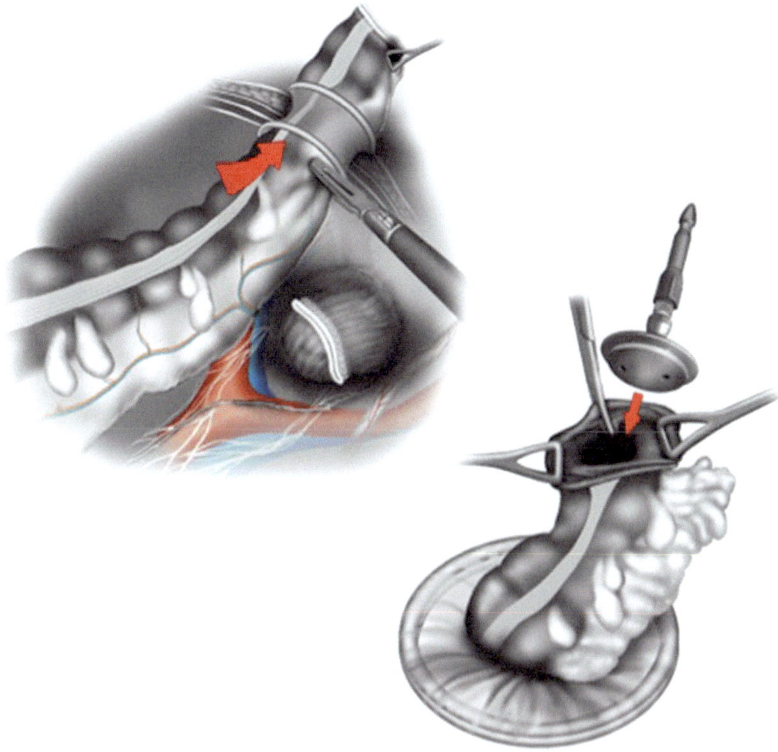

**Fig. 10.10** Exteriorization. (**a**, *Top*): after specimen extraction, the colon is drawn out through this site, keeping the wound protector in place. (**b**, *Bottom*): the anvil and center rod of the circular stapler are introduced into the bowel lumen and secured with a purse-string suture. *With permission from: Leroy J, Henri M, Rubino F, Marescaux J. Sigmoidectomy. In: Milsom JW, Böhm B, Nakajima K, eds. Laparoscopic Colorectal Surgery, 2nd ed. Springer, New York 2006*

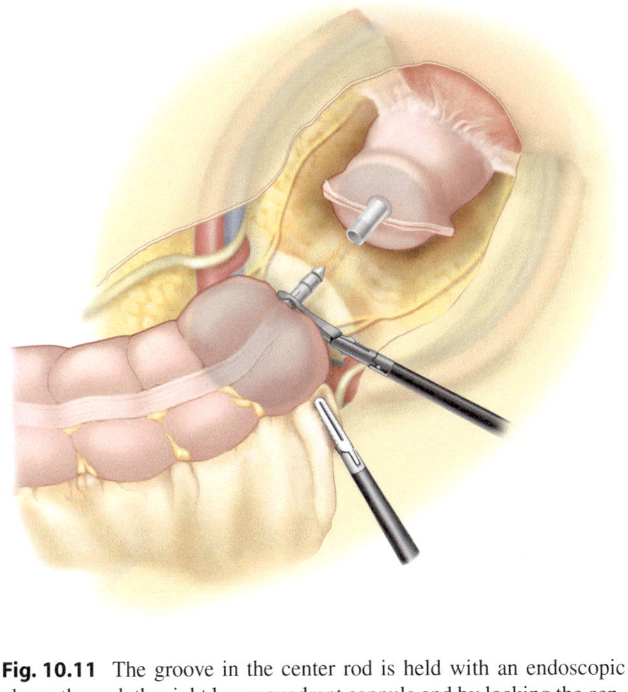

**Fig. 10.11** The groove in the center rod is held with an endoscopic clamp through the right lower quadrant cannula and by locking the center rod into the center post of the circular stapler. *With permission from Memorial Sloan Kettering Cancer Center*

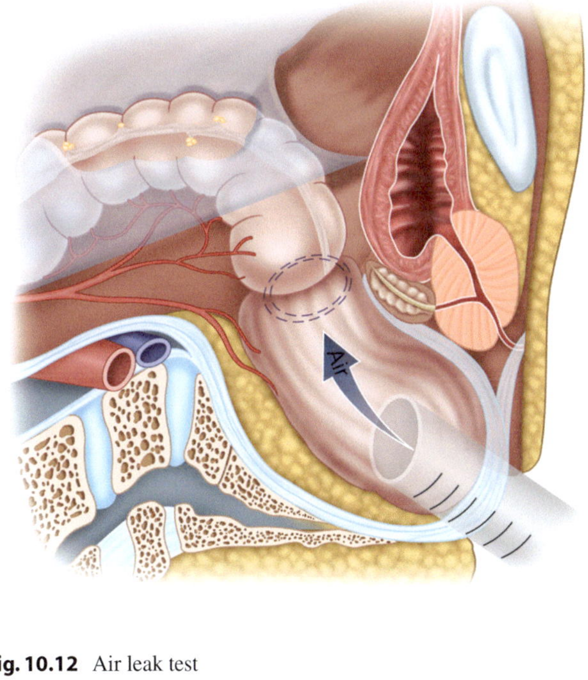


**Fig. 10.12** Air leak test

## Conclusion

A straight laparoscopic approach to rectal cancer can be successfully utilized as the surgical procedure of choice by those with appropriate expertise. While this approach can be technically demanding and requires advanced laparoscopic skills, in most cases, your patient will reap the benefits from a minimally invasive approach.

## References

1. Bipat S, Glas AS, Slors FJ, Zwinderman AH, Bossuyt PM, Stoker J. Rectal cancer: local staging and assessment of lymph node involvement with endoluminal US, CT, and MR imaging—a meta-analysis. Radiology. 2004;232:773–83.
2. Paty PB, Nash GM, Baron P, et al. Long-term results of local excision for rectal cancer. Ann Surg. 2002;236:522–9.
3. Bretagnol F, Rullier E, George B, Warren BF, Mortensen NJ. Local therapy for rectal cancer: still controversial? Dis Colon Rectum. 2007;50:523–33.

# Laparoscopic Hand-Assisted Low Anterior Resection

# 11

Govind Nandakumar and Sang W. Lee

**Key Points**

- The hand-assisted approach to LAR offers the same benefits as a straight laparoscopic approach while providing the added advantage of tactile feedback and use of the hand.
- A Pfannenstiel incision for the hand-assisted device is ideally suited for a low anterior resection.
- After placing the hand-assisted device, use your hand inside the abdomen to protect the intra-abdominal contents when placing your trocars.
- A sponge is extremely useful to aid in retraction, visualization, "drying" the operative field and cleaning the camera. Have a method in place to keep track of your sponges in addition to the routine counts.
- Ligation of the IMV near the ligament of Treitz provides additional length to help ensure a tension-free anastomosis.
- The hand-assisted device can be used in several methods to complete the total mesorectal excision (TME) from placing trocars through it or using the hand to pull up the specimen during posterior dissection.

## Background

Laparoscopy has been increasingly adopted for surgical resections of the colon and the rectum. While laparoscopy for colon cancer has been well studied and the short and long-term data have matured [1], rectal cancer surgery is technically more challenging, and the data for a laparoscopic approach in rectal cancer is not as robust. In this gap, hand-assisted laparoscopic colon surgery can offer several advantages, while retaining many of the benefits of traditional laparoscopy. This chapter focuses on the technical aspects of hand-assisted low anterior resection (HALAR) for the treatment of rectal and rectosigmoid cancer.

## Indications

A low anterior resection may be indicated for benign or malignant disease processes. This chapter focuses on HALAR for malignant disease. However, this technique could be used for benign indications such as sigmoid colectomy for diverticulitis or Crohn's disease, resection of large polyps, treatment of intermittent sigmoid volvulus, and resection with rectopexy for rectal prolapse.

## Preoperative Planning

### Patient History and Physical Findings

A complete history and physical focusing on the underlying pathology is essential. For patients with colon cancer and/or polyps, a detailed surgical history, personal cancer history, and family history are essential. Preoperative genetic counseling and testing may be considered based on age and family history.

- Prior abdominal surgery, distension and obstruction are important to elicit in the history and physical examination prior to making a decision regarding pursuing an open versus laparoscopic approach.
- History and physical examination should also evaluate the cardiovascular and respiratory systems to assess the ability to tolerate pneumoperitoneum.
- Nutritional status and recent history of major weight loss should be considered in the decision to perform a primary anastomosis and/or a diverting ostomy.

**Electronic supplementary material:** Supplementary material is available in the online version of this chapter at 10.1007/978-1-4939-1581-1_11. Videos can also be accessed at http://www.springerimages.com/videos/978-1-4939-1580-4.

G. Nandakumar, M.D. (✉) • S.W. Lee, M.D.
Division of Colon and Rectal Surgery, Department of Surgery, Weill Cornell Medical College, 525 East 68th Street, Box 172, New York, NY 10065, USA
e-mail: doctorgovind@gmail.com; sal2013@med.cornell.edu

H.M. Ross et al. (eds.), *Minimally Invasive Approaches to Colon and Rectal Disease: Technique and Best Practices*, DOI 10.1007/978-1-4939-1581-1_11, © Springer Science+Business Media New York 2015

## Imaging and Diagnostic Studies

- All patients with colon or rectal cancer and/or a polyp should have a complete extent of disease workup including carcino embryonic antigen (CEA), computed tomography (CT) of the abdomen and pelvic, chest x-ray or chest CT, colonoscopy and routine preoperative laboratory testing.
- The CT should be reviewed carefully to assess adjacent organ involvement, metastatic disease, and obstructive disease.
- An MRI of the pelvis or an endorectal ultrasound is important in staging the tumor to make a decision regarding neoadjuvant chemotherapy and/or radiation. In addition, this can provide information regarding a threatened circumferential margin and the need for an extended or en bloc resection.
- A laparoscopic approach may not be feasible in the presence of massive distension, adjacent organ involvement and obstruction.
- Advanced tumors, low rectal cancers, and adjacent organ involvement generally require neoadjuvant treatment. The hand-assisted approach is useful in these difficult cases as it permits the use of a combination of laparoscopy for mobilization and open techniques to complete the pelvic dissection.
- Colonoscopy and evaluation of the entire colon is important to ensure there are no synchronous lesions proximal or distal to the area of resection. In large obstructing tumors, preoperative colonoscopy may not be feasible. On the table, $CO_2$ colonoscopy and colonoscopy after neoadjuvant treatment are considerations. $CO_2$ rather than conventional air colonoscopy should be used intraoperatively in order to avoid prolonged colonic distension, which can hinder laparoscopy.
- We recommend endoscopic tattooing to be performed just distal to the tumor and in three quadrants. Tattooing is also important prior to neoadjuvant treatment as it identifies the location of the tumor if there is a complete response. Relying only on the distance from the anal verge, especially for more proximal lesions is fraught with the potential for error.
- A digital examination and proctoscopy by an experienced surgeon are very important in assessing the rectal cancer. The size of the tumor, distance from the dentate line, circumferential involvement, anterior versus posterior location, mobility, and tonicity of the sphincter are important in operative planning.
- Preoperative marking by a trained enterostomal therapist helps prevent common pouching difficulties should the patient need diversion.

## Surgical Management

### Preoperative Planning

- The patient receives a mechanical bowel preparation to facilitate handling of the colon and to facilitate intraoperative colonoscopy, if required. While the need for bowel preparation is controversial, the consequences of a leak may be more significant without preparation.
- The patient is seen and evaluated by the surgical and anesthesia teams in the preoperative area on the day of surgery.
- Most patients are offered and elect to have an epidural or intravenous catheter for patient-controlled anesthesia.
- A second- or third-general cephalosporin or ertapenem is used for antibiotic prophylaxis within 1 h of skin incision and re-dosed as needed. No antibiotics are administered postoperatively.
- Venodyne boots and 5,000 U of subcutaneous heparin are used for deep vein thrombosis prophylaxis.
- A Foley catheter is used in all patients and removed as early as possible.
- Ureteral stents are used selectively in cases of recurrent surgery, neoadjuvant chemoradiation therapy, and prior inflammatory conditions (i.e., abscess/leak).

### Positioning

- The patient is positioned in a modified lithotomy position with both arms tucked to the sides. It is essential to ensure that all pressure points, fingers, and calves are padded adequately.
- The use of a beanbag and cloth tape allows extreme positioning with decrease in possibility of patient sliding.
- Alternatively, the use of Gel Pads makes routine taping of patient not necessary.
- The practice of using shoulder braces should be avoided as they can cause brachial plexus injury.
- Prior to draping, the patient is placed in steep Trendelenburg and on either side to ensure that the patient is secured well on the operating table.
- It is essential to ensure that both knees are in line with the torso in order to avoid collision of instruments to patient's thighs when working in the upper quadrants of the abdomen.
- The abdomen is prepped from the nipples to the mid-thigh.
- Access to the anus is always maintained for possible intraoperative colonoscopy and assessment of the tumor and extent of dissection, and to perform the anastomosis.
- Figure 11.1 shows one possible setup for use of the hand port.

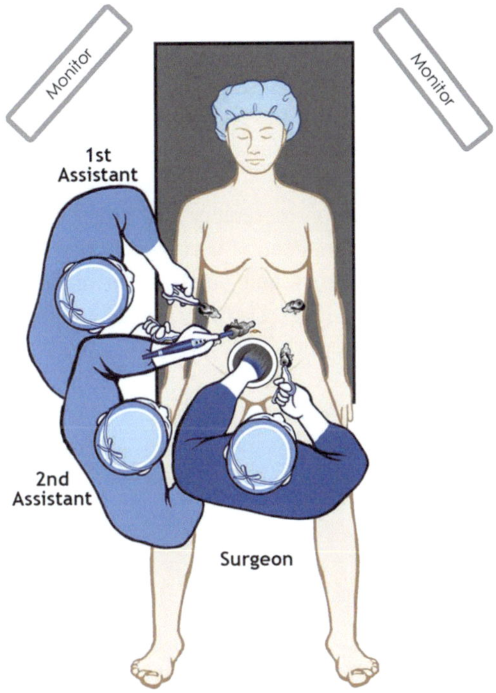


**Fig. 11.1** OR setup with the teaching surgeon using his hand and trainee operating. *With permission from Carter J, Whelan RL. Hand assisted laparoscopic anterior resection. In: Milsom JW, Bohm B, Nakajima K, eds. Laparoscopic colorectal surgery. Springer, New York 2006;pp:255-273. © Springer 2006*

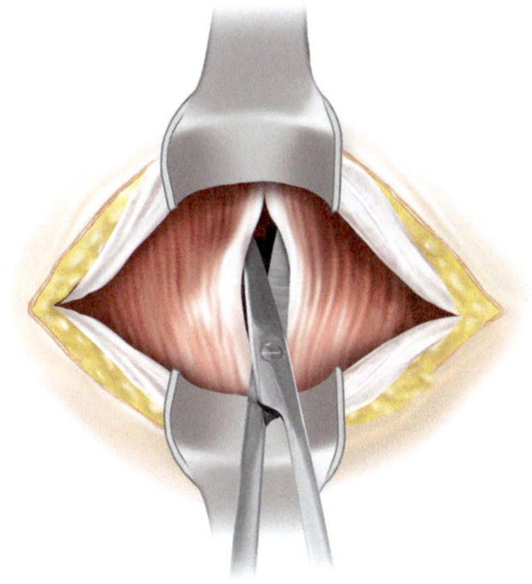

**Fig. 11.2** Pfannenstiel incision showing muscle separation along the midline. *With permission from Yuko Tonohira*

## Procedure

### Port Placement and Hand Device

The ideal features of a hand-assisted device have previously been defined [2]. The device needs to be flexible to allow for a wide range of motion of the surgeon's hand without permitting gas leakage. The device should also function as a wound protector and retractor for portions of the operation that will be performed through the hand-access device. The ergonomics of the device are also essential to ensure surgeon comfort and appropriate circulation to the surgeon's hand during long operations.

For a low anterior resection, a Pfannenstiel incision, opening the anterior fascia transversely and dividing the posterior fascia longitudinally without dividing the rectus, is well suited (Fig. 11.2). It is important to dissect the anterior fascia off the rectus superiorly almost to the umbilicus and inferiorly as far as possible. This maneuver is the key in achieving adequate retraction and exposure. This incision has a low incidence of hernia formation [3]. Perforating vessels should be carefully controlled to prevent a rectus sheath hematoma. One disadvantage of this incision is that conversion to an open may require a midline incision that will eventually lead to an inverted "T"-shaped incision. The actual length of the incision is usually dependent on the glove size of the surgeon. A general rule of thumb is to create an incision the same length as the surgeon's glove size in centimeters.

For cases where the likelihood of conversion to open surgery is high, a lower midline incision for the hand-access device is better suited. This incision allows for easy conversion to a midline laparotomy, should it be necessary.

After induction of anesthesia, the abdomen is draped in the usual fashion, and a Pfannenstiel incision is made 1–2 fingerbreadths above the top of pubis. After raising flaps as described earlier, the peritoneal cavity is entered with careful attention to protecting the bowel and the urinary bladder. Placing the patient in Trendelenburg position helps move the small bowel away from the pelvis. The flexible ring of the wound protector is inserted and flattened against the parietal peritoneum.

A 10 mm port is placed at the umbilicus under manual guidance through hand port. The lid of the hand-assisted device is placed and pneumoperitoneum is established. Exploratory laparoscopy is performed to rule out metastatic disease. The feasibility of a laparoscopic approach can also be established at this time.

Under direct visualization, two 5 mm ports are placed on the right side—lateral to the rectus muscle to avoid the inferior epigastric artery. The trocars should be one palm breath from each other and away from the anterior superior iliac spine. If a stoma is planned on the right side, our preference is to place trocars lateral and well away from stoma to avoid pouching difficulties with trocar sites. One or two 5 mm trocars are also placed on the left side (Fig. 11.3).

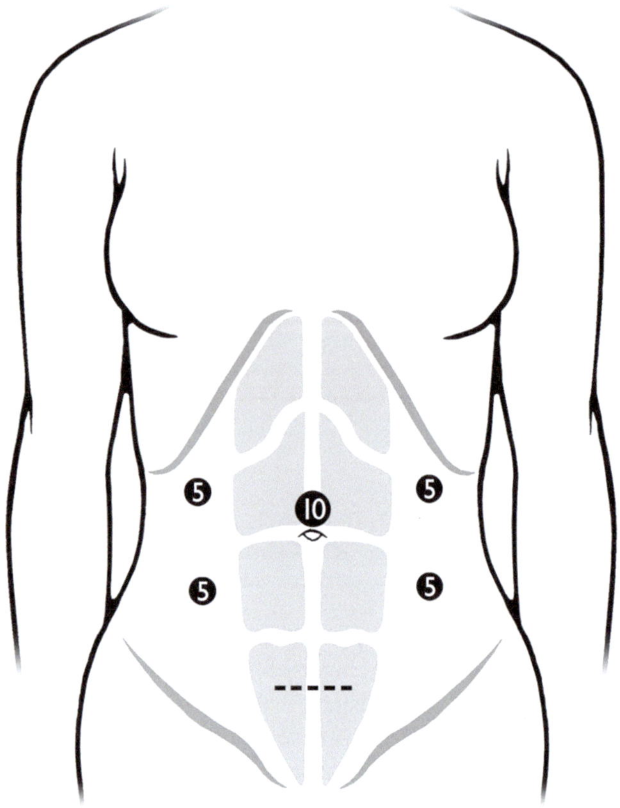


**Fig. 11.3** Suggested port placement. *With permission from Yuko Tonohira*

The monitors are positioned on both sides of the patient, with two monitors positioned on the left. The operating surgeon can stand on the right of the patient—using his/her right hand through the hand-assisted device and the left hand with a dissecting tool. A teaching surgeon may choose to stand between the legs and use either hand to expose for a trainee or operating surgeon.

The use of a moist laparotomy pad or a tagged towel placed intracorporeally through the hand-access device can facilitate retraction of the small intestines and cleaning of the laparoscope [4].

## Positioning and Alterations During Case

The patient is placed in the steep Trendelenburg position and left side up. The omentum is positioned superior to the transverse colon. The small bowel is moved to the right of the abdomen. At this point, there should be clear visualization of the mesentery of the left colon, the ligament of Treitz and the inferior mesenteric artery and vein. Placing the patient in reverse Trendelenburg may facilitate takedown of the splenic flexure.

## Technical Aspects

### Mobilization

- Place the greater omentum in the upper abdomen over the liver and the small bowel to the upper right quadrant of the abdomen (Fig. 11.4).
- Expose the left colon mesentery and inferior mesenteric artery and vein. The hand is used to identify and follow the sacral promontory and put traction on the inferior mesenteric artery (Fig. 11.5) by retracting the pedicle superiorly and anteriorly.

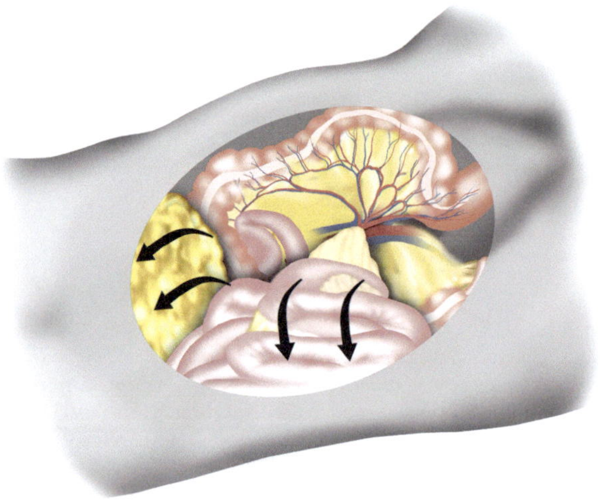

**Fig. 11.4** Exposure is achieved by placing the omentum in the upper abdomen and the small bowel in the right upper quadrant. *With permission* from *Leroy J, Henri M, Rubino F, Marescaux J. Sigmoidectomy. In: Milsom JW, Bohm B, Nakajima K, eds. Laparoscopic colorectal surgery. Springer, New York 2006;pp:145-169. © Springer 2006*

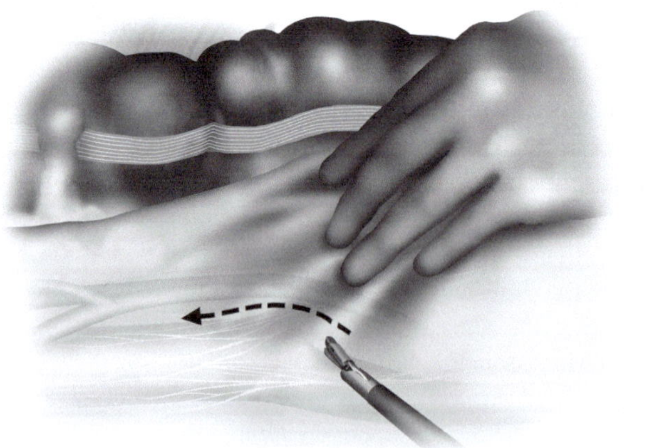

**Fig. 11.5** Lateral traction on the sigmoid colon exposes the inferior mesenteric artery. *With permission from Carter J, Whelan RL. Hand assisted laparoscopic anterior resection. In: Milsom JW, Bohm B, Nakajima K, eds. Laparoscopic colorectal surgery. Springer, New York 2006;pp:255-273. © Springer 2006*

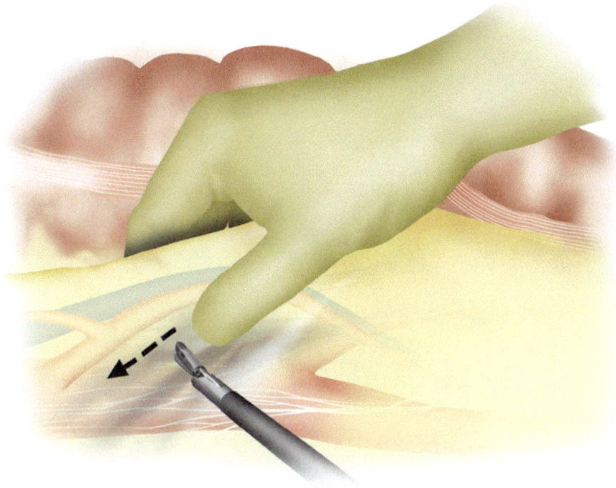

**Fig. 11.6** A peritoneal window is created to start the retromesenteric dissection. *With permission from Yuko Tonohira*

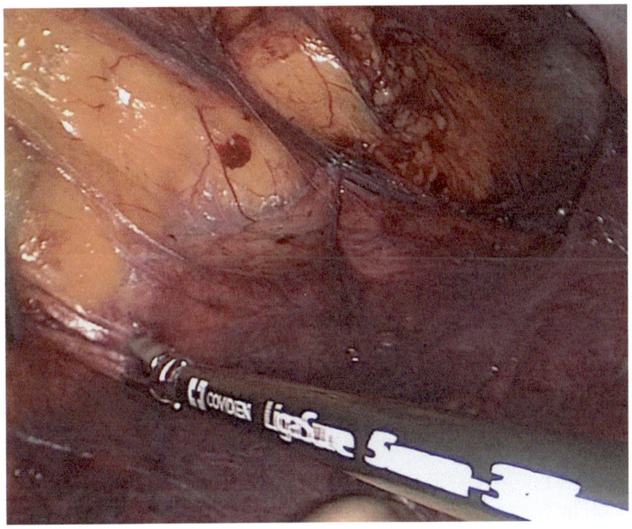

**Fig. 11.7** "Purple down" The retroperitoneal fascia (*purple*) is dissected off the mesentery (*yellow*)

- The peritoneum along the inferior aspect of the pedicle is incised sharply, starting at the sacral promontory and working toward the origin of the inferior mesenteric vessels (Fig. 11.6).
- The inferior mesenteric artery is isolated at its origin. Care is taken to protect the main trunks of the hypogastric nerves that run posterior along the aortic plexus and must be swept dorsally.
- Blunt retromesenteric dissection is started carefully ensuring that the retroperitoneal fascia (purple) is not lifted with the mesentery (Fig. 11.7).
- Using traction and countertraction, the retro-mesenteric plain is developed laterally and superiorly.
- It is critical to identify the left ureter prior to dividing any mesenteric vessels in order to avoid injury (Fig. 11.8).

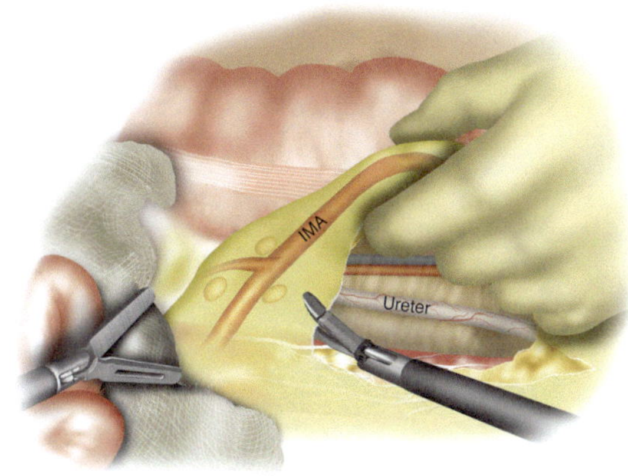


**Fig. 11.8** Identification of the ureter prior to dividing the vascular pedicle *With permission from Yuko Tonohira*

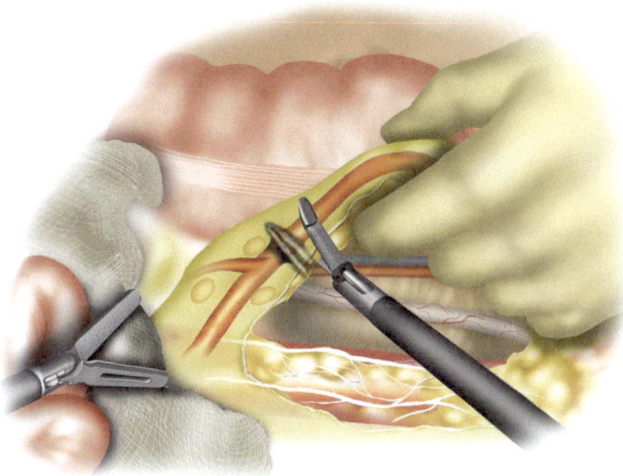

**Fig. 11.9** Division of the pedicle with an energy device preserving the left colic *With permission from Yuko Tonohira*

The left ureter is located medial to the gonadal vessels at this level and more distally at the level of the common iliac bifurcation. If the left ureter cannot be identified, a different surgical exposure method such as lateral-to-medial mobilization can be utilized. Alternatively, the ureter can be identified more proximally near the origin of the IMA. If all of the laparoscopic maneuvers fail to identify the ureter, open dissection through the Pfannenstiel incision can be attempted.

- The inferior mesenteric artery (IMA) is isolated, and a window is created around the vessel ensuring the ureter is not lifted up with the mesentery. All vessels are divided with a bipolar energy device with overlapping burns. Leaving a stump helps control unexpected bleeding (Fig. 11.9). In patients with calcified mesenteric vessels, either vessel loop ligator, clips, or laparoscopic stapler should be used for vessel ligation.

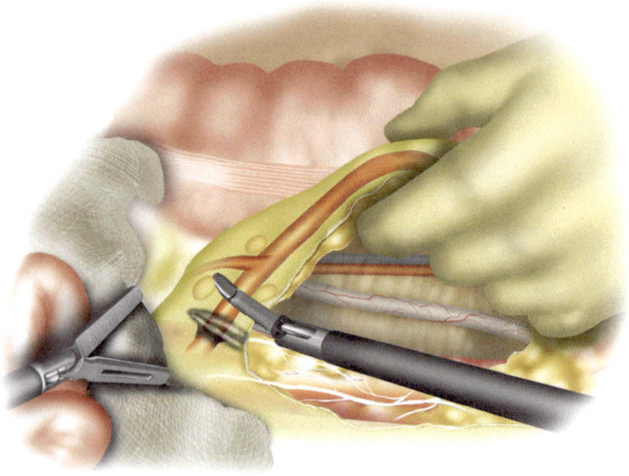

**Fig. 11.10** High ligation of the IMA (proximal to the left colic) *With permission from Yuko Tonohira*

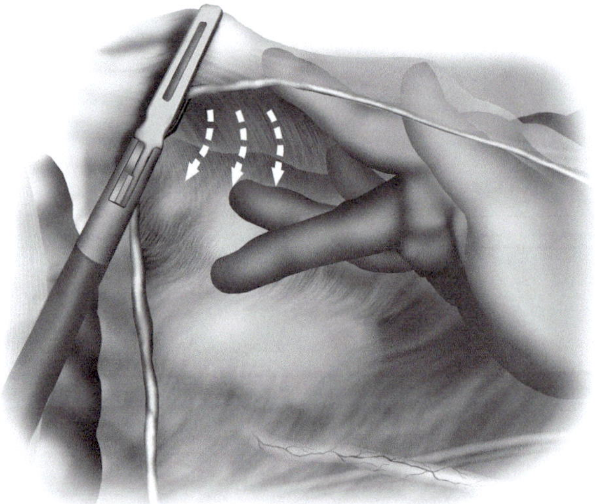

**Fig. 11.11** Retromesenteric dissection using traction and counter-traction *With permission from Carter J, Whelan RL. Hand assisted laparoscopic anterior resection. In: Milsom JW, Bohm B, Nakajima K, eds. Laparoscopic colorectal surgery. Springer, New York 2006;pp:255-273. © Springer 2006*

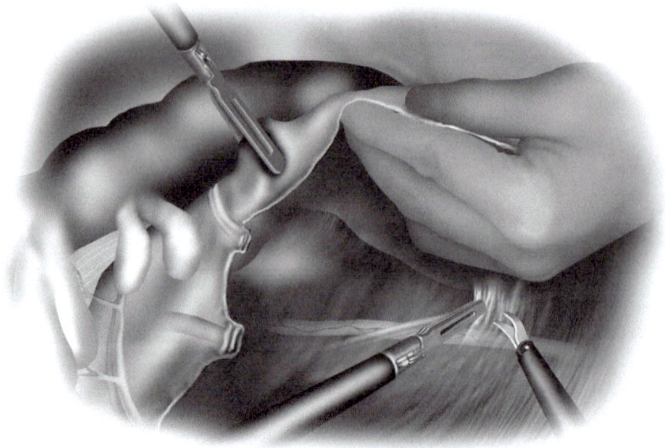

**Fig. 11.12** Retromesenteric dissection ensuring that the purple retroperitoneal fascia is kept down and the ureter is protected. *With permission from Carter J, Whelan RL. Hand assisted laparoscopic anterior resection. In: Milsom JW, Bohm B, Nakajima K, eds. Laparoscopic colorectal surgery. Springer, New York 2006;pp:255-273. © Springer 2006*

- Depending on the location of the tumor, the IMA can be divided high on the aorta (Fig. 11.10) or can be ligated distal to the take off of the left colic. Division distal to the left colic theoretically provides an extra source of arterial blood flow to the conduit without sacrificing oncological principles.
- Division of the IMA facilitates completion of the retromesenteric dissection (Figs. 11.11 and 11.12).
  - Medially to the root of the mesentery.
  - Laterally to the white line.
  - Superiorly to the inferior border of the pancreas.
- The inferior mesenteric vein (IMV) is divided. Of note, the ligament of Treitz may need to be partially released to obtain adequate exposure of the IMV, and there is an avascular plane just lateral (i.e., to the right) to its origin. The duodenum needs to be protected from inadvertent thermal injury. High division of the IMV at this location is critical to achieve good mobilization and a tension-free anastomosis in the low-lying pelvis.
- An alternative approach is to perform the IMV dissection first followed by the IMA dissection. The lesser sac can be entered anterior to the pancreas with this approach. Care should be taken to ensure that the mesentery to the transverse colon is protected.
- The lesser sac can also be entered by releasing the omentum from the transverse colon (Fig. 11.13). The gastrocolic attachments need to be divided to achieve adequate mobilization.
- The lateral attachments to the colon are taken down using the dissecting tool through the left-sided port (Figs. 11.14 and 11.15).
- At this point, the splenic flexure should be completely mobilized with the ability to perform a colo-anal anastomosis, if required.

## Total Mesorectal Excision (TME)

The principles of the total mesorectal excision remain the same irrespective of the specific technique used to complete this dissection. Some highlights include:

- Posterior dissection in the avascular plane preserving the mesorectal envelope, along with identifying and preserving the hypogastric nerves.

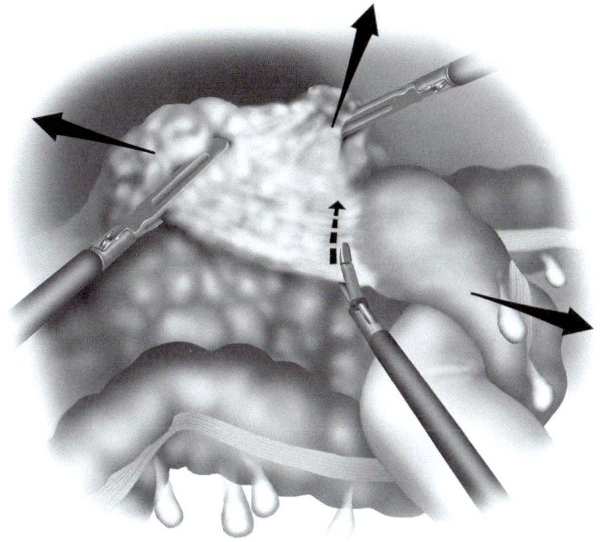

**Fig. 11.13** The omentum is released from the transverse colon. *With permission from Carter J, Whelan RL. Hand assisted laparoscopic anterior resection. In: Milsom JW, Bohm B, Nakajima K, eds. Laparoscopic colorectal surgery. Springer, New York 2006;pp:255-273. © Springer 2006*

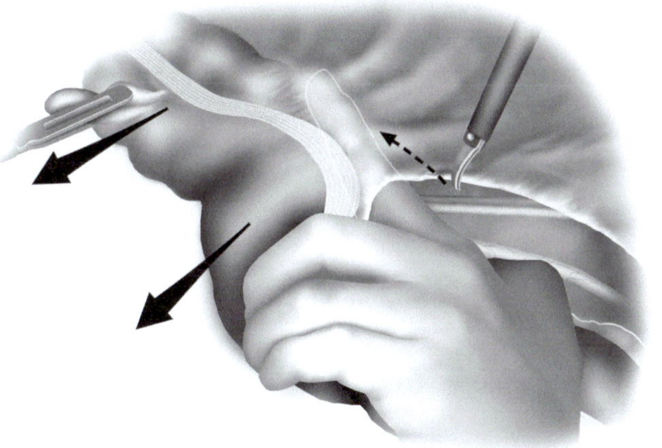

**Fig. 11.14** The lateral attachments are released along the white line. *With permission from Sonoda T. Hand assisted laparoscopic total abdominal colectomy. In: Milsom JW, Bohm B, Nakajima K, eds. Laparoscopic colorectal surgery. Springer, New York 2006;pp:274-294. © Springer 2006*

- Lateral peritoneal attachments are divided, and the lateral dissection is carried out close to the mesorectum while preserving its envelope.
- Anterior dissection with or without excision of the anterior fascia, depending on the location and the extent of the tumor.

The hand-assisted device offers multiple options in carrying out these aspects of the dissection. The specific technique used is dependent on the preference of the surgeon and the

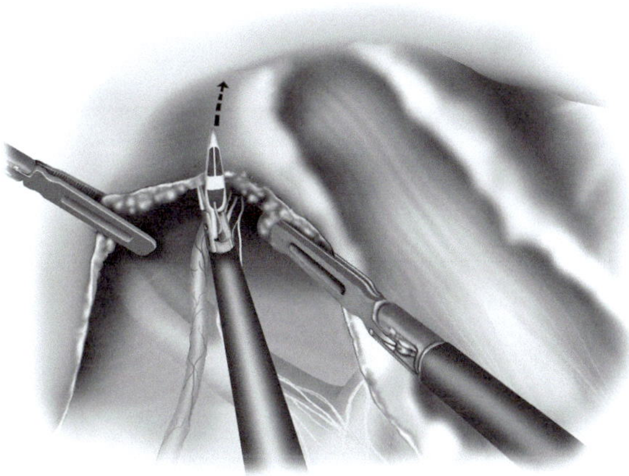

**Fig. 11.15** Takedown of lateral attachments. *With permission from Yuko Tonohira*

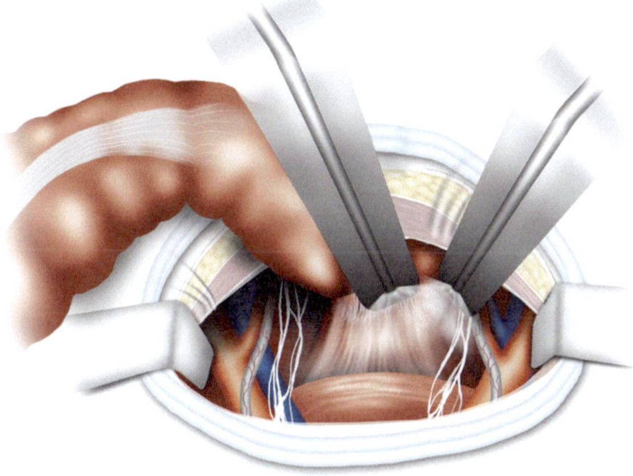

**Fig. 11.16** The lid of the hand-assisted device is removed, and the TME is performed similar to open surgery with the help of "bright tract" retractors *With permission from Yuko Tonohira*

specific characteristics of the patient and tumor. The following techniques can be used to complete the TME.

1. *Open technique through the hand-assisted port*
   (a) The lid of the device is removed and the wound retractor portion of it is retained for retraction (Fig. 11.16).
   (b) Laparotomy pads are used to pack the small bowel out of the pelvis.
   (c) The proximal colon is divided using a linear stapler 5–10 cm from the tumor ensuring that the point of division has pulsatile blood flow.
   (d) Two lighted retractors (long linear retractors with a lip) are used to provide tension and counter-tension to complete TME dissection as described above (Fig. 11.17). These retractors are better suited than the traditional St. Mark's retractors as they are less

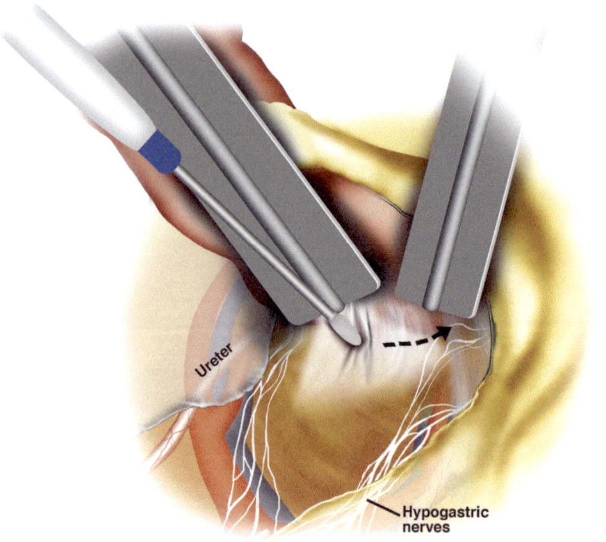


**Fig. 11.17** "Bright tract" retractors used to complete the TME *With permission from Yuko Tonohira*

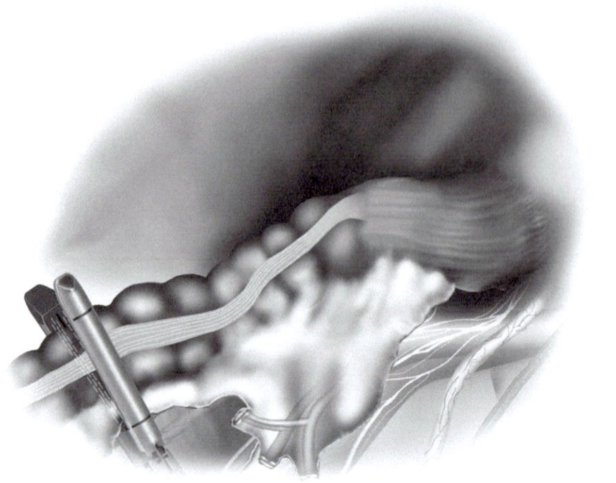

**Fig. 11.19** Laparoscopic stapler used to transect proximal bowel. *With permission* from *Leroy J, Henri M, Rubino F, Marescaux J. Sigmoidectomy. In: Milsom JW, Bohm B, Nakajima K, eds. Laparoscopic colorectal surgery. Springer, New York 2006;pp:145-169. © Springer 2006*

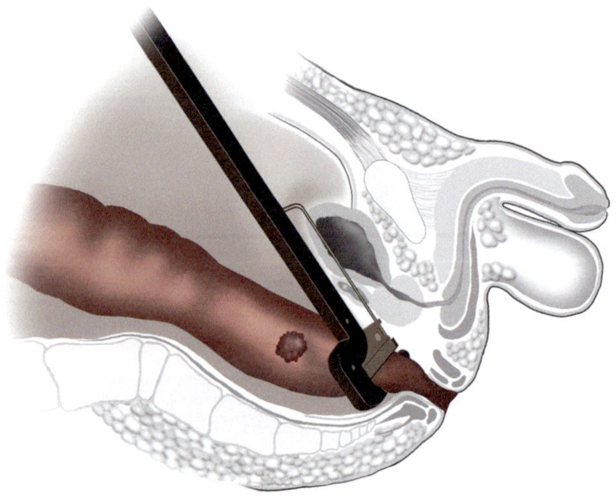

**Fig. 11.18** Open stapler used to transect distal rectum *With permission from Yuko Tonohira*

bulky and can be used as a pair through to provide adequate exposure.

(e) Proctoscopy is performed to ensure that the dissection has progressed beyond the tumor.

(f) Transection of the rectum distal to the tumor can be achieved with an open "TA" stapler through the Pfannenstiel incision (Fig. 11.18). Using two staplers can facilitate traction in difficult cases. The first stapler is placed proximally and used to provide traction to place the second stapler more distal. Staplers that can staple on either side and divide in the middle are also available, but can be bulky to use in a narrow pelvis. Prior to transection, the distal rectum may be washed out with Betadine or sterile water to clear any tumor cells that may have been dislodged during the dissection.

(g) Transanal dissection preserving the external sphincter can be used for very low tumors followed by a hand-sewn anastomosis. In this case, Gelpi retractors and the Lonestar device (Cooper Surgical, Trumbull, CT) are particularly useful.

2. *Laparoscopic TME*
   (a) The dissection is carried out laparoscopically with or without (Chap. 10) hand assistance.
   (b) The hand can be used as a retractor similar to the hand held retractors used in open surgery.
   (c) The proximal bowel can be divided with a laparoscopic linear stapler (Fig. 11.19) or performed more expeditiously with an open stapler through the hand-assisted device (Fig. 11.20).
   (d) An umbilical tape tied around the rectal stump can serve as a useful retractor.
   (e) A laparoscopic energy source is used to complete the dissection as described with the open technique.
3. *Laparoscopic TME using the hand-access device as a retractor* (Video 11.1)
   (a) The colon is divided through the Pfannenstiel incision at the proximal margin.
   (b) The divided colon stump is exteriorized through the hand-access device (Fig. 11.21).
   (c) The rectum is retracted out of the pelvis.

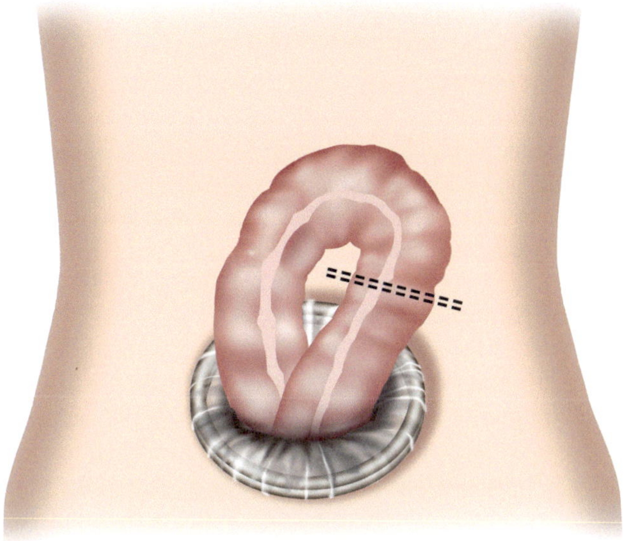

**Fig. 11.20** Use of the hand port facilitates division of the proximal bowel. *With permission* from *Watanabe M. Laparoscopic anterior resection for rectal cancer In: Milsom JW, Bohm B, Nakajima K, eds. Laparoscopic colorectal surgery. Springer, New York 2006;pp:170-187. © Springer 2006*

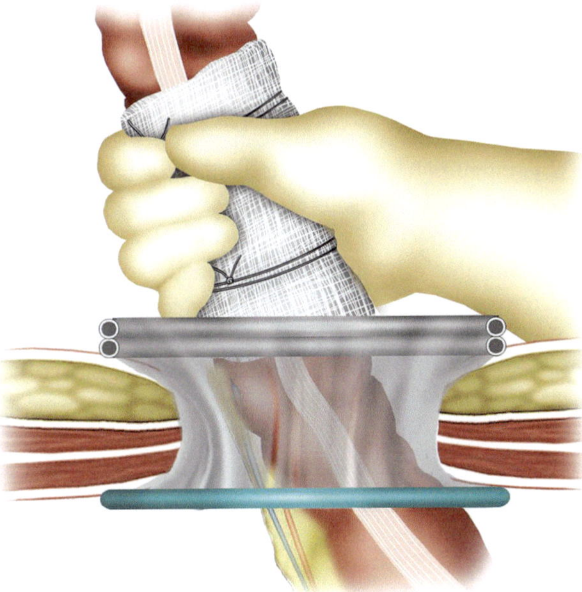

**Fig. 11.21** The colon can be brought out through the hand-port to provide traction and help complete rectal dissection. *With permission from Yuko Tonohira*

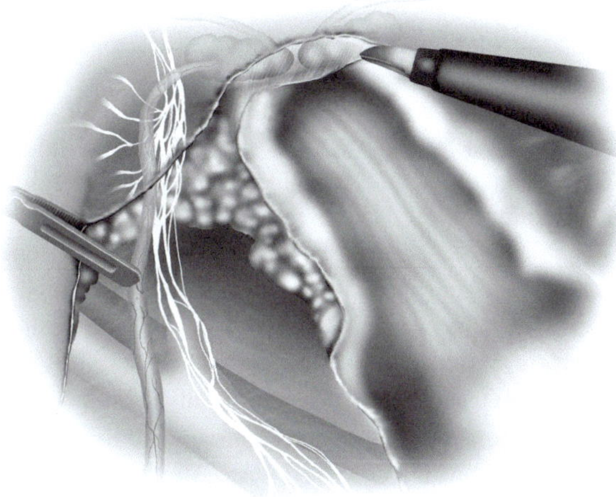

**Fig. 11.22** Anterior dissection in a male. *With permission* from *Watanabe M. Laparoscopic anterior resection for rectal cancer In: Milsom JW, Bohm B, Nakajima K, eds. Laparoscopic colorectal surgery. Springer, New York 2006;pp:170-187. © Springer 2006*

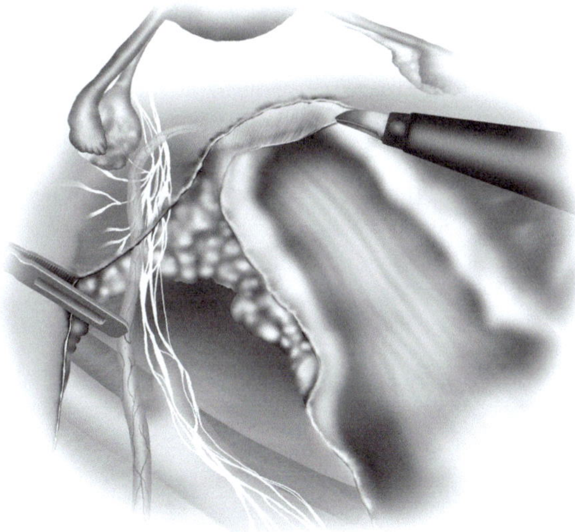

**Fig. 11.23** Anterior dissection in a female *With permission from Yuko Tonohira*

(d) A laparoscopic energy device can be used to complete the dissection sequentially as described with the prior technique; utilizing posterior dissection initially, followed by lateral dissection, and finally anterior dissection are carried out with cautery or an energy device (Figs. 11.22 and 11.23).

## Resection

The distal bowel is transected with a reticulating stapler after clearing the mesorectum at the appropriate level (note: this step can also be done through the hand port). Many surgeons feel that this is the rate-limiting step of a laparoscopic LAR with the currently available stapling technology. In this light, the hand-assisted approach retains many of the advantages of laparoscopy while permitting the use of an open technique to aid in this more difficult step of the operation.

## Anastomosis

The anastomosis is typically completed with a circular stapler. The hand port is very useful for this portion of the operation. The proximal bowel is prepared and checked for pulsatile blood flow. The anvil of an EEA stapler (typically 28 or 31 mm) is secured to the end of the bowel with a purse string. Alternatively, a side-to-end anastomosis can be performed by securing the anvil to the antimesenteric edge of the proximal bowel. The shaft of the EEA stapler is brought in transanally and the anastomosis completed. It is our preference that care is taken to ensure that the pin of the stapler is brought through the center of the TA staple line (Fig. 11.24).

After securing the anvil to the proximal bowel, pneumoperitoneum can be reestablished to perform the anastomosis laparoscopically.

The anastomosis is evaluated with a flexible sigmoidoscope. A leak text is performed with $CO_2$ insufflation, while the anastomosis is kept under saline. The flexible scope permits complete colonoscopy at this stage if the tumor was obstructive and preoperative complete colonoscopy was not possible. The hand-access device permits easy intervention should there be bleeding or a leak identified on colonoscopic evaluation. Reinforcing or hemostatic sutures can also be placed through the hand port under colonoscopic guidance, if required.

For very low tumors, the conduit can be positioned in the pelvis and a hand-sewn colo-anal anastomosis fashioned with interrupted absorbable sutures.

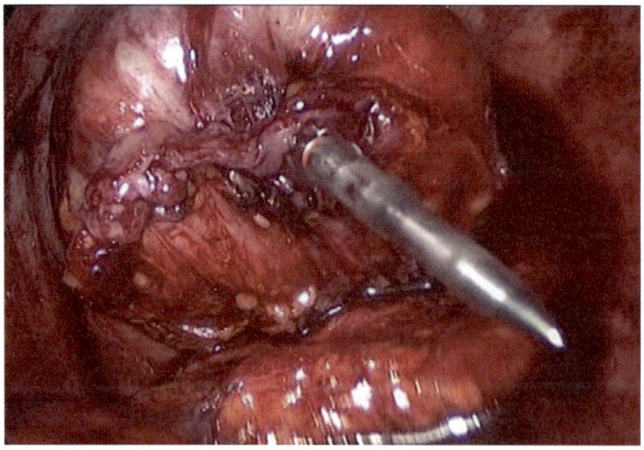

**Fig. 11.24** The anvil of the EEA stapler is brought through the middle of the transverse staple line

## Postoperative Care

### Complications

The routine complications associated with a low anterior resection and colorectal surgery are well described. This section focuses on specific complications as related to the laparoscopic hand-assisted LAR.

#### Wound Complications

Pfannenstiel incisions generally heal well with a low incidence of incisional hernia [3]. Our practice is to leave a small portion of the wound open to decrease the incidence of surgical site infection. Rectus sheath hematomas can occur and usually present as severe focal pain in the postoperative period. Careful attention to the perforating vessels when raising flaps can decrease the incidence of hematomas. Our practice is to close the posterior fascia to decrease the possibility of bowel herniating between the rectus muscles.

#### Operative Technical Complications

##### Bleeding

- Bleeding at the time of retro-mesenteric dissection is usually due to dissecting into the retroperitoneum or into the mesentery. If persistent bleeding is encountered, attempting dissection from an alternative approach may be useful.
- Bleeding from the pedicle can typically be controlled with clips. ENDOLOOPS (Ethicon, Cincinnati, OH) are useful to have available in all cases to control pedicular bleeding (especially with calcified vessels).
- Visualization can be easily maintained by placing a laparotomy pad or gauze through the hand-port to clean the field. This pad can also be used to keep the camera clean.
- Splenic injury can be avoided by dissecting away from the spleen and maintaining dissection in the plane close to the colon. Pressure and compression can easily be used to control splenic bleeding with a laparotomy pad through the hand-port, though hemostatic topical adjuncts may be required.

##### Ureter

- Ureteral injury should be rare if the ureter is identified prior to division of any vessels.
- Inability to find the ureter is an indication to convert to an open operation in difficult cases.
- Preoperative stents may help recognize an injury, but do not always prevent injury to the ureter.

### Bowel Injury

- Can be thermal secondary to the dissecting tool.
- Traction and tearing of the bowel are possible during mobilization and "running the bowel."
- Puncture injury from trocars and instruments is a concern and care should be taken to handle instruments under direct vision.

## Outcomes

Randomized control trials comparing open and hand-assisted colectomy have shown that the procedure is safe, has decreased blood loss, and is associated with a quicker postoperative recovery with a shorter length of stay [5]. Hand-assisted colectomy compared to open surgery has also been associated with a higher cost and longer operative times, especially in the early experience with this technique. There was no significant difference in the complication rate between the open and hand-assisted surgery. Of note, these studies included all colectomies and included benign and malignant disease.

There are several studies that have compared hand-assisted colectomy to straight laparoscopic colectomy. The HALS study was a multicenter study out of Europe and America that found no difference in outcome between the straight laparoscopic and hand-assisted techniques. However, the conversion rate was much lower in the hand-assisted group [6]. The Minimally Invasive Therapy and Technology (MITT) found a lower conversion rate with the hand-assisted technique. This study also found a decrease in operative time with the hand-assisted approach [7].

Tjandra et al. conducted a prospective non-randomized case-control study on ultralow anterior resection [8]. There was no difference in the number of lymph nodes harvested or the margin positivity. The operative time was shorter with the hand-assisted technique, while the need for postoperative narcotics and the time to flatus were slightly longer, with no difference in the length of stay. The clinical significance of these findings is unclear, however, this study showed that there might be some difference in recovery. In contrast, a study out of the Lahey Clinic did not find any difference in bowel function recovery [9].

In summary, studies comparing straight laparoscopic versus hand-assisted approached have found:

1. HALAR retains many of the benefits of a pure laparoscopic approach.
2. Comparable complication rate and length of stay.
3. Shorter operative time and lower conversion rate.
4. Longer incision compared to straight laparoscopy.
5. Increased level of inflammatory markers—though of unclear clinical significance.
6. Longer need for narcotics and longer time to flatus compared to straight laparoscopy—also of unclear clinical significance.

Overall, we feel it is clear that HALAR helps broaden the reach of laparoscopy to more complex patients such as obese patients and those with difficulty anatomy. The benefits of the hand-assisted device in teaching residents and fellows are also significant. A comparative study that looked at the benefit of the hand-assisted device in training found that less intervention was required by the attending surgeon in completing left-sided resection with the hand-assisted device (hand-assisted 72 % vs. laparoscopic 72 %, $P=0.06$) [10].

## Pearls and Pitfalls

### Hand-Access Device Placement

(a) The Pfannenstiel incision is, in general, preferred to the lower midline incision; however, especially early in your experience and for cases with a high likelihood of conversion, a lower midline incision may be preferred.
(b) The anterior fascia should be mobilized widely off the rectus as this permits retraction with the wound protector.
(c) Perforators from the rectus should be seen clearly and controlled to prevent a postoperative rectus sheath hematoma.

### Visualization

(d) Use of a tagged laparotomy pad or sponge can be very useful in cleaning the camera and retracting the small bowel out of the field.
(e) Positioning the patient in steep Trendelenburg and left side up is critical in achieving adequate exposure.
(f) Dexterity with the hand and ensuring that it does not obstruct the field of vision are a must. In general, keep the hand away from the camera, and use a "C-shape" configuration with your hand and maximal thumb-forefinger apposition for dissection.
(g) Use of laparotomy pads and lighted retractors are important for the pelvic portion of the operation (Fig. 11.16). Traditional St. Mark's retractors are difficult to use through a small incision.

### Splenic Flexure

(h) Posterior dissection to the inferior border of the pancreas followed by lesser sac dissection at the distal transverse colon prior to taking down the lateral attachments will help with difficult splenic flexure takedown.

(i) Positioning the patient in reverse Trendelenburg can help complete splenic flexure dissection.

(j) Traction and dissection towards the spleen rather than away from the spleen will prevent splenic trauma.

## Pelvic Dissection

(k) Using two lighted bright tract retractors to provide medial and lateral traction helps in a narrow pelvis.

(l) The uterus can be suspended to the abdominal wall or retracted using the ring of the hand-assisted device.

(m) Intraoperative proctoscopy is very useful in assessing the distal extent of the resection.

## Conclusion

Hand-assisted low anterior resection is a useful tool in the armamentarium of an experienced laparoscopic colorectal surgeon. It broadens the scope of laparoscopy to technically challenging cases and allows for a safe platform to train future colorectal surgeons. The operative time is often reduced without compromising the other benefits of straight laparoscopy. HALAR can also be used as a first step for surgeons who are new to the field and as a bridge prior to conversion to open following straight laparoscopy.

## References


1. Bonjer HJ, Hop WC, Nelson H, Sargent DJ, Lacy AM, Castells A, Guillou PJ, Thorpe H, Brown J, Delgado S, Kuhrij E, Haglind E, Påhlman L, Transatlantic Laparoscopically Assisted vs Open Colectomy Trials Study Group. Laparoscopically assisted vs open colectomy for colon cancer: a meta-analysis. Arch Surg. 2007;142(3):298–303.
2. Nakajima K, Lee SW, Cocilovo C, Foglia C, Kim K, Sonoda T, Milsom JW. Hand-assisted laparoscopic colorectal surgery using GelPort. Surg Endosc. 2004;18(1):102–5.
3. Sonoda T, Pandey S, Trencheva K, Lee S, Milsom J. Longterm complications of hand-assisted versus laparoscopic colectomy. J Am Coll Surg. 2009;208(1):62–6.
4. Nakajima K, Milsom JW, Margolin DA, Szilagy EJ. Use of the surgical towel in colorectal hand-assisted laparoscopic surgery (HALS). Surg Endosc. 2004;18(3):552–3.
5. Meshikhes AW. Controversy of hand-assisted laparoscopic colorectal surgery. World J Gastroenterol. 2010;16(45):5662–8.
6. HALS Study Group. Hand-assisted laparoscopic surgery vs standard laparoscopic surgery for colorectal disease: a prospective randomized trial. Surg Endosc. 2000;14(10):896–901.
7. Marcello PW, Fleshman JW, Milsom JW, Read TE, Arnell TD, Birnbaum EH, Feingold DL, Lee SW, Mutch MG, Sonoda T, Yan Y, Whelan RL. Hand-assisted laparoscopic vs. laparoscopic colorectal surgery: a multicenter, prospective, randomized trial. Dis Colon Rectum. 2008;51(6):818–26.
8. Tjandra JJ, Chan MK, Yeh CH. Laparoscopic- vs hand-assisted ultralow anterior resection: a prospective study. Dis Colon Rectum. 2008;51(1):26–31.
9. Chang YJ, Marcello PW, Rusin LC, Roberts PL, Schoetz DJ. Hand-assisted laparoscopic sigmoid colectomy: helping hand or hindrance? Surg Endosc. 2005;19(5):656–61.
10. Champagne BJ, Lee EC, Valerian B, Armstrong D, Ambroze W, Orangio G. A novel end point to assess a resident's ability to perform hand-assisted versus straight laparoscopy for left colectomy: is there really a difference? J Am Coll Surg. 2008;207(4):554–9.

# Laparoscopic Abdominoperineal Resection

# 12

Jennifer S. Davids and Justin A. Maykel

## Key Points

- For low rectal cancer, small randomized prospective controlled trials have shown that, compared to open APR, laparoscopic APR has equivalent oncologic outcomes and is associated with earlier postoperative recovery and shorter hospital stay.
- Although there are few absolute contraindications to laparoscopic APR, strategic patient selection is essential to a successful outcome.
- There are a variety of innovative approaches to laparoscopic abdominoperineal resection that can be used to individualize patient management.
- The overall principles of laparoscopic APR are the same as for open surgery; total mesorectal excision is the cornerstone.
- Conversion to an open procedure for any reason should not be considered a "failure."

## Introduction

### Indications

Regardless of the surgical approach, abdominoperineal resection (APR) is indicated primarily for the treatment of malignant diseases but may also be appropriate for benign disease in selected circumstances. In terms of malignancy, APR is performed for low rectal cancer, recurrent rectal cancer, as well as salvage therapy for anal cancer or melanoma. While adenocarcinomas involving the sphincter complex traditionally mandate APR, the technique of intersphincteric resection and coloanal anastomosis can be offered for patients who refuse a stoma and are willing to accept the risk of positive microscopic margins and compromised postoperative continence. Other patients are best treated with APR due to technical limitations in achieving an adequate distal margin and/or performing an anastomosis deep in the pelvis. Additionally, APR may provide better quality of life compared to low anterior resection (LAR) with primary anastomosis for patients who also have marginal baseline continence or are at risk for low anterior resection syndrome. There are a few indications for APR for benign disease. APR may be appropriate for selected patients with severe refractory anorectal Crohn's disease, although in one small retrospective study ($N=10$ patients) it was associated with increased likelihood of new severe proximal colonic disease [1, 2]. APR may be performed as a completion proctectomy in a patient with ulcerative colitis or Crohn's colitis who has undergone previous abdominal colectomy or who is not a candidate for or who does not desire a restorative procedure. Lastly, APR may improve quality of life and facilitate wound healing for patients with spinal cord injuries and/or sacral decubiti, who are already diverted but suffer from persistent mucous discharge.

### Outcomes

Large randomized multicenter trials have demonstrated that laparoscopic colectomy for colon cancer is associated with equivalent oncologic outcome to conventional open surgery and has the benefit of superior short-term outcomes including faster recovery, reduced length of stay, and less analgesic use [3–5]. For rectal cancer, current data is limited to two prospective randomized trials, with anticipation of more solid data upon completion of the American College of Surgeons Oncology Group (ACOSOG) Z6051 trial, which aims to enroll 650 patients by December 2013 [6, 7]. The United Kingdom Medical Research Council trial of conventional

**Electronic supplementary material:** Supplementary material is available in the online version of this chapter at 10.1007/978-1-4939-1581-1_12. Videos can also be accessed at http://www.springerimages.com/videos/978-1-4939-1580-4.

J.S. Davids, M.D. • J.A. Maykel, M.D. (✉)
Division of Colorectal Surgery of Colon and Rectal Surgery,
University of Massachusetts Memorial Hospital Center,
67 Belmont Street, Suite 201, Worcester, MA, USA
e-mail: Justin.maykel@umassmemorial.org

H.M. Ross et al. (eds.), *Minimally Invasive Approaches to Colon and Rectal Disease: Technique and Best Practices*,
DOI 10.1007/978-1-4939-1581-1_12, © Springer Science+Business Media New York 2015

versus laparoscopic-assisted surgery in colorectal cancer (CLASICC) trial compared short-term end points after laparoscopic ($N=253$) versus open ($N=128$) rectal resections for cancer (including both LAR and APR) and concluded that there was no statistically significant difference in intraoperative complications (14 % vs. 13 %) or 30-day postoperative complications (40 % vs. 37 %) [8]. The analysis included a subset of patients who underwent open ($N=36$) versus laparoscopic ($N=60$) APR. The two groups had similar rates of positive circumferential resection margins (20 % vs. 26 %). While these rates are quite high, equivalent 5-year overall survival rates (41.8 % open vs. 53.2 % laparoscopic, $P=0.310$), disease-free survival rates (36.2 % vs. 41.4 %, $P=0.618$), and distant recurrence rates (40.8 % vs. 35.7 %, $P=0.762$) were found [9].

A prospective randomized trial by Ng et al. specifically evaluated perioperative outcomes in patients with low rectal cancer undergoing open ($N=48$) versus laparoscopic ($N=51$) APR [10]. In this study, the laparoscopic group had earlier return of bowel function (3.1 days until flatus vs. 4.6 days until flatus, $P<0.001$), as well as improved time until independent ambulation (4.4 days vs. 5.9 days, $P=0.005$). They did note that the laparoscopic approach had a longer operative time (213 min vs. 163 min, $P<0.001$) and higher cost ($9,588 vs. $7,517, $P<0.001$). Lastly, in concordance with the CLASICC data, they also reported equivalent 5-year survival (75 % vs. 76 %, $P=0.20$).

In conclusion, the existing data on laparoscopic versus open APR suggests that, when performed by laparoscopic rectal cancer experts, this technique delivers equivalent oncologic outcomes with improved in-hospital recovery at the expense of longer operating room time and overall higher cost. The adequacy of oncologic resection remains unsettled due to high reported positive surgical margins. We anticipate that data from the ongoing larger trials will quantify outcomes pertaining to survival, morbidity, and cost, as well as sexual function and quality of life. These results will undoubtedly have the potential to impact policy, as current American Society of Colon and Rectal Surgeons (ASCRS) practice guidelines (last updated in 2005) note the uncertainty of the "oncologic effectiveness" of laparoscopic rectal cancer surgery given the absence of large prospective randomized controlled trials [11].

## Total Mesorectal Excision (TME)

The cornerstone of rectal cancer surgery is the total mesorectal excision (TME), popularized by Heald [12]. Early on, concerns regarding the potential to achieve a proper laparoscopic TME were fueled by the results of the CLASICC trial, in which patients who underwent laparoscopic low anterior resection ($N=129$ patients) had a higher rate of positive circumferential resection margin compared to the open procedure ($N=64$), although this did not reach statistical significance (12 % vs. 6 %, $P=0.19$) and did not translate to a difference in 5-year survival [8, 9]. Notably, as mentioned above, CRM rates were high, but equivalent for laparoscopic and open APR. Undoubtedly, these data reflect the technical challenges associated with laparoscopic low anterior resection with primary anastomosis. Inability to palpate the extent of the tumor to determine margins, as well as limitations on stapler angulation, can make distal transection challenging. Fortunately, neither of these technical constraints is relevant to laparoscopic APR. Particularly with the narrow male pelvis, the ability of the surgeon to access the plane of resection from both the abdominal and perineal approaches is a technical advantage of APR compared to LAR.

## Patient Selection and Preoperative Considerations

Patient selection for laparoscopic APR is the key to a successful operation and a good patient outcome. Candidates for laparoscopic APR should be fit enough to tolerate a larger, open surgery, should it be necessary. The only absolute contraindication to laparoscopic APR is the inability to tolerate pneumoperitoneum and steep Trendelenburg positioning. Relative contraindications include morbid obesity, prior pelvic surgery, and suspected or known dense intra-abdominal adhesions. In the obese patient with a narrow pelvis and foreshortened/thickened mesentery, it can be challenging to retract the small bowel out of the pelvis and maintain good visualization when entering the presacral space.

The surgeon must perform a thorough history and physical examination on all candidates for APR. The history should include preoperative bowel control and continence for patients who are being considered for LAR versus APR. For all malignancies, a careful digital rectal exam should be performed, focusing on tumor location relative to the sphincter complex, size, mobility, and response to neoadjuvant therapy. At the time of cancer diagnosis, patients should be staged with CT scans of the chest, abdomen, and pelvis. Blood work includes carcinoembryonic antigen (CEA) and a complete blood count. Imaging with MRI, endorectal ultrasound, or both is based somewhat on individual surgeon preference and expertise and will not be discussed in detail in this chapter. Pelvic imaging can give the surgeon additional information related to the tumor and adjacent structures, providing valuable data points to optimize operative planning.

A thorough preoperative evaluation is required for patients undergoing APR. This includes a complete blood count, electrolytes, coagulation studies, type and screen, urinalysis, and, if age appropriate, chest X-ray and EKG. Evaluation by a pulmonologist or cardiologist is recommended if the patient has baseline cardiopulmonary disease. Nutrition labs including albumin and prealbumin should be obtained if the patient is clinically malnourished. All patients should be seen by an enterostomal therapist preoperatively for counseling and site marking. Consultation preoperatively with a plastic surgeon should be considered if a large pelvic defect is anticipated (see section below on reconstruction of the defect). Lastly, ureteral stent placement should be considered for patients with bulky pelvic tumors, radiation therapy, or prior pelvic surgery. In colorectal surgery, ureteral stents have not been shown to decrease the likelihood of injury, but they do increase intraoperative injury identification, allowing for immediate repair [13]. Lighted stents in laparoscopic pelvic surgery have been described, but are not essential [14].

## Operative Technique (Video 12.1)

### Anesthesia, Prophylaxis, and Positioning

Prior to case, appropriate antibiotics are administered. The patient is initially in supine position. Venous thromboembolism (VTE) prophylaxis includes Venodyne boots placed before induction of general endotracheal anesthesia. The surgeon should consider administering either unfractionated or low-molecular-weight heparin subcutaneously preoperatively as well. In a large database study, laparoscopic proctectomy did not have decreased incidence of VTE compared to the open approach [15, 16]. Following intubation, an orogastric tube is placed.

The patient is moved into the lithotomy position, with legs in Yellowfin boots. Ureteral stents are placed at this time, if needed. Prior to prepping, the surgeon ensures there is adequate exposure of the anus and perineum off the edge of the bed. Bony prominences are carefully padded and legs are positioned in the boots to avoid pressure on the peroneal nerve. The Yellowfins are eventually brought downward, decreasing the amount of hip flexion, to maximize workspace with the laparoscopic instruments. Both arms are padded and tucked to the patient's side using a drawsheet. Next, the patient is secured to the table, in order to prevent shifting during steep Trendelenburg and left-right tilting. The upper body is secured at the chest and shoulders as a blue towel is folded into thirds, laid across the chest, and wrapped around the bed twice with 3-in. tape. In our experience, beanbag or inflatable devices add unnecessary bulk, lift the patient higher off the bed, and limit instrument mobility during the laparoscopic dissection. One-liter IV saline bags may be carefully placed parallel to the shoulders and are wrapped twice circumferentially around the bed with wide cloth tape (Fig. 12.1). In rare instances, with improperly placed shoulder supports coupled with prolonged time in the Trendelenburg position, shoulder supports have been associated with brachial plexus injuries [17] and should be used with caution. A Foley catheter is placed under sterile technique if ureteral stents are not used. The surgeon should perform a final digital rectal examination to confirm appropriateness of resection and to assess response to neoadjuvant therapy, if relevant. Residual stool may be evacuated from the rectum with enemas containing a Betadine-saline mixture. The anus is sewn closed with a 2–0 silk purse string suture to prevent contamination of stool (Fig. 12.2). The abdomen is then prepped with chlorhexidine and the perineum prepped with Betadine. Prior abdominal incisions are marked with a pen, and the stoma site can be confirmed and reinforced. The patient is draped, and the operation begins after a time-out is performed.

### Port Placement and Entry into the Abdomen

Entry into the peritoneal cavity can be accomplished using the Hasson or Veress technique in the infraumbilical position. If the patient is obese or has had previous surgery at the umbilicus (prior laparotomy, umbilical hernia repair), a safer alternative is to use the Veress or Visiport technique in the left upper quadrant. Pneumoperitoneum is established to 15 mmHg, and additional 5-mm ports are placed under

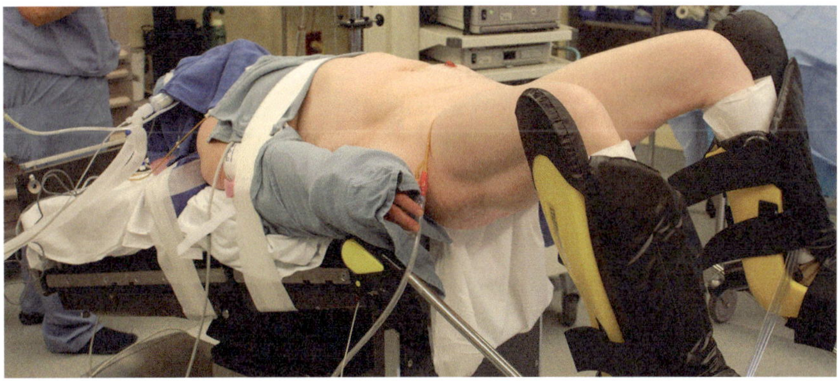

**Fig. 12.1** Supine OR positioning depicting patient secured to bed, shoulder rolls in place, in the lithotomy position, buttock off end of the bed, with thighs as parallel as possible to the abdomen

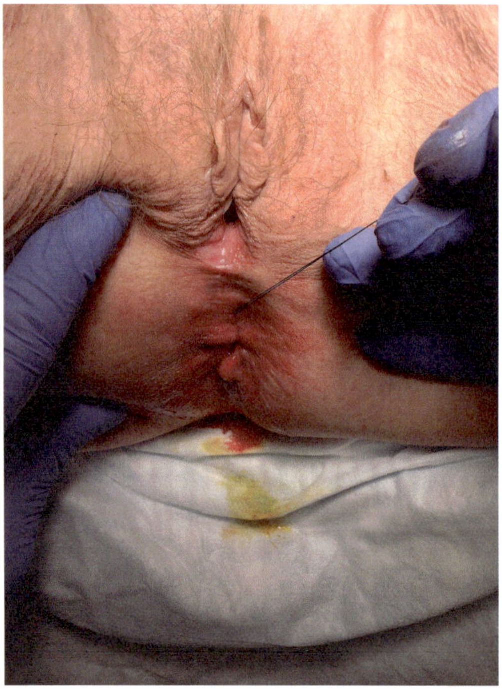

**Fig. 12.2** Anus sewn closed at initiation of case

direct vision in the following locations: suprapubic, right lower quadrant, and left mid-abdomen (future colostomy site) (Fig. 12.3). An additional trocar may be placed in the epigastrium if needed, taking care not to place it too far to allow laparoscopic instruments to reach the deep pelvis. The laparoscopic abdominal portion has also been described using single-port access, with a single-port device (SILS Port, Covidien, Inc., Norwalk, CT, or the GelPOINT Advanced Access Platform, Applied Medical, Rancho Santa Margarita, CA) [18], and positioned at the colostomy site, umbilicus, or Pfannenstiel location. Since the specimen can eventually be removed via the perineal incision, the laparoscopic APR procedure does not need any extension of abdominal incisions for specimen extraction, as required for laparoscopic colectomy procedures. This is another reason why we do not typically utilize the hand port routinely, although some surgeons find the insertion of the hand helpful for pelvic retraction (Fig. 12.4). A 5-mm or 10-mm 30-degree scope is used. The Olympus EndoEYE camera (Olympus, Central Valley, PA) may help facilitate visualization in the pelvis, particularly with the single-port laparoscopic approach. Once the ports are placed, both the surgeon and assistant may stand on one side of the patient, but we prefer to have the surgeon stand on the patient's right side and assistant on the left. Monitors are positioned to the patient's left and right at the foot of the bed. An additional monitor may be placed above the patient's left shoulder to facilitate splenic flexure mobilization, when needed.

## Colon Mobilization and Division of the Superior Hemorrhoidal Vessels

The liver and peritoneal surfaces are visually inspected for evidence of metastases. The patient is placed in steep Trendelenburg position with the right side down. The small bowel is swept out of the pelvis using 2 atraumatic graspers. The descending colon and sigmoid colon are mobilized from the sigmoid fossa along the white line of Toldt in a lateral-to-medial fashion, using Endo Shears (Covidien, Inc., Norwalk, CT) with cautery. An alternative approach is the medial dissection where the sigmoid is lifted, the peritoneum incised, and the plane between the mesorectal fascia and the retroperitoneum is created, taking particular care to leave the ureter in the retroperitoneum and sweep it down from the specimen. In most cases, the splenic flexure and proximal descending colon do not need to be mobilized in order to have sufficient length for the end colostomy. The sigmoid colon is grasped and retracted upward, and the superior hemorrhoidal vessels are identified within the mesentery. Using the Endo Shears and atraumatic grasper, windows in the mesentery are created around the superior hemorrhoidal vessels. After demonstrating once more that the ureters are out of the line of transection, the vessels are ligated at their origin. This maneuver can be performed with a 5- or 10-mm (depending on the amount of tissue to be divided) advanced bipolar device or laparoscopic stapler with white 2.5-mm staple cartridge (Fig. 12.5a, b). A grasper should be positioned and ready to obtain prompt control of the vascular stump, in the event of inadequate hemostasis.

## Total Mesorectal Excision

The presacral plane is further developed into the wispy areolar tissue, using either Endo Shears or the L-hook cautery. Alternative instruments such as ultrasonic energy devices (Harmonic Scalpel™, Ethicon, Cincinnati, OH) or articulating laparoscopic instruments (Cambridge Endo, Framingham, MA) may facilitate the exposure and dissection. The hypogastric nerves are visualized medially along the sacrum as well as laterally along the pelvic sidewall and are left intact (Fig. 12.6). The total mesorectal dissection proceeds into the pelvis to the pelvic floor (levators), first posteriorly and then laterally, and lastly the anterior plane is approached. The colon and rectum can be retracted out of the pelvis with the assistance of gravity, a laparoscopic grasper, or suture secured to the abdominal wall or trocar. In women, the uterus and adnexa can be suspended with a suture passed through the abdominal wall or by a uterine manipulator placed at the initiation of surgery. During the dissection it is imperative to identify and preserve both ureters, the pelvic sympathetic and parasympathetic nerves, iliac blood vessels, presacral

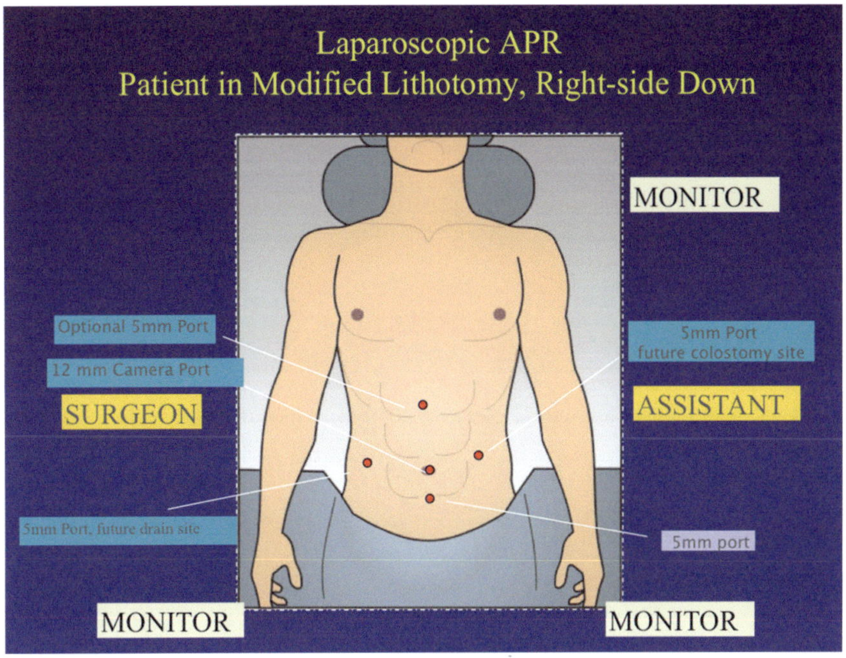


**Fig. 12.3** OR setup with trocar, surgeon, and monitor positioning

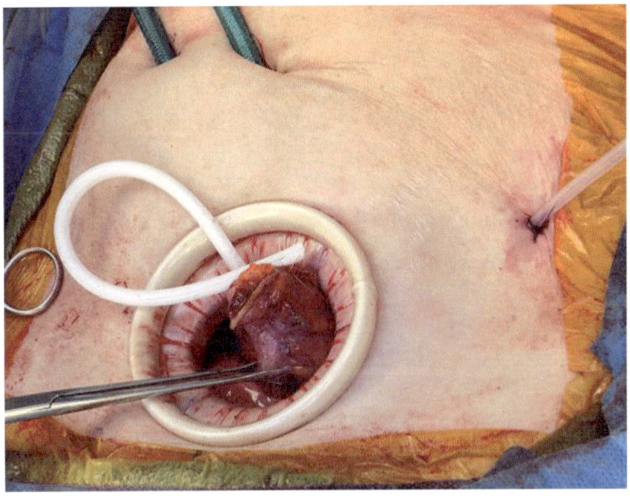

**Fig. 12.4** Laparoscopic APR through a hand port. JP sewn to specimen to pull through the perineal wound and leave the JP in the pelvis to drain

veins, vagina, seminal vesicles, and prostate. Of course, tumor involvement of any of these structures mandates en bloc resection. The posterior dissection will take you to and through Waldeyer's fascia and the anterior curve of the pelvis to the muscular pelvic floor. At this level, it is particularly important not to "cone in" on the specimen, taking care to leave a waist of muscle and adipose tissue covering the thinned rectum as it dives into the pelvic floor musculature (corresponding with the location of the majority of these low rectal tumors). The anterior plane is the most challenging, particularly below the anterior peritoneal reflection (see Fig. 10.8). Developing the posterior and lateral planes first allows for improved visualization of the proper anterior plane of dissection. The use of multiple graspers to create tissue tension helps find the correct plane. Rigid sizers placed in the vagina may help better retract and define the rectovaginal septum dissection in women. The laparoscopic suction irrigator is useful to remove smoke and fluid and as a deep pelvic retractor. Alternatively, there are cautery instruments with side ports for smoke evacuation controlled by the surgeon with trumpet valves.

Dissection anteriorly begins with opening of the peritoneal reflection in a horseshoe (i.e., upside down U) fashion. Maintaining cephalad retraction on the distal sigmoid and upper rectum allows the plane to be more easily delineated. This anterior reflection of the peritoneum is variable, though, in general, the lower one-third of the rectum is without a peritoneal covering. Just deep to this are the seminal vesicles in men, characterized by their white tubular appearance. Dissection continues caudally along the endopelvic fascia, also referred to as Denonvilliers fascia, with identification of the smooth posterior border of the prostate gland. The periprostatic plexus is located along this anterior dissection (see Fig. 10.8). This plexus contains both sympathetic and parasympathetic fibers that innervate the prostate, prostatic and membranous urethra, seminal vesicles, ejaculatory ducts, and bulbourethral glands. The neurovascular bundles are normally located anterolaterally along the pelvic sidewall prior to joining the plexus. Damage to these nerves can result in incomplete erection, lack of ejaculation, retrograde ejaculation, or complete impotence.

Controversy and differing opinions exist regarding the proper plane of dissection anteriorly, as well as the exact

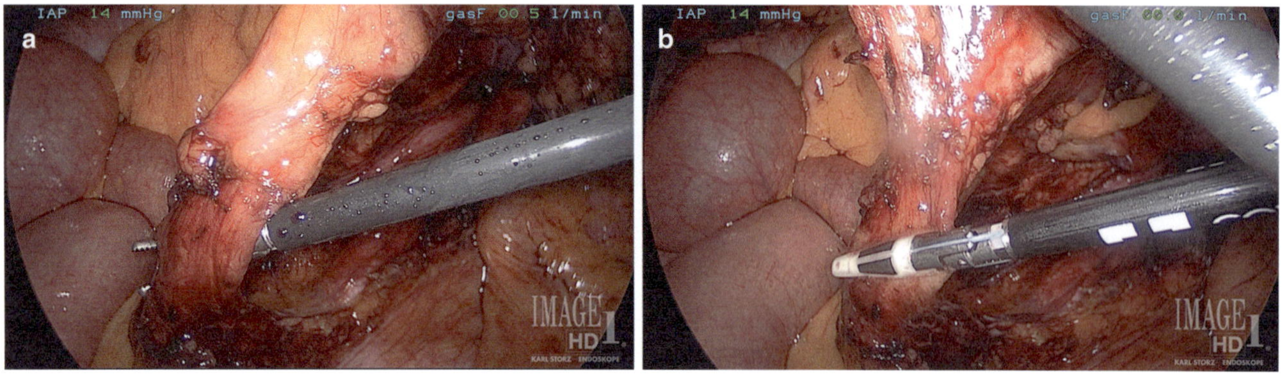


**Fig. 12.5** Intracorporeal exposure (**a**) and ligation (**b**) of the inferior mesenteric/superior hemorrhoidal vessels

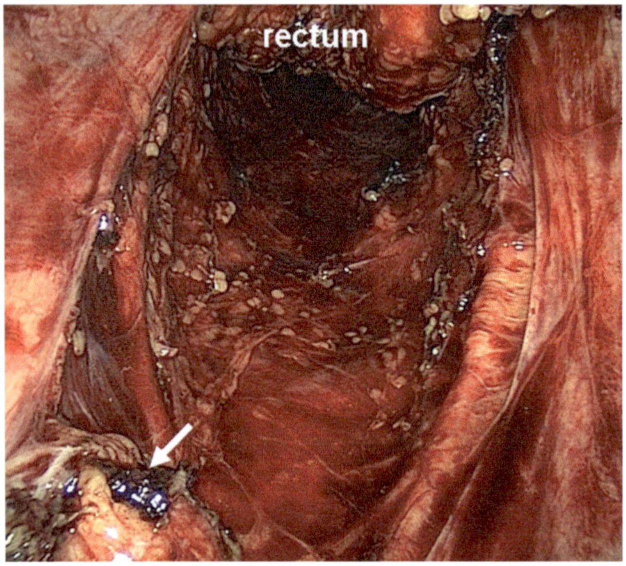


**Fig. 12.6** Dissection in the presacral plane. The *white arrow* indicates the superior hemorrhoidal artery (ligated) in a patient with Crohn's proctitis. Hypogastric nerves are visible laterally

location of Denonvilliers fascia. Many surgeons feel that Denonvilliers fascia is more adherent to the prostate than the rectum. Therefore, dissection immediately on the fascia propria of the rectum in the plane of the TME will allow for complete removal of an intact anterior mesorectum while leaving Denonvilliers fascia on the prostate and avoiding damage to the nerves. Others suggest that Denonvilliers fascia is more closely adherent to the rectum, without a plane posterior to it. In this case, the fascia will be removed along with the rectum during a standard TME dissection. In either light, most colorectal surgeons are aware of the loose areolar tissue immediately outside the fascia propria, providing familiar territory for initial dissection. The choice distally then remains whether to perform dissection on the rectal side or prostatic side of Denonvilliers fascia and to understand the potential consequences of each. Likely the optimal approach is to dissect on the prostate and seminal vesicles for large anterior tumors to minimize the risk of a positive anterior margin. This comes with the obvious increased risk of nerve damage. In women, a similar dissection should occur along the posterior vaginal wall.

## Division of the Sigmoid Colon and Ostomy Creation

The sigmoid colon is grasped and retracted toward the anterior abdominal wall, and a window is created in the mesentery that is sufficiently large to accommodate the 45-mm or 60-mm blue-load laparoscopic stapler. Two firings may be necessary to fully divide the colon. The remaining mesentery between the colon and the superior hemorrhoidal vessels is divided with the energy sealing device (Video 12.2). The proximal end is grasped with a ratcheted grasper. A 19-French round Jackson-Pratt drain is placed into the pelvis using the right lower quadrant port site and can be sutured to the specimen to assure it is pulled down into the pelvis during specimen extraction through the perineal wound. The end is brought through the abdominal wall at the right-sided port and secured to the skin with a nylon suture. Insufflation is maintained. The skin site for the ostomy is created centered at the left lower quadrant 5-mm port. A ring of skin and subcutaneous tissue is cored out using electrocautery. Army-Navy retractors are used for exposure. The anterior fascia is incised with a cruciate incision, the rectus is splayed using a large Kelly clamp, and the abdomen is entered by dividing the posterior sheath and peritoneum in a cruciate fashion using electrocautery. The proximal colon end is brought through the abdominal wall. The 12-mm umbilical port site is closed with a Vicryl suture through the fascia, and skin is closed on all ports with 4–0 Monocryl and either Dermabond or Mastisol and Steri-Strips. The staple line is excised from the end of the colon, and the colostomy is matured with 3–0 Vicryl sutures in a Brooke fashion. The stoma appliance is applied. Having completed the abdominal portion of the dissection, the team prepares for the perineal dissection.

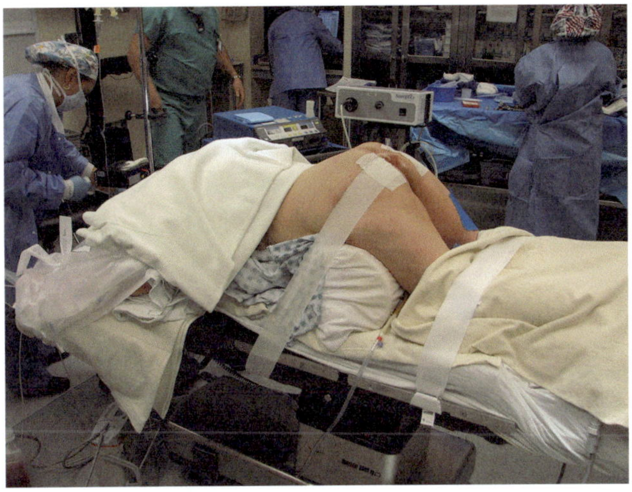

**Fig. 12.7** Patient positioning in the prone jackknife position. Chest and hip rolls in place and buttocks taped widely apart

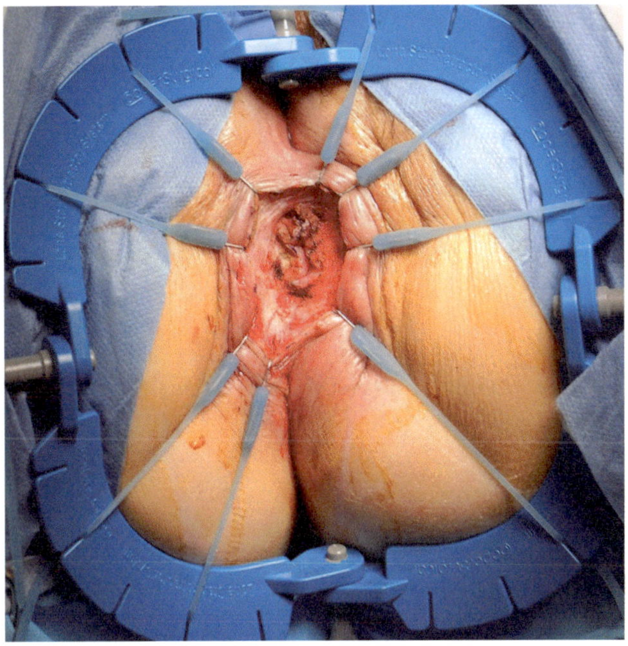

**Fig. 12.8** Starting the perineal dissection, the Lone Star Retractor has been set up and extrasphincteric plane is being developed

## Perineal Dissection

The patient is placed onto a second operating room table in the prone jackknife position (Fig. 12.7) over soft chest and hip rolls. Bony prominences are padded and the buttocks are taped apart using heavy cloth tape. Attention is focused on the colostomy, which should not have any direct pressure on it if positioned off the hip roll. The field is prepped with Betadine. The anus has already been sewn closed. After confirming the location of the coccyx posteriorly, the ischial tuberosities laterally, and the mid-perineum anteriorly, an elliptical incision is made circumferentially around the anus. The Lone Star Retractor™ (CooperSurgical, Trumbull, CT) is secured. The extrasphincteric plane is entered and followed to the levators (Fig. 12.8). The coccyx is palpated, and the anococcygeal ligament is divided posteriorly to enter the pelvis. The surgeon's finger is placed in this space and hooked around the levator muscles. A cylindrical dissection is performed, taking a circumferential portion of levator muscle with the specimen to avoid narrowing it and creating a "waist" [19, 20]. The specimen is exteriorized through the posterior space, and the more difficult anterior plane is better visualized and dissected. In men, the dissection proceeds just posterior to the prostate and urethra. In women, the plane is developed between rectum and vagina. The surgeon's finger can be placed in the vagina to help feel and expose this plane. Tumor involvement of the prostate or vagina mandates en bloc resection. In the case of a bulky tumor that cannot be exteriorized (or a narrow pelvis), the specimen is circumferentially dissected, disconnected, and pulled out through the pelvis. The surgeon may choose to open and examine the specimen on the back table or, ideally, in coordination with the pathologist to more accurately determine margin status.

The tip of the Blake drain is positioned deep in the pelvis. The perineal wound is thoroughly irrigated and hemostasis is ensured. The peritoneum is not closed primarily, as this creates a closed space in the pelvis, allowing for accumulation of blood and fluid that is at risk for becoming infected and contributing to perineal wound complications and pelvic abscess [21]. The wound is closed in layers, first using one to two layers of 0 Vicryl figure-of-eight interrupted sutures, and then one to two layers of 2–0 Vicryl figure-of-eight interrupted sutures, irrigating with saline between each layer. The skin is reapproximated with loosely spaced 2–0 Vicryl simple interrupted sutures. Local anesthetic (0.25 % marcaine with epinephrine) may be infiltrated. A dry sterile dressing is applied.

## Alternative Approaches

### Performing the Perineal Dissection First ("Abdominoperineal Resection")

The perineal dissection can be performed before the abdominal approach. The purported advantage of this approach is that the most challenging distal aspect of the laparoscopic pelvic dissection to the levators has already been performed from below [22]. With this approach, we recommend performing the perineal dissection in the prone position to facilitate exposure, retraction, and coordinated dissection with

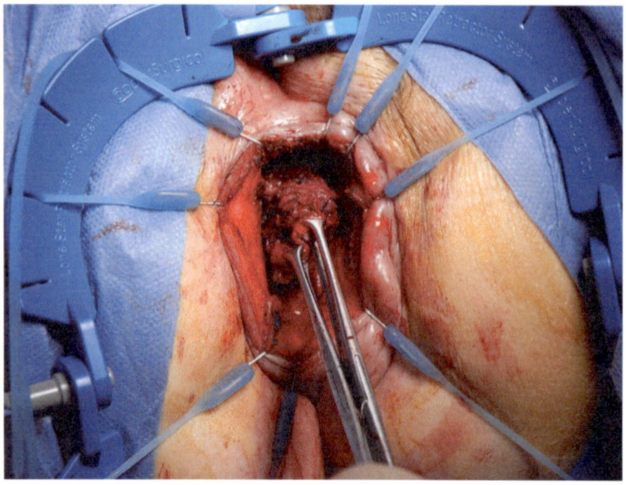

**Fig. 12.9** Initial dissection in the intersphincteric plane for a patient with Crohn's proctitis

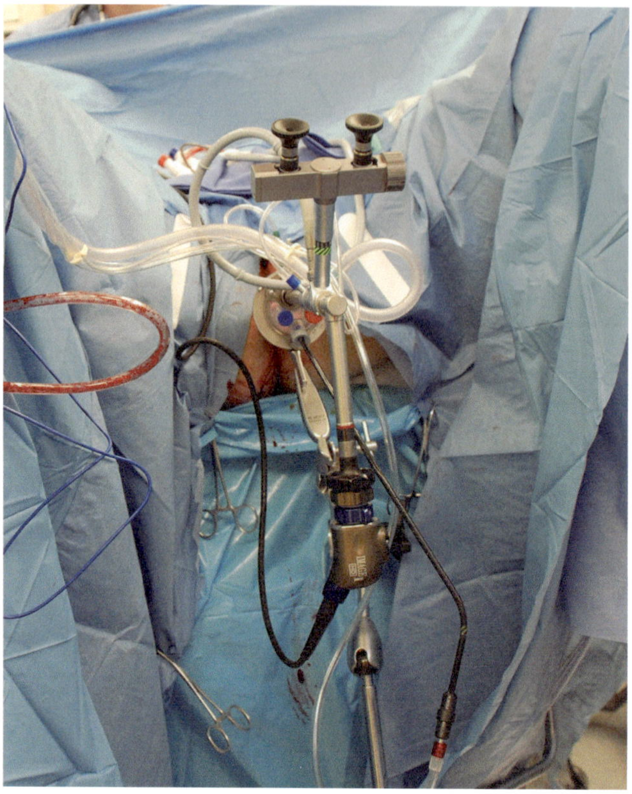

**Fig. 12.10** TEM setup through perineal incision. Alternatives include the GelPOINT system and SILS port

your assistant and proceeding similarly to the description above. The pelvis is entered circumferentially at the level of the levators, first in the posterior plane. As described above, a portion of levator is taken to avoid coning in on the specimen. Upon completion of the perineal portion, a lap pad is tucked into the wound, and it is covered with an occlusive dressing (Tegaderm, 3M, St. Paul, MN) to prevent insufflation gas from escaping during the abdominal portion of the case. The patient is repositioned and prepped and the abdominal phase begins.

## Laparoscopic Perineal Approach

The perineal portion of the operation can be approached via a laparoscopic technique as well. The traditional laparoscopic abdominal exposure and retraction in the deep pelvis remains challenging, as a result of bulky uterus and adnexa as well as redundant pelvic peritoneum, smoke accumulation, and overall visualization. These factors continue to limit the widespread application of minimally invasive proctectomy for both the laparoscopic and robotic approaches. The theoretical advantage of this retrograde method relates to the creation of the dissection plane in the pelvis within a plane beneath these other pelvic structures, so exposure is less impeded. In fact, with $CO_2$ insufflation of the plane outside of the mesorectal fascia, the dissection plane begins to create itself. At this time, the literature that describes the feasibility, safety, and oncologic outcomes with this approach remains in its infancy [23].

The patient is in lithotomy position. The anus is sewn closed as described previously. Dissection is initiated either in the intersphincteric (benign disease such as ulcerative colitis) or extrasphincteric plane (for malignancy) (Figs. 12.8 and 12.9). Once an adequate dissection has been completed, typically to just beyond the level of the levators, the GelPOINT Path port, SILS device, or TEM proctoscope (Richard Wolf, Vernon Hills, IL) is positioned within the dissected space and secured to the skin (Fig. 12.10). This securing maneuver helps prevent $CO_2$ leakage and movement or dislodgement of the access device. The space is insufflated to 15 mmHg, which will put the tissues on tension, thereby retracting the anus/rectum and helping to provide a working space with exposed wispy fibers in the mesorectal dissection plane (Fig. 12.11). Laparoscopic hook cautery or scissors is used for the dissection, and a suction irrigator is used both for smoke evacuation and countertraction. This small space fills easily with smoke, obscuring the surgeons view, and the working space quickly collapses with suction. This particular challenge can be addressed by connecting two separate $CO_2$ insufflation lines to the access device or by switching to a system that allows for continuous smoke evacuation and $CO_2$ exchange. The dissection proceeds to the level of the cervix in women and to the seminal vesicles in men or until the prior resection from above is reached. The specimen is then removed through the perineal defect.

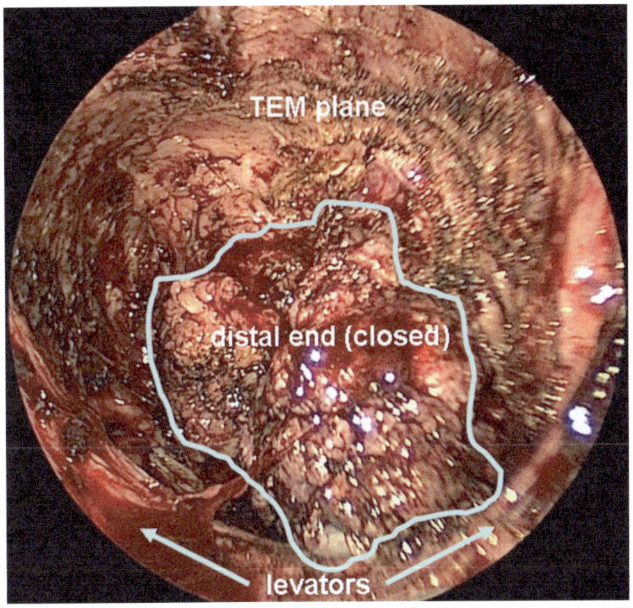


**Fig. 12.11** View of the laparoscopic total mesorectal excision dissection plane

## Reconstruction of the Perineal Defect

Preoperatively, consideration should be given to the potential need for reconstruction of the pelvic defect following abdominoperineal resection. Without reconstruction, the large pelvic dead space after APR may lead to perineal wound complications including infection, abscess, chronic draining sinus, fistula, or hernia. More specifically, reconstruction is indicated for extra-levator/cylindrical resections or pelvic exenterations for malignancy that result in large defects, particularly in the irradiated pelvis, which is associated with increased rate of wound complications [24]. Preoperative consultation with a plastic surgeon with expertise in this area is essential. The intent here is to provide a brief overview of the most common techniques.

## Myocutaneous Flaps

The main advantage of myocutaneous flaps is that they provide pelvic reconstruction with autogenous, nonirradiated, well-vascularized tissue (Fig. 12.12). Immediate flap reconstruction has been shown to significantly decrease perineal wound morbidity from APR after radiotherapy [25]. The three main options are flaps created from the following muscles: rectus abdominis (RAM), gracilis, and gluteus maximus. The RAM flap is based on the inferior epigastric artery pedicle, is rotated to fill the pelvic defect, and is generally oriented obliquely in the perineum. The gracilis flap is based on the profunda femoris artery, and the gluteus maximus flap is based on the inferior gluteal artery. These RAM flaps are typically harvested unilaterally opposite the site of the colostomy. It should be noted that these flaps do also increase operative time, have donor site morbidity, and also run the risk of flap necrosis.

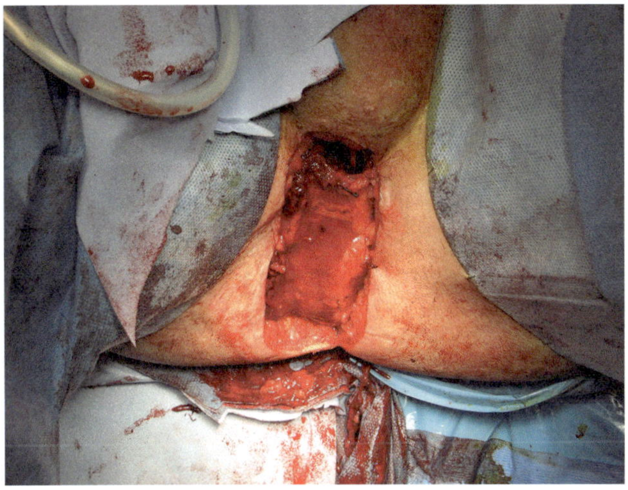

**Fig. 12.12** Myocutaneous flap in place following APR, flap mobilization, and placement

## Omentoplasty

Omentoplasty refers to the creation of a pedicled flap of omentum (based on the gastroepiploic artery) that is transposed down into the pelvis to fill the dead space. Omental flaps can be used alone or in combination with a myocutaneous flap. Risks of omental flaps are rare and include internal hernia formation, necrosis, and bleeding [26]. They may not be technically feasible if the omentum is congenitally small or has been previously resected, has tumor deposits, or is involved in an inflammatory process. Adequate length may not be obtainable with the laparoscopic approach. Small retrospective studies have shown decreased rates of perineal wound complications with omentoplasty with or without concomitant myocutaneous flaps [27].

## Mesh

Biologic mesh can be used to reconstruct the pelvis after APR (Fig. 12.13). These novel acellular materials are derived from porcine dermis, intestinal submucosa, or human acellular dermis. These materials act as scaffolding, promoting tissue ingrowth and neovascularization. Compared to myocutaneous flaps, biologic mesh is appealing because it is associated with decreased operating room time and can be placed without the need for a plastic surgeon.

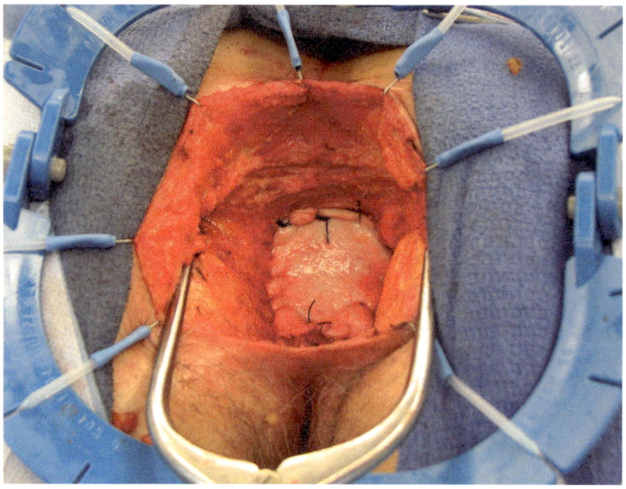

**Fig. 12.13** Reconstruction of pelvic floor using biologic mesh following APR

Biologic mesh has been shown to be safe for use in contaminated fields [28]. A drawback remains the significant cost, with prices as high as $30/cm$^2$ (compared to $2/cm$^2$ for polypropylene). Use of biologic mesh has largely supplanted synthetic mesh for pelvic reconstruction in the contaminated field, given the increased risk of bowel obstruction, bowel erosion and fistulization, and mesh infection. Both nonabsorbable (GORE-TEX) and absorbable (Vicryl) products have been used as well.

**Table 12.1** Potential complications of laparoscopic abdominal perineal resection

| |
|---|
| *Intraoperative* |
| Injuries to adjacent structures |
| • Ureters |
| • Urethra |
| • Prostate |
| • Seminal vesicles |
| • Vagina |
| Injuries to other abdominal/pelvic organs |
| • Spleen |
| • Small bowel |
| • Colon |
| Hemorrhage |
| • Iliac vessels |
| • Presacral venous plexus |
| *Postoperative* |
| Urinary retention |
| Pelvic abscess, hematoma |
| Perineal wound infection |
| Cardiopulmonary failure |
| Renal failure |
| *Long term* |
| Small bowel obstruction |
| Hernias |
| • Ventral |
| • Parastomal |
| • Perineal |
| • Colostomy prolapse |
| • Sexual dysfunction |
| Locally recurrent cancer |

## Perioperative Management and Complications

In our practice, patients are placed on a "fast-track" colorectal planner. Nasogastric tubes are not routinely employed. Patients are given clear liquids on postoperative day (POD) 1, full liquids on POD 2, and regular diet on POD 3 and beyond. Early ambulation is encouraged. Pain control is achieved with an intravenous patient-controlled anesthesia and ketorolac. The Foley catheter is removed on POD 3. The pelvic drain is usually removed prior to discharge or when output becomes minimal to prevent drainage and wound complications related to perineal incision. An enterostomal therapist visits the patient (and family if interested) and performs ostomy education prior to discharge. A visiting nurse is set up to see the patient to continue with stoma education and care. The first postoperative office visit is scheduled for 2 weeks postoperatively. Patients who underwent APR for malignancy require routine postoperative surveillance to monitor for local recurrence and distant metastasis.

Most of the intraoperative and postoperative complications for laparoscopic APR are the same as for the open procedure (Table 12.1). The main intraoperative complications include injuries to adjacent structures including the ureter(s), urethra, prostate, seminal vesicles, vagina, and iliac or presacral vessels. More remote structures such as the small bowel, colon, or spleen can be injured as a result of the laparoscopic approach (trocar injury, direct or capacitive coupling electrocautery injury, traction injury). These complications can often be controlled and repaired laparoscopically, but this may require laparoscopic expertise by other team surgeons such as urologists and vascular specialists. Of course, presacral hemorrhage is the most dangerous intraoperative scenario that may mandate immediate conversion to laparotomy. Perioperative complications include ileus, cardiopulmonary issues, urinary retention, renal failure, pelvic sepsis or hematoma, and perineal wound infection. More long-term complications include adhesive bowel obstructions, parastomal and perineal hernias, stoma prolapse, and sexual dysfunction. It should be highlighted that, ideally, the decision to convert to an open approach is made preemptively, before an intraoperative complication occurs. Significant dense adhesions, a thick sigmoid mesentery, inability to identify the ureters, and difficult visualization in the pelvis are all legitimate reasons to open. In many cases, much of the dissection has already been done laparoscopically, thereby minimizing the size of the open incision that needs to be made; often a small Pfannenstiel incision can be used to complete the abdominal approach. In the case of hemorrhage from the presacral veins or superior hemorrhoidal vessels, prompt lower midline laparotomy may be necessary to obtain adequate control.

## Conclusion

Laparoscopic APR has been shown in many series to be safe and feasible, with earlier postoperative recovery and decreased length of stay. Larger prospective randomized controlled trials are ongoing, but two smaller trials demonstrated equivalent oncologic outcomes between the laparoscopic and open approaches. Appropriate patient selection and preoperative evaluation and planning are critical to a good surgical outcome. There are a variety of laparoscopic approaches detailed in this chapter, and the surgeon can customize the approach for a particular patient. The fundamental steps of the laparoscopic approach are identical to the conventional open operation; therefore, conversion to an open procedure to accomplish these critical steps should be considered an exercise of good judgment and is not a failure. With many commonalities, the robotic approach will be discussed elsewhere in this textbook. Postoperative management typically follows a "fast-track" plan, and patients who do well are usually discharged within 3–5 days.

## References


1. Ng SS, Leung KL, Lee JF, et al. Surgical treatment of anoperineal Crohn's disease: can abdominoperineal resection be predicted? J Am Coll Surg. 1999;189(2):171–6.
2. de Buck van Overstraeten A, Wolthuis AM, Vermeire S, et al. Intersphincteric proctectomy with end-colostomy for anorectal Crohn's disease results in early and severe proximal colonic recurrence. J Crohns Colitis. 2013;7(6):227–31.
3. Lacy AM, García-Valdecasas JC, Delgado S, et al. Laparoscopy-assisted colectomy versus open colectomy for treatment of non-metastatic colon cancer: a randomised trial. Lancet. 2002;359(9325):2224–9.
4. Clinical Outcomes of Surgical Therapy Study Group. A comparison of laparoscopically assisted and open colectomy for colon cancer. N Engl J Med. 2004;350(2):2050–9.
5. Liang JT, Huang KC, Lai HS, et al. Oncologic results of laparoscopic versus conventional open surgery for stage II or III left-sided colon cancers: a randomized controlled trial. Ann Surg Oncol. 2007;14(1):109–17.
6. Fleshman J. American College of Surgeons Oncology Group (ACOSOG)-Z6051. A phase III prospective randomized trial comparing laparoscopic-assisted resection versus open resection for rectal. Cancer. http://clinicaltrials.gov/ct2/show/NCT00726622.
7. Row D, Weiser MR. An update on laparoscopic resection for rectal cancer. Cancer Control. 2010;17(1):16–24.
8. Veldkamp R, Kuhry E, Hop WC, et al. Laparoscopic surgery versus open surgery for colon cancer: short-term outcomes of a randomised trial. Lancet Oncol. 2005;6(7):477–84.
9. Jayne DG, Thorpe HC, Copeland J, et al. Five-year follow-up of the Medical Research Council CLASICC trial of laparoscopically assisted versus open surgery for colorectal cancer. Br J Surg. 2010;97:1638–45.
10. Ng SS, Leung KL, Lee JF, et al. Laparoscopic-assisted versus open abdominoperineal resection for low rectal cancer: a prospective randomized trial. Ann Surg Oncol. 2008;15(9):2418–25.
11. Tjandra JJ, Kilkenny JW, Buie WD, et al. Practice parameters for the management of rectal cancer (revised). Dis Colon Rectum. 2005;48(3):411–23.
12. Heald RJ, Husband EM, Ryall RD. The mesorectum in rectal cancer surgery—the clue to pelvic recurrence? Br J Surg. 1982;69(10):613–6.
13. da Silva G, Boutros M, Wexner SD. Role of prophylactic ureteric stents in colorectal surgery. Asian J Endosc Surg. 2012;5(3):105–10.
14. Redan JA, McCarus SD. Protect the ureters. JSLS. 2009;13(2):139–41.
15. Monn MF, Haut ER, Lau BD, et al. Is venous thromboembolism in colorectal surgery patients preventable or inevitable? One institution's experience. J Am Coll Surg. 2013;216(3):395–401.
16. Buchberg B, Masoomi H, Lusby K, et al. Incidence and risk factors of venous thromboembolism in colorectal surgery: does laparoscopy impart an advantage? Arch Surg. 2011;146(6):739–43.
17. Navarro-Vicente F, García-Granero A, Frasson M, et al. Prospective evaluation of intraoperative peripheral nerve injury in colorectal surgery. Colorectal Dis. 2012;14(3):382–5.
18. Gaujoux S, Bretagnol F, Au J, et al. Single port access proctectomy with total mesorectal excision and intersphincteric resection with a primary transanal approach. Colorectal Dis. 2011;13:e305–7.
19. Holm T, Ljung A, Haggmark T, et al. Extended abdominoperineal resection with gluteus maximus flap reconstruction of the pelvic floor for rectal cancer. Br J Surg. 2007;94:232–8.
20. West NP, Finan PJ, Anderin C, et al. Evidence of the oncologic superiority of cylindrical abdominoperineal excision for low rectal cancer. J Clin Oncol. 2008;26(21):3517–22.
21. Robles Campos R, Garcia Ayllon J, Parrila Paricio P, et al. Management of the perineal wound following abdominoperineal resection: prospective study of three methods. Br J Surg. 1992;79:29–31.
22. Marks JH, Frenkel JL. Laparoscopic abdominoperineal resection (APR). In: Wexner SD, Fleshman JW, editors. Master techniques in general surgery: colon and rectal surgery: abdominal operations. 1st ed. Philadelphia, PA: Lippincott Williams & Wilkins; 2012. p. 323–31.
23. de Lacy AM, Rattner DW, Adelsdorfer C, et al. Transanal natural orifice transluminal endoscopic surgery (NOTES) rectal resection: "down-to-up" total mesorectal excision (TME)-short-term outcomes in the first 20 cases. Surg Endosc. 2013;27(9):3165–72.
24. Chadwick MA, Vierten D, Pettitt E, et al. Short course preoperative radiotherapy is the single most important risk factor for perineal wound complications after abdominoperineal excision of the rectum. Colorectal Dis. 2006;8:756–61.
25. Nisar PJ, Scott HJ. Myocutaneous flap reconstruction of the pelvis after abdominoperineal excision. Colorectal Dis. 2009;11(8):806–16.
26. Nilsson PJ. Omentoplasty in abdominoperineal resection: a review of the literature using a systematic approach. Dis Colon Rectum. 2006;49(9):1354–61.
27. Butt HZ, Salem MJ, Vijaynagar B, et al. Perineal reconstruction after extra-levator abdominoperineal excision (eLAPE): a systematic review. Int J Colorectal Dis. 2013;28(11):1459–68.
28. Han JG, Wang ZJ, Gao ZG, et al. Pelvic floor reconstruction using human acellular dermal matrix after cylindrical abdominoperineal resection. Dis Colon Rectum. 2010;53(2):219–23.

# 13 Laparoscopic Proctocolectomy

David A. Etzioni and Tonia M. Young-Fadok

*"There are no big problems, there are just a lot of little problems."*

—Henry Ford

**Key Points**

- Laparoscopic proctocolectomy requires technical skills that extend beyond the more common segmental procedures and should be reserved for those surgeons with experience and expertise.
- While the steps may remain the same, the underlying indication for a total proctocolectomy dictates several unique aspects that need to be considered prior to and when performing the operation.
- Break up the case into several smaller operations (e.g., right colon, splenic flexure, etc.) and focus on what needs to be accomplished for that particular part of the procedure.

## Background

Within the spectrum of surgical procedures, laparoscopic proctocolectomy presents a distinct set of challenges for even experienced surgeons. The operation can seem formidable in terms of the time required to perform it and the potential for technical challenges and complications. In this chapter, we will review the decision-making regarding patient selection, timing of operation, and especially the technical aspects of the case.

**Electronic supplementary material:** Supplementary material is available in the online version of this chapter at 10.1007/978-1-4939-1581-1_13. Videos can also be accessed at http://www.springerimages.com/videos/978-1-4939-1580-4.

D.A. Etzioni, M.D., M.S.H.S. (✉)
T.M. Young-Fadok, M.D., M.S.
Division of Colon and Rectal Surgery, Mayo Clinic College of Medicine, 5777 E. Mayo Blvd., Phoenix, AZ 85054, USA
e-mail: etzioni.david@mayo.edu

## Epidemiology and Economics

While laparoscopic proctocolectomy is performed commonly in tertiary medical centers, it is not a common operation within the overall population. The most common indications for performing the procedure are ulcerative colitis, Crohn's disease, and familial adenomatous polyposis. It is quite unusual for the procedure to be performed for other indications, although in rare instances the operation is appropriate for other polyposis syndromes, cancer, or colitides. Unfortunately, it is very difficult to estimate accurately the number of laparoscopic proctocolectomies that are performed each year in the United States (US), as there is no specific code for laparoscopic proctocolectomy in the current International Classification of Diseases (ICD-9) coding scheme. The ICD code 45.81 (laparoscopic intra-abdominal colectomy) is the only code that reasonably correlates to the procedure.

Based on this code, a brief analysis of data from the 2011 Healthcare Cost and Utilization Project (HCUP) is revealing. The HCUP database represents a sampling of approximately 20 % of the discharges within the United States each year and therefore provides a powerful view into rates and patterns of surgical utilization. Using HCUP and the ICD codes listed above, we see that the operation is performed on 4,800 patients with underlying UC, 1,200 patients with Crohn's disease, and 1,300 with FAP.

Laparoscopic proctocolectomy also engenders a distinct burden to patients and payers. Costs for the operative episode of care are estimated to be between $43,000 [1] and $50,000 [2]. The rate of complications is significant, including anastomotic leakage, reoperation, obstruction, fistula, wound infection, and hemorrhage.

Given the cost and likelihood of complications, it needs to be remembered that proctocolectomy is not an entirely elective procedure. For many patients, their quality of life with IBD has deteriorated to the point that proctocolectomy, with either end ileostomy or reconstruction with an ileoanal

H.M. Ross et al. (eds.), *Minimally Invasive Approaches to Colon and Rectal Disease: Technique and Best Practices*, DOI 10.1007/978-1-4939-1581-1_13, © Springer Science+Business Media New York 2015

pouch, may be the only way to restore a reasonable quality of life. Also, the expense of surgery may be cost beneficial in the long term. In one study, the costs of care for patients after recovery from proctocolectomy were significantly lower than the costs of care prior to the procedure [2].

## Preoperative Considerations

Patients undergo proctocolectomy for several different indications, each of which mandate a different set of considerations when planning the procedure.

### Ulcerative Colitis

In general, patients with ulcerative colitis undergo proctocolectomy when there is a failure of medical management to control their disease. This can manifest in a number of ways, including worsening symptoms of abdominal discomfort, diarrhea, and neoplastic changes. The majority of these patients have been treated with an escalating regimen of medications, including powerful immunosuppressives. When a surgical approach is planned based on the results of a pathologic evaluation, it is critical that these results be reviewed by an experienced gastrointestinal pathologist (preferably two). Other indications include perforation and hemorrhage (which are relatively infrequent), side effects from medications, the wish to avoid medications in patients of childbearing age, and growth retardation in children and adolescents.

Once a decision has been made to proceed with proctocolectomy, several issues need to be resolved as part of the overall surgical plan. The first and most important issue is understanding the long-term goal for the patient's overall intestinal continuity. While an ileoanal pouch is the standard of care for patients with ulcerative colitis undergoing proctocolectomy, this is not a foregone conclusion. A very small number of patients may be candidates for a total colectomy and ileorectal anastomosis if the following criteria are met: (1) relative rectal sparing (although this should also prompt consideration of a diagnosis of Crohn's disease), (2) preserved rectal compliance, and (3) absence of rectal dysplasia/neoplasia. It is important to point out that restoration of gastrointestinal continuity is not necessarily a goal of care. Older patients, especially those with compromised sphincter function or limitations in mobility, may be better served by a plan for a permanent end ileostomy.

A second question in planning an operation for these patients is whether a proctocolectomy (with or without ileoanal pouch) or an abdominal colectomy (leaving the rectum behind) is the more appropriate *initial* operation. Fundamentally, the proctectomy portion of the operation is more complicated and more likely to engender short- and long-term complications. Therefore, a proctocolectomy is inappropriate in a patient who is metabolically depleted and malnourished, acutely ill/toxic, or otherwise unfit for surgery. Obesity may also render an attempt at proctocolectomy and J-pouch inadvisable until the patient has lost weight.

An area of emerging controversy is whether or not patients who are treated with biologic medications (e.g., infliximab, adalimumab, certolizumab) are at higher risk for postoperative complications. This topic has been meta-analyzed at least three times in the last 3 years [3–5], with mixed meta-results. Two of these studies found higher rates of postoperative complications [3, 5], and one found no higher risk [4]. Of note, the study which reported no greater risk with biologic therapy [4] calculated a risk of short-term infectious complications that was over two times greater (odds ratio = 2.24), but because of sample size issues, this was considered not statistically significant. At the current time, an accurate estimate of the magnitude of increased risk that is associated with biologic therapy is elusive. Given the significant rate/burden of complications inherent in laparoscopic proctocolectomy, it seems prudent to take steps to optimize the patient's condition, and toward this goal we recommend discontinuing biologic medications prior to laparoscopic proctocolectomy. Our practice is to stop these medications for 1.5–2 dosing intervals prior to surgery. In situations where a smaller scope of surgery and/or no anastomosis is required (e.g., colectomy/proctocolectomy with ileostomy), then this restriction can be relaxed. In situations where the patient's condition is clinically urgent and an interval period after the last dose of biologic medication is not feasible, then we consider the ongoing or recent use of biologic therapy to be a risk factor, which should prompt consideration of a three-stage operation.

### Crohn's Disease

Relative to ulcerative colitis, Crohn's disease is more heterogenous and often involves more nuanced surgical decision-making. As with ulcerative colitis, surgical treatment is called for when medical therapy fails or complications occur. Unlike ulcerative colitis, however, operating on one portion of the colorectum for Crohn's disease does not specifically mandate a proctocolectomy or even a total colectomy.

In terms of operative planning, the most important distinction between Crohn's disease and ulcerative colitis is that with Crohn's disease an ileoanal pouch is widely considered to be contraindicated. Rates of pouch failure and poorer quality of life are seen when an ileoanal pouch is used for a patient who is either known or subsequently discovered to have Crohn's disease [6–8].

As laparoscopic proctocolectomy will result in a permanent ileostomy for a patient with Crohn's, there are choices regarding how to manage the distal anal canal. The two main options are ultralow-stapled transection or intersphincteric proctectomy. A stapled transection is reasonable in the absence of perianal disease. This approach is the most technically expedient, but there is the risk of a staple line dehiscence and subsequent pelvic infection. Also, there is the possibility of perianal disease arising from residual anal mucosa. It does, however, preserve the sphincter, which some patients find reassuring when making the difficult decision to proceed with an operation. The alternative, an intersphincteric proctectomy, requires additional operating time but provides a more secure closure of the pelvic floor. These two approaches are likely equivalent—however, in patients with significant perianal disease, we recommend intersphincteric proctectomy with debridement of all active fistulas.

## Familial Adenomatous Polyposis (FAP)

The burden of polyps and the likelihood of progression to cancer in patients with true FAP is generally an indication for proctocolectomy. Diagnostic evaluation and operative planning for these patients should include a full colonoscopy, esophagogastroduodenoscopy (EGD), as well as computed tomography (CT) of the abdomen/pelvis. These evaluations are critical to planning appropriate treatment. Several issues regarding the patient's status need to be determined prior to surgery.

First, the presence of malignancy needs to be determined, especially rectal cancer. Given the innumerable polyps seen in the colorectum of a patient with FAP, it is often impossible to completely exclude cancer, but dominant masses should be biopsied.

Second, the extent of rectal polyposis needs to be closely evaluated. Patients with a minimal burden of polyp disease in the rectum may be candidates for total abdominal colectomy and ileorectal anastomosis. For highly selected patients, this option may provide better defecatory function and avoid the morbidity associated with proctectomy. The exact threshold, in terms of the burden of polyps, which mandates proctocolectomy (as opposed to ileorectal anastomosis) is hotly debated. No more than 10–20 polyps should be present, and if an ileorectal operation is planned, the rectum should be entirely cleared of polyps preoperatively. Even in patients with minimal polyp disease in the rectum, however, there will be a need for lifelong surveillance of the rectal remnant. The likelihood of a subsequent rectal cancer is still estimated at 5.5 % [9].

Third, the CT scan should be closely reviewed for the presence of neoplastic disease. This may manifest in the form of metastatic disease from undetected colon carcinoma or Gardner's syndrome with intra-abdominal desmoid tumors. Finally, the purpose of an EGD is to examine for the presence of duodenal adenomas, which are a significant source of morbidity for patients with FAP [10].

In taking care of these patients, it is highly important to consider that FAP is a hereditary disease, with an autosomal dominant mechanism of inheritance. The patient and family need to be counseled, and a referral to a genetics counselor is highly advisable.

## Site Marking

Any patient for whom an ostomy is being considered will benefit from preoperative consultation and stoma site marking with a trained ostomy nurse [11, 12]. It is important for the surgeon to communicate the planned type of ostomy with the ostomy nurse—often the surgeon is privy to pragmatic details about ostomy formation (e.g., hernia sites, thickened abdominal wall, etc.) that may affect planning.

Planned ostomy sites may be utilized for trocar placement, with obvious benefits. Often a temporary ileostomy site can be moved a few centimeters in order to allow for the area to also be used for a trocar. Alternatively, a trocar site that is close to the ileostomy does not pose a long-term problem—the trocar incision generally heals well even if it is under the ileostomy appliance.

## Stapled IPAA vs. Mucosectomy and Handsewn Anastomosis

In patients for whom an ileoanal pouch is planned, a decision needs to be made before operation—whether to perform a stapled anastomosis or a mucosectomy and handsewn anastomosis. The relative advantages of each of these approaches are partially intuitive/theoretical and partially based in evidence.

Intuitively, preservation of a cuff of 2–3 cm of rectal mucosa above the dentate line (including the transition zone) allows for better gastrointestinal function and quality of life after an IPAA. Four randomized trials have examined this belief, each with a relatively small sample size [9–12]. These trials were meta-analyzed by Schluender et al., and their findings were that the two approaches are essentially similar. It is worth noting, however, that these studies are quite small (total of 180 patients) and somewhat older. Also, two of these four studies demonstrated some evidence of improved function among patients with a double-stapled technique [11, 12]. These differences within single studies did not translate into an overall finding in meta-analysis, possibly because of nonuniformity of measured end points or issues with sample sizes. A systematic review comparing a broader spectrum of studies (both experimental and prospective/retrospective) found that the double-stapled technique conferred improved nocturnal continence and better physiological parameters of function [13–15]. It is the authors' belief that patient function is better with the double-stapled technique.

For patients with UC, preservation of a rectal cuff is not without costs. The residual mucosa can become a problem in patients with IBD or FAP as a result of either ongoing inflammation ("cuffitis") or subsequent development of dysplasia/neoplasia. Adenocarcinoma arising from the anal transition zone is rare, but reported after IPAA with double-stapled anastomosis for UC [16, 17]. The risk is small, but poorly quantifiable. Intuitively, the risk of dysplasia and subsequent carcinoma in patients with UC is the result of a "field defect," where dysplastic changes are driven by the ongoing pancolonic inflammation. Therefore, the risk of dysplasia in a rectal cuff (post-IPAA) is higher among patients who have distal colonic or rectal dysplasia. Lovegrove et al. propose an algorithm whereby patients with diagnosed dysplasia in the distal rectum are better served by a handsewn anastomosis with mucosectomy and those with more proximal dysplasia are still offered a double-stapled anastomosis [13]. This is the authors' practice.

The choice of double-stapled vs. mucosectomy and handsewn IPAA is especially important for patients with FAP. While cuffitis is not necessarily a consideration, the underlying risks of adenoma and carcinoma formation are higher in this group. Patients with FAP do seem to have a lower risk of adenoma/carcinoma with a handsewn technique [14, 15]. Unfortunately, even a mucosectomy and handsewn anastomosis is not a guarantee against adenoma/carcinoma formation. Islands of rectal mucosal cells have been found to exist under the distal pouch after mucosectomy in pathology specimens examined after pouch excision [16]. In the largest review of its kind, von Roon et al. found that after 10 years, the risk of adenoma formation was 22.6 % with mucosectomy and 51.1 % with handsewn anastomosis [19]. Additionally, there are multiple reports of a carcinoma developing in the anal canal of a patient with FAP, even after IPAA with mucosectomy [15, 17]. Regardless of technique, patients with FAP need lifelong surveillance of their pouch and anal canal after IPAA.

### Patient Positioning

The patient's position is best considered to be at least as useful as any surgical assistant during a laparoscopic proctocolectomy, and in order to make the best use of gravity, some planning is necessary. Without appropriate steps, extreme positioning can lead to patients sliding on the bed or even falling. While no one method is universally accepted to maintain position on the bed, the two main approaches are (1) foam padding on the bed, which generates significant friction and restricts slipping, and (2) a deformable "beanbag," which contours around the patient's back and shoulders, thereby cradling the patient. Regardless of how the OR bed is prepared, low lithotomy is, in all cases, the preferred position for laparoscopic proctocolectomy. The thighs should be in line with the patient's abdomen to prevent interference with the use of instruments in the lower abdominal ports during mobilization of the flexures.

## Technical Approach

### Trocar Placement

Our preferred approach is based on a diamond-shaped configuration used for port placement (Fig. 13.1). Initial access to the peritoneal compartment is achieved through a cutdown incision just above the level of the umbilicus. After the abdomen is entered, a 12 mm blunt port is inserted, and pneumoperitoneum is achieved. Following exploration of the abdominal cavity, three additional operating ports are inserted in the following locations: (1) a 5 mm port in the suprapubic midline, (2) a 5 mm port in the left lower quadrant, and (3) a disc of skin and subcutaneous fat are excised and a 12 mm port is placed through the planned ileostomy site in the right lower quadrant. Additional 5 mm ports may be placed as required. The mobilization of the splenic flexure may be facilitated through the addition of an additional 5 mm right upper quadrant trocar.

Some flexibility in port placement is also important. In obese patients, the umbilicus may be significantly more caudal relative to abdominal/pelvic structures, necessitating a more cephalad point of entry into the abdomen.

### Ordering the Elements of the Procedure

A laparoscopic proctocolectomy is essentially comprised of multiple smaller operations: (1) right colon mobilization, (2) hepatic flexure mobilization, (3) left colon mobilization, (4) splenic flexure mobilization, (5) rectal mobilization, (6) division of the anorectum, (7) transection of colon mesentery, (8) ileoanal pouch formation/anastomosis, and (9) ileostomy formation. There are many "correct" ways to order the elements of a laparoscopic proctocolectomy, several impractical ways (difficult to transect the rectum before mobilizing it!), and a few inadvisable ways.

We recommend against transecting the left colon/sigmoid mesentery before mobilizing the rectum, as these attachments provide important caudal retraction when the patient is in Trendelenburg position. It also is important to make

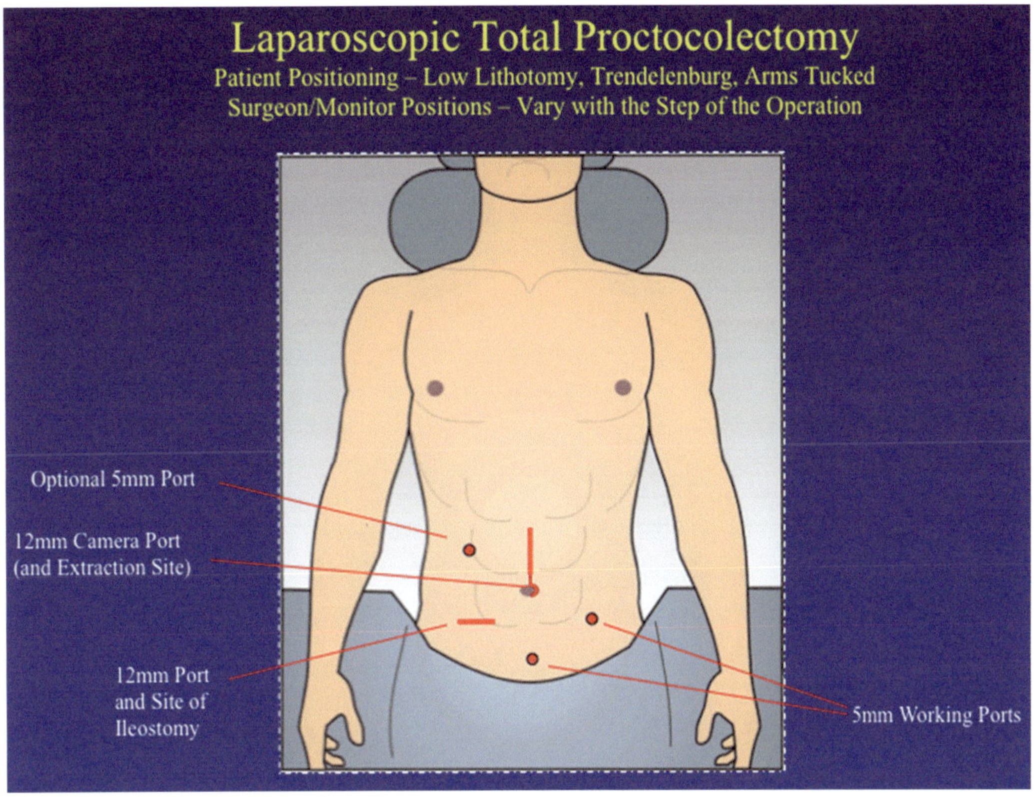


**Fig. 13.1** Port placement for a total proctocolectomy with IPAA

a strategic decision to divide transverse colon mesentery intra- vs. extracorporeally. If a vertical incision is planned, then this can facilitate an extracorporeal transection of the transverse colon mesentery, as well as pouch formation. Also, it is our preference not to divide major vascular pedicles early in the procedure, as this avoids an ischemic portion of colon remaining within the abdomen for extended periods of time. Hence we utilize a lateral-to-medial approach to mobilization of the intra-abdominal colon, which preserves the vascular pedicles. In general, however, the various elements of the case can be ordered according to surgeon preference.

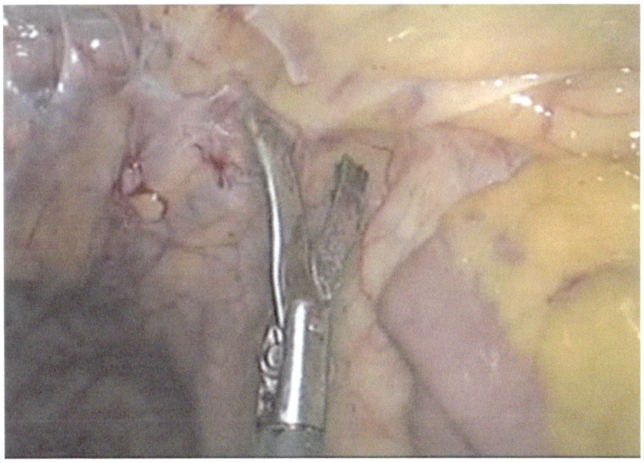

**Fig. 13.2** Mobilization of the terminal ileum. *Courtesy of Conor Delaney, MD, with permission*

## Right Colon Mobilization

For this maneuver, the OR table is placed in steep Trendelenburg, with the right side elevated. The small bowel is swept out of the pelvis and to the left using atraumatic techniques. The omentum is swept into the left upper quadrant. Commencing at the right pelvic brim, the peritoneal reflection bridging between the terminal ileum/cecum and the retroperitoneum is scored with the cautery scissors (Figs. 13.2 and 13.3). In patients with normal BMI, the ureter can often be visualized through the peritoneum, whereas in heavier patients this is more readily seen after opening the retroperitoneal plane. This dissection along the white line of Toldt continues superiorly and medially, taking care to remain in the correct plane anterior to Gerota's fascia (Videos 13.1 and 13.2). Throughout the dissection, care is taken to identify and protect the right ureter, inferior vena cava, and the duodenum. Some visual cues are useful here: (1) if the iliopsoas muscle is visualized, this implies that the dissection is too posterior, (2) the contour of the kidney should be seen

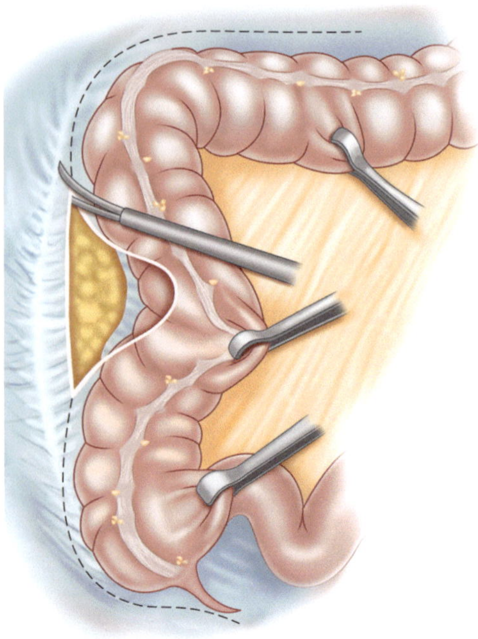

Fig. 13.3 Lateral-to-medial mobilization of the right colon

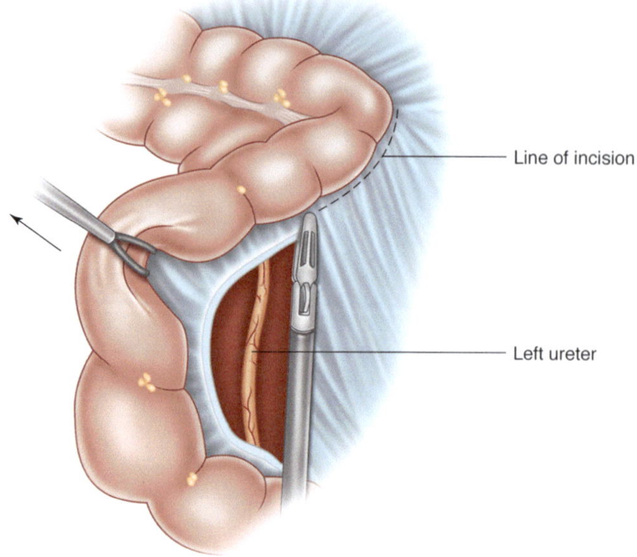


Fig. 13.4 Lateral-to-medial mobilization of the left colon

posterior (not medial) to dissection, and (3) the peritoneum of the right colon mesentery should not be breached—if the dissection is occurring through fatty tissue, this should prompt a reevaluation. Occasionally, due to scarring from inflammatory disease processes or prior surgery, this plane can be difficult to elucidate. In these cases, the right colon can be mobilized in a counterclockwise direction, starting at the level of the hepatic flexure and proceeding proximally. This portion of the dissection can be considered completed when inferior and anterior surfaces of the duodenum are exposed. The peritoneum around the base of the terminal ileal mesentery is fully dissected to the level of the duodenum to facilitate subsequent "reach" of the pouch, when a pouch-anal anastomosis is intended.

## Hepatic Flexure Mobilization

For this maneuver, the OR table is placed in steep reverse Trendelenburg, with the right side elevated. The operating surgeon, standing on the patient's left, can use the supraumbilical trocar to place caudal retraction on the hepatic flexure. With this retraction, the hepatocolic attachments between the superior margin of the colon and the inferior aspect of the liver are placed under tension and can be divided and swept off the underlying retroperitoneum. From the left abdominal trocar, an energy delivery device can be used to divide these tissues. Dissection continues posteriorly, inferiorly, and medially to expose the anterior surface of the duodenum and the interface between the duodenum and pancreas. This dissection should readily merge with the mobilization, which has already been performed of the right colon. As dissection moves medially (clockwise), the lesser sac is entered.

## Left Colon Mobilization

The mobilization of the left colon typically starts at the level of rectosigmoid. This area is a well-defined starting point for both more proximal and more distal dissection. The patient is placed in Trendelenburg position, with the left side elevated. The sigmoid colon is grasped and retracted medially using the right-sided trocar, and the lateral peritoneal attachments are taken sharply using the suprapubic trocar (Fig. 13.4). Gentle sweeping of the peritoneal reflection laterally with judicious cautery will reveal the underlying ureter and iliac vessels underneath the peritoneal covering (Video 13.3). The white line of Toldt "stays with the patient," i.e., the plane of dissection is immediately medial to the white line, and this is the most reproducible method of finding the ureter. This dissection proceeds distally to the pelvic brim and proximally to the splenic flexure (Video 13.4).

## Splenic Flexure Mobilization

Splenic flexure mobilization is a critical and frequently challenging technical element of a proctocolectomy. The mobilization can be challenging, primarily due to issues regarding exposure and the risk of injuring the splenic capsule, vessels within the splenocolic ligament, or the colon mesentery.

The flexure can be approached in one of two directions—clockwise or counterclockwise—usually both directions need to be undertaken in order to perform a complete mobilization.

The counterclockwise dissection is a natural continuation of the sigmoid and left colon mobilization (Video 13.5). For this portion of the maneuver, the operating surgeon can work either from the patient's right side or between the patient's legs. The OR table should be in steep reverse Trendelenburg position and tilted slightly to the right. Adequate tension must be maintained medially as the splenic flexure is approached, in order to avoid wandering into or behind the kidney. As the apex of the flexure is mobilized, the underlying pancreas should be identified in order to prevent injury. The splenocolic ligament and other attachments between the transverse colon mesentery and the retroperitoneum are best divided using an energy delivery device.

The clockwise dissection begins in the area of the mid- to distal transverse colon (Video 13.6). A decision needs to be made whether or not to remove the greater omentum with the specimen or preserve it. If the intent is to leave the omentum, then the lesser sac can be entered by dissecting the omentum from the anterior surface of the transverse colon and reflecting it into the upper abdomen. The left and inferior trocars can be used to retract the omentum cephalad and the colon caudal. Using the right trocar, an energy delivery device can be used to open the lesser sac, moving distally. Alternatively, the omentum can be removed en bloc with the transverse colon. In these cases, the greater omentum is incised just caudal to the gastroepiploic vessels, superior to approximately the midpoint of the transverse colon, and the lesser sac is entered. The colon and omentum are retracted caudally, and the lesser sac is opened by dividing the gastrocolic and splenocolic attachments, moving toward the spleen. Finally, the retroperitoneal attachments need to be divided to ensure complete mobilization of the splenic flexure. This is facilitated by caudal retraction on the colon, keeping the tension on the adhesions and dividing from the apex (Video 13.7).

Splenic flexure mobilization can be made difficult by previous surgery, body habitus, or anatomical variations. In these situations, the placement of an additional trocar in the right upper quadrant may be of use, especially during the clockwise dissection. A grasper placed through this trocar can facilitate with anterior/cephalad retraction and exposure of the lesser sac.

## Rectal Mobilization

Mobilization of the rectum begins with the caudal continuation of the sigmoid/left colon dissection. The OR table is placed in Trendelenburg position, with the left side elevated. Using the right trocar as a grasper, the rectosigmoid junction is retracted medially (Video 13.8). A dissecting instrument is placed through the suprapubic trocar, and this is used to incise the reflection between the mesorectum and the pelvic sidewall. Notably, this maneuver can be accomplished with the operating surgeon on either the patient's right or left side. While it may seem initially awkward, it is our preference to perform this maneuver with the operating surgeon standing on the patient's left, using an instrument placed through the left trocar as a retractor.

During the course of this dissection, great care needs to be taken to identify the appropriate plane that separates the mesorectum from retroperitoneum. The left ureter and superior hypogastric nerve should be clearly identified. Proceeding distally, the peritoneum between the mesorectum and the lateral pelvis should be incised. Careful inspection of the left side of the rectum should demonstrate "white tissue" (pelvic sidewall tissues) laterally and "yellow tissue" (mesorectum) medially. The line between these two types of tissues marks the appropriate point of entry into the presacral plane.

This left-sided dissection then continues as far as possible prior to moving to the right side. The right-sided dissection uses similar landmarks to divide the pelvic peritoneum, separating the mesorectum from the pelvic sidewall. Once again, care needs to be taken to identify the superior hypogastric nerve and ureter, although the right ureter is usually not endangered during this portion of the operation. Moving medially and distally, the plane of dissection joins with the dissection already performed on the left side. With the rectum elevated anteriorly, the dissection continues distally as far as possible, occasionally necessitating further attention to lateral attachments (Video 13.9).

With the posterior and lateral attachments of the rectum mobilized, attention can be turned to the anterior plane. In a male, this begins with incising the peritoneal reflection and dissection to expose the seminal vesicles and subsequently the prostate. In the course of exposing this anterior plane, the suprapubic instrument is the most useful in attaining effective cephalad retraction. Importantly, the patient should be in steep Trendelenburg positioning to maximize the use of gravity as a "second assistant." There is significant confusion regarding the anatomy of Denonvilliers fascia in this area, and the importance of removing it during the course of a proctectomy. In the absence of an anterior rectal cancer in this location, there is no need to fashion a plane of dissection that denudes the prostate or seminal vesicles (see Fig. 10.8).

In females, the peritoneal reflection is significantly deeper within the pelvis (Fig. 13.5). The uterus is frequently a significant barrier to visualizing the anterior reflection. If this is the case, then the uterus can be retracted anteriorly with either a transvaginal uterine retractor or a transabdominal suture. In order to suture the uterus out of the field of

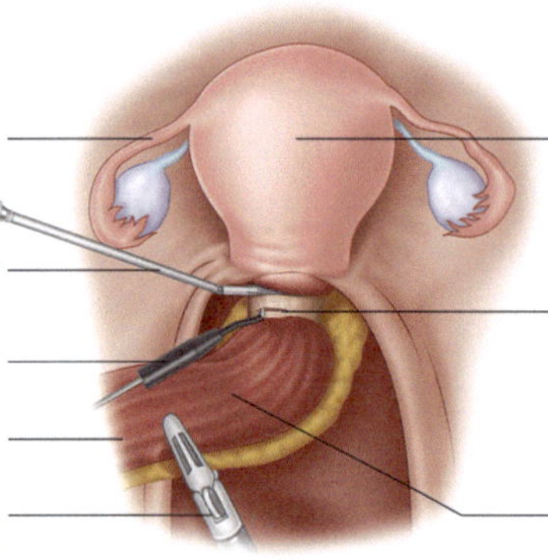


**Fig. 13.5** Anterior peritoneal reflection in a female patient

dissection, a straight needle is passed through the abdominal wall inferior to the suprapubic port, through the fundus of the uterus, then exited through the abdominal wall and tied.

## Division of the Anorectum

Several strategies are possible in choosing how to divide the anorectum. These include (1) intersphincteric proctectomy, (2) abdominoperineal resection, (3) laparoscopic stapled division, and (4) open stapled division.

Intersphincteric proctectomy (Fig. 13.6) is appropriate in patients who will have a permanent ileostomy. The benefit of an intersphincteric proctectomy over a stapled closure (ultralow Hartmann's) is the ability to completely remove the mucosa of the anorectum. This may be desirable, especially in patients with Crohn's disease or significant dysplasia within the rectum. The distal aspect of this operation is performed with the patient in high lithotomy, usually with the help of a self-retaining retractor.

It is unusual to perform an abdominoperineal resection as part of a proctocolectomy and is generally performed only in the context of invasive cancer close to the anorectal ring. In other cases, an intersphincteric proctectomy is preferable as it avoids the considerable morbidity, which accompanies the perineal wound closure.

The most common method for dividing the anorectum is using a laparoscopic linear stapler (see Video 10.2). Prior to performing this maneuver, the rectum should be dissected to the pelvic floor, circumferentially. Insertion of a finger into the anus is very helpful in assuring that the dissection is complete and that there are no areas of residual attachment/fixation. The thickness of the anorectum approaches the upper limit of what a laparoscopic stapler can safely encompass. Therefore, great attention needs to be paid to assuring that all surrounding tissues (mesorectum, areolar tissues, etc.) are cleared from the site of planned division. The laparoscopic staple must be articulating and can be introduced from either the suprapubic trocar (division in anterior-posterior orientation) or a right abdominal trocar position (division in oblique/horizontal orientation). The planned ileostomy site is a useful point of entry for an additional trocar. Staple height should be at least 4.0 (unformed staple length). A shorter cartridge length allows for better maneuvering (especially in narrow/male pelves) but may result in the need for multiple firings in order to completely transect the rectum.

Open division of the anorectum is an alternative to the laparoscopic approach. In order to accomplish this, a low abdominal incision (either Pfannenstiel or midline) is made, sufficient to allow a hand and a stapler to be inserted. Using a transverse stapler, the anorectum is divided just above/at the pelvic floor and the specimen is retrieved. The main advantage of this approach is the avoidance of multiple staple firings, which is associated with higher rates of anastomotic leakage [19, 20]. Depending on the planned operation, the low midline incision can be used to facilitate pouch formation and/or facilitate ileostomy formation.

## Transection of Colon Mesentery

Division of the colon mesentery is a significant portion of any laparoscopic proctocolectomy. We prefer not to divide the mesentery until the colon is completely mobilized, as ischemia ensues quite quickly. An ischemic colon is more fragile and also expands in size, making the operation more challenging if the mesentery is divided early in the operation. However, many surgeons who prefer a medial-to-lateral approach do divide the mesentery early in the procedure.

The most difficult part of the mesentery to divide is that of the transverse colon. Therefore, a specific decision needs to be made regarding specimen extraction and the division of this mesentery. If an incision is planned for specimen extraction, then an upper midline incision can be used for both specimen extraction and the division of the transverse colon mesentery. In cases where no incision is planned, then the entire colon mesentery can be taken intracorporeally.

Laparoscopic division of the colon mesentery generally begins after the anorectum is transected, when using the lateral-to-medial approach. The mesenteric division proceeds proximally, starting with the sigmoid colon (Fig. 13.7). Unless the operation is performed for known/suspected carcinoma, the level of the transection can be a "division of convenience," i.e., it can be fairly close to the colon wall (a high ligation of the inferior mesenteric artery or superior hemorrhoidal pedicle is not necessary). The mesentery of the sigmoid/left colon can be viewed and transected from a medial perspective (tenting up the colon) or pulled medially and transected from a lateral perspective.

Division of the transverse colon mesentery is challenging because (1) of its relationship to the stomach, duodenum,

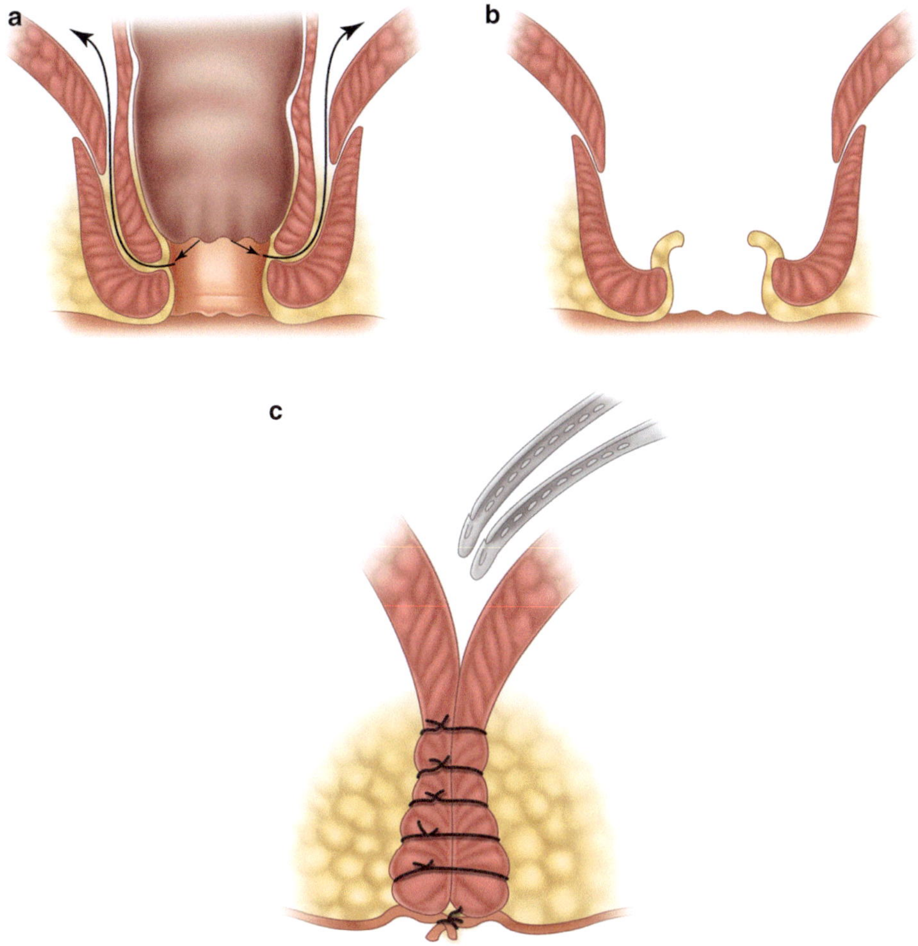


**Fig. 13.6** Intersphincteric proctectomy

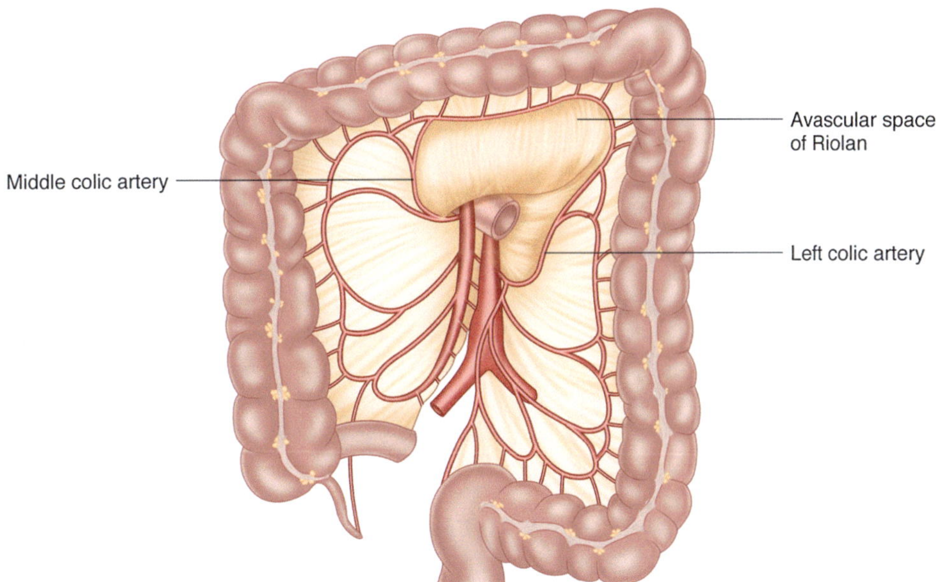


**Fig. 13.7** Major arterial blood supply to the colon

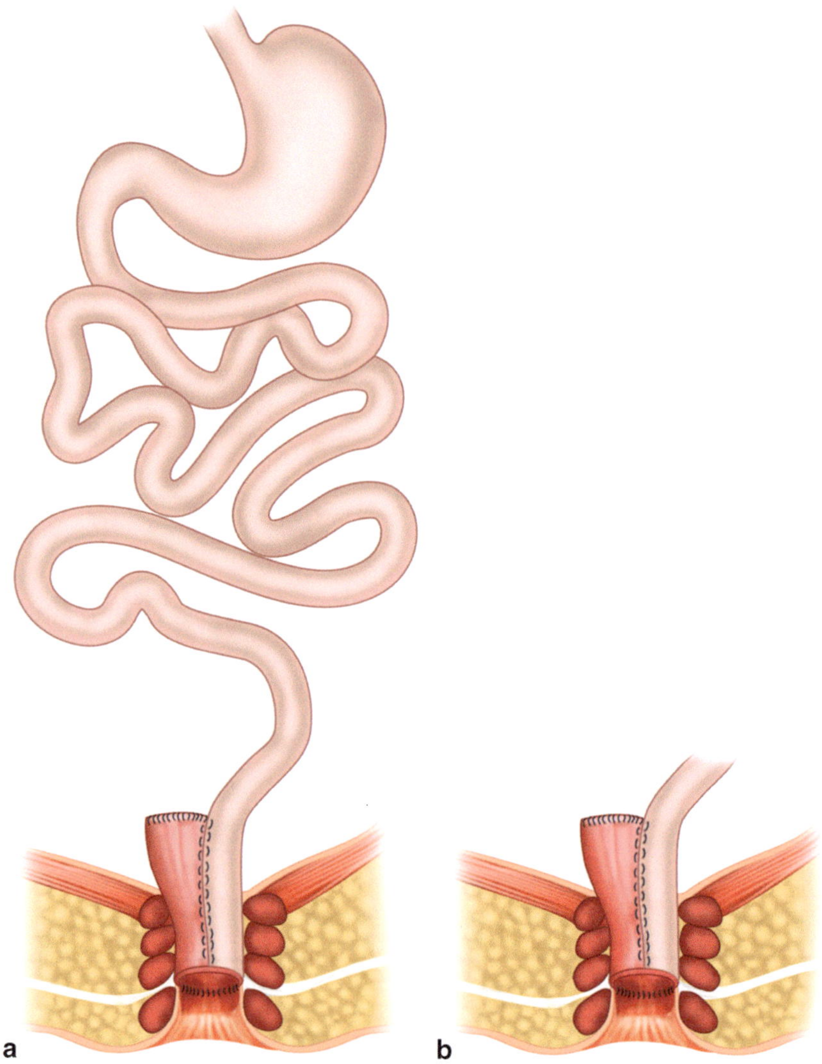


**Fig. 13.8** Schematic diagram of an ileal pouch-anal anastomosis

omentum, and proximal small bowel, (2) there is no cut end of colon nearby to use as a handle, and (3) the mesentery is relatively short. As with the left colon, the division of the mesentery can be approached from either the side of the lesser sac or from the inferior surface. Of note, as one proceeds proximally with this dissection, the ileocolic vessels are surprisingly close to the middle colic vessels. If the operative plan includes preservation of the ileocolic vessels (e.g., for ileoanal pouch), then the mesenteric dissection is essentially completed once the hepatic flexure is reached.

## Ileoanal Pouch Formation and Anastomosis

The indications and contraindications for ileoanal pouch formation are beyond the scope of this chapter, but we will briefly review some technical elements of pouch construction (Fig. 13.8). An ileoanal pouch, as part of an operation for ulcerative colitis, can be formed either through the planned ileostomy site or through an extraction incision either in the lower abdomen or periumbilical region. Forming the pouch through an ileostomy site can be challenging in patients who are not svelte, especially men. Generally the ileostomy site is only used as an extraction site in patients who are of normal body mass index, given the larger incision required for heavier patients and the difficulty in ascertaining reach of the pouch in patients with an obese abdominal wall or thick terminal ileal mesentery.

If a pouch is planned, then prior to making any incision in the abdomen, the small bowel needs to be completely mobilized. The most important area of fixation and loss of length occurs at the root of the terminal ileal mesentery, and this area of attachment between the small bowel mesentery and the retroperitoneum needs to be completely mobilized off the duodenum. To begin pouch formation, the terminal small bowel is exteriorized and examined for length. When exteriorized through an abdominal incision, the apex of a 15 cm pouch should be able to reach the inferior border of the pubis with minimal stretch. Earlier research [18] found that a reach of 6 cm below the pubis was necessary to ensure that all pouches reached the dentate line, but we find that this amount of reach is not a reasonable benchmark using an extraction incision (in any part of the abdomen).

If there is a concern over reach, then consideration should be given to pouch-lengthening maneuvers. There are many described means by which to achieve greater length, but the most effective are (1) incising the small bowel mesentery peritoneum [19], (2) dividing the superior mesenteric vessels, and (3) consideration of an alternative pouch configuration (e.g., S pouch). We refer to the algorithm for achieving appropriate reach as described in the review by Uraiqat et al. for a more detailed discussion regarding this important topic [20]. Our standard stapler size for pouch formation is 28 mm, and the anvil of this end-end anastomotic (EEA) stapler device is sutured into the apex of the pouch with 2-0 Prolene suture.

Once the pouch is created, it is returned to the abdomen, attempting to place it with correct orientation within the pelvis. The extraction incision is closed. The anastomosis is then fashioned with the benefit of laparoscopic visualization. The pouch mesentery is visualized along its length to ensure that the cut edge of the mesentery between the pouch and the second portion of the duodenum is straight. In placing the pouch into the pelvis, the pouch itself should be anterior to its corresponding mesentery, for maximal reach. The EEA device is placed into the anal canal, and the stapler pin is ejected in the middle of the anorectal cuff. Using laparoscopic instrumentation, the anvil is docked onto the stapler handle and closed. Prior to firing the EEA stapler, care must be taken to ensure that no twisting of the mesentery has occurred. Also, in a female patient, the posterior wall of the vagina should be palpated to verify that the stapler has not entrapped the wall during closure. After these checks have been performed, the stapler can be fired. The pouch orientation is checked one more time to ensure there is no twist (Video 13.10). We typically send the distal donut of tissue for pathologic evaluation, in addition to the main specimen. A transanal drain is placed in the pouch for decompression and removed 2–3 days later.

## Ileostomy Formation

An ileostomy can be formed during a laparoscopic total proctocolectomy as either (1) a permanent ileostomy or (2) a diverting loop ileostomy above an ileoanal pouch.

When the operation entails a permanent ileostomy, it is crucial to form an ileostomy, which is technically optimal. The technical elements that impact this goal primarily relate to (1) appropriate ostomy siting, (2) appropriate fascial aperture, and (3) appropriate ileostomy eversion. All patients undergoing elective surgery that involves ostomy formation should have a preoperative consult with a trained ostomy professional for education and site marking. The size of the fascial (and skin) aperture(s) should be only large enough to admit the ileostomy limb and accompanying mesentery.

When a temporary loop ileostomy is planned, the ileostomy is formed after the ileoanal anastomosis is completed and a drain has been placed in the pelvis (if desired). An aperture is made in the abdominal wall (if not already created) and sized appropriately for the ileostomy. A non-crushing clamp is placed through the aperture, and a loop of distal ileum is retrieved through the aperture. This loop of small intestine can be maintained extracorporeally while the abdomen is de-insufflated and the remaining trocars are removed under direct visualization. When all skin incisions are closed and sterile dressings have been applied, the loop ileostomy can be matured.

## Pearls and Pitfalls

- Using the ostomy sites for port placement has advantages; however, do not let this dictate placement if it will ultimately hinder your ability to perform the case.
- You need to be comfortable with both handsewn and double-stapled techniques, as invariably a situation will arise that will require you to use one or the other.
- Leave the major vascular pedicles alone early in the case. This will not only avoid leaving ischemic bowel in the abdomen for prolonged periods but also not burn any bridges up front. Focus on mobilization initially and determining the optimal method for completing each step.

## Summary

This chapter provides an overview of one form of approach to laparoscopic proctocolectomy, with or without IPAA, that we utilize in our practice. We acknowledge that there are multiple other approaches that also achieve good outcomes, for example, medial-to-lateral mobilization and use of hand-assisted approaches. We have more experience with the techniques outlined above. We have also found merit in a single incision approach in selected patients, but this is technically quite demanding, and we have chosen to describe the approach that is applicable to the majority of the patients in our practice.

## References


1. Ellis MC, Diggs BS, Vetto JT, et al. Trends in the surgical treatment of ulcerative colitis over time: increased mortality and centralization of care. World J Surg. 2011;35(3):671–6.
2. Holubar SD, Long KH, Loftus Jr EV, et al. Long-term direct costs before and after proctocolectomy for ulcerative colitis: a population-based study in Olmsted County, Minnesota. Dis Colon Rectum. 2009;52(11):1815–23.

3. Kopylov U, Ben-Horin S, Zmora O, et al. Anti-tumor necrosis factor and postoperative complications in Crohn's disease: systematic review and meta-analysis. Inflamm Bowel Dis. 2012;18(12):2404–13.
4. Yang Z, Wu Q, Wang F, et al. Meta-analysis: effect of preoperative infliximab use on early postoperative complications in patients with ulcerative colitis undergoing abdominal surgery. Aliment Pharmacol Ther. 2012;36(10):922–8.
5. Yang Z, Wu Q, Wu K, et al. Meta-analysis: pre-operative infliximab treatment and short-term post-operative complications in patients with ulcerative colitis. Aliment Pharmacol Ther. 2010;31(4): 486–92.
6. Richard CS, Cohen Z, Stern HS, et al. Outcome of the pelvic pouch procedure in patients with prior perianal disease. Dis Colon Rectum. 1997;40(6):647–52.
7. MacRae HM, McLeod RS, Cohen Z, et al. Risk factors for pelvic pouch failure. Dis Colon Rectum. 1997;40(3):257–62.
8. McIntyre PB, Pemberton JH, Wolff BG, et al. Indeterminate colitis. Long-term outcome in patients after ileal pouch-anal anastomosis. Dis Colon Rectum. 1995;38(1):51–4.
9. Aziz O, Athanasiou T, Fazio VW, et al. Meta-analysis of observational studies of ileorectal versus ileal pouch-anal anastomosis for familial adenomatous polyposis. Br J Surg. 2006;93(4):407–17.
10. Parc Y, Mabrut JY, Shields C. Surgical management of the duodenal manifestations of familial adenomatous polyposis. Br J Surg. 2011;98(4):480–4.
11. Reilly WT, Pemberton JH, Wolff BG, et al. Randomized prospective trial comparing ileal pouch-anal anastomosis performed by excising the anal mucosa to ileal pouch-anal anastomosis performed by preserving the anal mucosa. Ann Surg. 1997;225(6): 666–76. discussion 676–7.
12. Hallgren TA, Fasth SB, Oresland TO, et al. Ileal pouch anal function after endoanal mucosectomy and handsewn ileoanal anastomosis compared with stapled anastomosis without mucosectomy. Eur J Surg. 1995;161(12):915–21.
13. Lovegrove RE, Constantinides VA, Heriot AG, et al. A comparison of hand-sewn versus stapled ileal pouch anal anastomosis (IPAA) following proctocolectomy: a meta-analysis of 4183 patients. Ann Surg. 2006;244(1):18–26.
14. Wasmuth HH, Trano G, Myrvold HE, et al. Adenoma formation and malignancy after restorative proctocolectomy with or without mucosectomy in patients with familial adenomatous polyposis. Dis Colon Rectum. 2013;56(3):288–94.
15. von Roon AC, Will OCC, Man RF, et al. Mucosectomy with handsewn anastomosis reduces the risk of adenoma formation in the anorectal segment after restorative proctocolectomy for familial adenomatous polyposis. Ann Surg. 2011;253(2):314–7.
16. O'Connell PR, Pemberton JH, Weiland LH, et al. Does rectal mucosa regenerate after ileoanal anastomosis? Dis Colon Rectum. 1987;30(1):1–5.
17. Laureti S, Ugolini F, D'Errico A, et al. Adenocarcinoma below ileoanal anastomosis for ulcerative colitis: report of a case and review of the literature. Dis Colon Rectum. 2002;45(3):418–21.
18. Smith L, Friend WG, Medwell SJ. The superior mesenteric artery. The critical factor in the pouch pull-through procedure. Dis Colon Rectum. 1984;27(11):741–4.
19. Baig MK, Weiss EG, Nogueras JJ, et al. Lengthening of small bowel mesentery: stepladder incision technique. Am J Surg. 2006; 191(5):715–7.
20. Uraiqat AA, Byrne CM, Phillips RK. Gaining length in ileal-anal pouch reconstruction: a review. Colorectal Dis. 2007;9(7):657–61.

# Laparoscopic Rectopexy

**14**

Mia DeBarros and Scott R. Steele

**Key Points**

- Laparoscopic and open repairs have similar outcomes regarding recurrence and postoperative function.
- For patients with concomitant symptomatic constipation and a large redundant colon, consideration should be given to a sigmoid resection along with the prolapse repair.
- Posterior mobilization should be down to the pelvic floor, distal to the coccyx.
- Although various opinions exist, the authors' preference is to dissect anteriorly approximately 4 cm, or enough to allow the free edge of the mobilized anterior peritoneal reflection to reach the sacral promontory.
- Posterior mesh placement is best performed with sutures or tacks to the sacral promontory then secured to each side of the mesorectum with nonabsorbable sutures.
- Avoid ligation of the superior hemorrhoidal artery, when possible, with resection procedures.
- It is the authors' preference for a preoperative bowel preparation and postoperatively to place patients on an aggressive bowel regimen and short-term liquid diet to avoid constipation and straining in the early postoperative period.

**Electronic supplementary material:** Supplementary material is available in the online version of this chapter at 10.1007/978-1-4939-1581-1_14. Videos can also be accessed at http://www.springerimages.com/videos/978-1-4939-1580-4.

M. DeBarros, M.D.
Department of Surgery, Madigan Army Medical Center, Fort Lewis, WA 98431, USA

S.R. Steele, M.D., F.A.C.S., F.A.S.C.R.S. (✉)
University of Washington, Seattle, WA 9606, USA

Department of Surgery, Madigan Army Medical Center, Fort Lewis, WA 98431, USA

Colon and Rectal Surgery, Madigan Army Medical Center, Tacoma, WA, USA
e-mail: harkersteele@mac.com

## Introduction

Rectal prolapse or procidentia is a condition in which the rectal wall protrudes through the anus. If there is telescoping or incomplete protrusion that does not progress through the anus, this is referred to as occult rectal prolapse or rectal intussusception [1–4]. Full-thickness prolapse is a distressing and socially debilitating condition that occurs in a bimodal distribution, typically diagnosed before the age of 3 equally in both genders and after the fifth decade of life primarily in females (80–90 % of adult patients diagnosed) [1, 5]. The severity of this condition varies, and patients may present with a protruding mass that spontaneously reduces with standing or cessation of straining or one that has already progressed to continual prolapse. In rare cases, patients may initially present with incarcerated or strangulated prolapse. Most patients have anatomic or functional abnormalities in association with prolapse. Untreated chronic prolapse will result in problems with continence, constipation, and outlet obstruction. The goal of surgery is to control prolapse, restore continence when possible, and prevent constipation and impaired evacuation [1]. This is typically achieved by returning the rectum to its normal position in the pelvis by fixing it to the presacral fascia. This may be accomplished by two approaches: transabdominal or transperineal. The transabdominal approach is associated with lower recurrence rates (0–10 %) and is typically utilized in younger, fitter patients, while the perineal approach is associated with lower morbidity, shorter length of stay, and faster recovery but at the expense of less durable repair and higher recurrence rates of 5–40 % [1, 2, 6–8]. The most commonly performed abdominal procedures in the United States are rectopexy with resection, suture rectopexy, and mesh rectopexy. Another technique, ventral rectopexy, is utilized more often in the setting of rectal intussusception rather than full-thickness rectal prolapse. This approach involves the anterior mobilization of the rectum with mesh placed anteriorly on the rectum and fixation to the sacrum. The perineal approach

H.M. Ross et al. (eds.), *Minimally Invasive Approaches to Colon and Rectal Disease: Technique and Best Practices*, DOI 10.1007/978-1-4939-1581-1_14, © Springer Science+Business Media New York 2015

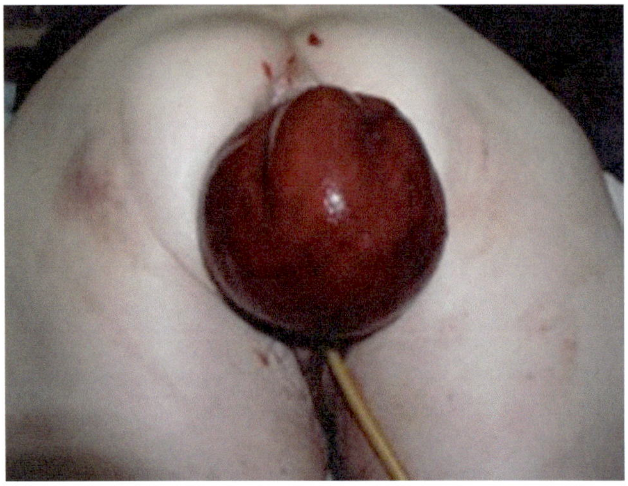

**Fig. 14.1** Incarcerated rectal prolapse *(Courtesy of Isaac Felemovicious, MD, with permission)*

is usually reserved for older, frailer patients with comorbidities that would prevent them from undergoing abdominal surgery and will not be described in this chapter.

Numerous studies and meta-analysis have shown that laparoscopic colorectal surgery is associated with reduced postoperative pain, early return of bowel function, and shortened length of stay; however, there is a paucity of randomized control trials examining laparoscopic rectopexy compared to the open approach [9–11]. The one randomized control performed by Solomon in 2002 found that the laparoscopic technique was associated with early return of bowel function, decreased postoperative pain, and decreased length of stay [12]. A Cochrane Review from 2008 confirmed this finding and noted that recurrence rates and functional outcomes were similar between the laparoscopic and abdominal approach [13]. In addition to the above benefits, laparoscopy has been utilized in a transabdominal approach for a more durable repair in patients that would otherwise have been unable to undergo a more morbid open procedure [14].

Current indications for laparoscopic rectopexy are similar to those of the open technique. Absolute contraindications include those patients who cannot tolerate pneumoperitoneum, required positioning and intraoperative repositioning (i.e., steep Trendelenburg) and incarcerated or strangulated rectal prolapse (Fig. 14.1). Relative contraindications include previous multiple pelvic surgeries and recurrent rectal prolapse following transabdominal rectopexy or inability to safely resect prior anastomosis.

## Preoperative Planning

Proper patient selection cannot be overemphasized. As with any operative procedure, patients should be medically fit and able to tolerate laparoscopy. All patients should undergo a detailed history and physical examination to include a thorough history of their bowel habits, abdominal or pelvic pain, and mucus discharge. The patient should be questioned carefully regarding the need to strain to initiate defecation, episodes of incomplete evacuation, and the use of digital maneuvers to aid in defecation. Physical examination should classically be performed in the left lateral (i.e., Sims) or squatting position, as prone jackknife may make it difficult for all but the most severe of prolapse cases. Examination should also include a digital rectal exam to assess sphincter tone, the presence of masses and concomitant pelvic floor pathology. Sphincter tone is assessed by asking the patient to actively tighten and relax the sphincter muscles. Pelvic floor muscles are assessed by asking the patient to both tighten his or her anal sphincter and "bear down" as if having a bowel movement. This simulates the action of defecation and allows for the assessment of proper contraction and relaxation of the pelvic floor muscles. The degree of prolapse is assessed by having the patient "bear down" while in the squatting or sitting position. It is important to determine if this is full-thickness prolapse with the presence of concentric rings and grooves or mucosal prolapse which has radially oriented grooves (Fig. 14.2a, b). The perineum is examined to identify increased perineal descent or bulging indicative of pelvic floor laxity. A vaginal exam on females may be appropriate to identify other concomitant anatomic abnormalities such as rectocele, cystocele, or uterine prolapse.

Preoperative testing and imaging should be completed on a selective basis. A colonoscopy is recommended in symptomatic patients, high-risk patients, and those >50 years of age if they are not up-to-date or have not had one to rule out malignancy as the cause of prolapse. In patients with severe constipation and infrequent bowel movements, a colonic transit study may be appropriate, as the patient may benefit from a resection as well as rectopexy. In patients with pelvic floor pathology on examination or the suggestion of pelvic floor pathology by history, cinedefecography or dynamic MRI is appropriate to exclude obstructive defecation or further classify the pelvic functional disorder. Anal manometry may be utilized in patients with incontinence to determine their baseline, but this rarely will change the operative approach. Anal ultrasound is another tool available to assess sphincter integrity in patients with fecal incontinence, though again, rarely changes the procedure aimed at addressing the prolapse.

As part of the preoperative preparation, patients should undergo a mechanical bowel preparation, which may be a full preparation or enemas the morning of surgery (according to surgeon preference and patient tolerance). It is our preference to use a full preparation, to avoid having a large stool burden and straining in the early postoperative period that may increase repair failures. Preoperative intravenous antibiotics are given at the appropriate time to ensure adequate

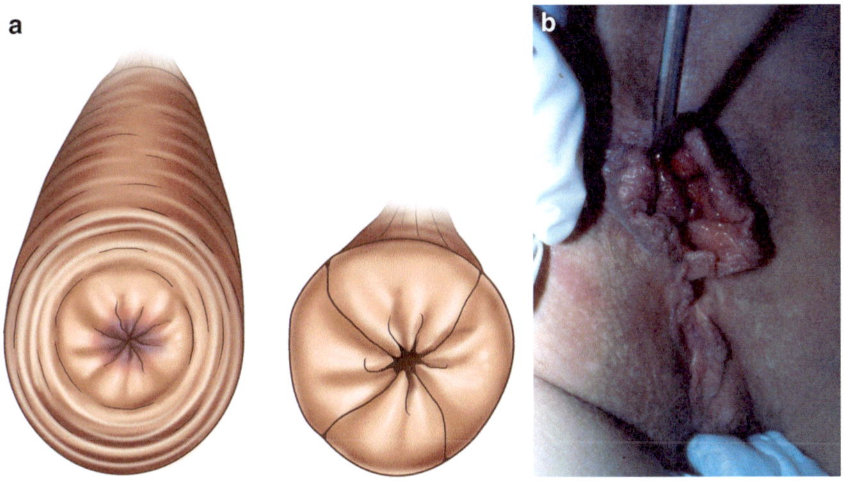


**Fig. 14.2** (**a**) Full thickness rectal prolapse vs. mucosal prolapse. Notice the radial folds with (**a**) mucosal (hemorrhoidal) prolapse and (**b**) mucosal prolapse (*Courtesy of Richard Billingham, MD, with permission*)

concentration during the initial skin incision. The use of oral antibiotics can also be considered, as there are studies that show that this will aid in decreasing the luminal bacterial load [15, 16] and surgical site infections in the setting of a concomitant resection. Deep venous prophylaxis should include the use of sequential compression devices and chemical prophylaxis (i.e., heparin or low molecular weight heparin).

## Procedure

### Setup

Once the patient has undergone general anesthesia, a Foley catheter and orogastric tube should be placed. The patient should then be placed in a modified lithotomy position to allow adequate access to the anus and rectum. The legs should be placed into padded stirrups and ensure that padding is adequate to prevent peroneal nerve injury. Both arms should be tucked to the sides. All bony prominences should be well padded. A sacral gel-pad can also be placed to provide additional decubitus support. The patient should be secured in the operating room table in such way to allow for table movement and steep angles such as Trendelenburg that may be required for laparoscopy without significant patient movement (Fig. 14.3).

The operating surgeon stands on the patient's right side with the assistant on the same or opposite side. Two monitors should be placed at the foot and left-side head of the patient (Fig. 14.4). An additional optional monitor may be placed at the head or foot on the right side for an assistant standing on the patient's left. All equipment for both laparoscopic and open procedures should be available in the event that a conversion to open or a resection and rectopexy is to be performed (Table 14.1). If a conversion is contemplated, the surgeon and first assistant may require the use of headlights to facilitate visualization. The use of ureteral stents are not

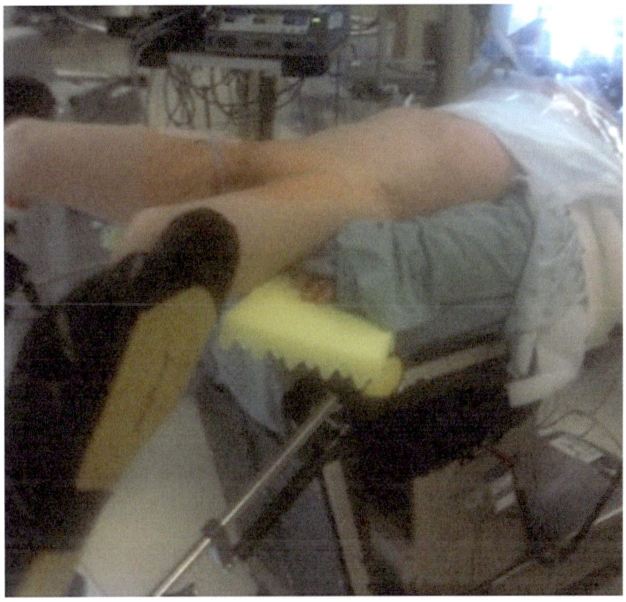

**Fig. 14.3** Patient positioning in the low-lithotomy position with arms tucked, and all bony prominences padded

routinely necessary, but should be considered in patients with prior pelvic or lower abdominal surgery, adhesive disease, or radiation to the pelvis. While this does not prevent intraoperative injury, it does allow for timely identification and repair. The abdomen should be shaved and prepped and draped in the usual standard fashion.

### Procedure Steps

#### Laparoscopic Rectopexy and Resection

**Port Placement (Fig. 14.4)**

- Initial access: We prefer to use a Hassan port in the infra- or supraumbilical position. For patients with extensive prior resection, a Veress needle may be

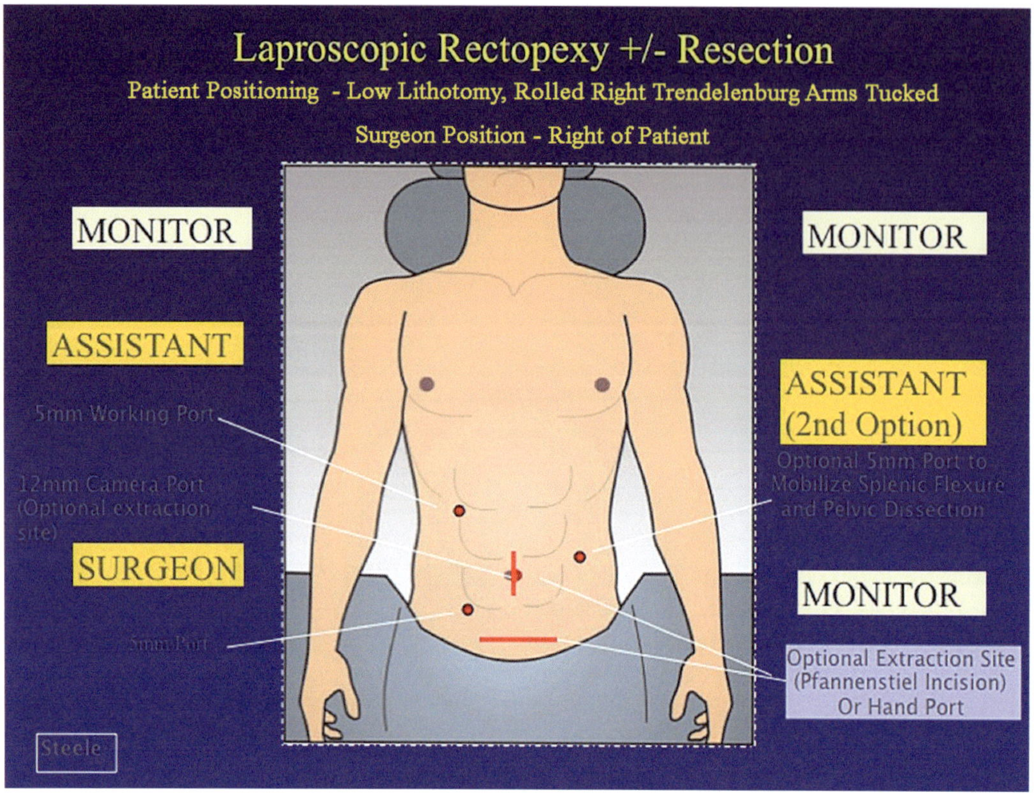


**Fig. 14.4** Suggested trocar and monitor placement for laparoscopic rectal prolapse repair

**Table 14.1** Equipment

| |
|---|
| Head lamps for surgeon and assistant (optional) |
| Laparoscopic monitors |
| 5- and 10 mm 30° laparoscope |
| Trocars (5 mm × 3), Hasson, 10–12 mm × 1, additional 5 or 10 mm trocars for optional ports |
| Laparoscopic blunt, atraumatic graspers, and scissors |
| Laparoscopic needle driver |
| Laparoscopic retractor (i.e., fan blade retractor, optional) |
| Electrocautery with extender tip (i.e., Bovie) |
| Laparoscopic energy device (surgeon preference) |
| Linear cutting stapler and appropriate staple loads |
| Circular cutting stapler (29–33 mm based on surgeon preference) |
| Sizers for circular cutting stapler |
| Nonabsorbable suture |
| Prosthetic mesh (optional) |
| Wound protector drape (optional for resection and extracorporeal anastomosis) |
| Proctoscope |

considered in the left upper quadrant or away from other prior surgical fields.

- Establishment of pneumoperitoneum: This is achieved through the umbilical port. Following adequate pneumoperitoneum, the 10 mm 30° camera is inserted. The abdomen is explored in all four quadrants, and any abnormalities are noted.
- Secondary trocar placement: An additional 10–12 mm trocar is placed in the right lower quadrant and a second 5 mm port in the right upper quadrant with emphasis on adequate triangulation. We attempt to have a minimum of a fist-size distance between each of these ports. If a rectopexy alone is the procedure, the 10–12 mm port will be changed to a 5 mm trocar.
- Optional trocars: (5 mm up to 12 mm in size) may be placed in the left paramedian position, lateral to the edge of the rectus in the left mid-abdomen to assist with sigmoid retraction. Additionally, a suprapubic 5 mm port may be useful in cases where the mesh or the mesorectum is secured to the sacrum with a tacking device.
- Optional hand-assist device placement: For surgeons who prefer to use a hand-assist device, this may be placed in the Pfannenstiel or midline position.

### Mobilization of the Sigmoid Colon and Rectum

- Mobilization of the sigmoid colon: A medial or lateral approach can be utilized depending on the comfort level and preference of the surgeon. Proximal mobilization typically involves only the section of redundant sigmoid and routine splenic flexure mobilization is not required. Further mobilization may result in more redundancy and possible recurrence of prolapse or constipation symptoms with a large "floppy" colon (see Fig. 13.4). The superior

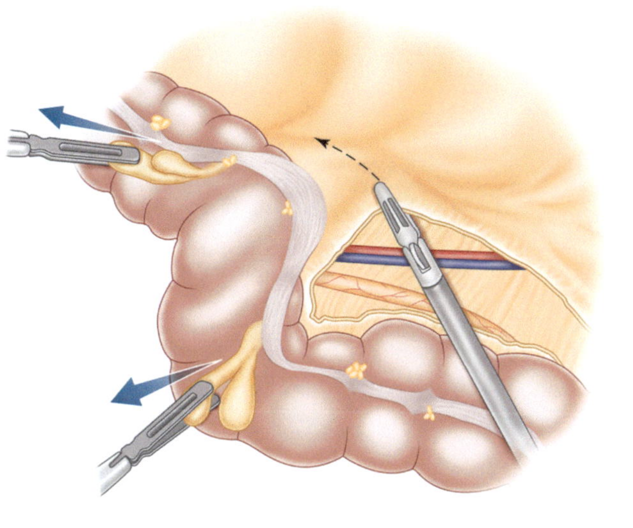

**Fig. 14.5** Takedown of the lateral attachments of the sigmoid

rectal/inferior mesenteric vessels should be preserved, if possible.

- Lateral approach: The left colon is retracted medially with blunt atraumatic bowel graspers, utilizing gravity by tilting the operating table to the patient's right and head down. An energy device or hook-electrocautery is then used to mobilize the sigmoid and descending colon away from left lateral abdominal wall (Fig. 14.5).
- Medial approach: The sacral promontory provides a uniform landmark to begin medial mobilization under the inferior mesenteric artery and access the avascular plane (Fig. 14.6).
    - ***Pearl: For either lateral or medial approach, the left ureter should be identified early and protected, typically as it courses over the bifurcation of the iliac vessels*** (Fig. 14.7).

- Rectal mobilization: The presacral space is entered at the sacral promontory, which is aided with anterior retraction on the rectosigmoid junction (Fig. 14.8). Care should be noted here to avoid transection of the hypogastric nerves that course medially in the retroperitoneum prior to forming two distinct trunks that course posteriorly and laterally in the pelvis (Figs. 14.9 and 14.10). Distally, mobilization continues down to the pelvic floor (Fig. 14.11). There are differing opinions regarding the extent of the lateral and anterior dissection.
    - Lateral dissection: We prefer to avoid extensive lateral dissection and do not divide the lateral stalks.
    - Anterior dissection: We dissect approximately 4 cm until the cut edge of the peritoneal reflection can be easily pulled back to the level of the sacral promontory (Fig. 14.12).
    - Alternative dissection: Others prefer to perform a complete rectal mobilization circumferentially down to the level of the pelvic floor.

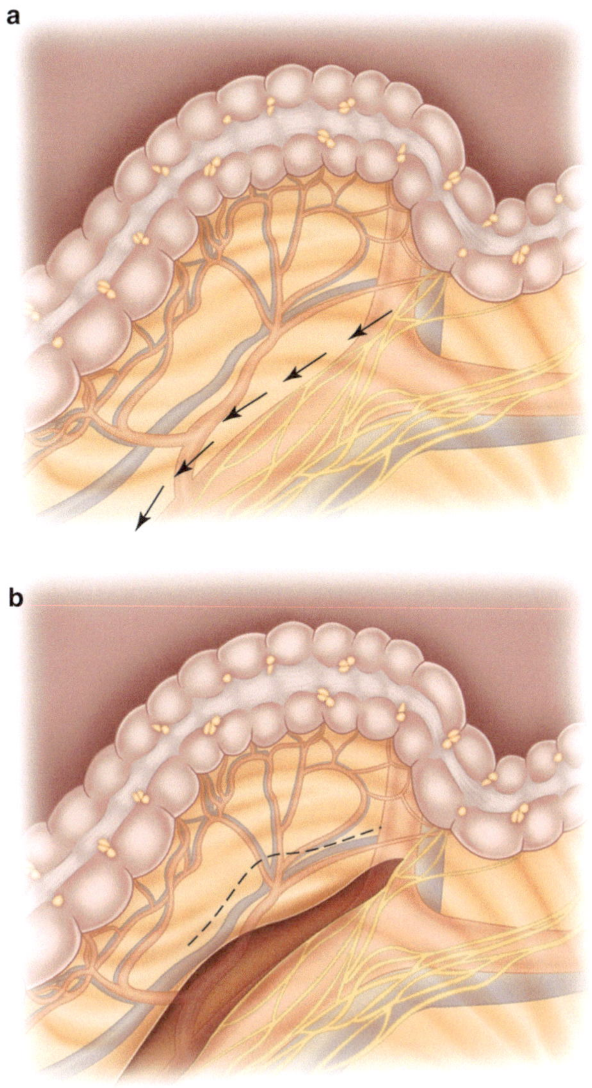


**Fig. 14.6** Mobilization line of dissection for a medial approach

## Resection of the Redundant Sigmoid Colon

- Distal division of sigmoid colon: A point is chosen for distal division past the point where the taenia splay using a cutting stapler (Fig. 14.13).
- Extra-corporealization of distal sigmoid colon: Once the distal portion of the bowel is transected, the bowel is brought out at either the umbilical port site or a small Pfannenstiel incision. The redundant sigmoid is delivered through the wound utilizing a wound protector (Fig. 14.14).
- Proximal division of sigmoid colon: Transection of the bowel with a laparoscopic linear cutting stapler is completed at a tension-free location that easily reaches the sacral promontory without redundancy.
- Placement of anvil: A purse-string suture is placed in the proximal bowel, and the anvil is secured. Sizers can then be used to determine the appropriate size of the circular stapler to be used. We almost exclusively use a 29 mm

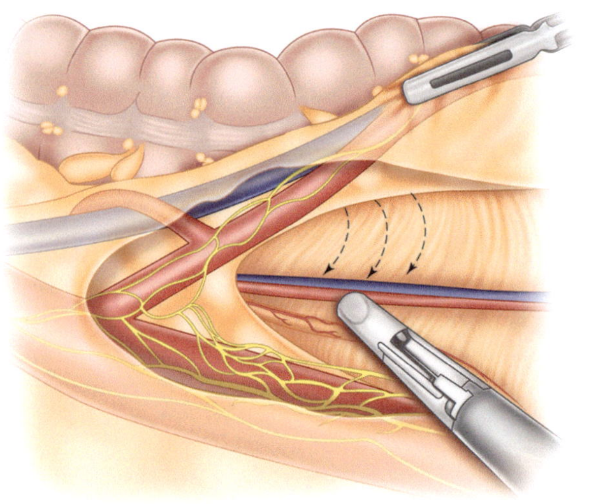

**Fig. 14.7** Most common location of identification of the left ureter as it crosses over the common iliac bifurcation

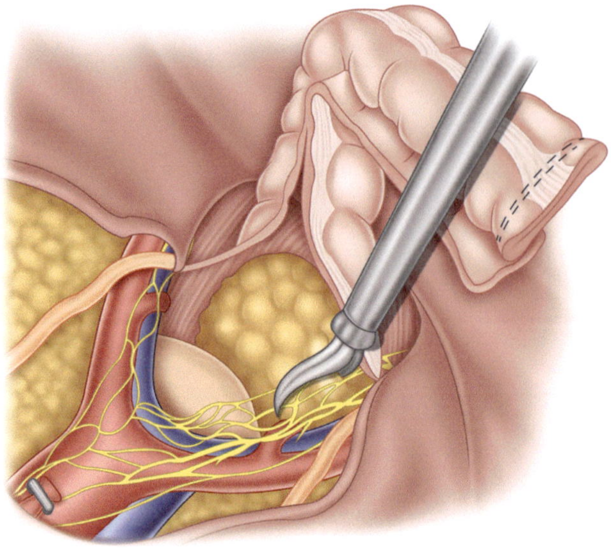

**Fig. 14.9** Hypogastric nerves at the level of the sacral promontory

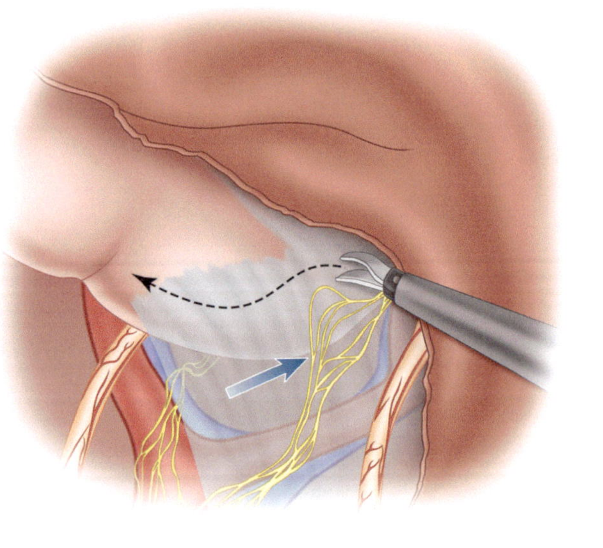

**Fig. 14.8** Accessing the presacral space

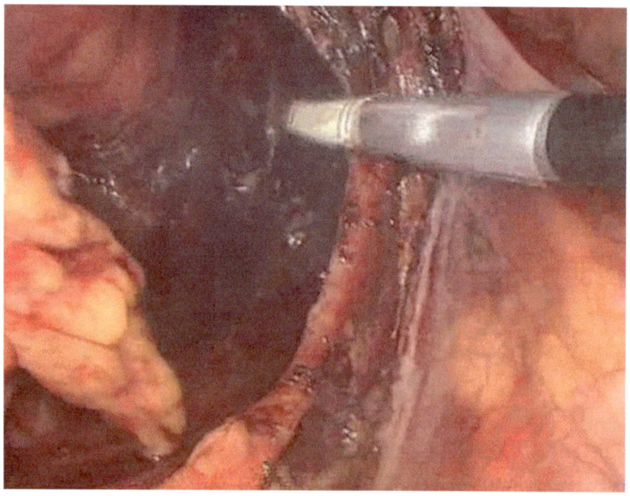

**Fig. 14.10** The right hypogastric nerve can be seen coursing posterior and into the pelvis

end-to-end stapler; however, sizing can be done according to surgeon preference.

  – ***Pearl: Remember that the diameter of the sizer is smaller than the corresponding stapler diameter when selecting the appropriate sized stapler.***

- Return of the colon to the abdomen: The descending colon can then be returned to the abdomen in preparation for anastomosis creation.

### Anastomosis Creation

- Anastomosis creation: The circular stapler is then placed into the anus to the level of the rectal stump. The trocar portion of the stapler is carefully advanced until the anvil is engaged. Prior to closing the stapler, the surgeon should confirm that there is no inclusion of extra tissue, twisting of bowel, or mesentery. The location of both ureters and vagina should be reconfirmed to ensure they are not included in the staple line. The stapler is then fired and tissue doughnuts should be removed and closely inspected to confirm circumferential integrity of the staple line.
- Inspection of anastomosis: The newly created anastomosis is carefully inspected for bleeding or ischemia as well as tension (Fig. 14.15). An air-leak test is performed using a proctoscope with endoluminal insufflation of air after the

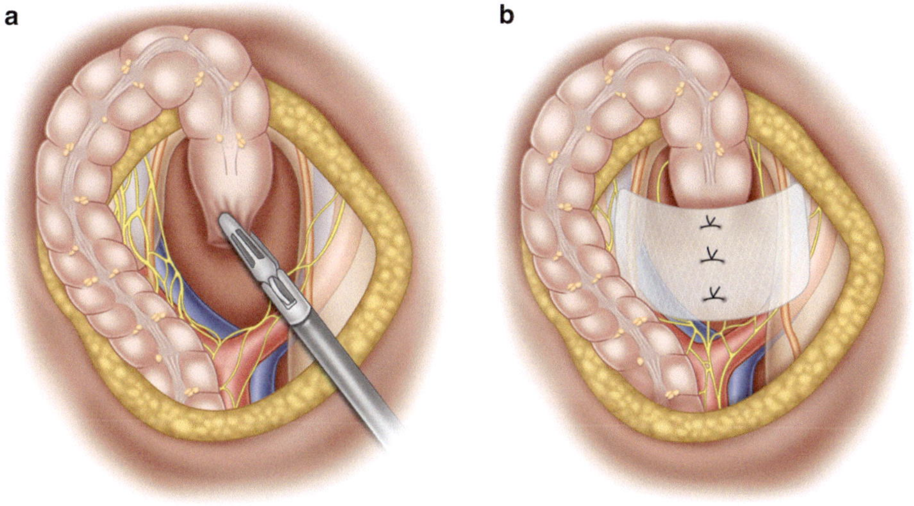


**Fig. 14.11** Posterior extent of mobilization down to the pelvic floor past the coccyx. Note that the mesh is secured to the sacral promontory

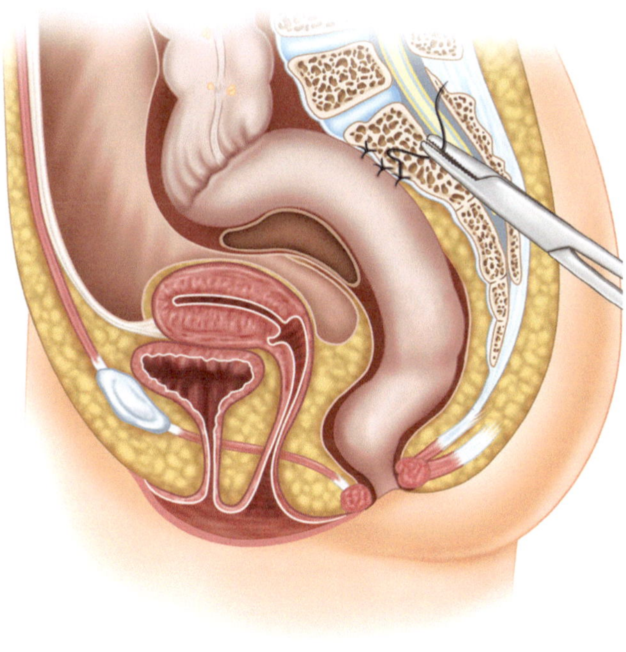

**Fig. 14.12** Cut edge of the anterior peritoneal reflection, which should reach back to the sacral promontory to ensure appropriate mobilization prior to rectopexy

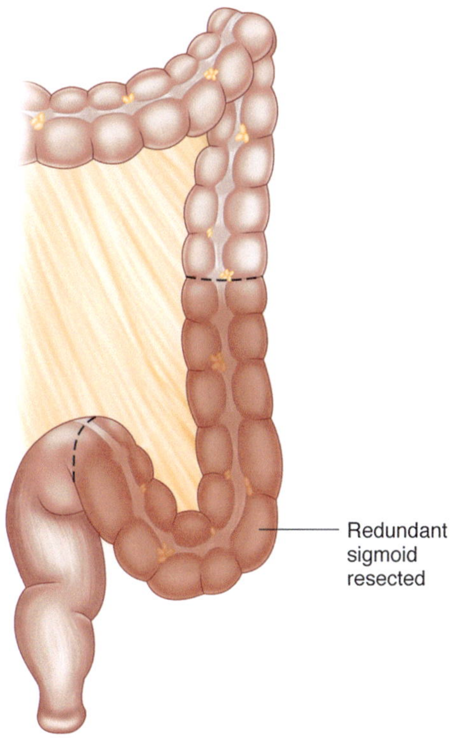


**Fig. 14.13** Extent of resection for redundant sigmoid delineated. Note the limited sigmoid mobilization with proximal mobilization

anastomosis has been submerged in warmed normal saline (see Fig. 10.12).

- Troubleshooting the anastomosis: Any leaks encountered should be reinforced with sutures or the anastomosis redone, and the air-leak test performed again. The use of a proctoscope also allows for endoluminal inspection of the anastomosis. If there is any evidence of tension or ischemia after anastomosis creation, further mobilization should be performed, and anastomosis should be taken down and recreated.

## Rectopexy

Rectopexy may be performed prior to creation of the anastomosis or after, though we prefer the latter. If the rectopexy is completed prior to the creation of the anastomosis, then pexy sutures should not be secured until after the creation of the anastomosis to ensure a tension-free anastomosis.

- Performing the rectopexy: Utilizing the previously created Pfannenstiel incision or the laparoscopic ports, the

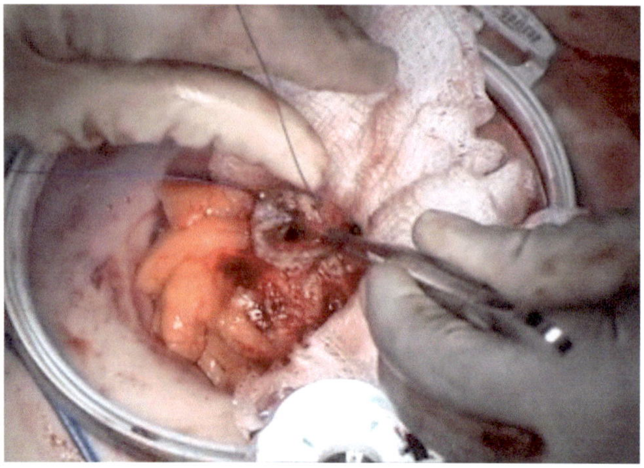

**Fig. 14.14** The proximal transection of the sigmoid colon has completed extracorporeally with the bowel brought out through a wound protector

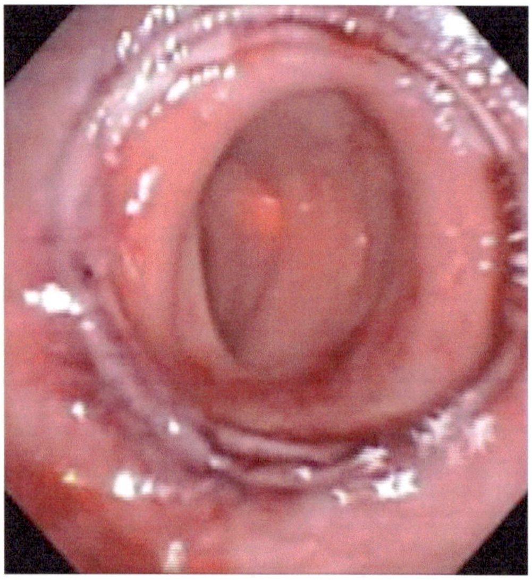

**Fig. 14.15** Anastomosis complete, endoscopic view

rectum is pulled posteriorly and superiorly toward the sacrum at a site of fixation approximately 1–2 cm below the sacral promontory. The rectum should be suspended without redundancy below the rectopexy sutures without excessive tension on the anastomosis. Two to three mattress sutures of nonabsorbable suture (0-Ethibond or 2-0 Prolene) are passed in an anterior to posterior fashion through the mesorectum adjacent to the bowel wall, through the presacral fascia and then back through the mesorectum in a posterior to anterior fashion approximately 1.5–2 cm form the initial bite (Figs. 14.16 and 14.17). Although some surgeons advocate for the bilateral placement of sutures, we prefer to place all the sutures on one side to avoid kinking at the site of rectopexy.

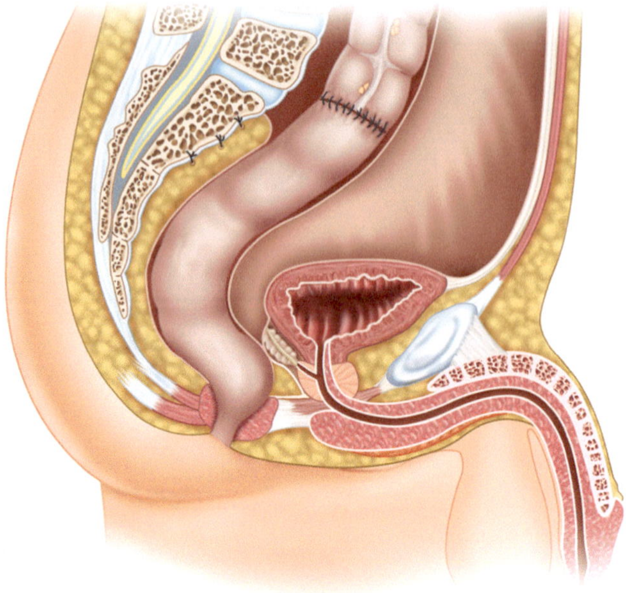

**Fig. 14.16** Mesorectal fixation using three horizontal mattress sutures unilaterally

  - Troubleshooting: Care should be taken to avoid injury in the presacral venous plexus and mesenteric vessels during placement of the suture. If presacral bleeding is encountered, the sutures should be tied down and direct manual pressure applied. If bleeding persists, more aggressive maneuvers such as thumbtacks or fibrin sealant may be utilized (Fig. 14.18).
- Closure of the abdomen: Once meticulous hemostasis is assured, then the Pfannenstiel incision is closed in layers (if utilized) and all port sites incisions are closed in the standard fashion. The placement of pelvic drains is not routine. The patient is placed back in the supine position, and the orogastric tube is removed at time of emergence from anesthesia. The Foley catheter should remain in place until postoperative day 1.

## Laparoscopic Rectopexy

### Trocar Placement (Fig. 14.4)

If rectopexy alone is indicated, similar port sites are placed as in the case of an additional resection.

- Trocar placement: A 5 mm trocar in the supra- or infra-umbilical position (camera port) followed by two 5 mm ports placed in each quadrant of the right hemi-abdomen at the lateral edge of the rectus muscle (Fig. 14.19).
- Optional ports may be placed to allow for self-retaining retraction instrument placement on the left side of the abdomen and in the suprapubic position.
- Surgeon's position is at the discretion of the operating surgeon, though we prefer to stand on the patient's right side, with the assistant on the left.

**Fig. 14.17** Lateral view of the sacral fixation

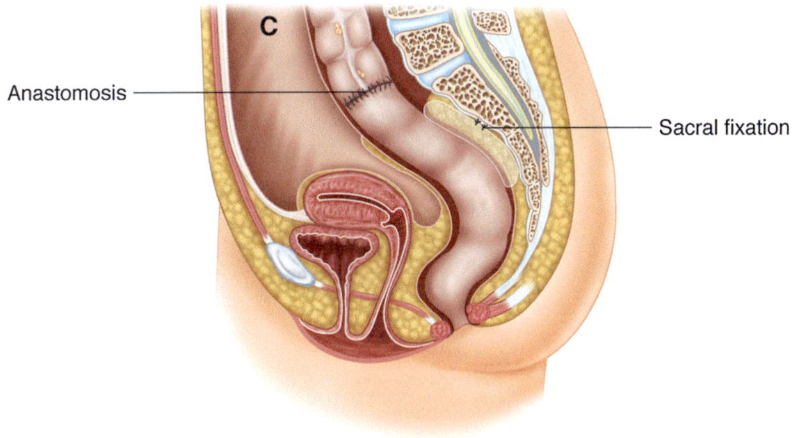


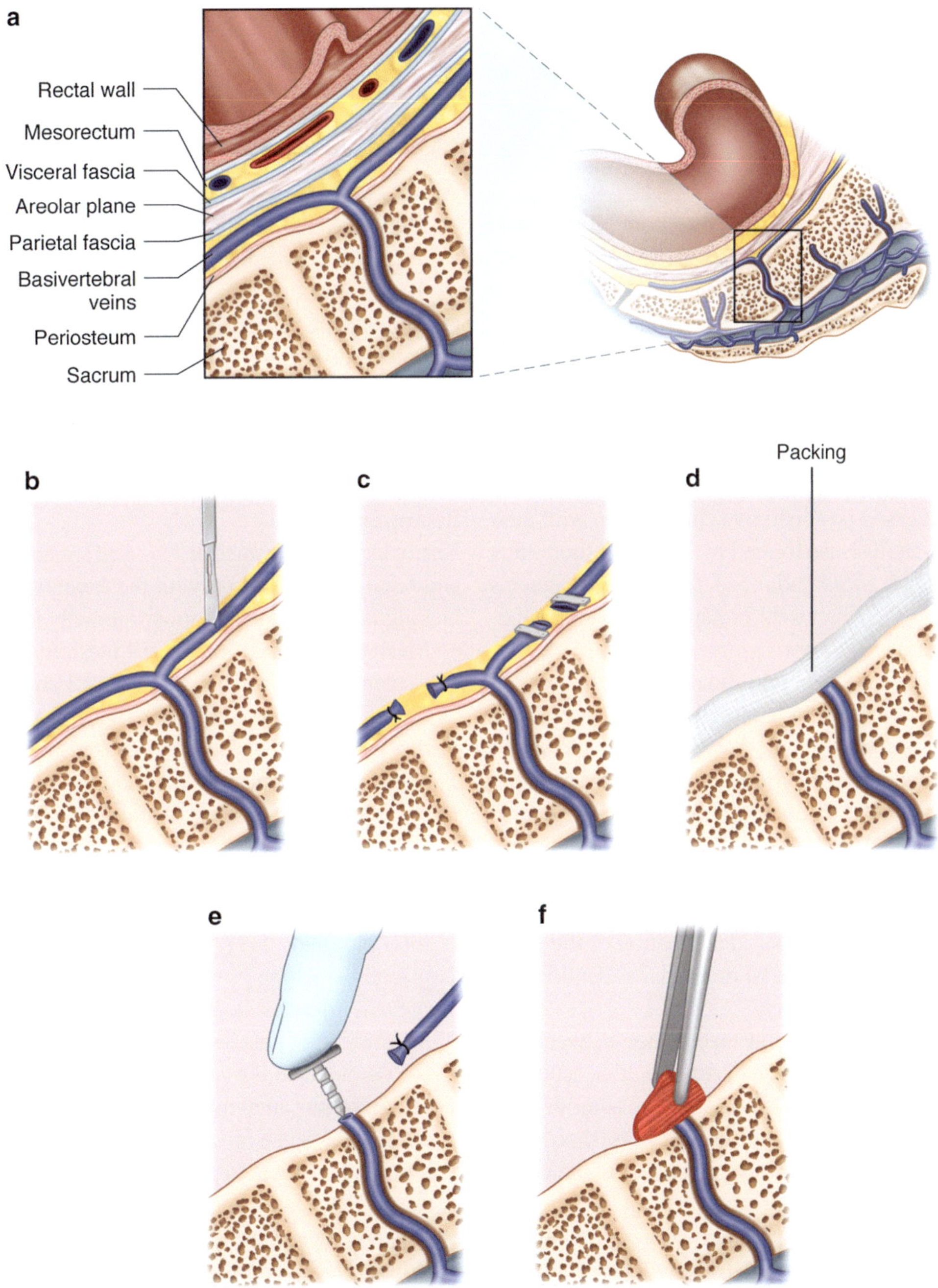


**Fig. 14.18** Optional bleeding control measures of muscle flap/thumbtacks

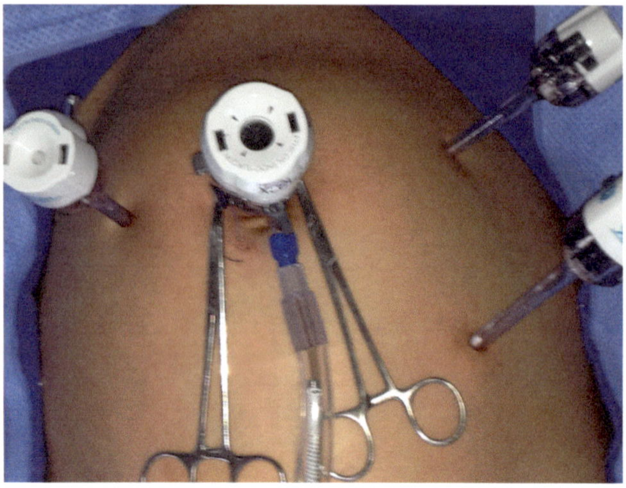

**Fig. 14.19** Trocar sites for straight laparoscopic rectopexy. The patient's feet are toward the top of the picture

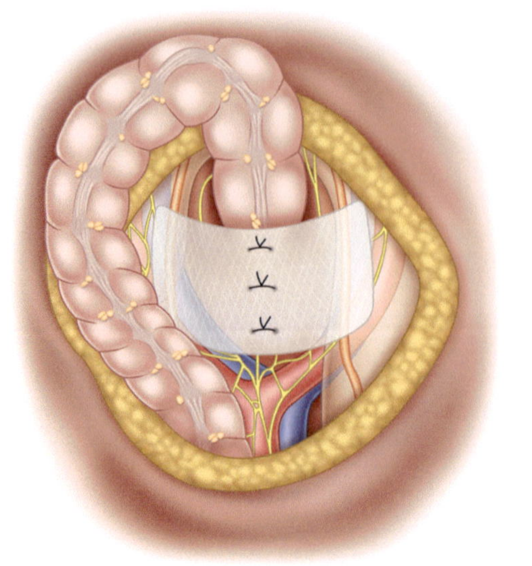

**Fig. 14.20** Rectopexy with mesh secured to the upper sacrum

### Rectum Mobilization

Similar to the resection rectopexy, rectal mobilization is carried down to differing levels (i.e., anterior vs. posterior vs. lateral) with rectopexy alone. The extent of anterior and lateral mobilization is again somewhat less defined. Whether or not the extent of anterior mobilization is efficacious in preventing recurrence or improving functional outcome is unknown. The argument for dividing the lateral ligaments is improvement in incontinence and decreased recurrence rates; however, proponents for preservation note that there are reports of increased postoperative constipation with their division. A meta-analysis performed by Tou et al. found that division, rather than preservation, of the lateral ligaments was associated with less recurrent prolapse but more postoperative constipation [13].

- Posterior dissection: Dissection should end at the level of the pelvic floor levators by continuing dissection in the anatomic mesorectum plane. Access to this avascular plane is reproducibly performed under the IMA at the level of the sacral promontory. The hypogastric nerves should be identified at the level of the sacral promontory and preserved. Injury or unintentional division of these nerves can cause sexual and urinary dysfunction. This can be avoided by ensuring proper identification of the avascular presacral plane that can be more easily identified by forward traction of the rectum.
- Anterior dissection: Dissection takes place between the anterior aspect of the rectum and the posterior aspect of the anterior pelvic structures by opening the anterior peritoneal reflection characterized by its horseshoe fold. Dissection may be aided by careful retraction of the uterus or bladder with the use of a laparoscopic fan blade retractor and countertraction on the rectum with the left laparoscopic blunt atraumatic grasper. The dissection is carried down to the level of the mid- to upper third of the vagina in females or seminal vesicles in males; more aggressive distal dissection especially in males can result in parasympathetic nerve injury.
- Lateral dissection: This involves the preservation or division of the lateral ligaments; however, there is a gathering evidence in the literature that these ligaments are not true anatomic structures.

### Rectopexy

Rectopexy is performed in the same manner as a resection and rectopexy procedure with the exception that suturing or tacking is accomplished intracorporeally (Video 14.1).

- Mesh placement: If the use of mesh for a sling procedure is planned, the mesh (size 5 cm × 2 cm) is rolled up and introduced into the abdominal cavity via the right lower quadrant port. The mesh is placed in a vertical fashion along the sacrum from the sacral promontory caudal into the pelvis and secured to the sacrum using endoscopic tackers or laparoscopic staplers. Suturing the mesh to the presacral fascia is possible but can be difficult due to the smaller size of the needles that can pass through the laparoscopic ports [17]. The tackers or staples should be placed below the promontory and close to the midline to prevent injury to the hypogastric nerves.
- Securing the lateral edges of mesh: The lateral edges are then secured to the rectal wall by nonabsorbable sutures utilizing an intracorporeal suturing technique. Care should be taken not to completely encircle the mesh around the rectum to prevent kinking or postoperative stenosis (Figs. 14.20 and 14.21 and Video 14.2).
- Closure: The placement of pelvic drains is not routine. When mesh is used, we prefer to close the peritoneum to

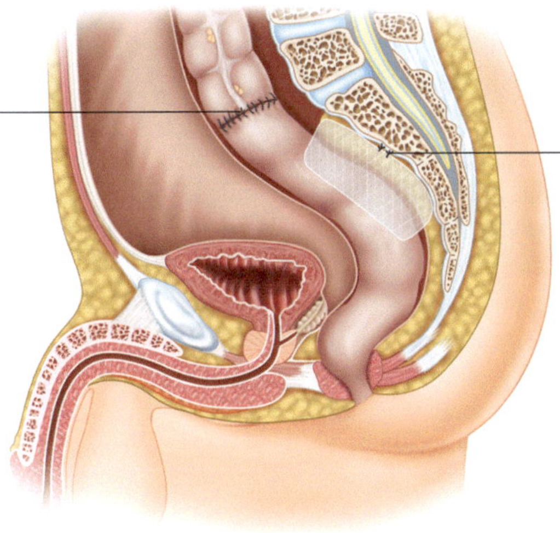


**Fig. 14.21** Sagittal view with mesh placement to the sacrum and the mesorectum

avoid leaving the mesh exposed. Meticulous hemostasis remains an important mainstay, and closure is achieved in the same manner as described previously.

## Postoperative Care

Standard postoperative management of these patients should include early ambulation and initiation of enteral feeding. Most patients may be started on a clear liquid diet on the day of the surgery and advanced as tolerated to solid foods on postoperative day 1, though some surgeons keep patients on a pureed or liquid diet for the first 7–10 days following repair. Pain control should be balanced to avoid exacerbation of ileus and can be achieved with the judicious use of narcotics and nonnarcotics such as ketorolac, acetaminophen, and ibuprofen, which are all available in the parenteral form. The bladder catheter is usually removed on postoperative day 1. Antibiotics should be discontinued within 24 h postoperatively unless there are specific indications to continue them. DVT prophylaxis should consist of early ambulation, sequential compressive devices while the patient is in bed, and chemical prophylaxis (heparin or low molecular weight heparin) until the patient is discharged from the hospital. We prefer an aggressive bowel regimen with the use of stool softeners (docusate) in combination with either an osmotic laxative such as polyethylene glycol 3350 (Miralax™) or a stimulant laxative (sennosides) to prevent postoperative constipation. Additionally patients should be counseled to avoid straining when at the commode to prevent early recurrence. Patients with rectopexy alone are typically discharged 1–4 days postoperatively, and those with resection and rectopexy are discharged 2–5 days postoperatively with planned clinic follow-up 7–10 days after the day of discharge.

## Complications

Complications may be divided into intraoperative and postoperative (Table 14.2). Intraoperative complications typically occur in <5 % and include inadvertent enterotomy, colotomy, ureteral injury, trocar placement injuries, and vascular injury. Enterotomies and colotomies should be repaired primarily if possible, and conversion to an open procedure should be done if the injury cannot be safely repaired. Ureteral injuries should be repaired intraoperatively if found

**Table 14.2** Complications of laparoscopic rectal prolapse repair

| Intraoperative |
|---|
| • Enterotomy |
| • Colotomy |
| • Ureteral injury |
| • Trocar placement injury |
| • Vascular injury |
| Postoperative |
| • Early |
| – Urinary tract infection |
| – Respiratory tract infection |
| – Surgical site infection |
| – Fecal impaction |
| – Anastomotic leak |
| – Deep space infection |
| – Hemorrhage |
| • Late |
| – Bowel obstruction |
| – Rectovaginal fistula |
| – Ureteral fibrosis |
| – Incontinence/constipation |

and typically involve consultation of a urologic surgeon when possible. Vascular injury is rare but can occur at several locations: epigastrics during placement of trocars, gonadal, and iliac vessels; during dissection and mobilization for resection and mesenteric vessels; and during mobilization and resection. Damage to the epigastrics is avoided by transilluminating the abdominal wall during trocar placement and direct vision for all secondary trocar placements. If damage does occur, direct pressure and electrocautery can be used with good success. Refractory bleeding can temporarily be stopped with a tamponade effect of a Foley catheter balloon introduced via the offending port site. The gonadal and iliac vessels are retroperitoneal structures and are avoided by early identification and careful dissection. If damage to these vessels does occur, direct manual pressure should be used and conversion to open should be considered depending on the extent and location of the injury. Mesenteric vessel injury occurs during mobilization and transection of the mesorectum and results from improper control prior to transection. All vessels should be identified and controlled prior to mesorectum transection.

Early postoperative complications include postoperative hemorrhage, fecal impaction, deep space infections, anastomotic leak, urinary tract infections, surgical site infections, and respiratory infections. Urinary tract infections can be avoided by sterilized technique and timely removal of the bladder catheter. Respiratory infections can be avoided by early postoperative recruitment of alveoli and avoidance of atelectasis with the use of incentive spirometry, deep breathing and coughing, and early ambulation. Surgical site infections are unfortunately not uncommon complications in all colorectal procedures, but their incidence can be minimized with the appropriate use of preoperative antibiotics, wound protectors (if resection is performed), and sterile technique, as appropriate. If a wound infection is encountered, it should be treated in the standard fashion with wound culture obtained to guide proper antibiotic treatment as necessary. Anastomotic leakage, although a feared complication, has a low incidence (<10 %). Leaks can be avoided by ensuring a tension-free, non-rotated connection with an adequate blood supply. If the anastomosis appears tenuous during the procedure, it should be taken down and re-created. If there is a suspicion for a leak postoperatively and the patient is stable, a CT scan with PO or rectal and IV contrast should be completed to determine the presence and location of the suspected leak. All patients with suspected leak that are unstable should undergo fluid resuscitation, the initiation of broad-spectrum antibiotics, and return to the operating room for exploration. Late postoperative complications include bowel obstruction, ureteral fibrosis, rectovaginal fistula formation, and worsening or new fecal incontinence or constipation.

## Outcomes

Most of the outcomes following rectal prolapse repair are reported in the open setting, though laparoscopic reports are similar. The major problem for most patients with rectal prolapse is fecal incontinence, with most series demonstrating up to 75 % of patients with some degree of incontinence. On the other side of the spectrum, 15–65 % of patients have concomitant constipation or evacuation disorders [13, 18]. Following successful repair of the prolapse, the literature reports wide ranges of improvement in fecal incontinence (11–100 %; mean 50 %) with resection and rectopexy. Some patients may have improvement but not complete resolution secondary to permanent damage to the sphincter mechanism or pelvic nerves from the chronic prolapse.

Improvement in constipation similarly has somewhat variable results, with some patients improving and others developing new onset or worsening symptoms. There appears to be better results when a resection is added to those patients with prolapse and severe preoperative constipation (18–80 %) [8, 10, 19–23]. Recurrence of prolapse following the open abdominal approach are reported at 0–10 % in most series [1, 10, 24]. There have been two prospective trials comparing the laparoscopic technique to the open technique with equivalent outcomes with respect to recurrence [12, 25]. Several other observational retrospective studies have evaluated laparoscopic rectopexy with and without resection and found equivalent recurrence rates, mortality and functional outcomes when compared to the open technique [26–29]. This was confirmed by meta-analysis in which laparoscopic rectopexy was associated with decreased length of stay and fewer postoperative complications despite longer operative times when compared to the open approach [13]. There are now reports that show a decrease in operative times as more experience is gained using laparoscopic techniques for colorectal procedures [12].

## Pearls and Pitfalls

- During the preoperative workup for prolapse, surgeons should look for significant pelvic floor abnormalities that may need to be addressed at the time of surgery. Pelvic floor disorders such as enterocele, cystocele, rectocele, and uterine and vaginal vault prolapse are present in up to 50 % of patients with rectal prolapse. The repair of these abnormalities in conjunction with prolapse repair is best performed with a multidisciplinary team that may involve a urologist, gynecologist, or urogynecologist, as well as a colorectal surgeon.
- Unexpected conversion to an open procedure is not a failure and should be considered if the procedure cannot

be performed safely secondary to dense adhesions or an injury that cannot be managed laparoscopically has occurred. Instruments for an open procedure should be available if conversion is required.

- Determining the appropriate amount of tension can be difficult. Use the peritoneal reflection as a guide, and don't hesitate to look endoscopically in the rectum to see if redundancy is still present when you feel your rectum is sufficiently mobilized prior to performing your rectopexy.
- When adding the resection to the rectopexy, mobilize the rectum first and then perform the resection and anastomosis (and leak test). Once this is complete, perform the rectopexy.
- Use sizers in the vaginal to help delineate the posterior vaginal wall from the anterior rectum to ensure you are in the correct plane of dissection.

## Summary

In conclusion, laparoscopic rectopexy with or without resection is a safe, effective procedure with equivalent functional outcomes, recurrence, and mortality rates when compared to open techniques (resection and rectopexy, suture rectopexy, and mesh rectopexy). The use of this approach also allows for the inclusion of patients who previously would not have tolerated the morbidity of an open abdominal approach and results in decreased postoperative pain, early return of bowel function, and decreased length of stay [29].

**Disclosures** Dr. Steele works as a consultant for Ethicon Endosurgery.

## References


1. Mandiba TE, Baig MK, Wexner SD. Surgical management of rectal prolapse. Arch Surg. 2005;140:63–73.
2. Jacobs LK, Lin YJ, Orkin BA. The best operation for rectal prolapse. Surg Clin North Am. 1997;77(1):49–70.
3. Felt-Bersma RJ, Cuesta MA. Rectal prolapse, rectal intussusception, rectocele, and solitary rectal ulcer syndrome. Gastroenterol Clin North Am. 2001;30(1):199–222.
4. Roig JV, Buch E, Alos R, Solana A, Fernandez C, Villoslada C, et al. Anorectal function in patients with complete rectal prolapse. Differences between continent and incontinent individuals. Rev Esp Enferm Dig. 1998;90(11):794–805.
5. Wassef R, Rothenberger DA, Goldberg SM. Rectal prolapse. Curr Probl Surg. 1986;23(6):397–451.
6. Azimuddin K, Khubchandani IT, Rosen L, Stasik JJ, Riether RD, Reed 3rd JF. Rectal prolapse: a search for the "best" operation. Am Surg. 2001;67(7):622–7.
7. Raftopoulos Y, Senagore AJ, Di Giuro G, Bergamaschi R. Group. RPRS. Recurrence rates after abdominal surgery for complete rectal prolapse: a multicenter pooled analysis of 643 individual patient data. Dis Colon Rectum. 2005;48(6):1200–6.
8. Kim DS, Tsang CB, Wong WD, Lowry AC, Goldberg SM, Madoff RD. Complete rectal prolapse: evolution of management and results. Dis Colon Rectum. 1999;42(4):460–6. discussion 6–9.
9. Delaney CP. Laparoscopic management of rectal prolapse. J Gastrointest Surg. 2007;11(2):150–2.
10. Steele SR, Goldberg JE. Rectal prolapse: In Acute Care Surgery and Trauma: Evidence-based Practice. (Ed Cohn.) Informa UK Ltd Publ, London 2009; (ISBN-10:1420075136); pp. 356–67.
11. Kuhry E, Schwenk WF, Gaupset R, Romild U, Bonjer HJ. Long-term results of laparoscopic colorectal cancer resection. Cochrane Database Syst Rev. 2008;2, CD003432.
12. Solomon MJ, Young CJ, Eyers AA, Roberts RA. Randomized clinical trial of laparoscopic versus open abdominal rectopexy for rectal prolapse. Br J Surg. 2002;89(1):35–9.
13. Tou S, Brown SR, Malik AI, Nelson RL. Surgery for complete rectal prolapse in adults. Cochrane Database Syst Rev. 2008;4, CD001758.
14. Carpelan-Holmstrom M, Kruuna O, Scheinin T. Laparoscopic rectal prolapse surgery combined with short hospital stay is safe in elderly and debilitated patients. Surg Endosc. 2006;20(9): 1353–9.
15. Bellows CF, Mills KT, Kelly TN, Gagliardi G. Combination of oral non-absorbable and intravenous antibiotics versus intravenous antibiotics alone in the prevention of surgical site infections after colorectal surgery: a meta-analysis of randomized controlled trials. Tech Coloproctol. 2011;15(4):385–95.
16. Cannon JA, Altom LK, Deierhoi RJ, Morris M, Richman JS, Vick CC, et al. Preoperative oral antibiotics reduce surgical site infection following elective colorectal resections. Dis Colon Rectum. 2012; 55(11):1160–6.
17. Zmora O, Khaikin M, Lebeydev A, Rosin D, Hoffman A, Gutman M, et al. Multimedia manuscript. Laparoscopic rectopexy with posterior mesh fixation. Surg Endosc. 2011;25(1):313–4.
18. Bachoo P, Brazzelli M, Grant A. Surgery for complete rectal prolapse in adults. Cochrane Database Syst Rev. 2000;2, CD001758.
19. Sayfan J, Pinho M, Alexander-Williams J, Keighley MR. Sutured posterior abdominal rectopexy with sigmoidectomy compared with Marlex rectopexy for rectal prolapse. Br J Surg. 1990;77(2):143–5.
20. Stevenson AR, Stitz RW, Lumley JW. Laparoscopic-assisted resection-rectopexy for rectal prolapse: early and medium follow-up. Dis Colon Rectum. 1998;41(1):46–54.
21. Tjandra JJ, Fazio VW, Church JM, Milsom JW, Oakley JR, Lavery IC. Ripstein procedure is an effective treatment for rectal prolapse without constipation. Dis Colon Rectum. 1993;36(5):501–7.
22. Luukkonen P, Mikkonen U, Jarvinen H. Abdominal rectopexy with sigmoidectomy vs. rectopexy alone for rectal prolapse: a prospective, randomized study. Int J Colorectal Dis. 1992;7(4):219–22.
23. Huber FT, Stein H, Siewert JR. Functional results after treatment of rectal prolapse with rectopexy and sigmoid resection. World J Surg. 1995;19(1):138–43; discussion 43.
24. Steele SR, Goetz LH, Miniami S, Madoff RD, Mellgren A, Parker SC. Management of recurrent rectal prolapse: surgical approaches influences outcome. Dis Colon Rectum. 2006;49(4):440–5.
25. Boccasanta P, Rosati R, Venturi M, Montorsi M, Cioffi U, De Simone M, et al. Comparison of laparoscopic rectopexy with open technique in the treatment of complete rectal prolapse: clinical and functional results. Surg Laparosc Endosc. 1998;8(6):460–5.
26. Heah SM, Hartley JE, Hurley J, Duthie GS, Monson JR. Laparoscopic suture rectopexy without resection is effective treatment for full-thickness rectal prolapse. Dis Colon Rectum. 2000;43(5):638–43.
27. Ashari LH, Lumley JW, Stevenson AR, Stitz RW. Laparoscopically-assisted resection rectopexy for rectal prolapse: ten years' experience. Dis Colon Rectum. 2005;48(5):982–7.
28. Kairaluoma MV, Viljakka MT, Kellokumpu IH. Open vs. laparoscopic surgery for rectal prolapse: a case-controlled study assessing short-term outcome. Dis Colon Rectum. 2003;46(3):353–60.
29. Wexner SD, Cera SM. In: Souba WW, Fink MP, Jurkovich GJ, Kaiser LR, Pearce WH, Pemberton JH, et al., editors. Procedures for rectal prolapse. 6th ed. London: BC Decker Inc; 2012.

# 15 Minimally Invasive Approach for Stoma Creation

Seth I. Felder, Zuri Murrell, and Phillip Fleshner

**Key Points**

- Laparoscopy for fecal diversion is safe, feasible, and effective.
- Laparoscopy does not change the indications for stoma construction [1–3] nor does it alter the basic surgical principles.
- In comparison with conventional stoma creation, the benefits of laparoscopic stoma creation may include decreased morbidity rates in the form of lower complication rates, reduction in postoperative analgesia, shorter hospitalization, comparable operating time, and improved cosmesis.
- Although most laparoscopic techniques for stoma construction use two or more port sites, single-port techniques have also been described with favorable outcomes.
- Stomas created for obstructing lesions create unique challenges such as creating adequate pneumoperitoneum to provide space and visualization.

## Introduction

As laparoscopy is increasingly adopted into the colorectal surgeon's practice, the application of minimally invasive techniques for stoma construction has gained added relevance [1–3]. Intestinal stomas are considered a vital element as either a permanent means for stool evacuation or as a temporary bridge in order to treat complicated abdominal problems or heal more distal anastomoses or wounds [4]. In comparison with conventional stoma creation, the benefits of laparoscopic stoma creation likely include decreased morbidity rates in the form of lower complication rates, reduction in postoperative analgesia, shorter hospitalization, comparable operating time, and improved cosmesis [5–11]. In addition, the entire abdominal cavity is easily accessible for inspection. Particularly in a healthcare climate emphasizing fast-track protocols [12] and cost containment, the implications of a minimally invasive approach promoting quicker return of bowel function and consequently time in the hospital, along with potential reductions in long-term adverse outcomes such as bowel obstruction due to surgical trauma resulting in adhesion formation, a laparoscopically created stoma may in time become regarded as the preferred, standard technique.

Laparoscopy does not change the indications for stoma construction [3] nor does it alter the basic surgical principles. The exteriorized bowel must be well vascularized without excessive mesenteric tension, pass through the rectus sheath and fascia properly oriented, and adequately reach the abdominal wall for maturation. A laparoscopic technique is ideally suited for stoma creation since it often does not require extensive dissection or specimen extraction [4]. Several intestinal sites may be chosen for stoma formation, although the terminal ileum and sigmoid colon are most commonly used. The decision regarding site placement depends on the operative indications as well as subsequent procedures planned [2]. Like other laparoscopic procedures, extensive intra-abdominal adhesions and comorbidities making general anesthesia prohibitive are relative contraindications. The creation of a laparoscopic stoma in the setting of an obstructing rectal cancer is dependent upon the degree of bowel distention as this directly impacts the ability to create adequate working space.

A variety of minimally invasive techniques for stoma creation have been described, demonstrating laparoscopy for fecal diversion to be safe, feasible, and effective. Although most laparoscopic stomas are created using two or more port sites, single-port techniques have also been reported with favorable outcomes [1, 10]. Laparoscopic stoma creation has been compared to open stoma creation in

**Electronic supplementary material:** Supplementary material is available in the online version of this chapter at 10.1007/978-1-4939-1581-1_15. Videos can also be accessed at http://www.springerimages.com/videos/978-1-4939-1580-4.

S.I. Felder, M.D. • Z. Murrell, M.D. • P. Fleshner, M.D. (✉)
Department of Colon and Rectal Surgery, Cedars-Sinai Medical Center, 8737 Beverly Boulevard, Suite 101, Los Angeles, CA 90048, USA
e-mail: pfleshner@aol.com

H.M. Ross et al. (eds.), *Minimally Invasive Approaches to Colon and Rectal Disease: Technique and Best Practices*,
DOI 10.1007/978-1-4939-1581-1_15, © Springer Science+Business Media New York 2015

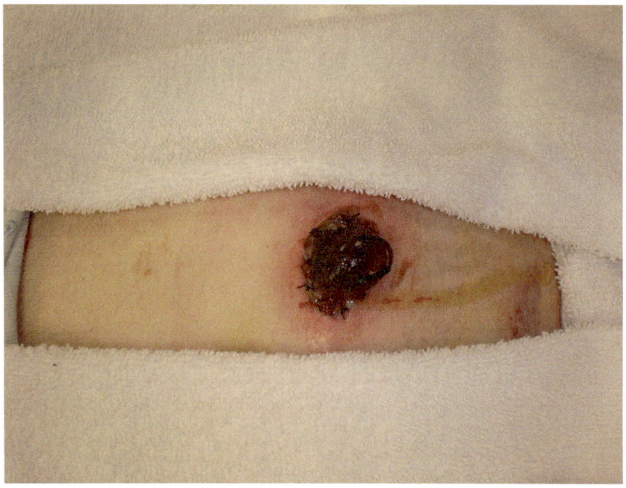

**Fig. 15.1** Ischemic ostomy. *Courtesy of Philip Y. Pearson, MD, with permission*

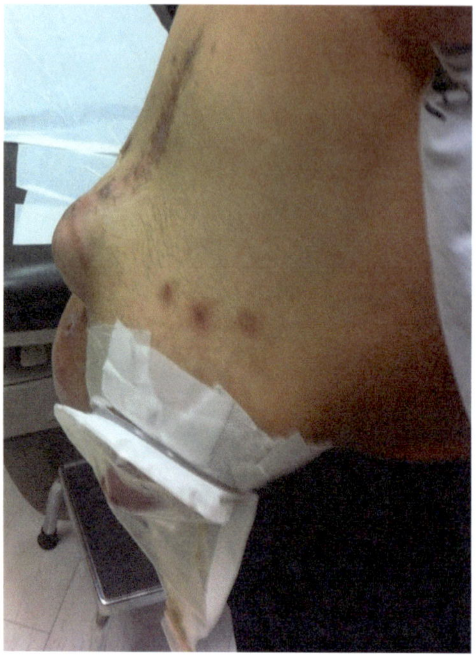

**Fig. 15.2** Parastomal hernia. *Courtesy of Peter Cataldo, MD, with permission*

several retrospective studies [5–11]; however, prospective trials have not yet been conducted. The available literature suggests that using a laparoscopic approach does not compromise functional outcomes, and the avoidance of a laparotomy and reduction in recovery time remain significant advantages.

Complications reported following laparoscopic stoma construction are similar to those following conventional, open construction. Stoma retraction, generally resulting from poor adhesion between the serosal surfaces of the everted stoma, stoma ischemia and necrosis due to excessive division of mesenteric blood vessels, tension on the stoma from inadequate mobilization or a tight fascial aperture, stoma stenosis (a consequence of postoperative ischemia), and stoma prolapse/hernia are all well-characterized postoperative complications (Fig. 15.1).

Parastomal hernia remains an especially significant problem following stoma creation (Fig. 15.2). In fact, the creation of a defect in the abdominal wall for a stoma by definition places a weakness in the abdominal wall where there once was complete continuity. Associated complications may be relatively minor, such as skin breakdown near the stoma site or difficulty fitting an appliance around the stoma, or can be life-threatening such as incarcerated intestine within the hernia [4]. Although seemingly a logical approach to reduce parastomal hernia, Level I evidence in support of prophylactic mesh placement at the time of open stoma construction is limited and comprised various types of mesh, placed in different abdominal positions [13–18]. A meta-analysis evaluating three of these studies included 128 patients and demonstrated a statistically significant reduction of parastomal hernia incidence between the mesh group (12.5 %) compared with the control group (53 %) without a difference in mesh-related morbidity. Beck et al. presented a prospective, randomized, controlled third-party blinded study of 113 patients comparing mesh inlay for parastomal reinforcement in patients undergoing surgery for permanent abdominal wall ostomies to standard end stomal construction at the 2013 American Society of Colon and Rectum Surgeons meeting [19]. Although reinforcement was found to be safe, the incidence of parastomal hernia formation was not statistically lower after 24-month follow-up [16]. However, studies evaluating prophylactic mesh placement in laparoscopically created stomas are extremely limited, with initial experiences demonstrating safety and feasibility and potentially favorable outcomes [17, 18]. Solid evidence for prophylactic placement of mesh in laparoscopic stoma construction is not yet available.

## Preoperative Planning

In the elective setting, preoperative stoma site selection and marking is essential. A stoma located incorrectly predisposes the patient to problems that cannot be managed conservatively (i.e., with changes in the stoma equipment). Since body habitus varies greatly between individuals, the ideal stoma site(s) must be modified, avoiding scars and skin creases [4].

To ensure skin folds do not interfere with appliance fitting, site selection should be done in supine, sitting, and bending positions, with attention also given to the individual's beltline [4]. The usual site in an average individual is on the apex of the subumbilical fat roll, in either the right or left iliac fossa (Fig. 15.3) [20]. Finally, the patient needs to be able to visualize the stoma in order to care for it.

## Operating Room Setup and Patient Positioning

Two video monitors are placed angling toward the patient at the shoulder level if constructing an ileostomy and placed toward the foot of the bed or the patient's knees if planning a sigmoid/descending colostomy. The procedure is performed with the patient in the supine position although a modified lithotomy position is also acceptable. If the latter position is utilized, the hips and knees are gently flexed to an angle no greater than 15° to avoid the patient's thighs interfering with the laparoscopic instruments. If an ileostomy is planned, the left arm is tucked to the side, and the surgeon stands on the left side of the patient or between the patient's legs (Fig. 15.4). If a sigmoid/descending colostomy is planned, the right arm is tucked, and the surgeon stands on the patient's right or between the legs. The site of peritoneal access is dependent upon the type of stoma being created and the patient's prior surgical history. For patients with prior abdominal surgery, accessing a "free" quadrant is usually the safest approach. After intra-abdominal access is obtained, the patient is placed in Trendelenburg position to augment visualization.

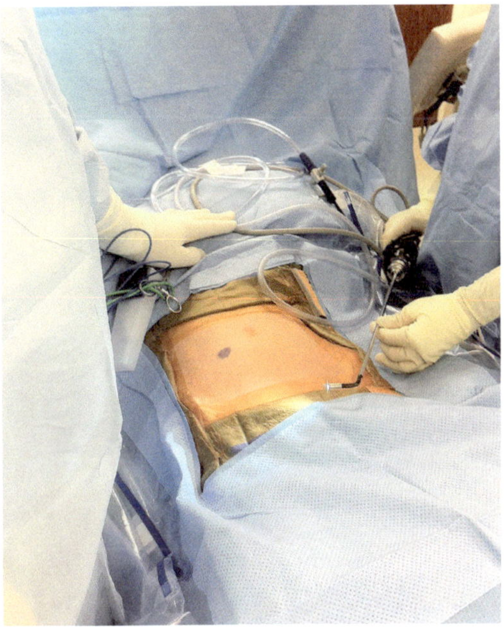

**Fig. 15.3** Stoma position marked on the abdomen

## Technique: Laparoscopic Ileostomy [1, 2, 4, 20]

Variations in multi-port placement positioning and sequence have been described; however, most approaches use 2 or 3 ports, taking advantage of the principle of trocar triangulation to facilitate exposure and mobilization. The first trocar inserted is a 5-mm cannula placed just inferior to the umbilicus. Once 15-mmHg pneumoperitoneum is established, a (30°) laparoscope is inserted to inspect the abdomen and direct the remaining port positions (Fig. 15.5). The patient is placed right side up in Trendelenburg position. The surgeon can visually ensure that the planned ostomy site is suitable and free of adhesions.

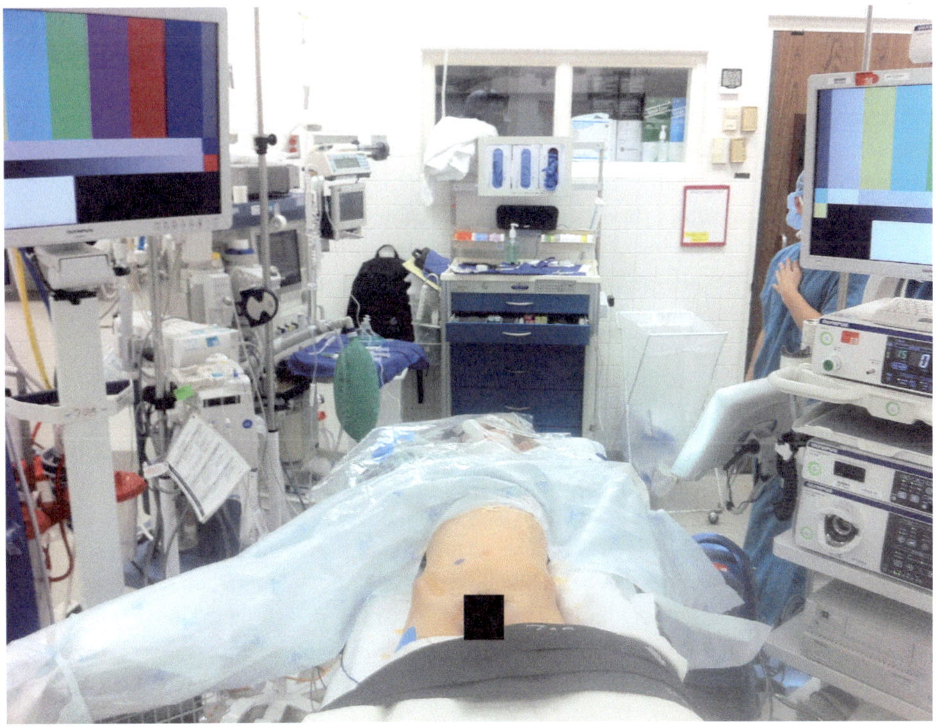

**Fig. 15.4** Room setup demonstrating monitor sites

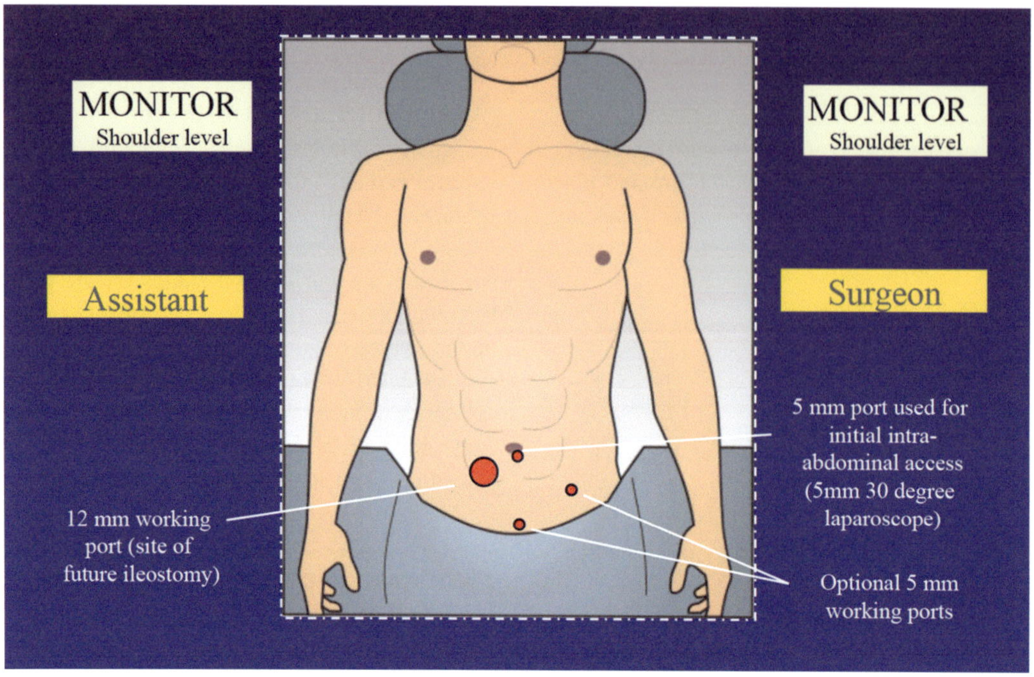


**Fig. 15.5** Ileostomy and port sites

If the previously selected right iliac fossa stoma site is acceptable, a 12-mm port is then placed after making a 2.5-cm incision at the predetermined stoma site, excising the skin and subcutaneous fat as a cone of tissue down to the anterior rectus sheath and then dividing the sheath in a cruciate fashion. The fibers of the rectus muscle are then split longitudinally by opening an instrument perpendicular to the line of the fibers. This procedure results in little or no bleeding unless the deep inferior epigastric vessels are encountered and divided deep to the rectus muscle. After the rectus muscle is split, the posterior rectus sheath is incised to accommodate the 12-mm trocar. The 12-mm trocar provides the ability to accommodate a laparoscopic stapler for intracorporeal division if creating an end ileostomy, rather than exteriorizing the intestines for extracorporeal division. If the ileum requires further mobilization not possible with a single working port, additional 5-mm trocar(s) may be placed either in the left lower quadrant, lateral to the rectus muscle and above the pelvic brim, or suprapubically.

The terminal ileum is located, and a point on the small bowel about 15–20 cm proximal to the ileocecal valve is identified laparoscopically. Visualization of the ligament of Treves, located on the antimesenteric border of the terminal ileum just proximal to the ileocecal valve, is also helpful in identifying the anatomy (Fig. 15.6). The terminal ileum is inspected for any pathology as well as length of mesentery available for loop stoma creation. The terminal ileum is usually supplied by two arcades of vessels, which join the ileocolic vessels adjacent to the cecum. These arcades must be divided as close to the ileocolic vessels as possible to preserve blood supply to the terminal ileum.

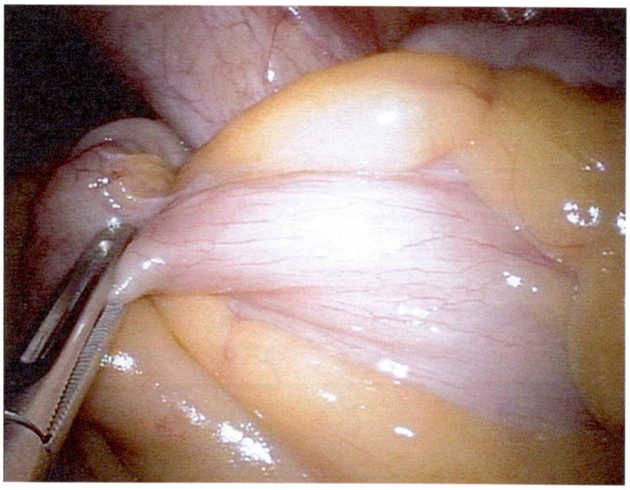

**Fig. 15.6** Terminal ileum with fold of Treves visible

The proximal side (1 serosal thermal burn) and distal side (3 serosal thermal burns) of the selected point on the small bowel are marked by using laparoscopic electrocautery. Alternatively, the future ileostomy site may be marked with different colored sutures for orientation. Once mobilized, the ileum can be grasped and divided with a laparoscopic stapler through the 12-mm port and brought through the abdominal wall or exteriorized through the fascial defect and divided extracorporeally (for an end stoma). If constructing a loop

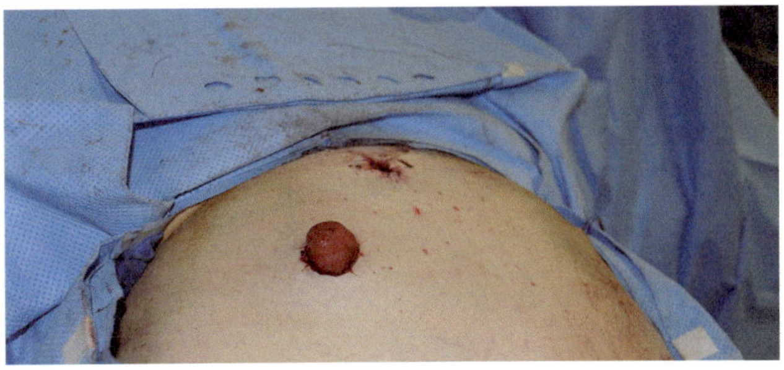

**Fig. 15.7** Completed stoma

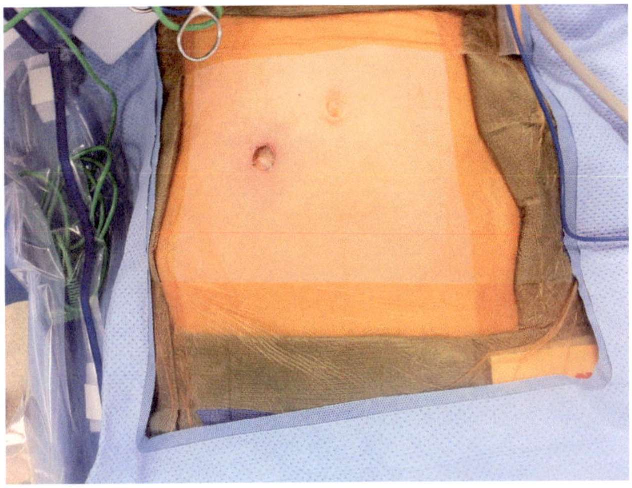

**Fig. 15.8** Anterior sheath

ileostomy, the ileum is grasped and brought through the fascia with attention to maintaining proper orientation. To exteriorize the ileum in both cases, the fascial defect within the posterior rectus sheath must be opened and enlarged over the trocar. Because the ascending colon usually tethers the ileocolic vessels to the right lower quadrant, optimal positioning of the stoma requires the placement of the proximal end along the inferior aspect of the stoma site in a loop ileostomy.

The ileostomy is then matured in the usual fashion (Fig. 15.7). The surgeon places an index finger both along the side of the stoma down to the fascia as well as into the stoma itself and beneath the peritoneum to ensure the fascial opening is not excessively tight and the stoma is not angulated.

For single-port laparoscopic ileostomy construction, a 2.5-cm incision is made in the right iliac fossa at the predetermined stoma site (Video 15.1). The incision is carried down to the anterior rectus sheath, which is then divided in a cruciate fashion. The skin and subcutaneous fat are excised as a cone of tissue down to the anterior rectus sheath (Fig. 15.8). The rectus abdominis muscle is spread in the direction of its fibers exposing the posterior rectus sheath and peritoneum, which are then divided in a cruciate fashion over a distance of 2.5 cm, wide enough to accommodate 2 fingers (Fig. 15.9).

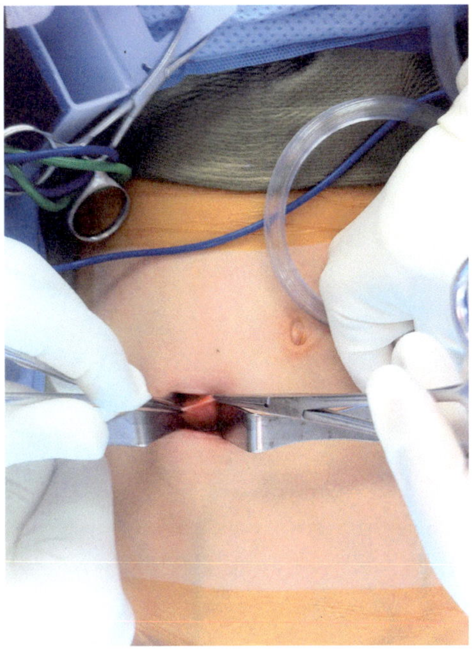

**Fig. 15.9** Posterior sheath: dissection down through the subcutaneous tissue, anterior rectus sheath, and rectus muscle, exposing the posterior rectus sheath

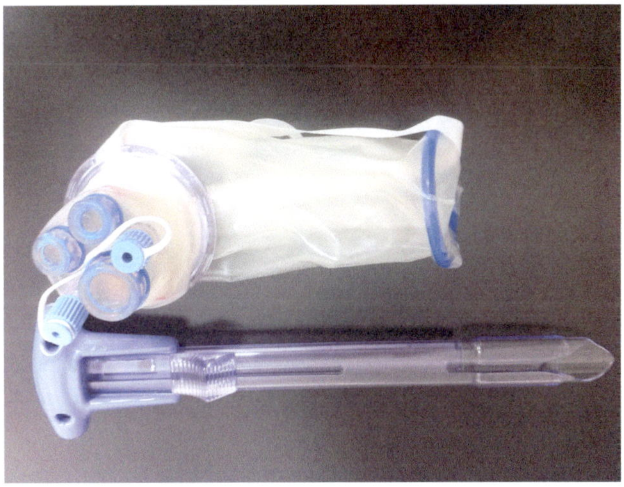

**Fig. 15.10** Single-port access system

The single-port access system is then inserted through this incision (Figs. 15.10 and 15.11). The abdomen is insufflated with $CO_2$ to 15 mmHg. A 5-mm laparoscope with a flexible steerable tip is used to visualize the abdomen. Single-incision laparoscopic instruments may be used, but standard laparoscopic instruments are suitable in most cases.

The terminal ileum is located, and a point on the small bowel about 15–20 cm proximal to the ileocecal valve is identified laparoscopically. The proximal side (1 serosal thermal burn) and distal side (3 serosal thermal burns) of this

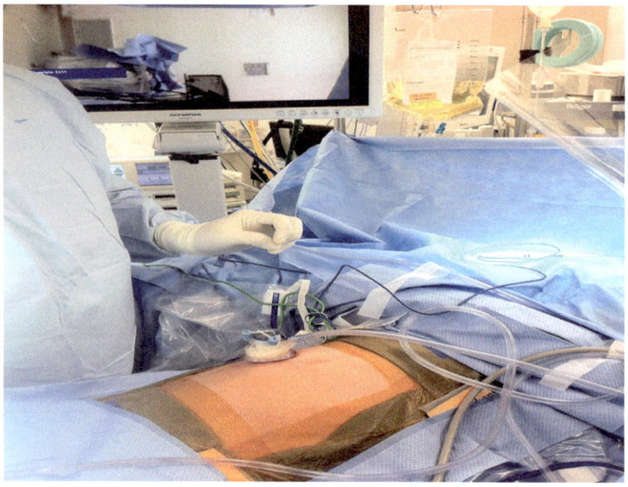

**Fig. 15.11** Single-port access system inserted through stoma site

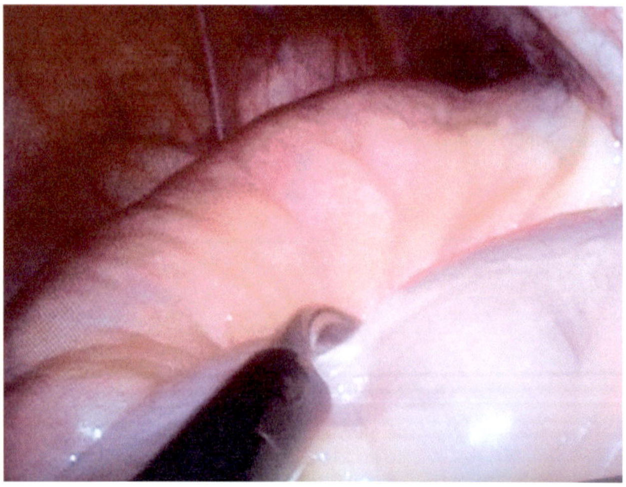

**Fig. 15.12** Marking distal and proximal ileum to maintain orientation of future stoma

point on the small bowel are marked by using laparoscopic electrocautery (Figs. 15.12 and 15.13). With a laparoscopic grasper (e.g., Babcock clamp), the bowel is delivered through the ileostomy incision and exteriorized, with particular attention directed to maintaining proper orientation. Because the ascending colon usually tethers the ileocolic vessels to the right lower quadrant, optimal positioning of the stoma requires the placement of the proximal end along the inferior aspect of the stoma site.

The single-port access system is removed (Fig. 15.14). The ileostomy is then matured in the usual fashion. The surgeon places an index finger both along the side of the stoma down to the fascia as well as into the stoma itself and beneath the peritoneum to ensure the fascial opening is not excessively tight and the stoma is not angulated.

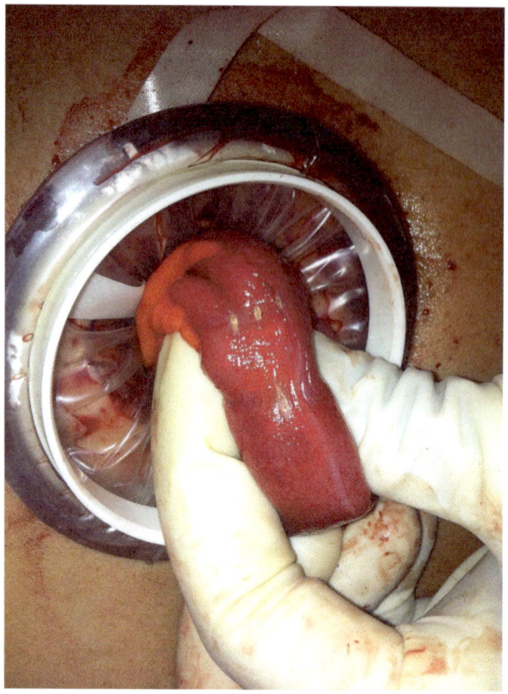

**Fig. 15.13** Ileum with laparoscopically created thermal burns indicating superior (distal) and inferior (proximal) orientation. The head of the patient is directed toward the *top* of the photo

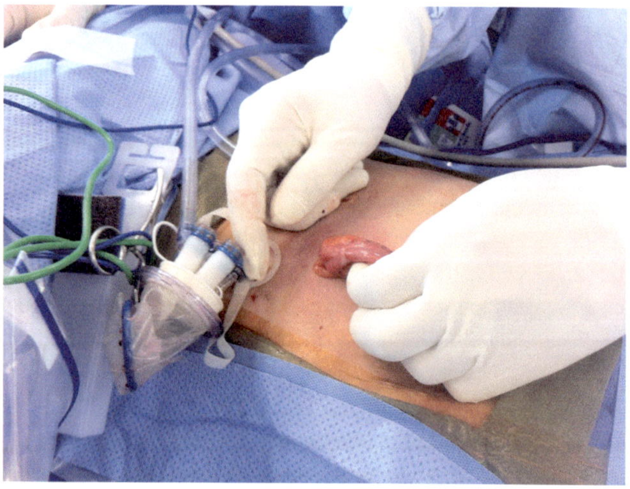

**Fig. 15.14** Ileum exteriorized from single-access port site

## Technique: Laparoscopic Colostomy [1, 2, 20, 21]

Variations in multi-port placement positioning and sequence have been described; however, most approaches use 2 or 3 ports, taking advantage of the principle of trocar triangulation to facilitate exposure and mobilization. The first trocar inserted is a 5-mm cannula placed just inferior to the umbilicus

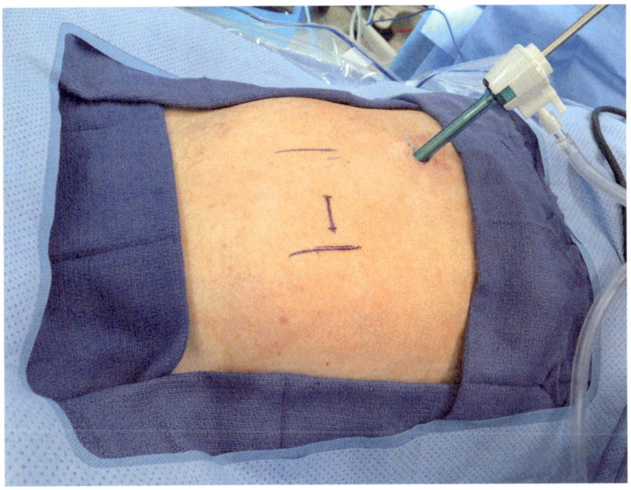

**Fig. 15.15** Placement of the initial 5-mm laparoscopic trocar at the umbilicus to enter and visualize the abdomen. *Blue marks*, from medial to lateral, represent the midline, the anticipated location of the colostomy, and the border of the rectus sheath

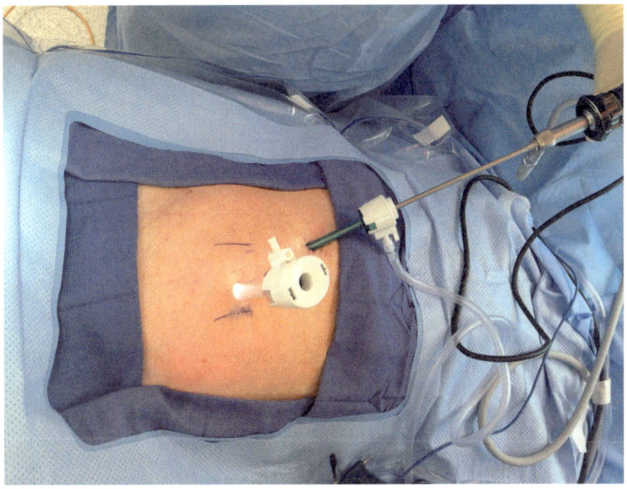

**Fig. 15.16** After the rectus muscle is split, the posterior rectus sheath is incised to accommodate the 12-mm trocar at the pre-marked ostomy site

(Fig. 15.15). Once 15-mmHg pneumoperitoneum is established, a (30°) laparoscope is inserted to inspect the abdomen and direct the remaining port positions. The patient is placed left side up in the Trendelenburg position. The surgeon can visually ensure that the planned ostomy site is suitable and free of adhesions.

If the previously selected left iliac fossa stoma site is acceptable, a 12-mm port is then placed after making a 2.5-cm incision at the predetermined stoma site, excising the skin and subcutaneous fat as a cone of tissue down to the anterior rectus sheath and then dividing the sheath in a cruciate fashion. The fibers of the rectus muscle are then split longitudinally by opening an instrument perpendicular to the line of the fibers. After the rectus muscle is split, the posterior rectus sheath is incised to accommodate the 12-mm trocar (Fig. 15.16). The 12-mm trocar provides the ability to accommodate a laparoscopic stapler for intracorporeal division if creating an end colostomy, rather than exteriorizing the intestines for extracorporeal division. A bowel grasper placed through the 12-mm trocar assesses bowel mobility by pulling the colon toward the abdominal wall. If the sigmoid or descending colon requires further mobilization not possible with a single working port, additional 5-mm trocar(s) may be placed either in the right lower quadrant, lateral to the rectus muscle and above the pelvic brim, or suprapubically.

The additional trocars allow for countertraction while the lateral attachments are mobilized using laparoscopic scissors connected to an energy source. Mobilization commences at the peritoneal reflection in the left paracolic gutter, and the dissection is carried medially in the avascular plane anterior to the gonadal vessels and the ureter. Mobilization should be sufficient to enable several centimeters of bowel to protrude without tension through the abdominal wall.

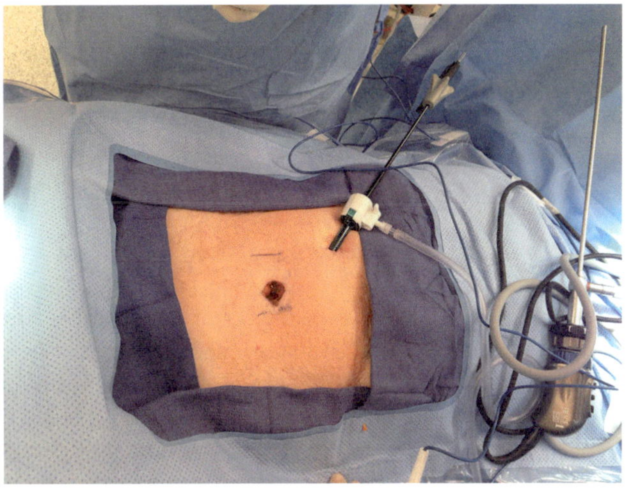

**Fig. 15.17** Once mobilized, the colon can be grasped and exteriorized through the 12-mm port site, with the fascial defect within the posterior rectus sheath opened and enlarged over the trocar to easily accommodate the colon

Once mobilized, the colon can be grasped and divided with a laparoscopic stapler through the 12-mm port or exteriorized through the fascial defect and then divided extracorporeally (Fig. 15.17). To exteriorize the colon in both cases, the fascial defect within the posterior rectus sheath must be opened and enlarged over the trocar. The opening in the abdominal wall should allow two average-sized fingers to pass through to the second phalanx. Before maturing the colostomy, pneumoperitoneum is reestablished to verify proper orientation and absence of twisting.

For single-port laparoscopic colostomy construction, a 2.5-cm incision is made in the left iliac fossa at the predetermined stoma site. The incision is carried down to the anterior rectus sheath, which is divided in a cruciate fashion. The skin and subcutaneous fat are excised as a cone of tissue down to the anterior rectus sheath. The rectus abdominis muscle is spread in the direction of its fibers exposing the posterior rectus sheath and peritoneum, which are then also divided in a cruciate fashion over a distance of 2.5 cm, wide enough to accommodate 2 fingers.

The single-port access system is then inserted through this incision, and a 15-mmHg pneumoperitoneum is established. A 5-mm laparoscope with a flexible steerable tip is used to visualize the abdomen. Single-incision laparoscopic instruments may be used, but standard laparoscopic instruments are suitable in most cases.

Using laparoscopic scissors connected to an energy source, the lateral attachments are mobilized as needed. The proximal side (1 serosal thermal burn) and distal side (3 serosal thermal burns) of the chosen point of colon are marked using laparoscopic electrocautery. When an end stoma is indicated, intracorporeal mesenteric division may be performed either with laparoscopic clips or an endoscopic vascular linear stapler, if necessary.

To avoid stapling of the afferent limb, the lithotomy position allows for intraoperative proctosigmoidoscopy and air insufflation, which can identify the distal colon by distention when the colon at the site of the anticipated stoma is occluded. With a laparoscopic grasper, the colon is delivered through the stoma incision and exteriorized, with attention to maintaining proper orientation in the case of loop colostomy.

The single-port access system is removed. The colostomy is then matured in the usual fashion, either as an end or loop ostomy. The surgeon places an index finger along the side of the stoma down to the fascia to ensure the fascial opening is not excessively tight and down the stoma to ensure the bowel is not angulated.

## Gaining Length When It Would Not Reach [4]

If standard mobilization fails to create a tension-free colostomy, several operative maneuvers can help to obtain left colon length. Following division of the lateral attachments, the splenic flexure should be completely mobilized. Further measures include transection of the medial peritoneal attachments at the base of the colon mesentery, transection of the inferior mesenteric artery proximal to the left colonic arterial takeoff to decrease tethering, and creation of "windows" in the peritoneum overlying the colonic mesentery just below the stoma to gain mesenteric length. If an end stoma was initially intended, but unable to easily reach the proposed stoma site, a loop stoma can be constructed to provide additional length, if necessary.

## Pearls and Pitfalls

- Pearls to ensuring adequate mobilization include full mobilization of sigmoid attachments in the pelvic, sufficient incision of the lateral peritoneum of the descending colon, and sufficient medial mobilization sigmoid colon. Before exteriorization, the proposed site of the stoma should be pulled up to the site of the stoma on the abdominal wall. If the bowel reaches this site without tension, there will be more than adequate length to reach the skin once the pneumoperitoneum is released.
- Prior to ligating any major vessels, ensure you have adequate collateral blood flow to avoid ischemia of the stoma.
- Prior to maturing the stoma, it is recommended to laparoscopically visualize the stoma to ensure proper orientation of the proximal and distal limb and that there is no twist in the mesentery.
- For a diverting-loop ileostomy, ensure you are not too close to the ileocecal valve. This will lead to the subsequent anastomosis being adjacent to the valve at the time of takedown.

## Summary

Laparoscopy is well suited for stoma creation, as neither extensive dissection nor specimen extraction is usually necessary. Although a variety of laparoscopic techniques have been described, the basic tenets remain the same—visualizing the appropriate intestinal segment, mobilizing the segment, and ultimately exteriorizing through the abdominal wall in a proper orientation. When considered relative to a conventional, open technique, laparoscopic stoma construction appears to be as safe and encourage quicker recovery without compromising functional outcomes.

## References

1. Zaghiyan KN, Murrell Z, Fleshner PR. Scarless single-incision laparoscopic loop ileostomy: a novel technique. Dis Colon Rectum. 2011;54(12):1542–6.
2. Lee S. Laparoscopic stoma formation. In: Milsom JW, Böhm B, Nakajima K, editors. Laparoscopic colorectal surgery. New York: Springer; 2006. p. 304–13.
3. Orkin BA, Cataldo PA. Intestinal stomas. In: Wolff BG, Fleshman JW, Beck DE, Pemberton JH, Wexner SD, Church JM, et al., editors. ASCRS textbook colon rectal surgery. New York, NY: Springer; 2007. p. 622–42.
4. Sands LR, Marchetti F. Intestinal stomas. In: Beck DE, Roberts PL, Saclarides TJ, Senagore AJ, Stamos MJ, Wexner SD, editors. ASCRS textbook colon rectal surgery. New York, NY: Springer; 2011. p. 517–33.
5. Hollyoak MA, Lumley J, Stitz RW. Laparoscopic stoma formation for faecal diversion. Br J Surg. 1998;85(2):226–8.

6. Young CJ, Eyers AA, Solomon MJ. Defunctioning of the anorectum: historical controlled study of laparoscopic vs. open procedures. Dis Colon Rectum. 1998;41(2):190–4.
7. Liu J, Bruch HP, Farke S, Nolde J, Schwandner O. Stoma formation for fecal diversion: a plea for the laparoscopic approach. Tech Coloproctol. 2005;9(1):9–14.
8. Oliveira L, Reissman P, Nogueras J, Wexner SD. Laparoscopic creation of stomas. Surg Endosc. 1997;11(1):19–23.
9. Nguyen HML, Causey MW, Steele SR, Maykel JA. Single-port laparoscopic diverting sigmoid colostomy. Dis Colon Rectum. 2011;54(12):1585–8.
10. Atallah S, Albert M, Larach S. Technique for constructing an incisionless laparoscopic stoma. Tech Coloproctol. 2011;15(3):345–7.
11. Schwandner O, Schiedeck TH, Bruch HP. Stoma creation for fecal diversion: is the laparoscopic technique appropriate? Int J Colorectal Dis. 1998;13(5–6):251–5.
12. Li M, Xiao L, Wu W, Yang S, Li S. Meta-analysis of laparoscopic versus open colorectal surgery within fast-track perioperative care. Dis Colon Rectum. 2012;55(7):821–7.
13. Hammond TM, Huang A, Prosser K, Frye JN, Williams NS. Parastomal hernia prevention using a novel collagen implant: a randomised controlled phase 1 study. Hernia. 2008;12(5):475–81.
14. Serra-Aracil X, Bombardo-Junca J, Moreno-Matias J, Darnell A, Mora-Lopez L, Alcantara-Moral M, et al. Randomized, controlled, prospective trial of the use of a mesh to prevent parastomal hernia. Ann Surg. 2009;249(4):583–7.
15. Jänes A, Cengiz Y, Israelsson LA. Randomized clinical trial of the use of a prosthetic mesh to prevent parastomal hernia. Br J Surg. 2004;91(3):280–2.
16. Shabbir J, Chaudhary BN, Dawson R. A systematic review on the use of prophylactic mesh during primary stoma formation to prevent parastomal hernia formation. Colorectal Dis. 2012;14(8):931–6.
17. Janson AR, Jänes A, Israelsson LA. Laparoscopic stoma formation with a prophylactic prosthetic mesh. Hernia. 2010;14(5):495–8.
18. López-Cano M, Lozoya-Trujillo R, Quiroga S, Sánchez JL, Vallribera F, Martí M, et al. Use of a prosthetic mesh to prevent parastomal hernia during laparoscopic abdominoperineal resection: a randomized controlled trial. Hernia. 2012;16(6):661–7.
19. Beck D, Fleshman J, Wexner S, Ellis N, Bauer J, Hyman N, Fleshner P. A prospective, multicenter, randomized, controlled, third party-blinded study of Strattice® fascial inlay for parastomal reinforcement in patients undergoing surgery for permanent abdominal wall ostomies. Podium abstract and presentation at ASCRS meeting; 2013.
20. Lavery IC. Techniques of Colostomy construction and closure. In: Fisher JE, Bland KI, Callery MP, Clagett GP, Jones DB, etitors. Mastery of surgery. Philadelphia, PA: Lippincott Williams and Willcott; 2007;1439–1448.
21. Byrn J. Laparoscopic colostomy. In: Soper NJ, Scott-Conner C, editors. The SAGES Manual: Volume 1 Basic Laparoscopy and Endoscopy. New York, NY: Springer; 2012;403–412.

# 16 Laparoscopic Stoma Reversal

Emre Gorgun

**Key Points**

- Laparoscopic surgery is now widely used in performing colectomies both for benign and malignant conditions.
- Laparoscopic colorectal surgery has short-term benefits over open colorectal surgery.
- Laparoscopic and open stoma reversals are challenging.
- Laparoscopic reversal of Hartmann's procedure may be associated with shorter hospital stay.
- The authors endorse preoperative bowel preparation for laparoscopic Hartmann's reversal.
- Preoperative flexible sigmoidoscopy reveals useful information regarding the length of the distal segment and thus facilitates operative planning.
- Initial access is gained by mobilizing the stoma from the surrounding tissue and placing a purse-string suture in the proximal bowel, which also helps to prevent stool or mucous from spilling through the end of the bowel.
- The utilization of the hand-assisted approach is an alternative to a primary technique or to a conversion to manage intra-abdominal adhesions and difficulties with visualization that would preclude the straight laparoscopic approach.

## Introduction

Since the introduction of laparoscopic surgery for the management of symptomatic cholelithiasis, the surgical approach for many intra-abdominal diseases has dramatically changed. Laparoscopic colectomy, for both benign and malignant conditions, is now widely performed. The collective experience with laparoscopic colon surgery has demonstrated that patients who undergo laparoscopic procedures have less pain, decreased incidence of ileus, and a shorter hospital stay. These trends have led some experienced surgeons to apply their laparoscopic skills to colostomy closure after Hartmann's procedure, in an attempt to decrease operative trauma—and possibly hospital stay as well—in this select group of patients. Additionally, some advanced laparoscopic surgeons have begun to apply their skills and available technology to performing minimally invasive re-operative surgery, including both complex lysis of adhesions and ileostomy takedown, with ileocolonic or ileorectal anastomosis.

Laparoscopic stoma reversal is technically demanding due to intraoperative difficulties caused by existing abdominal adhesions and, in many cases, a difficult pelvis. This added challenge can lead to longer operative times and a potential increase in complications, especially if such procedures are performed by inexperienced laparoscopic surgeons. By using laparoscopy, however, the operative trauma usually associated with laparotomy can be minimized and postoperative hospital stay potentially reduced. For example, colostomy closure after Hartmann's procedure is associated with a high morbidity of 15 to 34 percent and a prolonged hospital stay of 13 to 15 days [1, 2]. If complication rates after Hartmann's procedure could be reduced, then it is likely that the percentage of patients left with permanent stomas would decline (Fig. 16.1). Therefore, Hartmann's reversal may benefit from a laparoscopic approach.

## Preoperative Planning

Proper patient selection is crucial to preoperative planning, and patients should be both medically fit and able to tolerate laparoscopy. All patients should undergo a detailed history and physical examination, including a thorough review of their surgical history. Such preparation is especially important if the original stoma creation was performed in a different

**Electronic supplementary material:** Supplementary material is available in the online version of this chapter at 10.1007/978-1-4939-1581-1_16. Videos can also be accessed at http://www.springerimages.com/videos/978-1-4939-1580-4.

E. Gorgun, M.D., F.A.C.S., F.A.S.C.R.S. (✉)
Department of Colon and Rectal Surgery, Digestive Disease Institute, Cleveland Clinic, 9500 Euclid Avenue/A, Cleveland, OH 44195, USA
e-mail: gorgune@ccf.org

H.M. Ross et al. (eds.), *Minimally Invasive Approaches to Colon and Rectal Disease: Technique and Best Practices*, DOI 10.1007/978-1-4939-1581-1_16, 

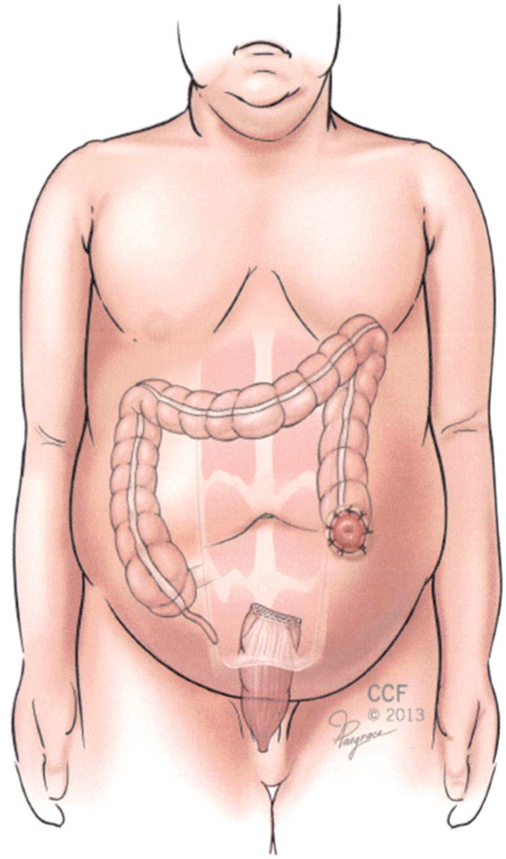


**Fig. 16.1** Hartmann's procedure. *With permission from Cleveland Clinic Foundation*

center from where the reversal will be performed. Physical examination can reveal important hints regarding the potential severity of intra-abdominal adhesions. A soft abdomen, with good anterior abdominal wall mobility as determined by bimanual examination, is usually indicative of a more favorable anatomy. On the other hand, a massive midline scar that is found to be sunken and possessing minimal mobility on bimanual examination is classically associated with underlying dense adhesions and restriction of the abdominal wall to accommodate. Patients in the latter group are usually not good candidates for the laparoscopic approach.

Preoperative colonoscopy and flexible sigmoidoscopy is especially recommended for high-risk and IBD patients or those who had a previous bowel perforation due to diverticulitis. Flexible sigmoidoscopy reveals useful information regarding the length of the distal segment (i.e., a rough estimation of above or below the promontory) and thus facilitates operative planning. As part of the preoperative preparation, patients with a colostomy should undergo a mechanical bowel preparation, ensuring the distal stump is clear of stool with one or two enemas. In our practice, however, patients undergoing ileostomy closure with bowel anastomosis are not usually given a mechanical bowel preparation. Preoperative intravenous antibiotics are given within 30–60 min of the incision time, to ensure adequate concentration at the outset, and later readministered in cases taking longer than 3–4 h. Deep venous prophylaxis should include the use of sequential compression devices as well as chemical prophylaxis (preoperative heparin).

## Procedure

### Setup

After informed consent is obtained, IV induction is given, followed by endotracheal intubation. A Foley catheter and an orogastric tube are placed. The patient is routinely placed in the modified lithotomy position (Fig. 16.2), which allows access to the anus. This position also allows an intraoperative $CO_2$ colonoscopy to be performed with ease, when required. The lithotomy position also provides additional space for the surgical team, especially when operating in the upper quadrants of the abdomen, by standing between the patient's legs (Fig. 16.3). Padded stirrups or yellow fins are used, and attention is given to preventing peroneal nerve injury. Both arms are tucked at the patient's sides. A gel pad on the operating table can provide additional decubitus support and stability against gravity with tilting. Additionally, we prefer to secure patients on the operating table with a strong tape placed over the chest to prevent patients from sliding during steep Trendelenburg and right or left tilt. For closure after Hartmann's procedure, the operating surgeon stands on the patient's right side, with the assistant either on the opposite or same side, as needed. Two monitors are placed on both sides of the table.

## Procedure Steps

### Laparoscopic Reversal of Colostomy After Hartmann's Procedure

#### Port Placement

- Initial access: Usually, the colostomy site can be taken down first. An incision is made at the mucocutaneous junction, and the colostomy is freed from the surrounding attachments. A purse-string suture is placed in the proximal bowel and the anvil is secured. This technique also helps to prevent stool or mucous spillage from the end of the colon (Fig. 16.4). After the colostomy has been completely mobilized, the bowel segment proximal to the anvil is returned to the abdomen and peritoneal access is gained. However, it is often necessary to place the anvil in the proximal bowel after adequate mobilization is performed. If so, the proximal colon can be closed with sutures or staples prior to returning it to the abdomen. In this approach, sealing can be achieved in different ways: Our general preference is to use Alexis bundle

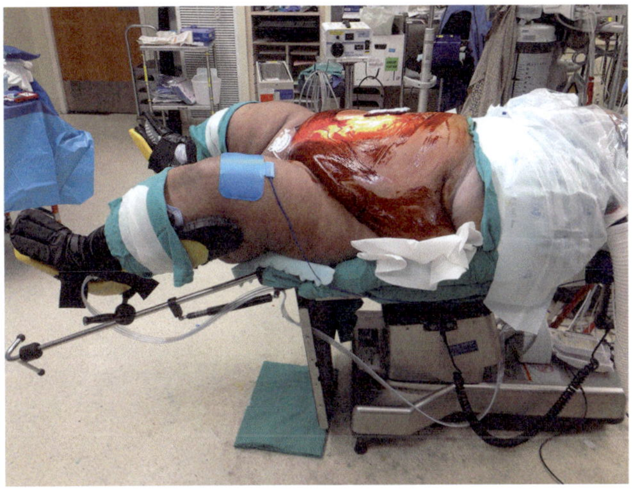

**Fig. 16.2** Modified lithotomy position

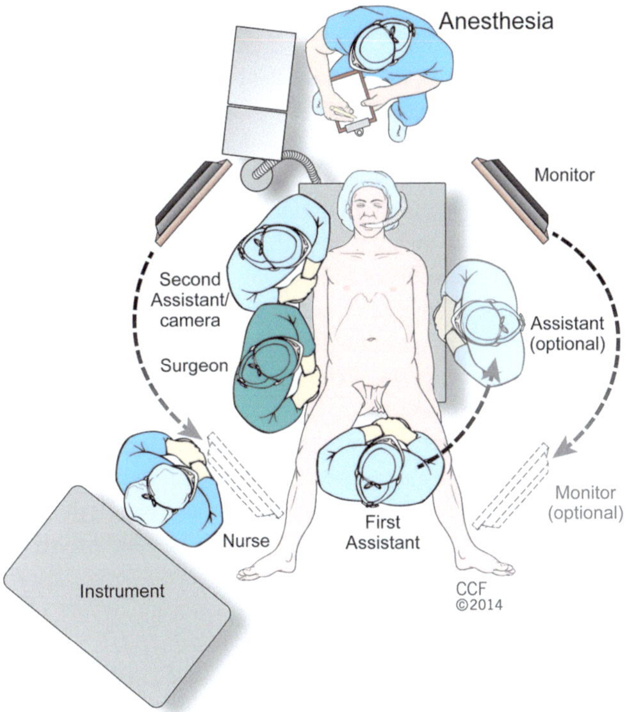


**Fig. 16.3** Room setup for a laparoscopic stoma reversal. *With permission from Cleveland Clinic Foundation*

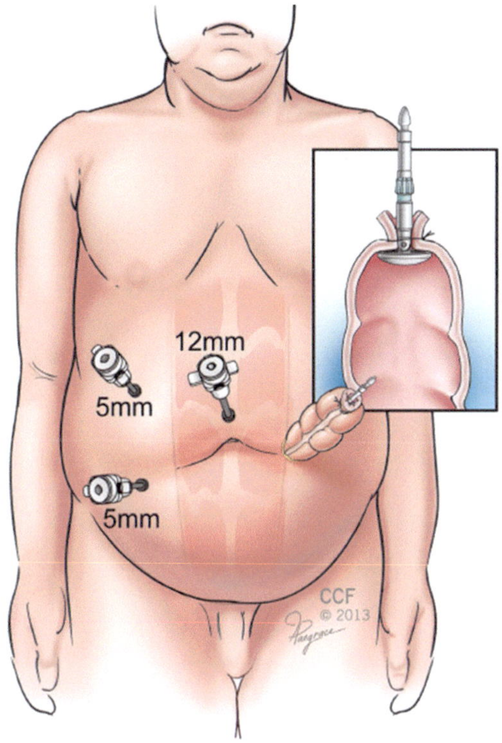


**Fig. 16.4** Initial port placement and peritoneal access. *With permission from Cleveland Clinic Foundation*

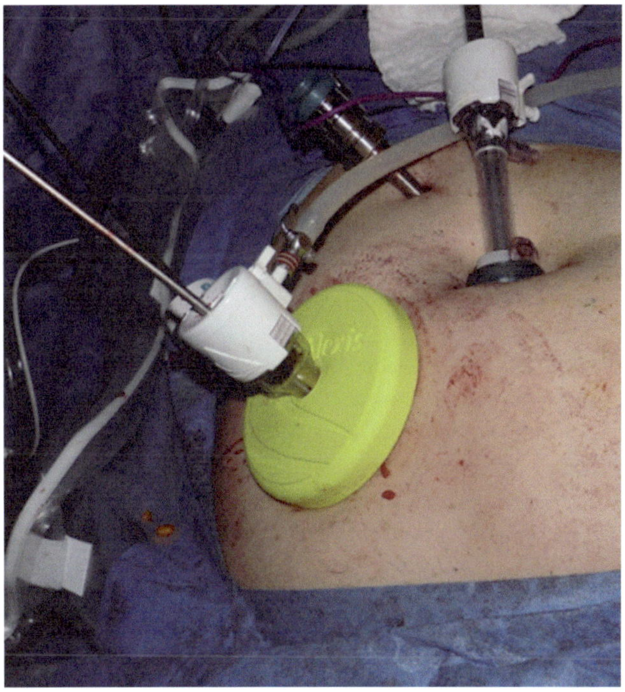

**Fig. 16.5** Alexis bundle wound protectors with "a cap" and trocar

wound protectors with "a cap" (Alexis laparoscopic system with Kii Fios First Entry, Applied Medical, Rancho Santa Margarita, CA), which helps maintain the pneumoperitoneum (Fig. 16.5). A 5–12-mm port is situated in the middle of the cap, which also enables a laparoscopic approach before and after specimen retrieval. This approach thus converts the stoma site into an additional working port, with 12-mm trocar. This port can subsequently be used as an access port for endoscopic staplers as well as a port site where specimens can be removed when necessary. Additionally, the operating surgeon can utilize this trocar by standing between the patient's legs and take down the splenic flexure when needed. Alternatively, single-port access laparoscopic Hartmann's reversal can be performed. When using this approach, a similar circumferential incision around the colostomy is

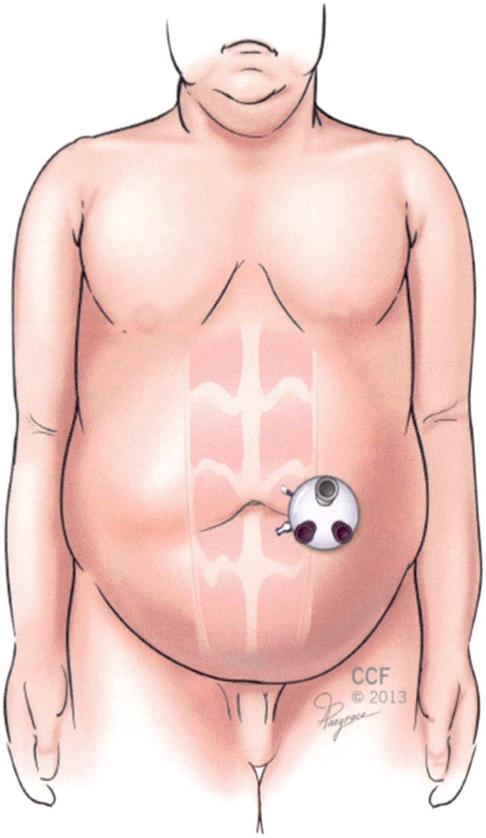


**Fig. 16.6** Single-port access laparoscopic Hartmann's reversal. *With permission from Cleveland Clinic Foundation*

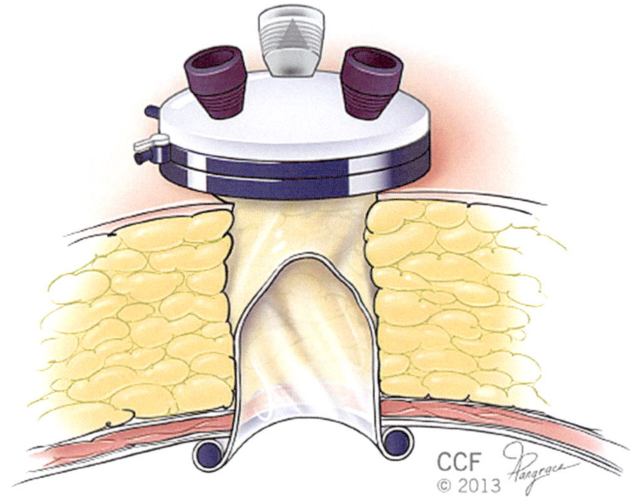


**Fig. 16.7** Side view of the single-port access device. *With permission from Cleveland Clinic Foundation*

made, followed by disconnection of the stoma from the mucocutaneous border. After the proximal bowel with the anvil is returned to the abdomen, a single-port access device (GelPOINT, Applied Medical, Rancho Santa Margarita, CA) is inserted into the abdomen (Figs. 16.6 and 16.7).

- Alternatively, an open Hasson technique may be used and access to the peritoneal cavity gained through an incision just above the umbilicus, in cases where initial stoma takedown is not preferred.
- After insufflation, two 5-mm trocars (Fig. 16.8) can be placed under direct vision on the right side, lateral to the rectus. A minimum of a fist-sized distance is left between the 5-mm ports. This room provides superior freedom to each of the instruments during dissection and manipulation.
- Hand-assisted approach: The utilization of the hand-assisted approach allows the surgeon the ability to assess the intraoperative findings prior to committing to the costs of opening the laparoscopic equipment. A hand port can be created in the suprapubic position, and via the open incision, the presence of adhesions and the state of the pelvis can be assessed (Fig. 16.9). If favorable, the laparoscopic equipment can be opened and the case can proceed. If conditions are not favorable, the incision can be extended and the case approached in an open fashion.
- Establishment of pneumoperitoneum: This step is achieved via insufflation through either the umbilical port or colostomy side port. Following adequate pneumoperitoneum, the camera is inserted first through the colostomy side port, and then, according to the density of adhesions, more space is created through further adhesiolysis or with the insertion of additional trocars as described above. All four quadrants of the abdomen are then explored and any abnormalities noted.
- Optional trocars: A 5-mm trocar may be placed in the left paramedian position, lateral to the edge of the rectus in the left upper quadrant. This placement can assist both with sigmoid retraction and small bowel adhesiolysis on the right side of the abdomen.

### Mobilization of the Proximal Colon

- Once the adequate pneumoperitoneum is established and the peritoneal cavity is adequately assessed, the proximal colon needs to be mobilized. The decision to perform a lateral-to-medial or medial-to-lateral approach is dependent upon the surgeon's preference and the intraoperative conditions. A lateral-to-medial dissection is usually satisfactory for mobilizing the remaining descending colon. In cases where, during the initial operation, perforectomy alone (i.e., resection of the perforated segment only) was performed and a long distal sigmoid colon was left behind, a more extensive descending colon mobilization will be required. At this stage the distal sigmoid colon will be mobilized down to the rectum. We generally prefer a medial-to-lateral approach; however, depending on the comfort level of the surgeon, a lateral approach can also be utilized. The superior rectal/inferior mesenteric vessels

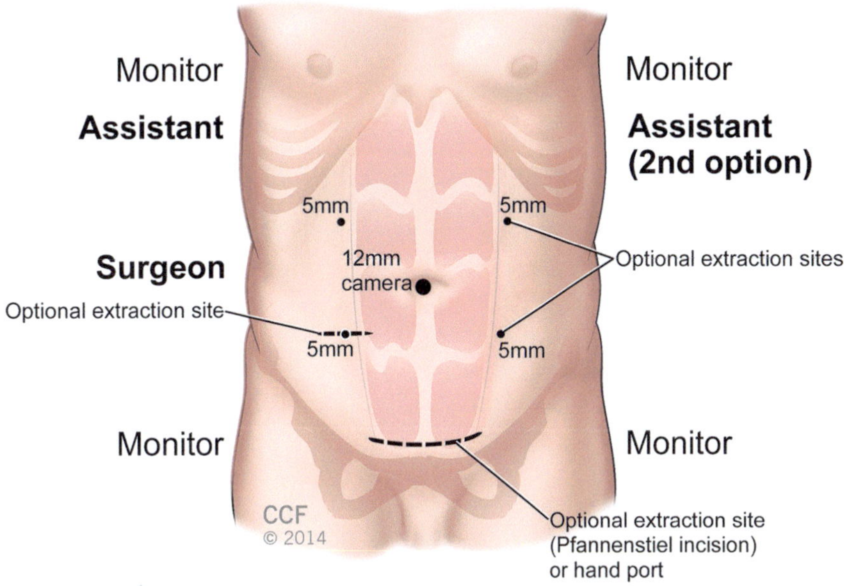


**Fig. 16.8** Port sites for straight laparoscopic or hand-assisted stoma reversal. *With permission from Cleveland Clinic Foundation*

can be identified and ligated after the left ureter is visualized and preserved. Ligation of the inferior mesenteric vein just below the level of the pancreatic body gives additional mobility to the proximal colon segment. Once the colon is adequately mobilized, it will need to be exteriorized for resection and insertion of the stapling anvil. The colon can be exteriorized via the stoma site or a suprapubic incision.

## Mobilization of the Hartmann's Pouch and Rectum

- The goals of this step are to achieve visualization of the pelvis and mobilize both the descending colon and the Hartmann's pouch. Laparoscopic adhesiolysis may be required, in order to free the left lower quadrant small bowel of adhesions. Additional mobilization of the descending colon or rectal stump may be required. The goal here is to create a tension-free anastomosis; however, any remaining sigmoid colon on the colostomy or rectal stump must be resected if the Hartmann's procedure was initially performed for perforated diverticulitis. Resection should be extended all the way down to the top of the rectum. In these cases, a formal splenic flexure takedown may be required before a tension-free reach and anastomosis can be achieved.
- In our experience, we prefer to implant the rectal stump above the fascia and just under skin, at the lower aspect of the incision, at the time of the primary operation. This practice makes finding the rectal stump significantly easier, and the potential for rectal scarring and small bowel adhesion formation around the stump itself is minimized (Fig. 16.9).

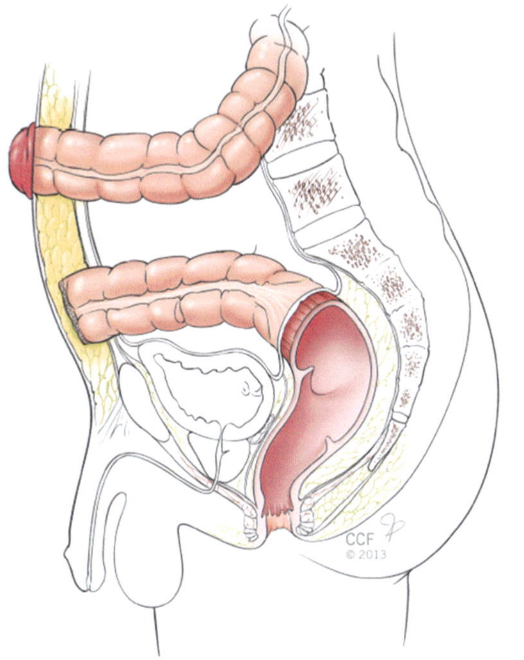


**Fig. 16.9** Hartmann's procedure with implantation of the rectal stump above the fascia. *With permission from Cleveland Clinic Foundation*

## Resection of the Distal Sigmoid Colon

- Distal division of the sigmoid colon: If the distal sigmoid colon is not resected during the index operation, this step must be completed, since this area is usually described as the "high-pressure zone" and recurrent diverticulitis attacks may be observed if this bowel segment is left behind. Therefore, a distal division point is chosen where the taenia splays, ensuring that transection is performed

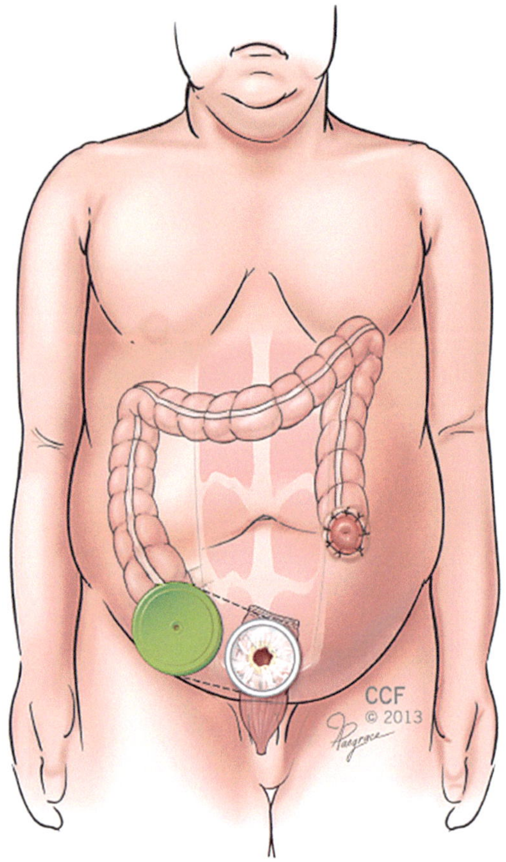


**Fig. 16.10** Maintaining pneumoperitoneum using wound protector at the Pfannenstiel incision. *With permission from Cleveland Clinic Foundation*

on the rectum. The bowel is then transected at this point, utilizing a laparoscopic linear cutting stapler. Endocutter stapler can be introduced either through the right lower quadrant or the stoma side port. Usually, one firing of the stapler is satisfactory to staple and cut across the bowel at this level of the rectum, provided the mesentery is meticulously prepared.

- Extra-corporealization of the distal sigmoid colon: Once the distal portion of the bowel is transected, the resected bowel segment is removed from the previous colostomy side or Pfannenstiel incision, through the wound protector (Fig. 16.10). If the remaining rectal stump is short and previous resection of the bowel was performed right at the top of the rectum, further stapling may not be required. In these circumstances we usually prefer to use "rectal sizers" and make sure the stump is adequately mobilized from the pelvic adhesions. This step also allows us to advance the circular stapling gun easily to the end of the bowel.

### Anastomosis Creation

- Creation of the anastomosis: A curved circular stapler is advanced through the anus to the level of the rectal stump. We generally bring the spike of the stapler to one corner of the rectal stump (Video 16.1). This way, only one corner is left behind on the rectal stump, rather than two, which could potentially act as "dog-ears." The spike portion is then engaged with the anvil. This step is best achieved by using the special disposable or reusable anvil graspers, for easier stapler-anvil engagement. Prior to closing the stapler, the surgeon should confirm that the proximal bowel is not twisted and that the mesentery is straight. The small bowel should also be retracted from the retroperitoneum and should not be trapped under the mesentery, which is best achieved by placing the patient in the Trendelenburg position and tilting the operating table to the right. The stapler is then fired and tissue doughnuts removed and closely inspected, to confirm the circumferential integrity of the staple line.
- Inspection of anastomosis and leak test: We routinely use $CO_2$ colonoscopy to carefully inspect the anastomosis and perform a leak test. The proximal bowel is clamped using an atraumatic bowel grasper and the pelvis is filled with saline. A leak test is performed by $CO_2$ insufflation. If any visible or pulsating vessel is seen, immediate endoclipping can be performed until absolute hemostasis is reached.
- Closure of the abdomen: After achieving complete hemostasis, all port sites larger than 10 mm are closed using absorbable suture. We do not routinely use abdominal or pelvic drains. The orogastric tube is removed at the time of emergence from anesthesia. The Foley catheter is discontinued on postoperative day one.

## Laparoscopic Reversal of Ileostomy with Ileorectal Anastomosis

### Port Placement

- Initial access: Disconnection from the skin is usually accomplished with a circumferential mucocutaneous junction incision around the ileostomy similar to the previously described with the colostomy. The surrounding attachments are sharply and bluntly freed and access to the peritoneal cavity gained. A purse-string suture is placed in the proximal bowel and the anvil is secured. This technique prevents ileostomy contents or mucous from spilling from the end of the stoma. After the ileostomy has been taken down, the proximal bowel segment with the anvil is returned to the abdomen, and the peritoneal opening is sealed. Sealing can be achieved in different ways. Our preference is to use Alexis bundle wound protectors (Alexis laparoscopic system with Kii Fios First Entry, Applied Medical, Rancho Santa Margarita, CA), which can be caped to maintain pneumoperitoneum. This device provides a good seal, and a 5–12-mm trocar in the middle can be used as an access port. This port can subsequently be used as an access port for endoscopic staplers, as well as a port site, where specimens can be removed as needed.

- After insufflation, a 5-mm trocar is placed under direct vision in the right upper quadrant, lateral to the rectus. A minimum of a fist-sized distance (Fig. 16.7) is left between the old ileostomy side port and the 5-mm ports. If the ileostomy was in the left lower quadrant, two 5-mm ports are placed on the right side of the abdomen, lateral to the rectus muscle. A minimum of a fist-sized distance is then left between the two 5-mm ports, which enables superior freedom of movement during dissection and manipulation, for each instrument.
- Optional hand-assist device placement and rectal stump mobilization: For surgeons who prefer to use a hand-assist device, this may be placed at the Pfannenstiel or midline position. For ileostomy reversal cases, the rectal stump may be implanted under the Pfannenstiel incision and above the fascia during the initial operation. This practice is our preference for patients with complex IBD, in whom subtotal colectomy with end ileostomy is created. We prefer to implant the rectal stump above the fascia to potentially avoid stump blowout within the pelvis. In these circumstances, at the time of the reversal operation, adding a hand port can ease surgical complexity and significantly shorten operative time. Additionally, if the incision where the rectal stump was implanted is too small to place a hand port, an additional XS or small wound protector can be added to achieve a seal and maintain pneumoperitoneum.
- Establishment of pneumoperitoneum: This step is achieved via insufflation through either the umbilical port or colostomy side port. Following adequate pneumoperitoneum, the camera is inserted. All four quadrants of the abdomen are explored and any abnormalities noted.
- Optional trocars: A 5-mm trocar may be placed in the left paramedian position, lateral to the edge of the rectus, in the left lower or upper quadrant, as needed. This added measure can assist both with distal sigmoid colon retraction as well as mobilization of the rectal stump. The assistant surgeon can utilize this trocar by standing on the left of the patient and using it to assist with retraction, or to further dissect the rectal stump.
- Alternatively, single-port access laparoscopic ileostomy reversal can be performed. For this purpose, a similar circumferential incision around the ileostomy is made, followed by disconnection of the stoma from the mucocutaneous border (Video 16.2). After the proximal bowel with the anvil is returned to the abdomen, a single-port access device (GelPOINT, Applied Medical, Rancho Santa Margarita, CA) is inserted into the abdomen (Fig. 16.11). Intra-abdominal adhesions are then divided using the GelPOINT system and three trocars. Laparoscopic adhesiolysis is then performed to obtain sufficient access to the abdominal and pelvic cavities. For the purpose of ileorectal anastomosis, the rectal stump is mobilized. A tension-free ileorectal anastomosis is ensured with a standard circular stapling device, which is inserted transanally and then tested for leaks. Single-port access may offer cosmetic advantages beyond the well-recognized benefits of multi-port laparoscopic surgery and can be performed with the use of standard straight instruments.

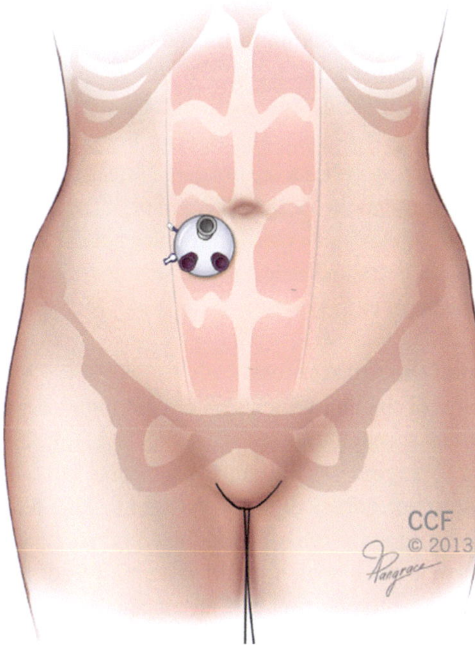


**Fig. 16.11** Laparoscopic ileostomy reversal with ileorectal anastomosis using single-access port: external view. *With permission from Cleveland Clinic Foundation*

### Mobilization of the Small Bowel

- Once adequate pneumoperitoneum is created and the abdomen is evaluated, the small bowel needs to be mobilized to ensure reach into the pelvic and proper orientation. This usually requires that most intra-loop adhesions be lysed and the small bowel mesentery be mobilized off the retroperitoneum. This often requires the superior mesenteric artery to be mobilized up to the level of the duodenum. To ensure there is no twisting of the small bowel mesentery, the small bowel should be placed in the left side of the abdomen and the cut edge of the mesentery should face the patient's right side.

### Mobilization of the Rectum

- The goals of this step are to achieve pelvic visualization and mobilize the rectal segment where the anastomosis will be created. Adhesiolysis may be needed, in order to free the bowel segment (Video 16.3). If ileorectal anastomosis will be created, the left gutter and the pelvic brim must be free of any small bowel.

### Rectal Resection

- Division of rectal stump: If the end of the rectal stump is not even and hard, the top of the rectum may need to be freed up from pelvic adhesions and then stapled in order to ensure a safer anastomosis. The bowel can be transected utilizing either a laparoscopic linear cutting stapler inserted through the GelPOINT port or, if the rectal stump is long enough, can be pulled through a small Pfannenstiel incision and stapled using a TX stapler (transverse stapler), in an open fashion.

### Creation of the Anastomosis

- Creation of the anastomosis: A curved circular stapler is advanced through the anus, to the level of the rectal stump. We again generally bring the spike portion of the stapler to one corner of the rectal stump. This placement allows us to leave only one of the rectal stumps behind, rather than two, which could potentially act as "dog-ears." The spike portion is then engaged with the anvil. This process is best achieved by using disposable or reusable anvil graspers. Prior to closing the stapler, the surgeon should confirm that the proximal bowel is not twisted and that the mesentery is straight. The small bowel should also be retracted from the retroperitoneum and should not be trapped under the mesentery. The stapler is then fired and tissue doughnuts should be removed and closely inspected to confirm circumferential integrity of the staple line.
- Inspection of anastomosis and leak test: We routinely use $CO_2$ colonoscopy to carefully inspect the anastomosis and perform a leak test. The proximal bowel is clamped using an atraumatic bowel grasper and the pelvis is filled with saline. An air leak test is performed by $CO_2$ insufflation. If any pulsating vessel is found, endoclipping is performed immediately or a vasoconstrictive agent is injected.
- Closure of the abdomen: After complete hemostasis is achieved, all port sites larger than 10 mm are closed using absorbable sutures. We do not routinely use abdominal or pelvic drains. The orogastric tube is removed at the time of emergence from anesthesia. The Foley catheter is discontinued on postoperative day one.

## Postoperative Care

Early ambulation and enteral feeding are part of our standard postoperative management. Most patients are started on a clear liquid diet on the day of surgery and advanced to solid food on postoperative day one, as tolerated. Pain control is usually achieved by narcotic, intravenous patient-controlled analgesia (PCA). Narcotic use in patients with ileus should be limited, and nonnarcotics such as ketorolac, acetaminophen, and ibuprofen should instead be administered parenterally. Foley catheter is usually removed on postoperative day one. Prophylactic antibiotic usage is limited to 24 h postoperatively. DVT prophylaxis consists of early ambulation, sequential compressive devices, and chemical prophylaxis (SQ heparin) until the patient is discharged from the hospital. Patients with laparoscopic stoma reversal and bowel anastomosis are typically discharged 3–4 days postoperatively, with planned clinic follow-up 4 weeks after the day of discharge.

## Complications

The use of the laparoscopic technique for the reversal of ostomies appears to offer distinct advantages over the open approach. In a comparative analysis between laparoscopic and open colostomy reversal, Rosen et al. found that the laparoscopic technique resulted in less operative blood loss, decreased complications, quicker return of bowel function, and a shorter hospital stay [3]. Patients with ostomies may have significant intra-abdominal adhesions. As a result, gaining access to the peritoneal cavity may cause inadvertent bowel injury. These adhesions are often centered under the previous midline incision as well as within the pelvis. During open stoma reversal, the previous midline incision is typically reentered, which may increase the likelihood of bowel injury, as these adhesions are most dense at the site of the previous incision. In the laparoscopic approach, however, the abdomen is entered at a site remote from any previous intra-abdominal scarring. As described above, the abdomen is entered through the stoma, and an incision at the previous scar site is thus avoided. Initial trocar placement is conducted at the stoma site by mobilizing the colostomy or ileostomy, and the peritoneum is accessed with an open cut-down technique, a maneuver that decreases the risk of bowel injury. Additionally, eliminating the laparotomy incision can decrease the incidence of postoperative wound complications.

Other complications may include inadvertent enterotomy or colotomy at the stoma site, ureteral injury, trocar placement injury, and vascular injury. Enterotomies and colotomies should initially be repaired, if possible, and conversion to an open procedure undertaken only if the injury cannot be safely repaired laparoscopically. Unexpected conversion to an open procedure is not a failure and should be considered an option if the procedure cannot be performed safely due to dense adhesions or an injury that cannot be managed laparoscopically. Open procedure instruments should be kept at hand, in the event that conversion is required. If found, ureteral injuries should be repaired intraoperatively and typically require the consultation of a urologic surgeon. Vascular injury is rare but can occur at several locations: epigastric vessels during trocar placement, gonadal and iliac vessels during dissection and mobilization prior to resection, and mesenteric vessels during mobilization and resection.

**Table 16.1** Complications of laparoscopic stoma reversal

| |
|---|
| Intraoperative<br>• Enterotomy<br>• Colotomy<br>• Ureteral injury<br>• Trocar placement injury<br>• Vascular injury |
| Postoperative<br>• Early<br>o Early Ileus<br>o Surgical site infection<br>o Urinary tract infection<br>o Respiratory tract infection<br>o Anastomotic leak<br>o Organ space infection<br>o Hemorrhage<br>o Small bowel obstruction<br>• Late<br>o Bowel obstruction<br>o Stoma closure side hernia<br>o Incisional hernia |

Damage to the epigastric may be avoided by transilluminating the abdominal wall during trocar placement or by placing the trocars lateral to the rectus muscles. If damage does occur, direct pressure and electrocautery can be implemented with good success. Refractory bleeding can be stopped temporarily by the tamponade effect of a Foley catheter balloon introduced via the offending port site. Because the gonadal and iliac vessels are retroperitoneal structures, they may be avoided by early identification and careful dissection. If damage to these vessels does occur, direct manual pressure should be used and conversion to open should be considered, depending on the extent and location of the injury.

Early postoperative complications include hemorrhage, deep space infections, anastomotic leak, urinary tract infection, surgical site infection, and respiratory infection (Table 16.1). Urinary tract infections can be minimized by implementing sterilization techniques and removing the Foley catheter by postoperative day one. Respiratory infections can be prevented by introducing early postoperative respiratory exercises. Atelectasis may also be avoided with the use of incentive spirometry, deep breathing, coughing, and early ambulation. Unfortunately, surgical site infections are not an uncommon complication in any colorectal procedure, but their incidence can be minimized with the appropriate use of preoperative antibiotics and wound protectors and by adopting a culture of operative infection prevention, which includes rules such as changing gloves prior to skin closure, irrigation of the wound with saline, etc. If a wound infection occurs, it should be treated in the standard fashion, with wound culture obtained to guide proper antibiotic treatment, as necessary. Anastomotic leakage, although a feared complication, has a low incidence. Anastomotic leaks can be avoided by ensuring a tension-free, non-twisted anastomosis with an adequate blood supply. If the anastomosis appears tenuous during the procedure, it should be taken down and re-created. If there is suspicion for a leak postoperatively and the patient is stable, a CT scan with PO or rectal and IV contrast should be completed, to determine the presence and location of the suspected leak. All patients with suspected leaks that are unstable should undergo fluid resuscitation and initiation of broad-spectrum antibiotics and return to the operating room for exploration.

## Outcome

Open Hartmann's reversal is technically challenging and has been associated with significant morbidity (13–50 %) and mortality (5–10 %). Once the Hartmann's is created, intestinal continuity may be restored but, due to its high perioperative risk and complication rates, up to 60 % of patients never have their stomas reversed [4–7]. A recent study from the UK, regarding trends in the Hartmann's procedure and Hartmann's reversal, showed that only 23 % of patients had their stoma reversed within a 4-year period after their primary operation. Increasing age and the presence of comorbid disease are the most common risk factors for nonreversal. If complication rates after open Hartmann's procedure could be reduced, it is likely that the number of stoma reversals after Hartmann's procedure would increase and the percentage of patients left with a stoma would potentially decrease.

Open stoma reversal has also been associated with a hospital stay of 13–15 days [8, 9]. Studies examining the results of laparoscopic colon resections have shown that the laparoscopic approach results in less postoperative pain, decrease postoperative ileus rates, and reduced length of hospital stay. These findings have led some surgeons to believe that patients may benefit from a minimally invasive approach, and performing laparoscopy for the purpose of stoma reversal was explored. The role of laparoscopy in colostomy reversal, however, has been little studied since it was first reported [10]. A small case series reported conversion rates as high as 25 % because of multiple and dense adhesions and difficulty in identifying the rectal stump. Such a procedure is indeed technically challenging and requires an experienced laparoscopic surgeon. Generally, the main reported reasons for conversion were dense abdominal and pelvic adhesions secondary to diffuse peritonitis at the time of the primary operation, as well as difficulties with identifying the rectal stump. In our experience, we prefer to implant the rectal stump above the fascia and just under skin, at the lower aspect of the incision, at the time of the primary operation. This practice makes finding the rectal stump significantly easier, and the potential for rectal scarring and small bowel adhesion formation around the stump itself is minimized.

Hand-assisted techniques have also been described with good results [11]. During laparoscopy, the operating surgeon may be surprised to find how few adhesions exist, especially when the time interval between the procedures is more than 6 months. Therefore, we feel it is worth introducing a laparoscope in all patients, to assess the feasibility of a laparoscopic approach. This conclusion was confirmed by a meta-analysis analyzing 8 studies with a total of 450 patients. In this study, 193 patients had laparoscopic surgery and 257 had open surgery. Laparoscopic reversal resulted in significant reductions in complication rates, intraoperative blood loss, and length of hospital stay, when compared to the conventional approach. No difference was found in leak rates [12].

## Pearls and Pitfalls

- Do not be afraid of converting early if the adhesions are too dense.
- The most difficult part of the case is often locating the staple line in the pelvis. Many times, it is stuck down to the sacrum posteriorly. Beware of the adjacent venous plexus when attempting to mobilize the stump.
- Placing an EEA sizer though the anus can aid in identifying the proximal end of the stump. Additionally, in women, a sizer in the vagina can help identify the posterior vaginal wall and plane between the rectum and vagina/vaginal cuff.
- Excessive force with the EEA stapler may traumatize the rectal stump. If stapling gun cannot be advanced easily further, mobilization and resection of the rectal stump be required.
- The hand-assisted approach allows for preliminary assessment of intra-abdominal adhesions and the condition of the pelvis in cases of concern for a hostile abdomen. It also offers an alternative for conversion to full laparotomy.

## Summary

Laparoscopic reversal results in decreased morbidity and mortality. The published studies so far have shown that laparoscopic reversal is associated with less intraoperative blood loss, shorter hospital stay, lower wound infection rates, less postoperative pain, and lower incidences of pelvic abscess, anastomotic leak, and incisional hernia, when compared to open reversal. Further advantages include faster patient convalescence, time to the first bowel movement, and return to oral feeding.

The laparoscopic reversal of stomas therefore seems to not only be safe but also to result in fewer complications than open surgery. However, randomized controlled trials are needed to strengthen the growing body of evidence, which seems to point in favor of this approach. In conclusion, the laparoscopic approach for stoma reversal and the restoration of intestinal continuity may be the procedure of choice for select patients requiring stoma closure with an anastomosis.

## References

1. Roe AM, Prabhu S, Ali A, Brown C, Brodribb AJ. Reversal of Hartmann's procedure: timing and operative technique. Br J Surg. 1991;78:1167–70.
2. Mosdell DM, Doberneck RC. Morbidity and mortality of ostomy closure. Am J Surg. 1992;162:633–7.
3. Rosen MJ, Cobb WS, Kercher KW, Heniford BT. Laparoscopic versus open colostomy reversal: a comparative analysis. J Gastrointest Surg. 2006;10(6):895–900.
4. Pearce NW, Scott SD, Karran SJ. Timing and method of reversal of Hartmann's procedure. Br J Surg. 1992;79:839–41.
5. Wigmore SJ, Duthie GS, Young IE, et al. Restoration of bowel continuity following Hartmann's procedure: the Lothian experience 1987–1992. Br J Surg. 1995;82:27–30.
6. Kunin N, Letoquart JP, La Gamma A, et al. Restoration of colonic continuity after Hartmann's operation. J Chir (Paris). 1992;129: 526–30.
7. Keck JO, Collopy BT, Ryan PJ, et al. Reversal of Hartmann's procedure: effect of timing and technique on ease and safety. Dis Colon Rectum. 1994;37:243–8.
8. David GG, Al-Sarira AA, Willmott S, et al. Use of Hartmann's procedure in England. Colorectal Dis. 2009;11:308–12.
9. Riansuwan W, Hull TL, Millan MM, et al. Nonreversal of Hartmann's procedure for diverticulitis: derivation of a scoring system to predict nonreversal. Dis Colon Rectum. 2009;52:1400–8.
10. Gorey TF, O'Connell PR, Waldron D, et al. Laparoscopically assisted colostomy closure after Hartmann's procedure. Br J Surg. 1993;80:109.
11. Lucarini L, Galleano R, Lombezzi R, et al. Laparoscopic-assisted Hartmann's reversal with the Dexterity Pneumo Sleeve. Dis Colon Rectum. 2000;43:1164–7.
12. Siddiqui M, Sajid M, Baig M. Open vs laparoscopic approach for reversal of Hartmann's procedure: a systematic review. Color Dis. 2010;12:733–41.

# Laparoscopic Parastomal Hernia Repair

# 17

Joshua A. Tyler and Matthew G. Mutch

**Key Points**

- Have a solid plan in place ahead of time to decide on local repair, relocation, use of mesh, as well as the ability to convert to open, if necessary.
- Safe entry into the abdomen is the initial key step with this approach.
- Expect to have to perform an extensive lysis of adhesions around the hernia sac.
- You must carefully reduce all of the hernia sac contents. Avoid the urge to simply start pulling bowel loops out of the sac, as this will often lead to inadvertent serosal tears or full-thickness bowel injury.
- Prior to repair or relocation, you should only be looking at the afferent limb of the stoma and the fascial defect (i.e., all of the other loops of bowel must be reduced).
- You will need both tacking and transfascial sutures for a successful repair.

## Background

Parastomal hernia occurs when abdominal contents herniate across the fascial defect through which an ostomy passes. The incidence of parastomal hernia (PH) ranges from 5 to 80 %, and the rate variance is due to differences in the classification of PH. Factors impacting the classification depend on whether the diagnosis is made clinically, radiographically, or at the time of surgical repair [1]. As of 2003, there were nearly half a million ostomates living in the United States, with 120,000 new stomas created annually [2]. Stoma presence alone has a significant impact on quality of life, and this impact may be exacerbated when a PH is present. Symptoms associated with PH include abdominal pain, inability or impaired ability to apply stoma devices, bulging, and intestinal obstruction or strangulation.

Risk factors for the development of PH include obesity, smoking, nutritional impairment, steroid use, emergent nature of case at stoma creation, infection, underlying inflammatory bowel disease or malignancy, and chronically elevated intra-abdominal pressure (COPD, BPH). Of these, obesity is likely the greatest risk factor (Fig. 17.1) [3]. Indications for surgical repair include pain, difficulty or inability to pouch the stoma, and obstructive symptoms such as acute incarceration or strangulation (Fig. 17.2). Surgical repair can be technically difficult and plagued with high recurrence rates. As a result, asymptomatic hernias are often carefully watched after appropriate patient counseling. Options for repair of the PH include local or primary repairs, mesh repairs, and re-siting the stoma. Primary or local repairs with or without the use of mesh have largely fallen out of favor due to unacceptably high recurrence rates on the order of 70 % [4]. Historically, open repairs with mesh had a 30 % recurrence rate and carried the risks of a major operation and mesh infection. However, with the widespread adoption of laparoscopic approaches to parastomal hernias, the risk of recurrence has decreased significantly. The more commonly used mesh repair techniques include the Sugarbaker and keyhole techniques using either synthetic or biologic mesh implants. The Sugarbaker technique has had the best results with recurrence rates ranging from 9 to 15 %. In this chapter, we will review the technical aspects and potential challenges associated with a laparoscopic repair of parastomal hernias.

**Electronic supplementary material:** Supplementary material is available in the online version of this chapter at 10.1007/978-1-4939-1581-1_17. Videos can also be accessed at http://www.springerimages.com/videos/978-1-4939-1580-4.

J.A. Tyler, M.D.
Chief, Colon and Rectal Surgery, Department of General Surgery, Keesler Medical Center, 301 Fisher St, Keesler AFB, MS 39534, USA
e-mail: Joshua.tyler.1@us.af.mil

M.G. Mutch, M.D., F.A.C.S., F.A.S.C.R.S. (✉)
Section of Colon and Rectal Surgery, Barnes-Jewish Hospital, Washington University School of Medicine in St. Louis, 660 South Euclid Ave., Campus box 8109, St. Louis, MO, USA
e-mail: mutchm@wustl.edu

H.M. Ross et al. (eds.), *Minimally Invasive Approaches to Colon and Rectal Disease: Technique and Best Practices*, DOI 10.1007/978-1-4939-1581-1_17, © Springer Science+Business Media New York 2015

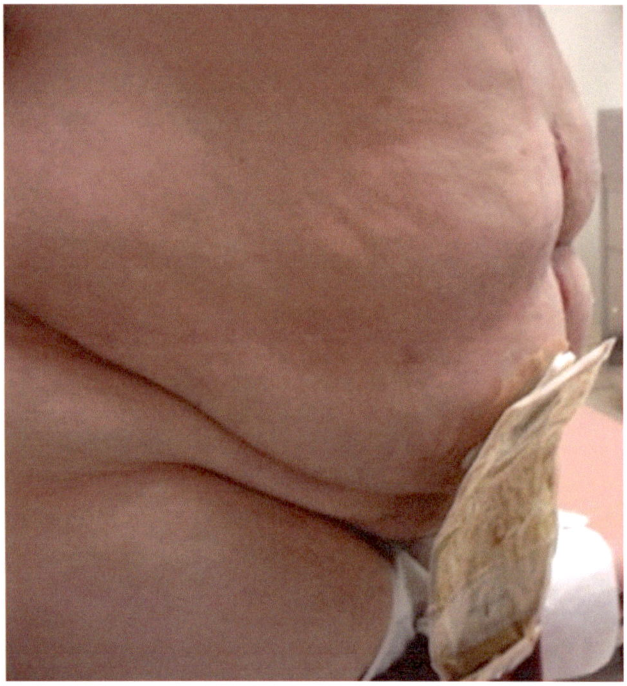

**Fig. 17.1** Stoma in a patient with morbid obesity. Notice the large bulge around the stoma indicating the possible presence of a parastomal hernia

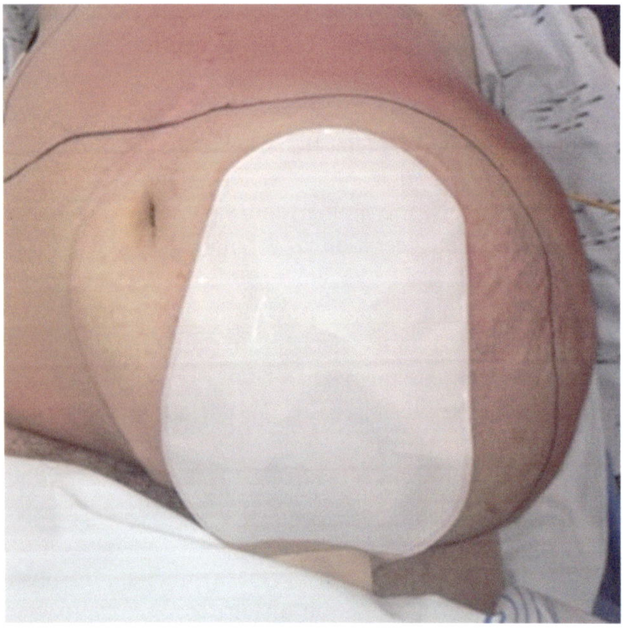

**Fig. 17.2** Strangulated parastomal hernia with associated cellulitis

## Preoperative Planning

As with most surgical procedures, patients offered PH repair should have an appropriate surgical indication and should be cleared as good operative candidates from a

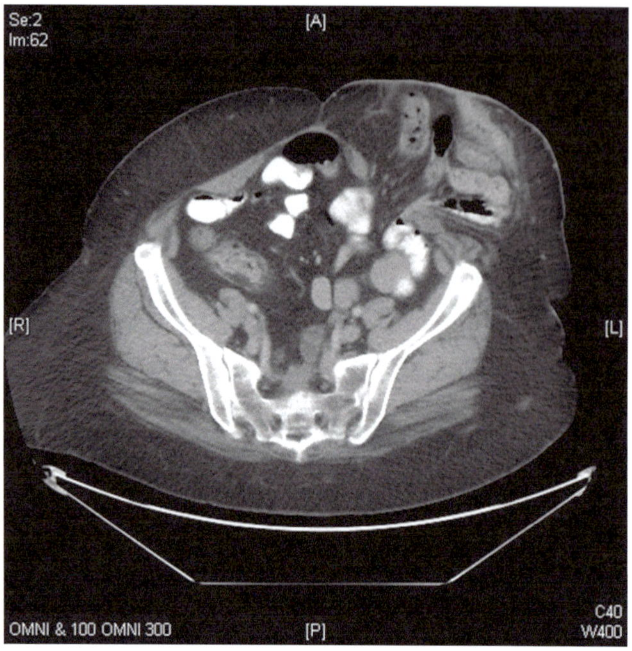


**Fig. 17.3** CT demonstrating a large fascial defect with a moderate-sized parastomal hernia

cardiopulmonary risk standpoint. Physical examination often reveals the presence of a hernia, and this may be better defined by asking the patient to Valsalva. It is important to note if the hernia is reducible. Cross-sectional imaging is often helpful in preoperative planning, especially in defining hernia anatomy, elucidating presence of hernia in patients whose exam is limited due to habitus, as well as accounting for the presence of other hernias in the vicinity of the PH that may impact the repair or size of mesh used (Fig. 17.3). In addition, patients should be up-to-date on their colonoscopic screening, as well as any cancer surveillance that might impact the operative plan. Controllable hernia risk factors should be emphasized when PH repair occurs in the elective setting to optimize success of the repair and decrease recurrence risk. These factors may include smoking cessation, weight loss, cessation of steroids (if possible), and control of medical factors that cause frequent Valsalva such as benign prostatic hyperplasia (BPH) and chronic cough or obstructive pulmonary disease. In preoperative holding, deep venous thrombosis chemoprophylaxis and broad-spectrum intravenous antibiotics to cover both skin and enteric flora within one hour of incision are given. A thorough discussion with the patient should occur regarding the operative plan and the risks of conversion to an open repair, need for relocation, or substitution of biologic for permanent mesh. A successful laparoscopic approach is dependent upon safe access to the peritoneal cavity, adhesiolysis, and reduction of the hernia contents. The presence of an associated incisional hernia also increases the risk of conversion or need for relocation.

## Procedure

### Setup

After induction and intubation, an orogastric tube and Foley catheter should be placed. The patient may be positioned at the discretion of the operating surgeon either in supine or in low lithotomy position. Generally, the arms should be tucked with pressure points padded, but this may not be necessary on all cases. The patient should be well secured to the operating room table to allow for intraoperative positioning changes such as Trendelenburg position that may be necessary during the procedure.

The operating surgeon stands on the contralateral side of the PH to allow maximal working room in the abdominal cavity. The assistant may stand either on the same or opposite side. Two monitors should be utilized—one directly across from the operating surgeon to allow for in-line tissue manipulation and visualization and a second for the assistant to view. The approach to PH repair is quite variable as stomas may be right or left sided and have associated incisional hernias. Principles described here are general guidelines, but the operating surgeon must be comfortable with some variation in monitor and port placement to allow for variation based on patient anatomy. All equipment for both a laparoscopic and open procedure should be in the room in the event that the procedure must be converted. The abdomen should be shaved and prepped and draped in the usual standard fashion. The stoma appliance should be removed and the stoma prepped into the field and then covered with gauze and an occlusive dressing to control effluent during the case (Fig. 17.4 a, b). This will help minimize the exposure of enteric contents and contamination to the mesh while it is being introduced into the abdomen.

## Procedure Steps

### Insufflation and Port Placement

After the patient has been prepped and draped, and the laparoscopic equipment has been passed onto the field and situated, a time-out is completed, and intraperitoneal access is established. This is accomplished based on surgeon preference, typically with a 12 mm camera port placed first either with an open Hasson technique or after insufflation with a Veress needle usually placed in an abdominal quadrant deemed to have the fewest adhesions and is far enough away from the hernia to provide good visualization for dissection and mesh placement (Fig. 17.5). The abdomen should be insufflated to a pressure of 15 mmHg. The working ports are typically 5 mm in size, and generally 2–3 ports are required. Ports should be triangulated to the location of the hernia. A third port for the assistant is not always necessary, but can facilitate tissue retraction for the operating surgeon. This also helps if an extensive adhesiolysis is necessary prior to hernia reduction, and often some adhesions must be taken down to facilitate port placement. It must be kept in mind that the dissection of the hernia and its contents requires exposure of all 360° around the stoma and hernia.

### Adhesiolysis and Hernia Reduction

Once adequate space has been cleared to facilitate port placement, attention is directed at completing an intra-abdominal survey for unexpected pathology, extent of adhesions, and the hernia and its contents. The hernia should be identified (Fig. 17.6) and reduced, taking care to protect the stoma. If adjacent small bowel or omentum is within the hernia, this can often be reduced with firm traction. However, first ensure that any adhesions to the stoma or the hernia sac are lysed, which may be accomplished sharply with laparoscopic

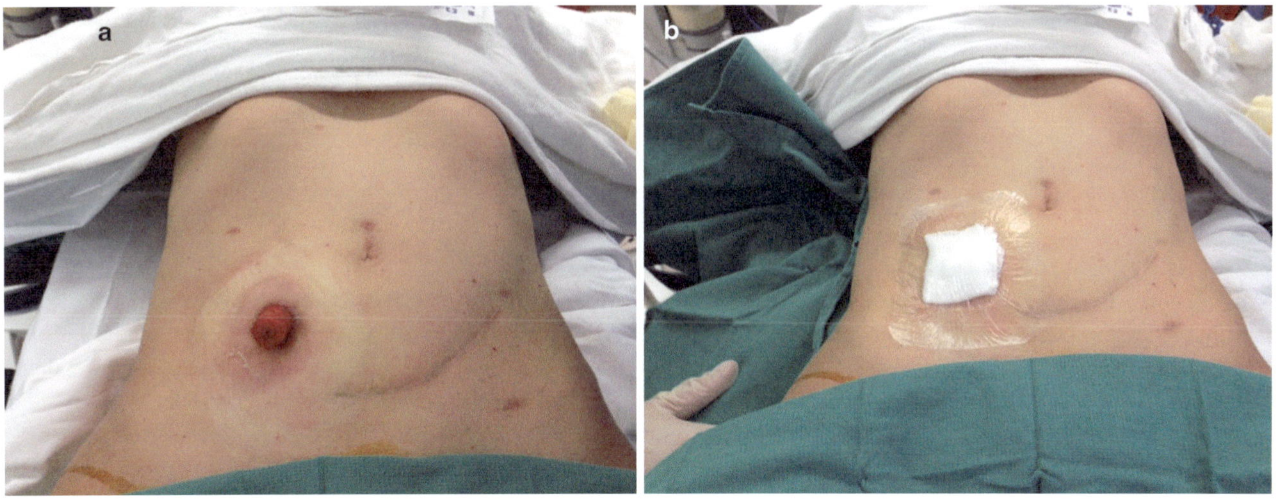

**Fig. 17.4** Prepping and draping of the stoma. (**a**) The appliance is removed and the area around the stoma is cleaned. (**b**) The site is covered with a gauze and occlusive dressing. *Courtesy of Joshua Bleier, MD, with permission*

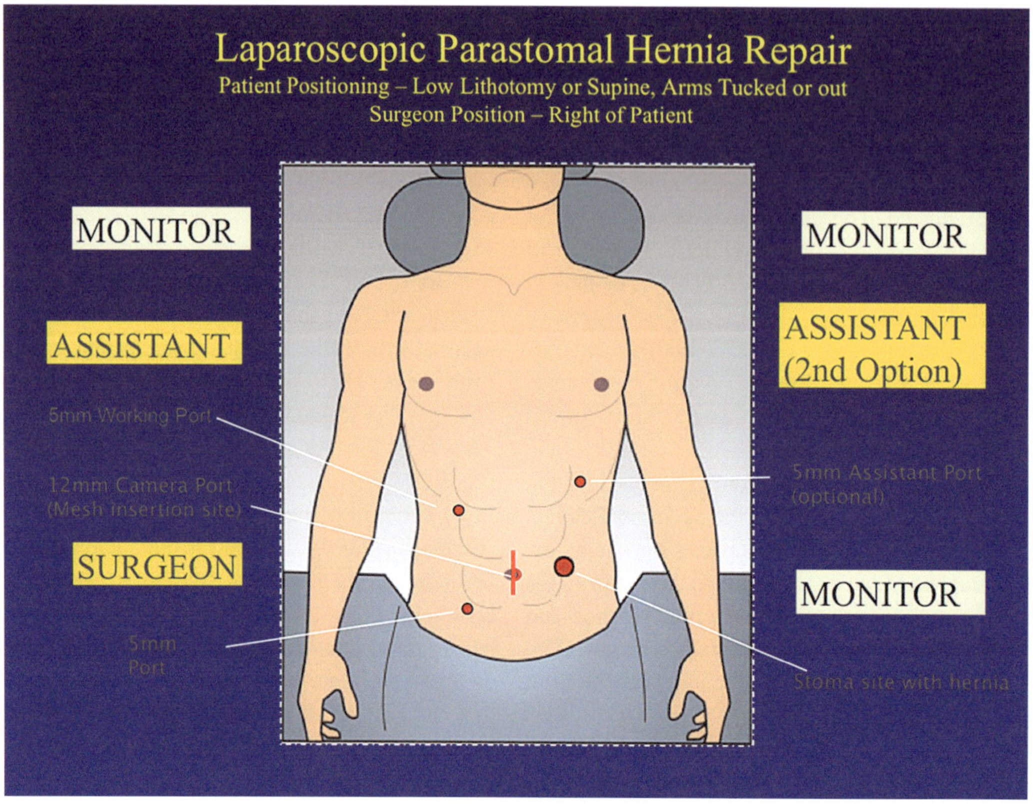


**Fig. 17.5** Port placement and patient positioning for laparoscopic parastomal hernia repair

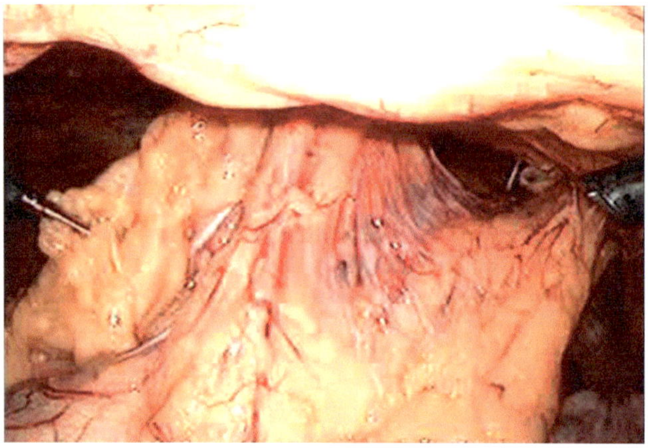

**Fig. 17.6** Initial appearance of hernia following port placement

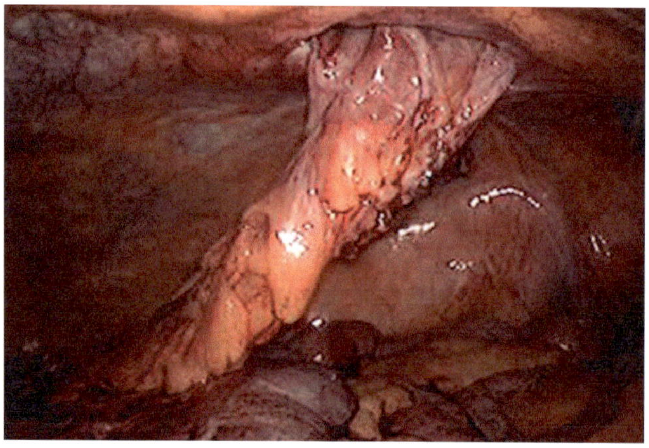

**Fig. 17.7** Hernia appearance after reduction of hernia contents and adhesiolysis

scissors with or without monopolar cautery or an alternative energy device can be used. Care should be taken to identify the bowel proximal to the stoma as well as to avoid any enterotomies. Omentum and small bowel may often be adherent to the stoma limb and adhesions in this area may be dense, so sharp dissection without energy is preferred in this scenario. The hernia contents should be reduced completely, and the limb to the stoma should be mobilized as completely as possible. Once this is complete, all that should remain is the afferent limb to the stoma and the fascial defect (Fig. 17.7).

## Mesh Measurement and Preparation

At this point, the size of the hernia defect should be measured. This may be accomplished intracorporeally using a measuring device or with an open grasper as an estimate of size (an open grasper is typically 3–4 cm). Alternatively, a spinal needle can be passed transabdominally at the medial, lateral, cephalad, and caudad aspects of the defect and size measured in this fashion (Fig. 17.8). Once the defect has been measured, a piece of mesh should be selected to allow for 4–5 cm of overlap in all directions of the defect. If additional

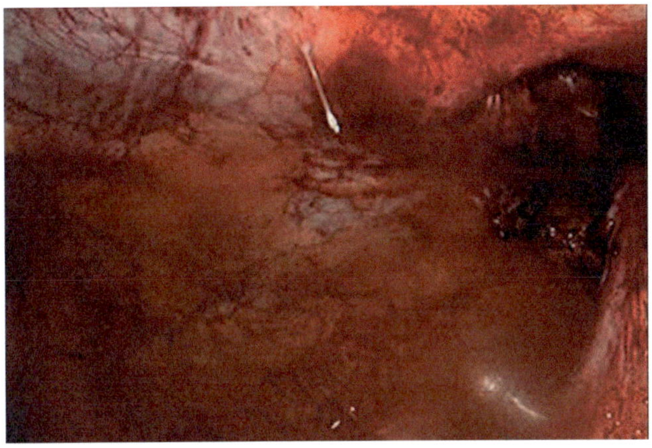

**Fig. 17.8** Measurement of hernia defect with needle to determine mesh size

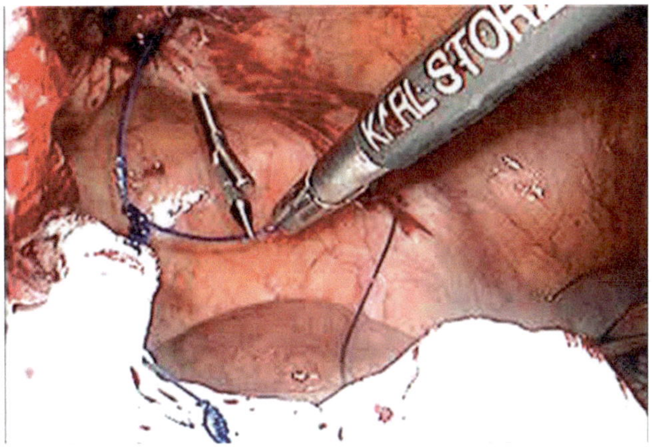

**Fig. 17.9** Placement of first transfascial suture (lateral side, caudad to stoma)

defects are present, the mesh must be enlarged to accommodate coverage of all defects. Any mesh shape may be used (round, oval, square, or rectangular), but it is crucial to ensure that the overlap is adequate. As long as no enterotomies have been made, synthetic mesh may be used. If synthetic mesh is used, it should have an anti-adhesion barrier on the dorsal side of the mesh that will be exposed to the abdominal contents. If an enterotomy is made, the risk of mesh infection is increased, and synthetic mesh should be avoided. In this case, a biologic mesh is an acceptable alternative.

Once the mesh has been selected, it should be prepared according to the manufacturer's package insert if it needs to be manipulated prior to use (i.e., saline hydration). Once ready for use, the mesh should be laid flat extracorporeally, and the transfascial sutures should be placed. For the Sugarbaker technique, transfascial sutures should be placed at the cephalad and caudad aspects of the lateral side of the mesh far enough apart to allow the stoma to exit the from the mesh, and then circumferentially from there approximately every 5 cm. Generally a nonabsorbable monofilament suture (1 Prolene) is used, and these should be tied in the mid-point of the suture to allow for long tails of equivalent length on each side. For a Sugarbaker repair typically six to eight transabdominal fixation sutures are used. On the lateral aspect of the mesh, the gap should be left large enough to allow the stoma limb to pass between the mesh and anterior abdominal wall without causing obstruction. Once all transfascial sutures have been placed, the sutures are laid in the middle of the mesh and the mesh is rolled like a cigar and inserted through the 12 mm camera port. It is often helpful to label the fixation sutures and mark the anterior surface of the mesh to help facilitate intraperitoneal orientation.

## Mesh Securement

### Sugarbaker Technique (Videos 17.1 and 17.2)

Once inserted, the mesh should be unrolled and oriented in its planned position. At this point, it is helpful to desufflate the abdomen to a pressure of around 10 mmHg to take tension off the abdominal wall and allow the mesh to lay as it will when the abdomen is completely desufflated. If the mesh is secured at full insufflation pressure, it will become undulated upon desufflation, often leading to mesh laxity and the appearance of a hernia recurrence over time. The lateral sutures are fixated first. Starting with the caudad-most suture to the stoma (Fig. 17.9), a suture-passing device (i.e., Carter-Thompson needle) is placed transabdominally through a small stab incision. One of the tails is passed intracorporeally into the suture device and it is extracted and secured with a clamp. This is repeated for the second tail of the suture, with care taken to pass the suture-passing device through the same skin stab wound but a separate fascial puncture site. This second tail is delivered and secured with a clamp but not tied. Attention should then be directed to the cephalad-most suture to the stoma on the lateral side of the mesh (Fig. 17.10), which should be secured next. By securing the cephalad and caudad sutures, this allows for proper mesh orientation, making the remainder of the sutures more

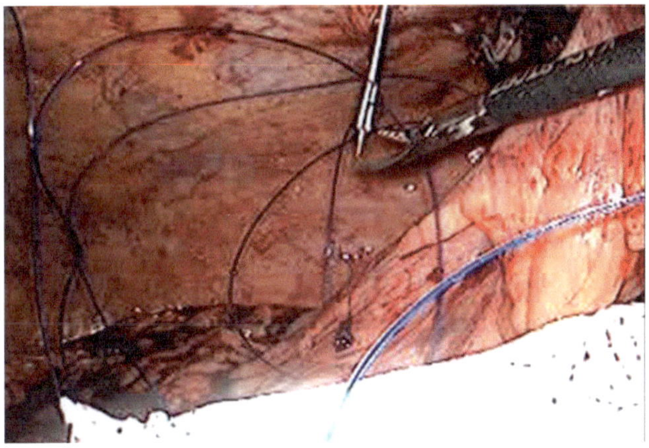

**Fig. 17.10** Placement of second transfascial suture (lateral side, cephalad to stoma)

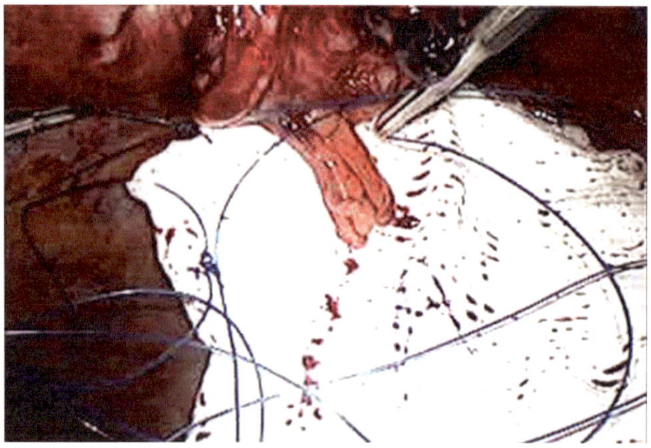

**Fig. 17.11** Mesh appearance while maintaining traction on the two transfascial sutures closest to stoma

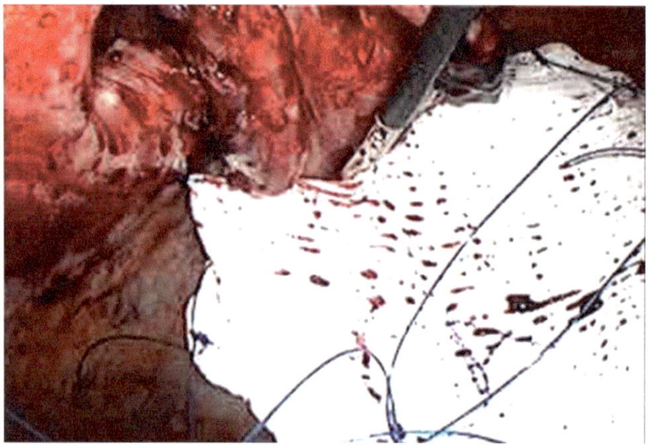

**Fig. 17.12** Checking suture placement with a grasper to ensure adequate space for stoma to pass lateral to mesh

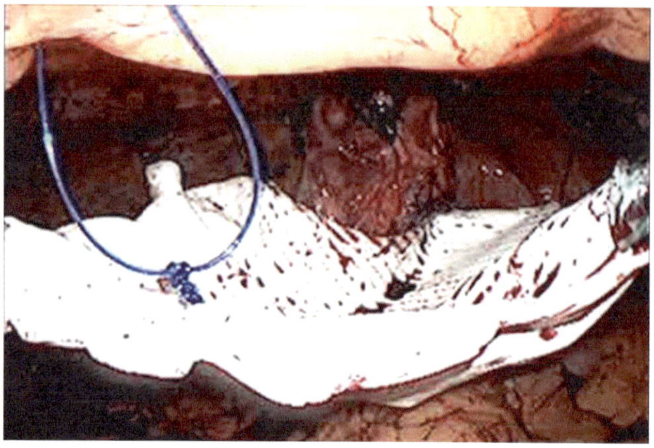

**Fig. 17.13** Securing remaining transfascial sutures

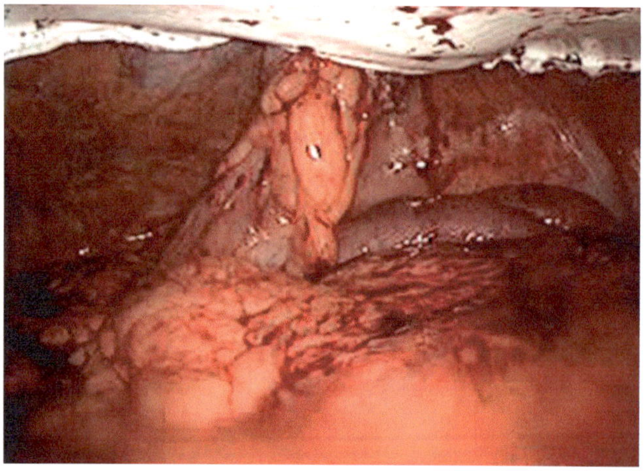

**Fig. 17.14** Final appearance of mesh with all sutures tied

easily positioned, and sets the gap where the stoma exits the mesh. It is of utmost importance that the transfascial sutures closest to the afferent limb of the stoma not be too close or tied so tight that it causes an obstruction of the stoma at the level of the mesh. If need be these sutures can be adjusted to give stoma adequate space between the mesh and abdominal wall (Fig. 17.11). This may be checked by ensuring a grasper can fit between the mesh and the stoma while maintaining tension on the transfascial sutures (Fig. 17.12). Once the cephalad and caudad sutures are placed, the remainder of sutures are secured starting farthest from the camera position and working circumferentially around the mesh leaving the sutures closest to the camera position for the end (Fig. 17.13). The mesh should be oriented so that the stoma deviates around the lateral side of the mesh and then back medially towards the stoma fascial defect in a Sugarbaker fashion. At any point if an undesirable suture position has been created, the sutures can be delivered back into the abdomen, and a separate position chosen by repeating the same procedure. It is important to note that none of the sutures are tied until all have been passed transabdominally. This allows for ensuring adequate coverage and tension on the mesh and avoidance of buckling or areas of poor coverage. Once all sutures are delivered, traction can be placed on each suture simultaneously to check for optimal mesh positioning as well as to ensure that neither the sutures nor mesh will cause a bowel obstruction. If the mesh is acceptably positioned, each suture can be tied at this point (Fig. 17.14). Once each suture has been tied, the remainder of the circumference of the mesh can be secured approximately every centimeter with a laparoscopic tacking device with care taken to avoid the afferent limb of the stoma. Either metal or absorbable tacks may be used based on surgeon preference. Some surgeons also prefer to tack in the middle portion of the mesh as long as care is taken to avoid both the stoma and the hernia defect.

### Keyhole Technique

For the keyhole technique, a slit is created in the middle of the cephalad border of the mesh. Again, a sublay position is utilized with a mesh that consists of an anti-adhesive barrier on the intra-abdominal side. The slit is carried to the middle of the mesh where a cruciate incision is made to allow for a large enough opening for the stoma. The transabdominal fixation sutures are placed circumferentially around the mesh as previously described. Once the mesh is passed intracorporeally, it is positioned so the slit is passed around the stoma. The fixation sutures are passed transabdominally in the same fashion as the Sugarbaker technique, and the gaps between the sutures are closed with an endoscopic fascial tacking device. The slit in the mesh is then closed by intracorporeal suturing using a heavy, monofilament, permanent suture. The first stitch is placed to create an appropriate opening for the stoma to pass through the mesh. Given that this stitch sits in the hernia defect, it cannot be fixated to the fascia. Additional sutures are then placed to close the slit in the mesh in the same fashion.

## Repairing the Hernia with Stomal Relocation

A laparoscopic approach may also be utilized even if the stoma is relocated. If this is planned, one method to do this is to initially lyse the adhesions and reduce the contents of the hernia sac laparoscopically as previously discussed. An endoscopic stapler may then be used to divide the bowel at the level of the fascia (i.e., leaving the matured portion that runs through the abdominal wall intact). The bowel is then mobilized to ensure adequate length is available for the stoma to reach its new location. The skin is opened at the new site and (after opening the subcutaneous tissue and bluntly dividing the rectus muscles as described in the chapter by Dr. Fleshner in Chap. 15) the bowel passed through the abdominal wall for maturation at the completion of the case. The abdomen is then desufflated, the remaining portion of the "old" stoma is resected from abdominal wall, and an "open" incisional hernia repair with mesh is performed per the operating surgeon's preference. We then re-insufflate, evaluate the repair, ensure adequate hemostasis and mesh coverage of the hernia defect, and inspect the abdomen for proper orientation of the new stoma and any other abnormalities. After the trocars are removed, the new stoma site can be matured in standard fashion.

## Postoperative Care

Patients progress along our institution's standard postoperative care pathway, including early ambulation and full liquids the night of surgery. Nasogastric tubes are not routinely used, and the Foley catheter is removed postoperative day 1. Diet is advanced to regular diet on postoperative day 1 provided that the patient has tolerated liquids without issue. Depending on the amount of adhesiolysis, these patients may be more prone to ileus, and their diet should be advanced accordingly. Early and frequent ambulation is important, and we also utilize standard chemoprophylaxis for deep venous thrombosis.

Pain control is a major factor in the postoperative setting and usually contributes to the ultimate length of stay requirements. Given that these patients may be prone to ileus, pain adjuncts to minimize narcotics including ketorolac and acetaminophen should be employed. In addition, regional pain control may be considered in the form of an epidural, liposomal bupivacaine, or regional pain catheters if desired. We routinely utilize a narcotic patient-controlled anesthetic device and transition to oral narcotics once the patient tolerates oral intake.

## Complications

Intraoperative complications are relatively infrequent (<5 %) and may occur in the form of enterotomy or bleeding. Enterotomy may occur if an extensive adhesiolysis is required and can usually be repaired primarily if present. Depending on surgeon comfort, this can usually be done laparoscopically, but if conversion to open is required, this should be performed. Consideration should also be given to utilization of biologic mesh rather than synthetic in this situation. Bleeding is usually rare but may occur during adhesiolysis or due to injury of the epigastric vessels during port or transfascial suture placement. Injury to the epigastric vessels may occur with trocar placement or with the transfascial suture device. It is normally successfully managed laparoscopically by performing suture ligation with the suture-passing device.

Postoperative complications may be grouped into early and late categories. Early complications include ileus, surgical site infection, respiratory and urinary tract infections, and hemorrhage. If with postoperative hemorrhage, the patient should be taken back to the OR for identification and control of the bleeding source if determined to be necessary. Ileus may be managed with limitation of narcotics through the use of pain adjuncts, and if emesis occurs, nasogastric decompression may become necessary. Ileus will resolve with time and narcotic limitation but should raise the question as to if the mesh or sutures may be causing iatrogenic bowel obstruction. This situation may be further delineated with cross-sectional imaging to look for a mesh-level obstruction with decompressed distal bowel between the mesh and the stoma site or a contrast study through the stoma. Deep surgical site infection is rare with this procedure provided that no enterotomies are made. Superficial surgical site infection may be treated with opening and packing of surgical wounds, with or without antibiotics. If the stoma is relocated as part of the procedure, the wound from the old stoma site may simply be packed daily with dry gauze

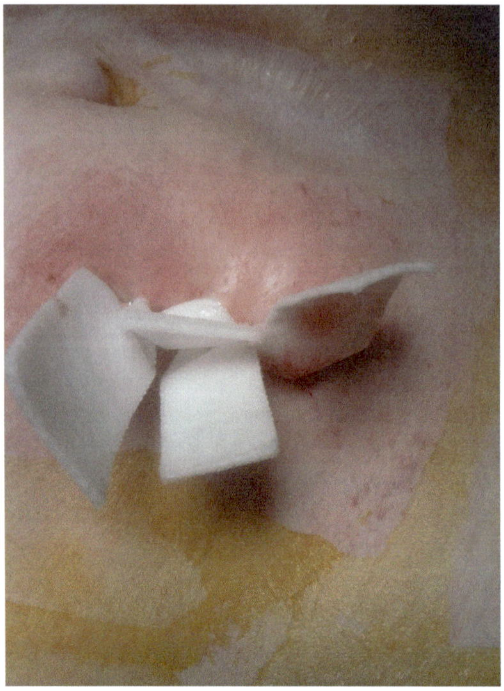

**Fig. 17.15** Stoma site after relocation closed with staples and wicks between staples

to heal by secondary intention. Another option is to approximate the skin loosely with 2–3 skin staples, with Telfa wicks placed in between (Fig. 17.15). These wicks are removed prior to hospital discharge (usually by postoperative day 3). Urinary tract infection may be avoided with careful Foley placement sterile technique, as well as early removal. Respiratory tract infection may be mitigated with early ambulation and incentive spirometer use, as well as effective pain control to avoid limited or shallow breathing due to pain.

The most common late complication is hernia recurrence. There is a wide range reported in the literature (6–46 %) depending on the type of repair, mesh used, comorbidities of the patient (i.e., obesity, COPD), and experience of the surgeon. Additionally, a number of factors can limit this, starting with patient selection. While parastomal hernias may be common in ostomates, surgeons must carefully weigh risk and benefit of repair coupled with the patient characteristics. Modifiable factors should be controlled to the extent possible, such as encouraging patient weight loss and smoking cessation. Utilization of mesh rather than primary repair will also limit hernia recurrence. Most surgeons will limit patient activity and lifting for 6–8 weeks after surgery, and some surgeons routinely employ abdominal binders in the postoperative setting, although data on benefit of binders has been lacking. Meticulous technique in mesh placement is critical to recurrence prevention, ensuring adequate overlap on all sides of the defect. Mesh infection is relatively rare but can be a devastating complication, as it requires the mesh to be excised.

## Outcomes

Multiple techniques have been described for parastomal hernia repair. These repairs have traditionally been done open, but with the advent and ever-increasing utilization of laparoscopic surgery, laparoscopic parastomal hernia repair has been shown to be safe and technically feasible, with the added benefits of laparoscopic over open surgery. The benefits of laparoscopic surgery have been shown to translate to PH repair, to include shorter operative time and length of stay, as well as to lower overall morbidity and surgical site infection [5].

Repair options include open primary repair, stoma re-siting, and laparoscopic keyhole and Sugarbaker techniques. Although little prospective randomized data exist, several meta-analyses and cohort studies have shown that mesh repair is superior to primary repair, with primary repair nearly nine times more likely to recur [4]. Data comparing keyhole versus Sugarbaker techniques are variable, with some studies showing no difference in recurrence rates between the two [1], although most studies show lower recurrence rates with the Sugarbaker technique (Sugarbaker 0–29 % recurrence rate vs keyhole 58–72 %) [3–8]. Over 40 % of patients undergoing PH repair also have incisional ventral hernias, which have been shown to be simultaneously successfully repaired [9]. Data on the use of biologic mesh in PH repair show similar recurrence rates to synthetic mesh; however, data are limited by their small retrospective nature and short length of follow-up [10]. No study has demonstrated a superior type of biologic over another (cross-linked vs non-cross-linked, bovine vs human scaffolding).

Given the incidence of parastomal hernia and difficulty in their repair, many surgeons have looked to a means of prevention. There are some data from a meta-analysis of several randomized trials to suggest biologic mesh reinforcement at the time of permanent ostomy creation may decrease recurrence rates [11]. Other prospective randomized trials have not shown benefit to this technique. While encouraging, this technique has not been widely adopted and should be studied in larger randomized prospective trials.

## Pearls and Pitfalls

Several key points may optimize PH repair. Preoperative identification of other ventral hernias is critical in operative planning and mesh selection. This will allow for successful repair of the PH, as well as any concomitant incisional hernias. Additionally, it cannot be overstated that utmost care must be taken to ensure that the lateral aspect of the mesh provides adequate overlap of the defect, yet not be so tight so as to occlude the afferent limb of the stoma. Mesh selection and appropriate suture placement on the mesh are imperative.

This should always be assessed prior to final tying of the transfascial sutures. Finally, ensuring the mesh remains sterile and is not contaminated is of paramount importance to the success of the repair.

## Conclusion

Parastomal hernia is a common problem in ostomates and is challenging to repair. Laparoscopic repair of PH is safe and effective, with numerous benefits compared to open repair to include shorter length of stay and decreased overall morbidity and surgical site infection. Surgical technique is a critical component of successful PH repair, and the Sugarbaker technique may provide the lowest recurrence rate compared to other techniques.

## References


1. Helgstrand F, Rosenberg J, Kehlet H, Jorgensen LN, Wara P, Bisgaard T. Risk of morbidity, mortality, and recurrence after parastomal hernia repair: a nationwide study. Dis Colon Rectum. 2013;56(11):1265–72.
2. Turnbull GB. Ostomy statistics: the $64,000 question. Ostomy Wound Manage. 2003;49(6):22–3.
3. Asif A, Ruiz M, Yetasook A, Denham W, Linn J, Carbray J, Ujiki MB. Laparoscopic modified Sugarbaker technique results in superior recurrence rate. Surg Endosc. 2012;26(12):3430–4.
4. Hansson BM, Slater NJ, van der Velden AS, Groenewoud HM, Buyne OR, de Hingh IH, Bleichrodt RP. Surgical techniques for parastomal hernia repair: a systematic review of the literature. Ann Surg. 2012;255(4):685–95.
5. Halabi WJ, Jafari MD, Carmichael JC, Nguyen VQ, Mills S, Phelan M, Stamos MJ, Pigazzi A. Laparoscopic versus open repair of parastomal hernias: an ACS-NSQIP analysis of short-term outcomes. Surg Endosc. 2013;27(11):4067–72.
6. Pastor DM, Pauli EM, Koltun WA, Haluck RS, Shope TR, Poritz LS. Parastomal hernia repair: a single center experience. JSLS. 2009;13(2):170–5.
7. Craft RO, Huguet KL, McLemore EC, Harold KL. Laparoscopic parastomal hernia repair. Hernia. 2008;12(2):137–40.
8. Muysoms EE, Hauters PJ, Van Nieuwenhove Y, Huten N, Claeys DA. Laparoscopic repair of parastomal hernias: a multi-centre retrospective review and shift in technique. Acta Chir Belg. 2008;108(4):400–4.
9. Hansson BM, Morales-Conde S, Mussack T, Valdes J, Muysoms FE, Bleichrodt RP. The laparoscopic modified Sugarbaker technique is safe and has a low recurrence rate: a multicenter cohort study. Surg Endosc. 2013;27(2):494–500.
10. Slater NJ, Hansson BM, Buyne OR, Hendriks T, Bleichrodt RP. Repair of parastomal hernias with biologic grafts: a systematic review. J Gastrointest Surg. 2011;15(7):1252–8.
11. Wijeyekoon SP, Gurusamy K, El-Gendy K, Chan CL. Prevention of parastomal herniation with biologic/composite prosthetic mesh: a systematic review and meta-analysis of randomized controlled trials. J Am Coll Surg. 2010;211(5):637–45.

# Part III

# Technical Challenges and Tips

# Overcoming Technical Challenges: The Abdomen

# 18

Eric K. Johnson

**Key Points**

- Gravity is an ally in laparoscopy. Exploit it to your advantage.
- Don't be afraid to add a port. Assistance with traction/countertraction is invaluable in laparoscopy.
- Use of hand assistance may avoid conversion to an open procedure.
- Splenic flexure mobilization can be challenging. Be familiar with several techniques and be prepared to combine them.
- Transverse colon mobilization and division of the middle colic vessels can be the most challenging part of laparoscopic colectomy.
- High ligation of the main blood supply to the colon facilitates mobilization, requires less division of the mesentery, and is sound from an oncologic standpoint. Take care to preserve the marginal artery to ensure adequate blood supply to the distal colon/anastomosis.

## Introduction

The utilization of laparoscopy in colorectal surgery has increased exponentially since the publication of the COST trial in 2004 [1]. While laparoscopy was beginning to become mainstream in general surgery in the early 1990s, the technique didn't immediately catch on with colonic procedures. There are several reasons for this, not the least of which was the technical difficulty associated with performing a colonic resection using laparoscopic instruments.

**Electronic supplementary material:** Supplementary material is available in the online version of this chapter at 10.1007/978-1-4939-1581-1_18. Videos can also be accessed at http://www.springerimages.com/videos/978-1-4939-1580-4.

E.K. Johnson, M.D., F.A.C.S., F.A.S.C.R.S. (✉)
Associate Professor of Surgery, Uniformed Services University of the Health Sciences and Madigan Army Medical Center, Joint Base Lewis, McChord, WA 98431, USA
e-mail: doktrj@gmail.com

Patients come in all shapes and sizes, and the presence of obesity, large amounts of intra-abdominal adipose tissue, and difficult anatomy can make a laparoscopic approach quite challenging. These factors, coupled with a lack of technique familiarity, a lack of data, and some poor initial outcomes, slowed the adoption of laparoscopy in this setting. While techniques and instrumentations have improved over time, laparoscopic colectomy continues to present several challenges and pitfalls. The learning curve of the surgeon also plays a big part in the successful utilization of the laparoscopic approach. This is a twofold phenomenon, as the initial phase is ascending the learning curve and the second phase is the more comfortable the surgeon feels, the more willing they become to take on more difficult cases. It is the aim of this chapter to assist the reader in these specific areas.

## Positioning and Restraining the Patient

Performing effective laparoscopic surgery depends heavily on the use and exploitation of gravity. Because nature has only equipped us with two hands and we are handling organs of significant mass with 5- and 10-mm instruments, we must allow gravity to assist us with retraction during the procedure. Clever use of gravity may allow a surgeon to operate with fewer ports, or it may ensure that we are not forced to convert a case to a laparotomy. The surgeon must use Trendelenburg and reverse Trendelenburg positions with both right and left tilt. Often, many or all of these positions are used in a single case to ensure adequate exposure. The low lithotomy position not only provides access to the perineum and anus, but it also allows the surgeon or assistant to stand between the patients legs to operate, which may ease flexure mobilization and aid in ergonomics by keeping the surgeon and assistant in line with the direction of dissection and camera point of view.

It is not infrequent for very steep positioning to be required. Placement of a beanbag on the operating table

H.M. Ross et al. (eds.), *Minimally Invasive Approaches to Colon and Rectal Disease: Technique and Best Practices*, DOI 10.1007/978-1-4939-1581-1_18, © Springer Science+Business Media New York 2015

prior to positioning the patient assists in securing the patient so that steep positioning may be used. This is very important, especially when using the low lithotomy position, as the patient may slide up or down the table when steep positions are utilized. This can easily lead to nerve compression against a stirrup and its attendant morbidity. Many surgeons utilize two- or three-inch silk tape and wrap it around the patient's chest three times to secure them to the operating table. This is helpful, but care must be taken when wrapping the chest to ensure that the wrap is not too tight. There is at least one proprietary device designed to prevent patient slippage during steep positioning. Tucking the arms at the patient's side allows both the surgeon and assistant to stand on one side of the patient, typically away from the site of pathology for unilateral disease. Often, however, the surgeon and assistant may need to switch to the other side of the table. It is important not to be fixed in one location, as simply moving locations may significantly improve dissection. Increasing the hip angle or extending the hip so that the thigh is parallel to the floor will assist in ensuring that instrument motion is not limited by the patient's knee. "Setting the table" well will place the surgeon in the best position to get the most out of their instruments during the procedure.

## Traction/Countertraction

One of the biggest challenges of laparoscopy is taking a 2-dimensional image and converting it to a 3-dimensional working space. This is most evident when providing exposures. It is important to ensure the use of adequate traction and countertraction during any laparoscopic procedure. This is particularly important during the steps of transverse colon and splenic flexure mobilization. When exposure and visualization are poor, it is likely related to a lack of adequate traction. Take action to improve the traction on the structure of interest. Often all that is required is a change in the vector of retraction, which can be in any of the three dimensions (up, down, right, left, toward the camera, or away from the camera). If changing the direction of traction/tension does not improve exposure, do not hesitate to insert an additional 5-mm port. It adds little additional morbidity and can make all the difference in easing the difficulty of the procedure. Surgeons in training are often reluctant to use adequate traction on the abdominal viscera. Concern for possible injury to a hollow viscous is sound, but one is often able to use more traction than they consider safe. When grasping bowel, take a large bit as the pressure of the jaw is distributed over a larger area and the risk of tearing the serosa or bowel is much less than with a small bit. This is a skill that is developed over time.

## Hand-Assisted Laparoscopy

The use of hand-assisted laparoscopic surgery (HALS) was greeted with the same resistance seen by pure laparoscopy in its early days. As devices were developed and improved by industry, HALS began to see common adoption. Despite resistance from some purists, studies confirmed that outcomes for HALS colectomy were no different than those performed purely laparoscopically [2]. The hand is essentially the best atraumatic retractor that we have in laparoscopy, and it can be the difference between performing a case laparoscopically or openly.

Because the hand is large in relation to laparoscopic instruments and occupies quite a bit of working space, the surgeon must learn to position the hand such that it becomes a low-profile structure. This typically involves flexing, extending, or rotating the wrist at angles that can be somewhat uncomfortable (Figs. 18.1, 18.2 and 18.3). Not only is the hand a great retractor, it is also useful for finger dissection (Video 18.1), thinning out soft tissue structures, and palpating structures that are not easily seen on camera. The hand can be a tremendously useful tool with some of the challenging tasks that will be discussed.

## The Difficult Splenic Flexure

There are several factors that make splenic flexure mobilization a challenging task. The following are common variants that increase the technical difficulty associated with flexure takedown: a very high flexure, a flexure intimately attached

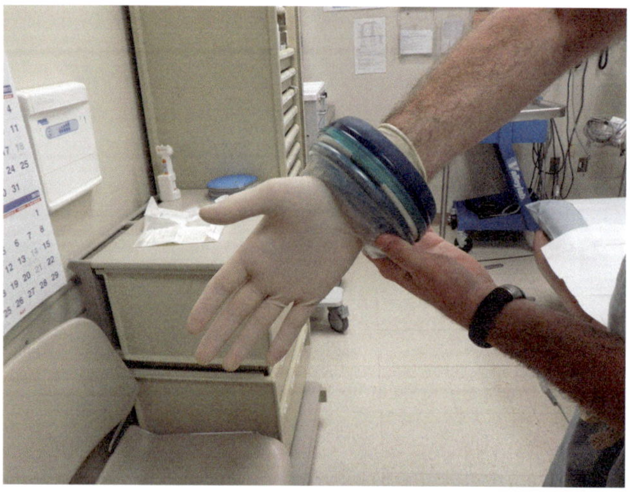

**Fig. 18.1** This image shows the hand after placement through the HALS port in a natural anatomic configuration. This position will rarely be used

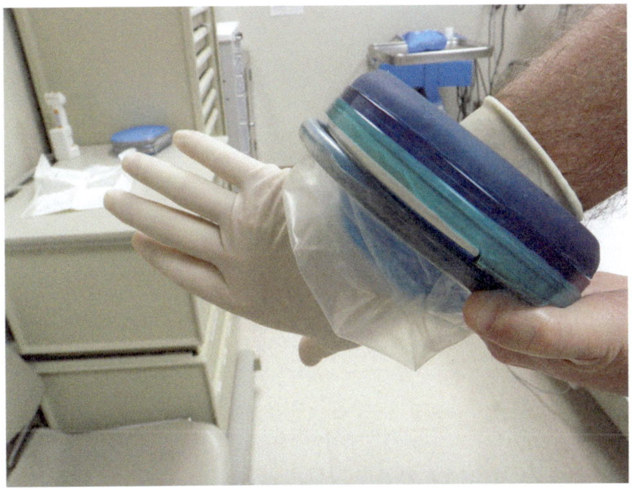

**Fig. 18.2** The wrist has been flexed or extended to place the hand in a useful position that will facilitate a better camera view

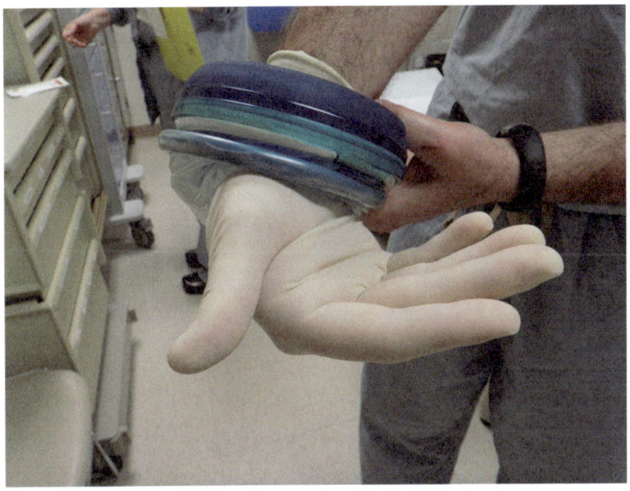

**Fig. 18.3** The wrist has been flexed or extended to place the hand in a useful position that will facilitate a better camera view

to the spleen via a short and vascular lienocolic ligament, association with a very fatty and heavy omentum, association with extensive congenital omental attachments to the left colon, and complex fusion between the omentum and the transverse mesocolon. For all of these reasons, it is helpful to get as good of an understanding of the anatomy or course of the splenic flexure before beginning a dissection.

There are a few approaches available to the surgeon, and often the use of a combination of approaches may be the easiest method to achieve a safe flexure mobilization. Often taking a "splenic flexure first" approach can be helpful. Especially if you know the flexure will definitely have to be taken down. Since this is often a more challenging portion of the case, saving it for the end can lead to the temptation to cut corners and perhaps omit this step in cases where the need for flexure takedown is questionable. Starting flexure takedown prior to violation of other planes may be helpful. For those that prefer a medial-to-lateral approach to the left colon, this approach can simply be extended up to the splenic flexure. The patient is initially positioned in Trendelenburg and tilted toward their right side. The mesocolon is grasped and elevated toward the anterior abdominal wall, and dissection continues in a lateral and cephalad direction. This will bring the surgeon underneath the inferior mesenteric vein (IMV), which affords one the opportunity to perform a high ligation of this vessel (Fig. 18.4). This serves to assist in gaining length on the left colon for anastomosis, it aids in ensuring an adequate lymphadenectomy, and it brings the surgeon underneath the splenic flexure itself.

Another option, if the medial approach is not continued, is to turn your attention to the lateral and cephalad attachments of the flexure. At this point, positioning is changed to reverse Trendelenburg, while tilt toward the patient's right side is maintained. Because a significant amount of medial mobilization has been performed, a "darker" color (Fig. 18.5) can be seen through the lateral and cephalad attachments. These attachments can easily be divided in the proper plane and direction using the medial dissection as a guide. Because of potential vascularity in the lienocolic ligament and surrounding tissues, it is often helpful to use an advanced bipolar or ultrasonic energy device in dividing these tissues (Video 18.2).

A third alternative is to start at the mid-transverse colon and separate the omentum from the transverse colon to enter the lesser sac. Once the lesser sac is accessed, the dissection continues out toward the splenic flexure to separate the omentum from the transverse colon and divide any adhesions of the omentum to the transverse colon mesentery in the lesser sac. All of these maneuvers increase the mobility of splenic flexure, so it is often helpful to incorporate all of them to get it mobilized safely.

Care must be exercised at the cephalad portion of the dissection when choosing the "sub-IMV" approach, as dissection in this area will be very close to the inferior border of the pancreas. It is very easy for those less familiar with this territory to find oneself underneath the tail of the pancreas, often heralded by dissection behind the splenic vein. This occurs because of the peritoneum overlying the pancreas and transverse colon mesentery on the lesser sac side. It may be difficult to visualize the pancreas, especially in an obese patient, and the structure may be injured during this dissection. If the pancreas is encountered and injury is suspected, it is wise to leave a closed-suction drain behind in the pancreatic bed. To avoid this, once the IMV is dissected, the surgeon should look "up" at the backside of the left colon and distal transverse mesocolon mesentery to identify the subtle avascular plane between the pancreas and mesocolon. Dissection in this plane will keep the pancreas down in the retroperitoneum, avoid damage and any resultant morbidity, and allow access to the lesser sac.

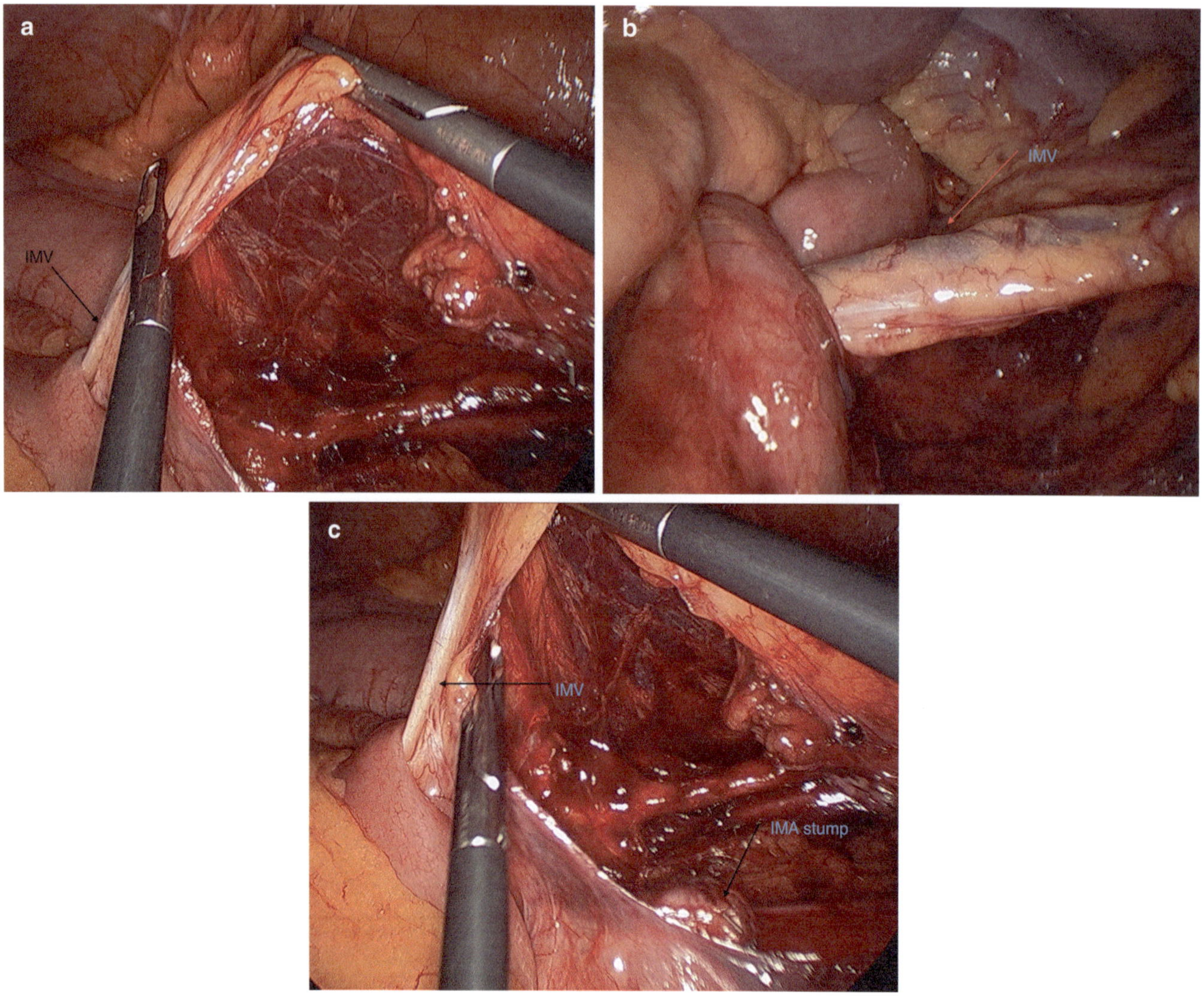


**Fig. 18.4** (a, b, c) In these images the inferior mesenteric vein is shown after being approached from the medial side. The vessel is elevated and placed on gentle traction

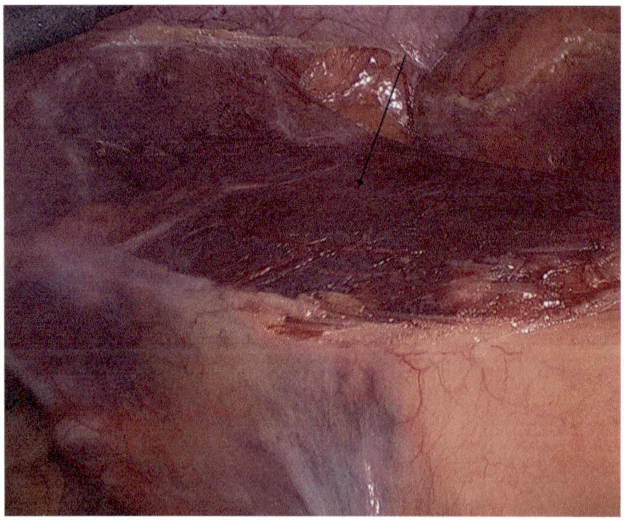

**Fig. 18.5** When a previously dissected plane is encountered after being approached from another direction, the surgeon will be able to appreciate this darker appearance. It often assists in confirming that the dissection plane is correct

Complete splenic flexure mobilization requires dissection onto and mobilization of the distal transverse colon. If one encounters difficulty with the "sub-IMV" or lateral and retrograde approach to the flexure, it is often helpful to abandon these approaches and begin dissection of the transverse colon (Fig. 18.6). The omentum can be reflected cephalad over the anterior surface of the stomach. Changing position again to Trendelenburg will allow gravity to assist in maintaining cephalad positioning of the omentum. A window is then created where the omentum attaches to the transverse colon. This line of dissection can be extended toward the splenic flexure, effectively detaching the omentum from the distal transverse colon. This opens the lesser sac and allows better definition of the transverse mesocolon that can now be divided from its retroperitoneal attachments. If dissection becomes difficult, the surgeon may work back and forth between the medial, lateral, and transverse colonic approaches dissecting what seems easy until complete mobilization has been achieved. If required, hand assistance can be invaluable in mobilizing a difficult splenic flexure and can be utilized in all of the above-described techniques.

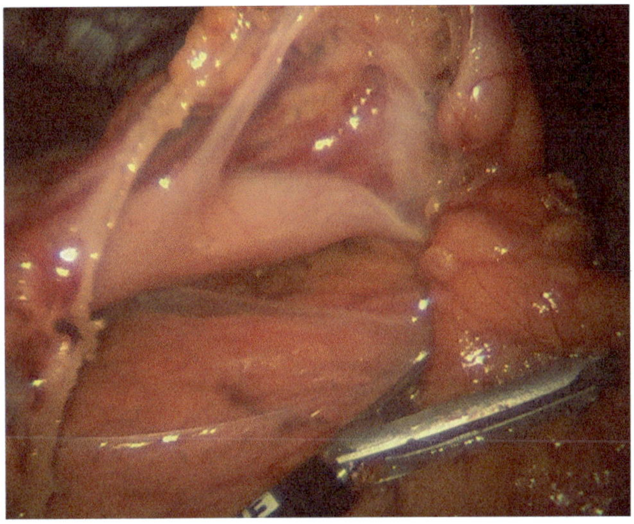

**Fig. 18.6** In this image, the splenic flexure is approached along the transverse colon from a medial direction. The greater omentum has been opened along the border of the colon and the lesser sac is entered. The posterior wall of the stomach and the pancreas are clearly seen

## The Transverse Colon

The transverse colon is a relatively mobile structure at its midpoint and can be quite redundant. Mobilization of the transverse colon and division of its vasculature can be one of the most challenging tasks to perform laparoscopically. In most scenarios, the transverse colon is approached after mobilization and division of the vasculature of the left or right colon as a part of an extended right or left colectomy, as a method of colonic mobilization to perform a tension-free anastomosis, or as a part of total abdominal colectomy or proctocolectomy. It is unusual to perform an isolated segmental transverse colectomy, and that will not be discussed.

## From the Right

The approach to the transverse colon is typically determined by whether a left- or right-sided resection is being performed. If approaching from the right, it is wise to take down the hepatic flexure of the colon (Video 18.3) and gain access to the lesser sac by dividing the lesser omentum. This is more easily achieved on the right than the left. Because of the vascularity of these areas, it may be easiest to divide these tissues with an advanced energy device. Locating the middle colic artery can be challenging, especially in the obese patient. This can be performed from above or below the transverse mesocolon—or via a "medial-to-lateral" approach versus a classic approach. If the ileocolic artery has already been divided from a medial approach, one can simply continue this approach medially and cephalad until encountering the middle colic vessels. The middle colic can then be divided with a stapler or energy device, which will result in a highly mobile segment of transverse colon. One potential pitfall of this approach occurs when the patient has a true right colic artery arising from the superior mesenteric artery (SMA), which is rare and is seen in only 10 % of individuals [3]. In this case, the right colic would be divided with the middle colic only being encountered during continued dissection across the transverse colon. While this would tend to be a necessary step in the operation anyway, it can lead to confusion about vascular anatomy and concern for division of the SMA itself. Another potential pitfall for the medial approach to the middle colic vessels is the adhesions or attachments of the omentum to the transverse colon mesentery in the lesser sac. This can make isolation and visualization of the middle colic vessels challenging. Completely opening up the lesser sac by dividing the lesser omentum or separating the omentum from the transverse colon before approaching the vasculature can be helpful. By having the lesser sac completely open, the potential for obscure bleeding or inadvertent injury to adjacent structures is minimized.

Approaching the middle colic vessels from above the transverse colon is more consistent with the classically described open procedure and is relatively simple from the right-hand side. One must take care to beware of injuring the duodenum, head of the pancreas, and gallbladder during this step. Again, once the lesser sac is entered, the transverse mesocolon can be divided by lifting it off of the retroperitoneal structures, clearly visualizing the anterior and posterior surfaces, and properly using a stapler or energy device. As a note of caution, if utilizing an energy device, take care to clearly visualize the entire extent of the vessel being divided, and apply the device completely across and perpendicular to the vessel (Video 18.4). Failure to perform these steps may result in significant delayed bleeding (Video 18.5). Because the middle colic vessels may be short with a high origin, a loss of control of these vessels can be problematic. This is a high rent district with the pancreas, stomach, duodenum, and superior mesenteric vessels all in this area, so great caution must be used to prevent and control bleeding.

## From the Left

If the approach is associated with a left-sided resection, the anatomy may be a bit more challenging. The advantage here is that one may not have to deal with the middle colic vessels. Because the fusion plane between the omentum and the transverse mesocolon tends to complex near the splenic flexure, it tends to be easier to begin to develop this plane at the mid-transverse colon. As mentioned earlier, the omentum may be retracted cephalad, exposing its attachment to the transverse colon. This attachment is opened and the lesser sac is entered. If there is a desire to preserve the

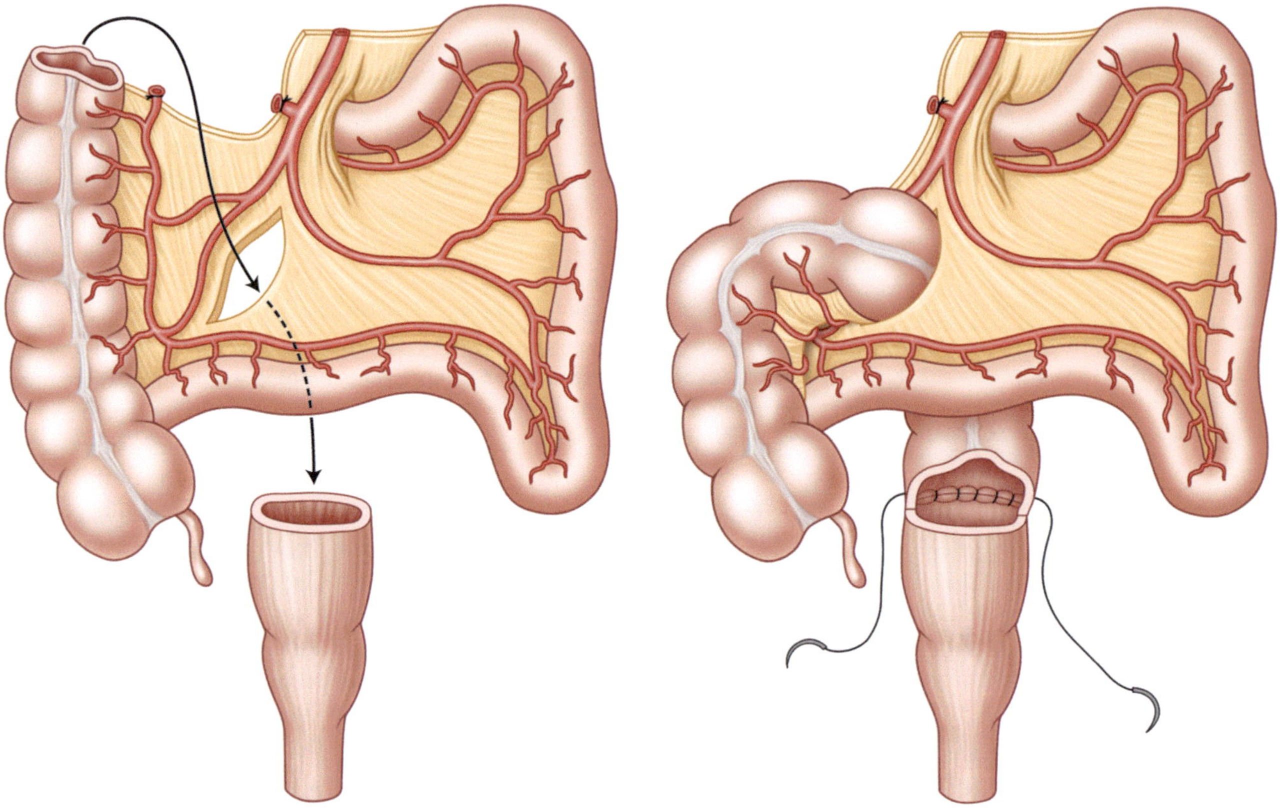

**Fig. 18.7** This drawing shows how a window is created in the right colonic mesentery under the ileocolic artery facilitating a shorter path for the proximal transverse colon or hepatic flexure to reach the pelvic brim in order to perform a colorectal anastomosis

greater omentum, it should be detached completely from the transverse colon in this same plane. In this case, the attachment is right adjacent to the bowel wall, though there is a clear avascular area to begin dissection. If omental preservation is not a goal, then the omentum can be divided above the transverse colon using an energy device once the lesser sac is entered. This dissection can also begin above the transverse colon by opening the lesser omentum and continuing to the left. It is wise to mobilize as much of the left colon as possible prior to performing the above. If the splenic flexure can be taken down with ease, then one will already be in the proper plane to perform this dissection, and the surgeon can simply continue to progress from the patient's left to as far medial as necessary. Often, because of difficulty with omental fusion proximal to the splenic flexure, this area is approached from both sides until it is completely freed from surrounding tissues.

When performing a true extended left colectomy, the middle colic vessels will be divided and the majority of the transverse colon will be resected. This may present difficulty with gaining enough colonic length to reach the upper rectum for a tension-free anastomosis. A useful technique in this setting is to mobilize the hepatic flexure completely, create a window in the mesentery of the small bowel/right colon between the ileocolic artery and the last major branch of the SMA, and bring the colon through for anastomosis (Fig. 18.7) [4]. This will reliably facilitate reach without tension.

## Gaining Colonic Length/Mobilization

Many of the strategies used to gain colonic length have been described above, but this topic deserves recognition on its own. We speak of gaining colonic length in three typical scenarios: gaining length to perform an extracorporeal anastomosis during a right-sided resection, gaining length to mature a stoma, and gaining length to perform a tension-free colorectal or coloanal anastomosis.

Gaining length on the right is needed so that enough colon can be exteriorized through the extraction incision such that an adequate resection can be performed while leaving enough length of colon and small bowel for extracorporeal anastomosis. This tends to rely on three key maneuvers: adequate mobilization of the right colon off of the retroperitoneum from the right iliac fossa to the duodenum (Fig. 18.8), mobilization of the hepatic flexure, and mobilization of the terminal ileum from the right iliac fossa and occasionally the right pelvic sidewall.

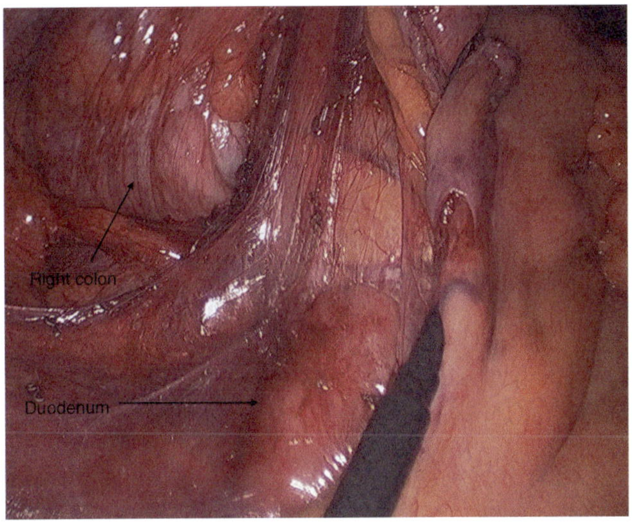


**Fig. 18.8** This image shows the right colon after complete mobilization up to the level of the duodenum. The colon is retracted anteriorly and cephalad with the duodenum in clear view

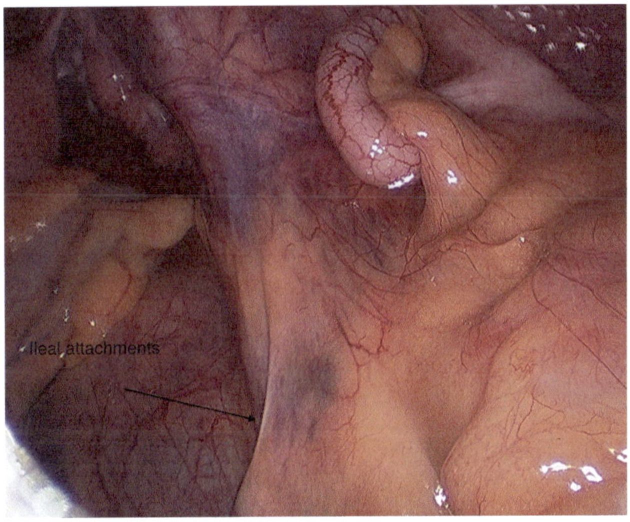


**Fig. 18.9** This image shows the normal congenital attachments of the terminal ileum to the right iliac fossa. These must be taken down to facilitate mobilization of the right colon and TI. They can sometimes extend down into the pelvic with intimate attachments to the right pelvic sidewall

High ligation of the ileocolic artery facilitates right colonic mobilization and should be performed in the majority of cases. For cancers of the right colon, ligation of the right branch of the middle colic vessels is required. In a thin patient, this can easily be ligated extracorporeally, but for an obese patient, it is safer to ligate it intracorporeally to avoid avulsion during extraction. It is not uncommon to encounter significant congenital adhesions of the terminal ileum to the right iliac fossa and right pelvic sidewall (Fig. 18.9). These must be taken down to ensure that the small bowel will reach an extraction incision. If the colon has been extracted and there is not adequate mobilization of the transverse colon, separation of the omentum from the distal transverse colon often provides enough extra mobilization for resection and anastomosis. Gaining length on the left is required in the setting of colostomy creation and colorectal/coloanal anastomosis. There are several maneuvers that assist with this that include: high ligation of the inferior mesenteric artery (IMA), high ligation of the IMV at the base of the pancreas, mobilization of the splenic flexure, detachment of the omentum from the transverse colon, and division of the transverse mesocolon near its retroperitoneal attachments. It is essential during any of these steps to stay high or central on the vessels/mesentery such that the marginal artery remains intact, thereby ensuring a healthy blood supply to the distal colon. It is best to ensure adequate length before making an extraction incision. If one is faced with inadequate length at the time of extraction, then the fascia has to be closed to resume laparoscopic mobilization, or a hand port must be employed to maintain a pneumoperitoneum.

## Potpourri

### Conversion

It goes without saying that we will all encounter a situation where we must convert to an open procedure. Sometimes this occurs emergently, but many times it is simply a result of a failure to progress in the case. In this particular scenario, it is often helpful to pause and consider what parts of the case can be completed laparoscopically before converting. Many hurdles of dissection can be overcome by alternating the approach of dissection to the medial, lateral, inferior, or superior directions. If some of the difficult portions of the case can be completed prior to conversion, you may ultimately be able to use a smaller incision and still confer some of the benefits of laparoscopy to the patient. Always remember, patient outcomes are better with preemptive conversion rather than reactive conversions for bleeding or injury to adjacent structures.

### Avoiding the "Twist"

It is imperative when creating an ileocolonic anastomosis that the free edges of the ileal and colonic mesentery line up from the root of the mesentery to the mesenteric edge of the bowel. This ensures that no volvulus is present. While this is easy to do in an open procedure, it can be challenging when creating an extracorporeal anastomosis after laparoscopy. While exposure of the root of the mesentery may be limited through an extraction incision, it is usually possible. This is one disadvantage to the use of a Pfannenstiel incision as an extraction site. If clear visualization is not possible through the incision, then the bowel edges may be opposed with Lembert sutures, the bowel can be returned to the peritoneal cavity, and laparoscopy can resume to ensure no volvulus is present. It is unusual to require this step. Occasionally, the use of a hand port and hand assistance will simplify this situation (Video 18.6). The anastomosis should be inspected laparoscopically after completion, again to ensure the absence of a volvulus. While it is not required to close the remaining mesenteric defect [5], this is often easily achieved through the extraction incision and is another way to ensure the absence of volvulus.

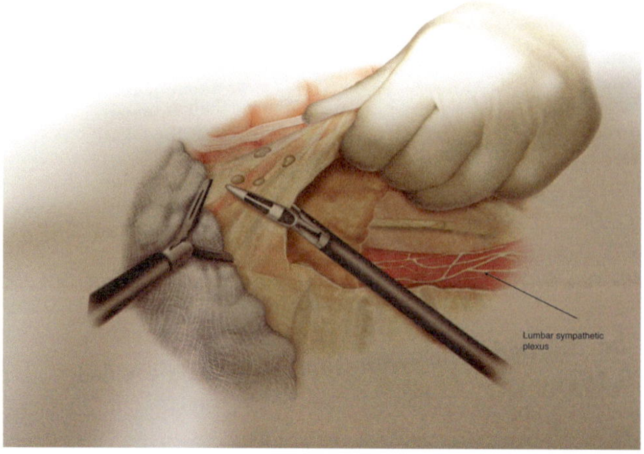


**Fig. 18.10** This image is a drawing that depicts the lumbar sympathetic nerve plexus and its relationship to surrounding structures

## Bloody Operative Field

Despite one's best efforts, the operative field may become bloody. Even a small amount of blood can impair the surgeon's view and it "soaks" up the light from the laparoscope making the operative field appear darker. It can be difficult to clear the field of blood using a suction-irrigation device, not to mention the effect on the pneumoperitoneum. It can be very helpful to insert a small sponge or "Ray-Tec" through a 12-mm port that can be used for absorptive purposes or for tamponade. When using a hand-assist device, it is easy to insert minilaparotomy pads into the field, which have even better absorptive capacity. As with any device inserted into the peritoneal cavity, we must account for what is used and ensure operative counts are correct at the time of closure.

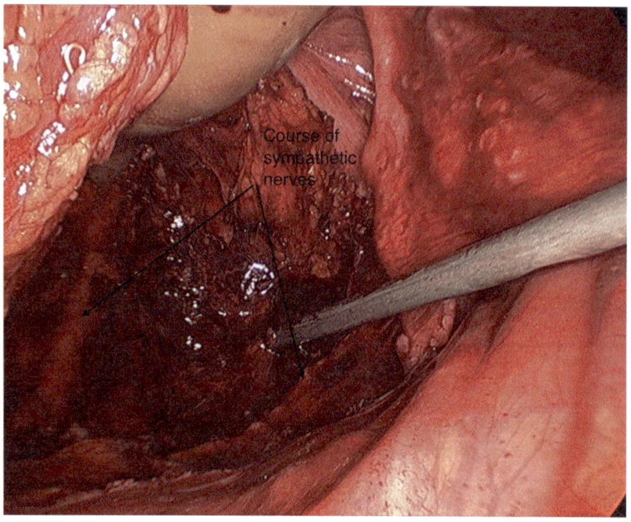


**Fig. 18.11** Image showing the SRA retracted toward the anterior abdominal wall in order to expose for dissection in the presacral space. The left and right branches of the lumbar sympathetic nerve plexus can be seen

## Sparing the Sympathetics

As the medial-to-lateral/vascular ligation first approach has gained popularity in laparoscopic colectomy, we have had to become more aware of protecting the lumbar sympathetic nerve plexus (Figs. 18.10 and 18.11). Typically the mesosigmoid is scored/opened just beneath the superior rectal artery when performing a sigmoid or left colectomy. The superior rectal artery (SRA) is retracted anteriorly, and dissection is carried under the sigmoid mesentery (Fig. 18.12). Dissection proceeds in a cephalad direction and the IMA is ligated highly (Fig. 18.13). The sympathetic plexus can be injured during any portion of this dissection—as well as dissection into the pelvis. Typically the SRA is pliable and can be easily retracted anteriorly. If it is difficult to lift the vessel, it is likely because the dissection began closer to the retroperitoneum than it should have. If this occurs, abandon the plane of dissection and march slightly closer to the SRA. Once a clear plane is entered, it can be followed up to the IMA without placing the nerves in jeopardy and risking retrograde ejaculation in the male patient. One potential approach that may assist in avoiding nerve injury is to start dissection under the SRA at the pelvic brim. If the upper presacral plane is entered early, it can be easier to continue in the correct plane of dissection in the cephalad direction.

## Finding the Ureter

Clear visualization and protection of the ureter is most important on the left side. This should be done early in the course of dissection. The technique differs based on the approach, aka medial or lateral. When taking a medial approach, as stated above, the retroperitoneum is entered beneath the SRA. The left ureter should come into view

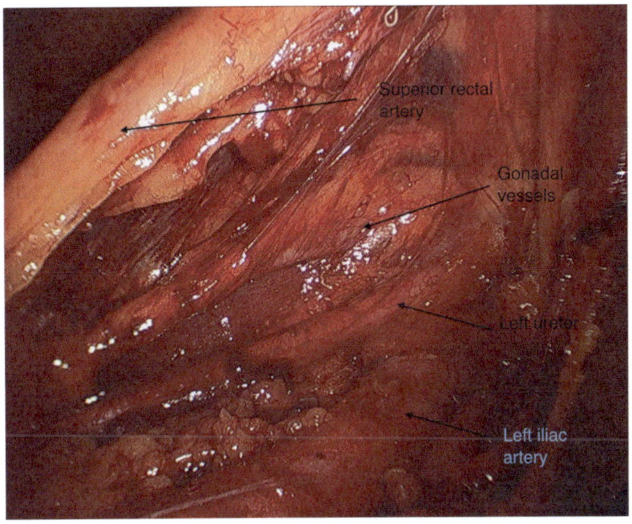


**Fig. 18.12** Image showing the SRA retracted anteriorly to expose the left ureter and the root of the IMA

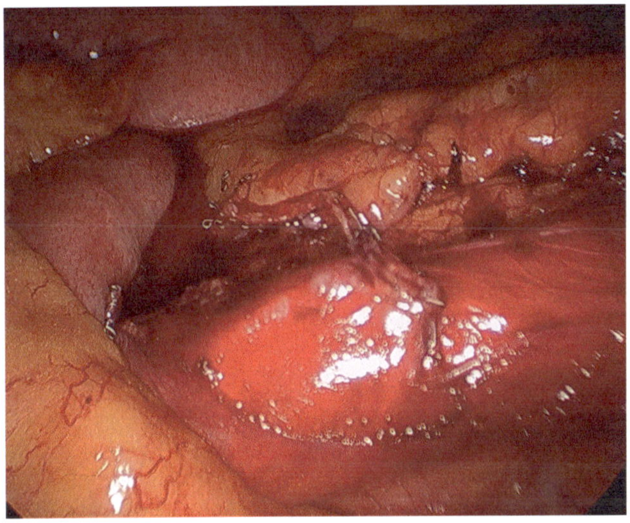

**Fig. 18.13** Image showing the IMA divided at its origin

quickly if dissection proceeds in the appropriate plane. If the psoas muscle is seen before the ureter is visualized, dissection has gone too far and should be stopped. Most likely the ureter and gonadal vessels are superior to the dissection plane, and the camera should be positioned to view a more superior plane. Back up and begin to sweep the overlying tissues downward toward the retroperitoneum, and the ureter will come into view. The ureter and gonadal vessels should be swept downward, and then dissection can continue in a lateral direction. The ureter should be clearly visualized prior to and when ligating the IMA to ensure its safety. If the ureter is still not identified, access the retroperitoneum at the level of the IMV. Once the correct plane is accessed, the dissection can then be carried caudad to the previous plane of dissection.

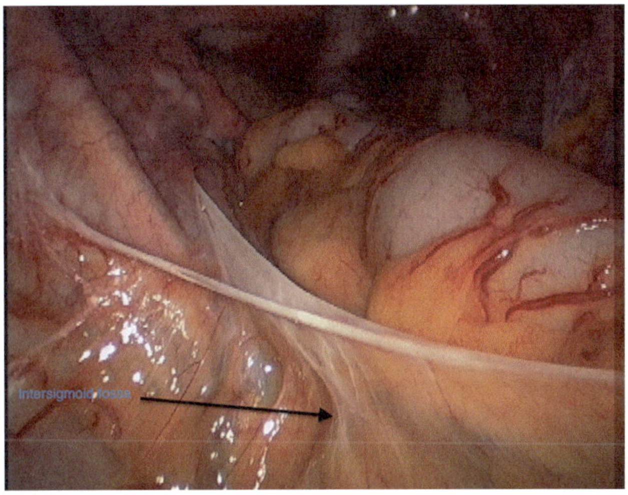


**Fig. 18.14** This image depicts the intersigmoid fossa—a structure that is often overlooked. It can be more apparent in some individuals—but typically appears as a dimple lateral to the rectosigmoid colon near the pelvic brim. It is created by congenital fusion of tissue planes and is simply a part of the distal white line of Toldt. It is a useful anatomic structure, as it marks the site of the ureter in those with unaltered anatomy

When taking a lateral approach, dissection is carried along the white line of Toldt. Avoid moving lateral to the white line. In fact, it is best to err just slightly on the colonic side of the line of Toldt. The ureter crosses the iliac artery at the pelvic brim and may be just beneath the lateral colonic attachments. Congenital fixation of the colon to the retroperitoneum results in the formation of a structure known as the intersigmoid fossa (Fig. 18.14). It is a small depression that is actually part of the white line and often goes unnoticed. The sigmoid will often be adherent to the left iliac fossa through attachments that are not part of the white, but must be taken down in order to truly visualize the line of Toldt. If the intersigmoid fossa is viewed, the ureter will reliably be located just beneath it, unless the area has been distorted by tumor or prior surgery. If there is preoperative concern about difficulty with locating the ureter, presence of severe inflammation, or concern for tumor adherence, placement of ureteral stents can be employed [6]. Some of these stents are colored or lighted to assist with their identification during laparoscopy.

## Fatty Mesentery

Mesentery that is very fatty or thick from inflammation can make standard laparoscopic techniques difficult. The mesentery is typically divided using staplers or advanced energy devices. A mesentery that is markedly thickened secondary to Crohn's disease can make these devices useless. When the problem is simply obesity, the mesentery may be divided with an energy device, layer by layer, ultimately exposing the vessels so they can be divided under direct vision. Inflamed mesentery in the Crohn's patient often cannot be addressed with staplers or available energy devices. The only viable option in this setting is either laparoscopic mobilization of the bowel with extracorporeal division of the mesentery using traditional clamps and ligatures or simply an open procedure. Blind stapling of the mesentery or division using an energy device will almost certainly result in immediate bleeding in this setting.

## Reoperative Surgery (Prior Colectomy, Vascular Anatomy)

A history of prior surgery or colectomy is no longer a contraindication to laparoscopic colectomy, and it is not unusual to encounter the patient who requires a second resection. It is imperative to have a definitive understanding of the details of their prior operation, especially as they pertain to the remaining vascular supply to the colon. CT scanners have become so good that a scan with intravenous contrast can be reconstructed much like an angiogram, clearly defining the remaining vascular supply. When prior ligations of major vessels like the ileocolic, middle colic, and IMA have been performed, we must ensure that one major vessel remains to provide adequate blood flow after a second resection. Solid preoperative planning and imaging as well as intraoperative attention to the vasculature are required. There are newer proprietary systems being marketed that facilitate intraoperative confirmation of perfusion in the bowel [7]. These systems are reported to be more accurate than measurement of Doppler flow as well as visualization of fluorescein with a Wood's lamp—both of which are difficult to perform laparoscopically. The above methods may augment simple observation of the bowel in this complex circumstance.

## Intraoperative Colonoscopy

In some cases, it may be required to perform a colonoscopy during a laparoscopic procedure. This will result in bowel distention that may obscure the view and make laparoscopy quite difficult. If this is required, it is helpful to use $CO_2$ to obtain gaseous distention of the colon. This requires a specific CO2 insufflator, which is not always available. Carbon dioxide is highly soluble and is rapidly absorbed from the bowel lumen resulting in near total decompression of the colon in minutes.

## Pearls and Pitfalls

- Have a variety of tools at your disposal during a laparoscopic case. Not all of them have to be open, but varying lengths, different cameras, and especially options to control bleeding (clips, ENDOLOOP) should be readily available if needed.
- While you may be a "straight-lap only" surgeon, the hand remains the best tool we have, and you may need it one day. Develop the skills and become comfortable—it may mean the difference between continuing laparoscopically and a semi-urgent open procedure.
- The transverse colon is a difficult portion of the case. Even trying to mobilize the omentum, it is easier than you think to inadvertently divide the mesocolon. Understand the anatomy, especially of the middle colic vessels, and take your time during this part of the procedure.
- There is a generally straight plane from the avascular area underneath the IMV to the sacral promontory when performing a medial approach that can often help in identifying the proper plane of dissection for the IMA. Starting by the ligament of Treitz and working caudally will take you on the superior (cephalad) portion of the IMA, while starting at the sacral promontory and working superiorly will take you on the inferior portion of the IMA pedicle. By dissecting from both sides, this often not only helps to identify the proper plane of dissection and vessel but also the left colic branch as well.
- Do not hesitate to alter the approach of the dissection as it often requires multiple angles to tackle a difficult dissection.

## Summary

Laparoscopic colon resection can be one of the most challenging procedures to perform in the realm of minimally invasive surgery. A detailed understanding of colonic anatomy and its variations is essential to achieving success in these procedures. As with most tasks that surgeons perform, there are multiple approaches that can be utilized. Understanding of several approaches as well as potential pitfalls associated with the most challenging aspects of these procedures will ensure a high likelihood of success with the minimally invasive approach.

## References

1. The Clinical Outcomes of Surgical Therapy Study Group. A comparison of laparoscopically assisted and open colectomy for colon cancer. N Engl J Med. 2004;350:2050–9.
2. Marcello PW, Fleshman JW, Milsom JW, Read TE, Arnell TD, Birnbaum EH, et al. Hand-assisted laparoscopic vs. laparoscopic colorectal surgery: a multicenter, prospective, randomized trial. Dis Colon Rectum. 2008;51:818–28.
3. Garcia-Ruiz A, Milsom JW, Ludwig KA, Marchesa P. Right colonic arterial anatomy. Implications for laparoscopic surgery. Dis Colon Rectum. 1996;39:906–11.
4. Le TH, Gathright JB. Reconstitution of intestinal continuity after extended left colectomy. Dis Colon Rectum. 1993;36:197–8.

5. Causey MW, Oguntoye M, Steele SR. Incidence of complications following colectomy with mesenteric closure vs no mesenteric closure: does it really matter? J Surg Res. 2011;171:571–5.
6. Senagore AJ, Luchtefeld M. An initial experience with lighted ureteral catheters during laparoscopic colectomy. J Laparoendosc Surg. 1994;4:399–403.
7. Pacheco PE, Hill SM, Henriques SM, Paulsen JK, Anderson RC. The novel use of intraoperative laser-induced fluorescence of indocyanine green tissue angiography for evaluation of the gastric conduit in esophageal reconstructive surgery. Am J Surg. 2013; 205:349–53.

# Overcoming Technical Challenges: The Pelvis

19

M. Shane McNevin

**Key Points**

- Defining the anatomy is crucial to staying out of trouble in the pelvis.
- The sacral promontory is a great landmark even in patients with higher BMIs.
- Beware of the hypogastric nerves at the pelvic inlet.
- Key structures (i.e., ureters) tend to medialize with prior pelvic surgery.
- When you cannot find the ureter, use a systematic approach first to identify it starting with ensuring you have not inadvertently kept it elevated with the mesentery to the left colon.

## Introduction

With the advent of improved instrumentation and refinement of surgical technique, minimally invasive approaches to pelvic pathology are commonplace [1–3]. In contrast to abdominal exploration, working within the fixed pelvic space and adjacent to major vascular and pelvic anatomic structures makes laparoscopic pelvic surgery more challenging. Despite that, the same basic principles of exposure and precise anatomic definition common to both open and laparoscopic surgery are consistent [4, 5]. This chapter will review techniques for left colon mobilization, vascular division, and rectal dissection.

**Electronic supplementary material:** Supplementary material is available in the online version of this chapter at 10.1007/978-1-4939-1581-1_19. Videos can also be accessed at http://www.springerimages.com/videos/978-1-4939-1580-4.

M.S. McNevin, M.D. (✉)
Sacred Heart Hospital, 105 W 8th, Suite 7010, Spokane, WA, USA
e-mail: skmcnevin@comcast.net

## Accessing the Abdomen/Port Configuration

A myriad of different techniques for accessing the peritoneum and port placement to facilitate dissection have previously been described. Access to the peritoneal cavity can be gained with either the Veress needle "closed" technique or the "semi-open" technique using the Hassan trocar, based on the operating surgeon's preference. Although not definitively proven, blind placement of instruments within the peritoneal cavity risks inadvertent injury to abdominal structures and should be minimized, or better yet avoided. For mobilization of the left colon, the modified "anchor" configuration is commonly utilized with an infraumbilical Hassan trocar and two 5-mm trocars in the RLQ and suprapubic abdominal space (Fig. 19.1). An additional 5-mm trocar can be placed in the LLQ for added retraction and can be helpful for the obese abdomen or when adhesive disease is encountered. While these configurations provide excellent access for colonic mobilization, an additional 5-mm trocar in the midaxillary line of the RUQ of the abdomen is often needed for rectal dissection. Specimen extraction can be performed via either a low midline or preferably a Pfannenstiel incision through the suprapubic 5-mm trocar site (Fig. 19.2). Considerably better pelvic exposure can be had by utilizing the Pfannenstiel incision.

An angled video or flexible-tip laparoscope is required for adequate exposure of relevant anatomic structures during left colon and rectal mobilization. Atraumatic instruments should be used, though careful vigilance for inadvertent injuries to abdominal structures even with these instruments should be maintained. The dissection can be accomplished in a number of different methods but is most commonly performed with a bipolar energy device or monopolar electrocautery and vascular staplers or clips. What is used is probably less important than the surgeon consistently using a technique that is reproducible, reliable, and comfortable. One important pearl to keep in mind in choosing a dissecting instrument is selecting one instrument that allows for both

H.M. Ross et al. (eds.), *Minimally Invasive Approaches to Colon and Rectal Disease: Technique and Best Practices*, DOI 10.1007/978-1-4939-1581-1_19, © Springer Science+Business Media New York 2015

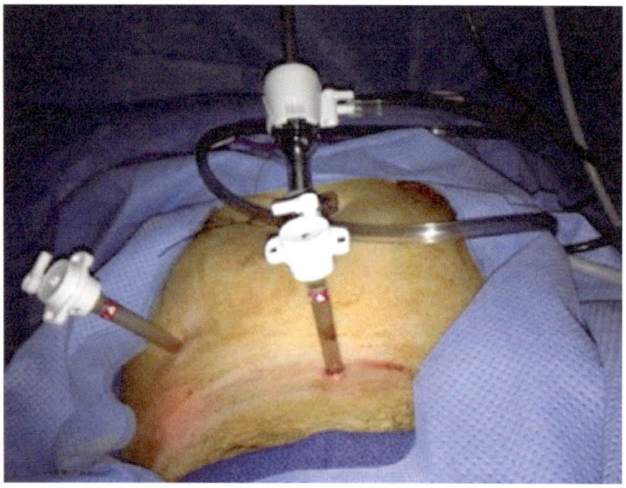

**Fig. 19.1** Modified anchor trocar placement for pelvic surgery

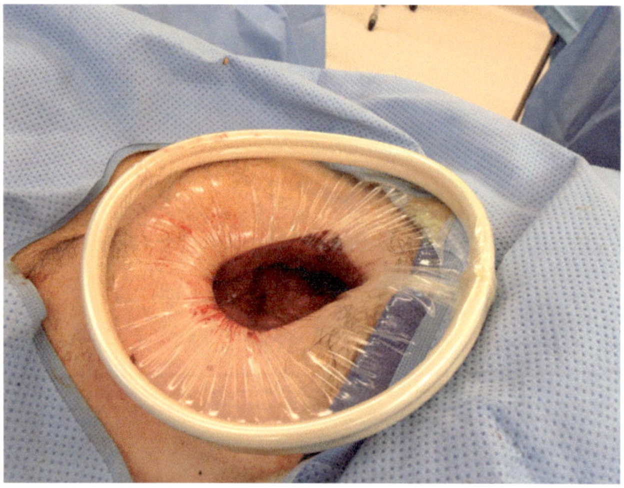

**Fig. 19.2** Extraction site with wound protector in place

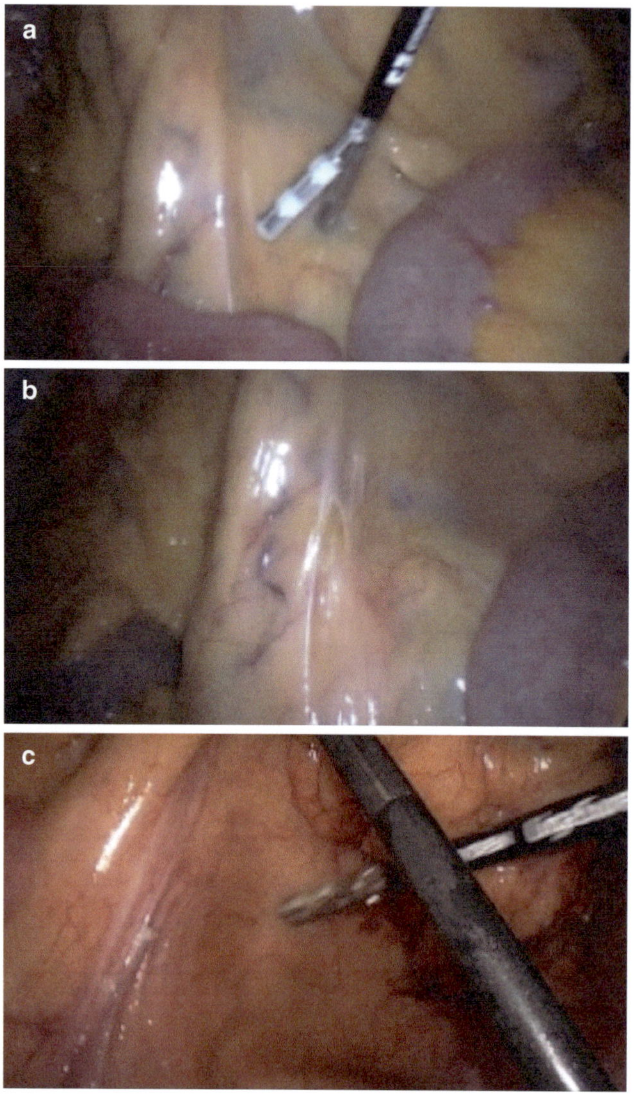

**Fig. 19.3** Medial-to-lateral mobilization. (**a**) Elevation of the IMA/SRA toward the abdominal wall; (**b**) scoring the peritoneum overlying the vessel; (**c**) caudal (i.e., pelvic) traction places the vessel on stretch and allows it to be clearly seen to identify the correct plane

dissection and vascular division that will significantly ease the case flow and increase the speed of the procedure by minimizing the number of instrument exchanges.

## Medial-to-Lateral Left Colonic Dissection

The most common and easiest technique employed for mobilization of the left colon is the medial-to-lateral approach and will be discussed in detail. Many other techniques have been described including the lateral-to-medial and sub-IMV to accomplish the same goals. As the surgeon becomes facile with the medial-to-lateral approach, it is beneficial to add these other techniques to the surgical repertoire. There will be occasions, especially as the surgeon gains experience and begins to utilize minimally invasive techniques for more difficult cases, where these other techniques may provide the only approach that can allow successful completion of a laparoscopic procedure.

## Retroperitoneal Exposure/Critical Anatomy

The initial step in the medial-to-lateral dissection is identification of the inferior mesenteric (IMA) and superior rectal arteries (SRA), as this will allow entry to the avascular retroperitoneum. Grasping the mesenteric edge of the mid-sigmoid colon and elevating it superiorly and caudally most easily accomplish this (Fig. 19.3a–c). The video laparoscope can be angled inferiorly (down) to best expose this anatomy.

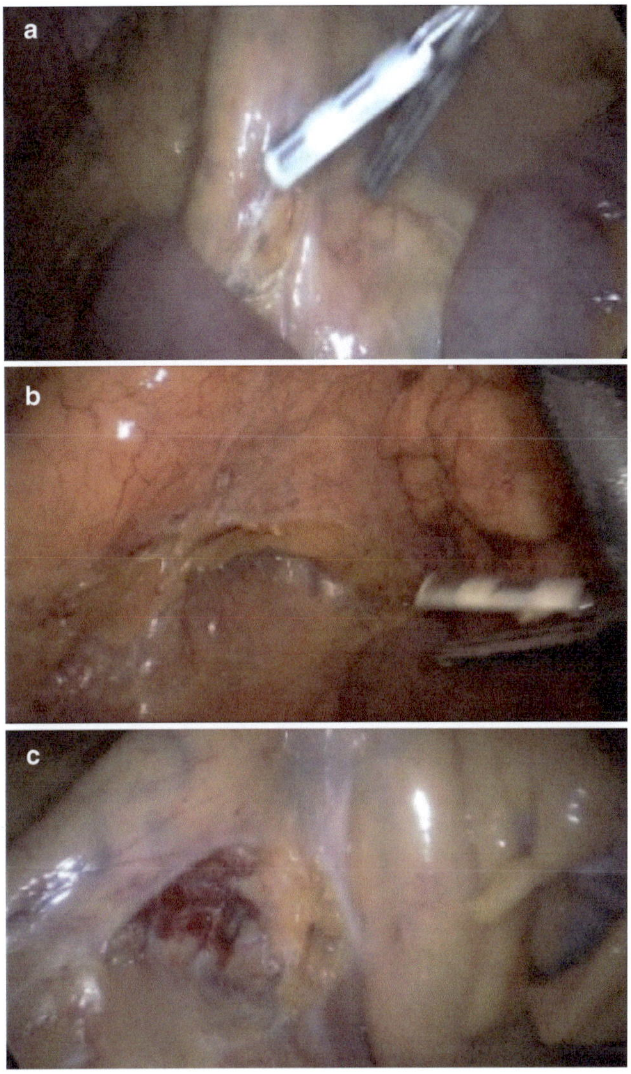


**Fig. 19.4** Base of the sigmoid mesentery. (**a**) Scoring over mesentery, (**b**) broad opening of a plane toward the sacral promontory, (**c**) deeper medial-to-lateral dissection

The base of the sigmoid mesentery can then be incised accessing the retroperitoneum (Fig. 19.4a–c).

After incising the retroperitoneum, the next step is identification of the hypogastric (sympathetic) nerves and left ureter and gonadal vessels. The hypogastric nerves are typically apparent running just inferior to the superior hemorrhoidal artery. These structures can be bluntly dissected inferiorly into the retroperitoneum away from this vessel and the root of the IMA (Fig. 19.5a, b). After this is performed, the surgeon then identifies the left ureter and gonadal vessels (Fig. 19.6). It is important to remember that the retroperitoneum curves anteriorly or away from your line of vision as the dissection progresses laterally. The surgeon must sweep the retroperitoneal tissue off the inferior aspect of the colonic mesentery to avoid mobilizing the ureter and gonadal vessels superiorly with the colon. The exposure, visualization, and dissection is facilitated by creating as large of an opening as possible underneath the SRA, as this greatly increases the mobility of the SRA and sigmoid colon mesentery. The video laparoscope can be angled superiorly (upward) to peer under the SRA and expose this plane. Additionally, the

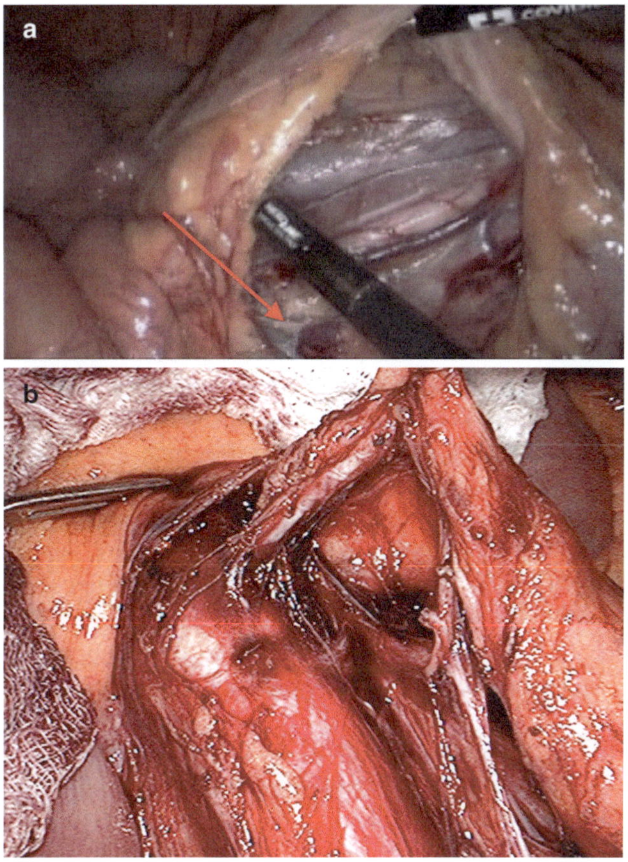


**Fig. 19.5** (**a**) Hypogastric nerves (*arrow*) swept posteriorly to the retroperitoneum near the base of the IMA. (**b**) Another view of the hypogastric nerve at the base of the IMA. *With permission from Jeffrey W. Milsom, Bartholomäus Böhm, and Kiyokazu Nakajima. Laparoscopic Anatomy of the Abdominal Cavity. In: Jeffrey W. Milsom, Bartholomäus Böhm, and Kiyokazu Nakajima, eds. Laparoscopic Colorectal Surgery. Springer, New York, 2006:pp104. © 2006 to Springer*

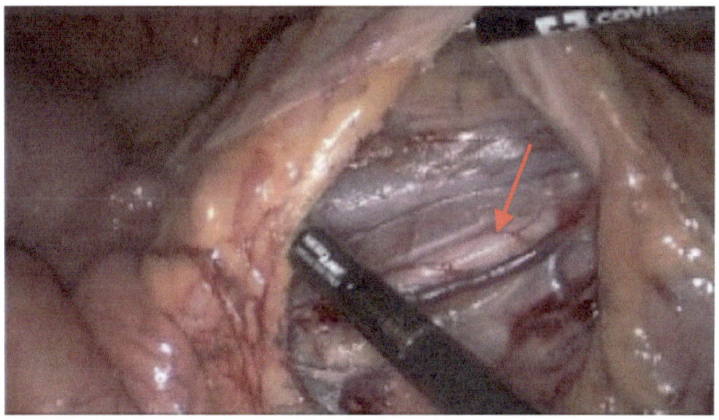

**Fig. 19.6** Left ureter (*arrow*) coursing medially to the gonadal vessels

proper technique to minimize trauma and bleeding in the retroperitoneum is to dissect in the superior-inferior plane and not laterally. Dissecting in the lateral plane (i.e., tangential to the retroperitoneum) often results in tearing of retroperitoneal structures and causes nuisance bleeding.

Utilizing these techniques often results in easy identification of the relevant retroperitoneal structures; however, on occasion the left ureter can be difficult to find. In this case, several maneuvers can be helpful. First, carefully examine the inferior aspect of the colonic mesentery to ensure that the left ureter has not been mobilized off the retroperitoneum. Second, clear the lateral aspect of the base of the IMA and then carefully dissect laterally away from this vessel in the retroperitoneum. Finally, carry the dissection inferiorly to the pelvic brim to the level of the common iliac artery bifurcation and identify the ureter as it crosses this vessel. If the ureter cannot be identified using these maneuvers, the dissection can be altered to access the retroperitoneum at the level of the inferior mesenteric vein or by the lateral-to-medial approach. Finally, if the ureter still cannot be identified, then conversion to open is likely indicated.

## Vascular Pedicle Division/Proximal Colonic Mobilization

After the left ureter and gonadal vessels are identified, safe vascular division can be performed. This is most typically performed with bipolar electrocautery, vascular staplers, or endoclips. Angling the video laparoscope to peer leftward often facilitates this exposure. The majority of surgeons use the bipolar energy device to both dissect and divide vasculature, thereby speeding the overall procedure (Fig. 19.7). Once the IMA is divided, then the mesentery can be elevated off the retroperitoneum with blunt dissection in the superior-inferior plane. The anatomic structure guiding this dissection is Gerota's fascia (Fig. 19.8), which can be bluntly dissected inferiorly to ensure that the left kidney is not mobilized off the retroperitoneum. Importantly, as the surgeon develops the plane over the superior aspect of the left kidney, it is important to consciously continue the dissection superiorly and not follow the curve of the kidney inferiorly. This will ensure that inadvertent injury, i.e., bleeding, resulting from injury to the left adrenal gland or its vasculature does not occur. Additionally, it ensures that the dissection will continue superiorly to the pancreatic tail (Fig. 19.9), thus dividing the retroperitoneal attachments to the splenic flexure, which is important for gaining colonic length and avoiding problematic bleeding in the retro-pancreatic space. Also, the plane should be developed lateral to the body of the colon to facilitate detachment of the colon from its lateral attachments performed later in the procedure (Fig. 19.10). Maintaining tension is the key to this dissection as it is an avascular plane and separates easily with adequate tension.

During proximal mobilization of the colonic mesentery off the retroperitoneum, the mesentery is typically divided concomitantly to facilitate exposure. It is important to consciously divide the mesentery at its root and not stray superolaterally toward the mesenteric edge of the left colon (Fig. 19.11). This will facilitate gaining added colonic length

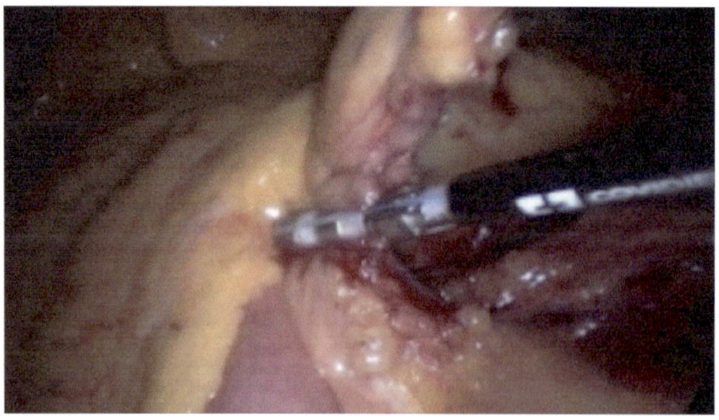

**Fig. 19.7** Division of the IMA pedicle using an energy vessel sealing device

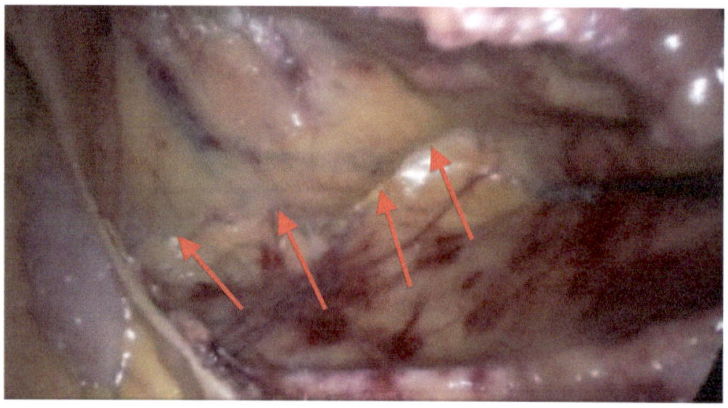

**Fig. 19.8** *Arrows* marking the line of dissection between the retrocolonic mesentery and the retroperitoneum and Gerota's fascia

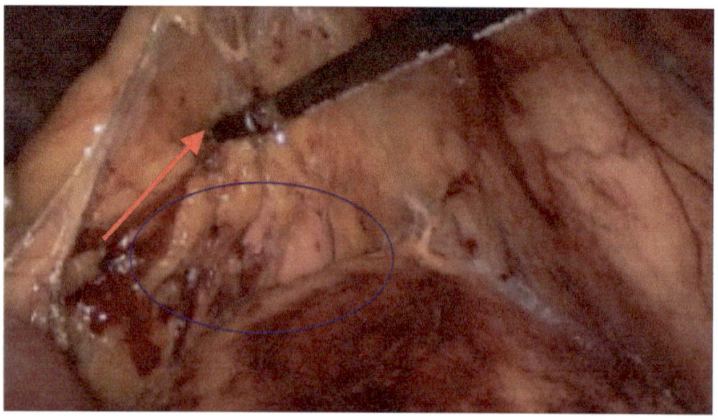

**Fig. 19.9** Cephalad mobilization from a medial approach. The pancreatic tail can be seen in the *blue oval*. The proper plane of dissection is highlighted by the *arrow* and the instrument

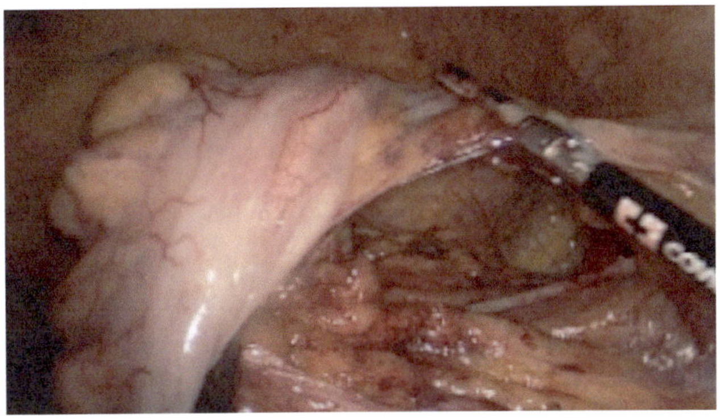

**Fig. 19.10** Dividing the lateral attachments of the left colon

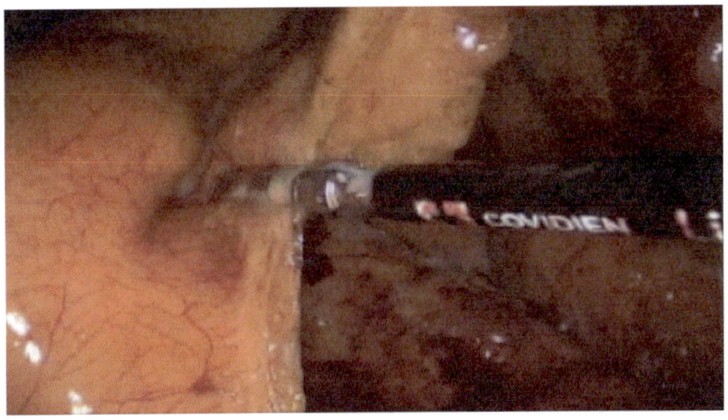

**Fig. 19.11** Division of the mesentery to the left colon

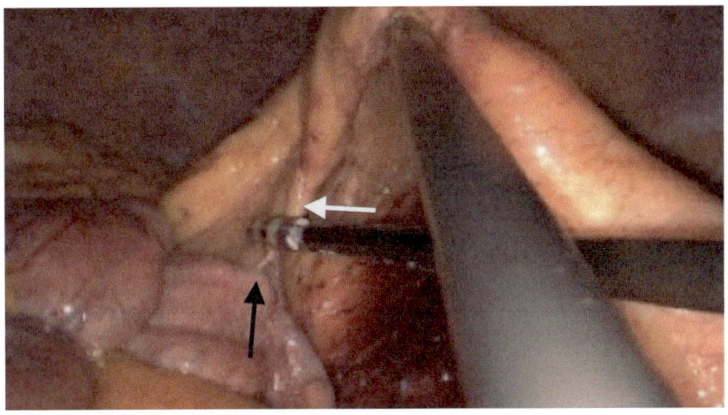

**Fig. 19.12** Progression of dissection. The ligament of Treitz can be seen by the *black arrow* while the *white arrow* points to the IMV

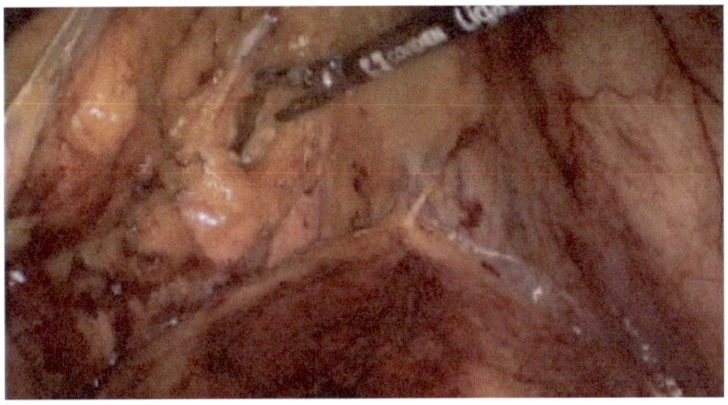

**Fig. 19.13** Attachments of the splenic flexure overlying the pancreas are divided allow access into the lesser sac

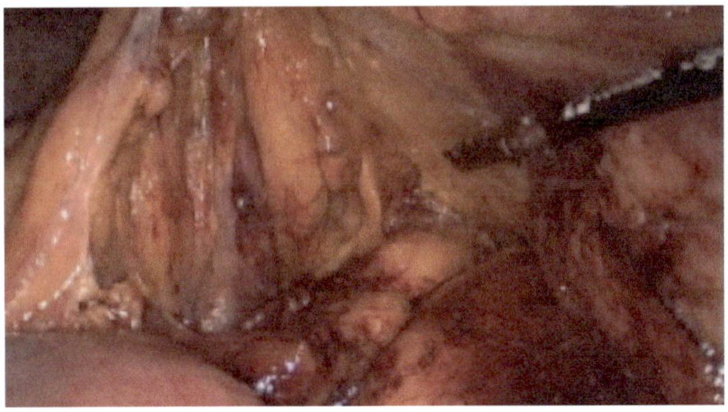

**Fig. 19.14** Completion of the medial dissection of the splenic flexure demonstrating the division of all the retroperitoneal attachments

by ensuring dissection in the proper plane and not risk inadvertent devascularization of the left colon by damaging the marginal artery.

## Inferior Mesenteric Vein Division/Splenic Flexure Mobilization

After division of the inferior mesenteric artery, the next major vascular structure encountered is the inferior mesenteric vein (IMV), which can be identified coursing laterally beneath the ligament of Treitz (Fig. 19.12). It can be argued whether this vessel needs to be divided or whether the splenic flexure even needs to be mobilized as a routine maneuver during left colonic dissection. There are three main advantages to routine performance of this maneuver. First, an anastomosis at or below the peritoneal reflection will be difficult to construct due to inadequate colonic length if this is not done. Second, once the incision for extraction is made and diseased bowel resected, the surgeon may find that even a more proximal colorectal anastomoses may still be under tension without splenic flexure mobilization. While it is not impossible to gain additional length at this point without converting to an open procedure, it is more difficult and time-consuming and often requires positional changes and loss of exposure. Finally, like everything we do, our skills depend upon repetition. Routine division of the IMV and splenic flexure mobilization ensure that this skill is available to the surgeon when it is critical to performance of the procedure. After division of the IMV, the splenic flexure is next mobilized starting by incising the medial aspect of the lieno-colic ligament just superior to the midbody of the pancreas thereby entering the lesser sac (Fig. 19.13). The remainder of the lieno-colic ligament is then divided laterally, mobilizing the pancreatic tail inferiorly (Fig. 19.14).

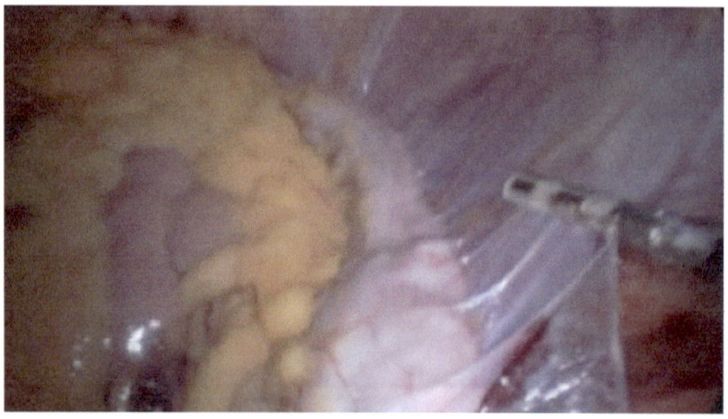

**Fig. 19.15** Division of the lateral attachments. Notice the *dark hue* demonstrating the avascular plane due to prior medial dissection

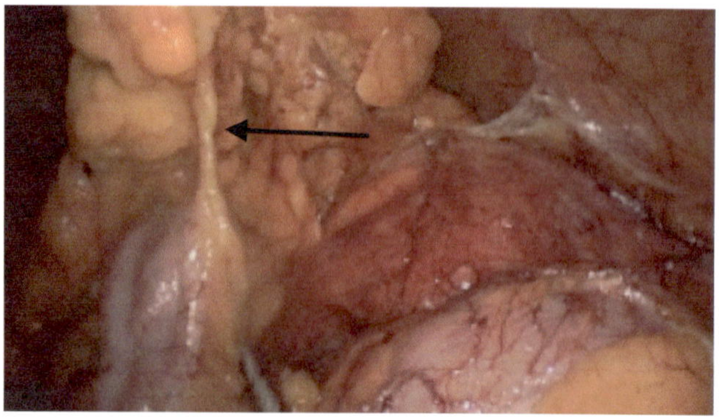

**Fig. 19.17** Omental attachments to the transverse colon (*black arrow*)

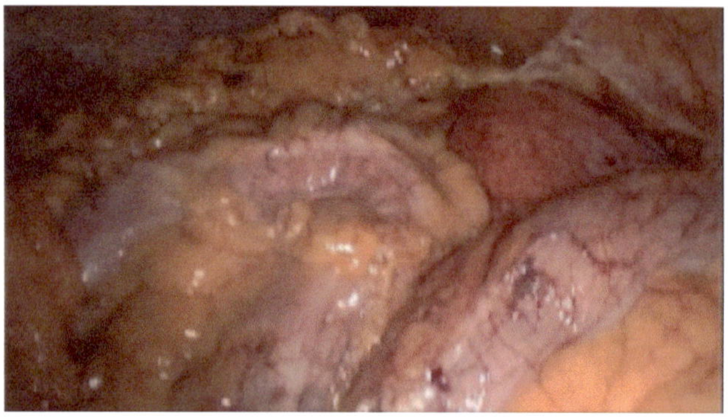

**Fig. 19.16** Splenic flexure with omental attachments still in place

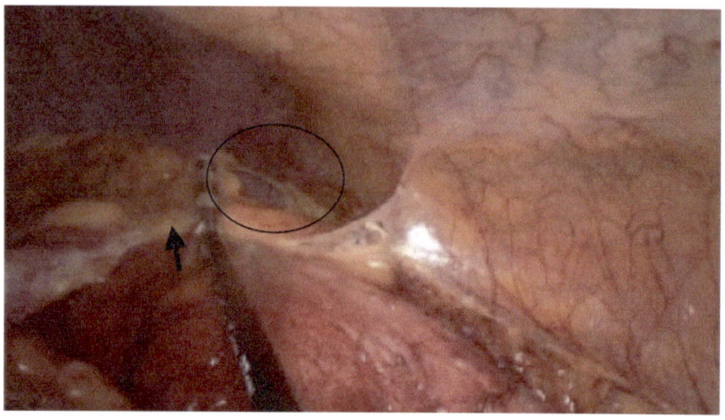

**Fig. 19.18** Final attachments of the splenic flexure (*black arrow*). The spleen can be seen in the background (*oval*)

The medial-to-lateral mobilization is now complete, and the colon can then be mobilized away from its lateral peritoneal attachments. Attention is directed back to the mid-sigmoid colon, which can be grasped and pulled medially. If the retroperitoneum has been mobilized lateral to the body of the colon, then the surgeon will see the proper dissection plane identified by a dark hue beneath the white line of Toldt (Fig. 19.15a, b). The peritoneum is then divided superiorly up to the splenic flexure. If the lieno-colic ligament has been adequately mobilized, the remaining attachment of the splenic flexure is only the greater omentum. The greater omentum can then either be mobilized away from the flexure and transverse colon, or the gastrocolic omentum can be divided taking the omentum inferiorly with the colon (Figs. 19.16 and 19.17). Finally, it is important to go back and ensure you don't have any last fibers that will need to be divided to allow for complete mobilization of the splenic flexure (Fig. 19.18).

## Rectal Mobilization/Bowel Division (Video 19.1)

After the proximal colon has been mobilized, attention can be turned to mobilization of the rectum. This can either be accomplished intra- or extracorporeally according to surgeon's preference. With either approach, this is accomplished by gaining access to the presacral space by reflecting the rectum anteriorly and under direct vision mobilizing the rectum respecting the mesorectal envelope. As in open surgery, this can be accomplished with either sharp dissection or monopolar cautery, and blunt dissection is discouraged. The video laparoscope can be angled superiorly (upward) to facilitate this exposure, and the dissection can be quite easily carried posteriorly to the levator ani if needed. Importantly, the three-dimensional anatomy of the sacrum needs to be kept in mind. The proper anatomic plane will initially be in the anterior-posterior projection and curve caudally in its inferior extent at the level of the upper coccyx just prior to the levator ani coming into view. Proper attention to exposure and traction-countertraction usually facilitates this anatomy and avoids injury to pelvic vascular structures.

## Identifying and Avoiding Damage to the Nerves

The hypogastric nerves typically course anterolaterally around the rectum just below the pelvic inlet and as they had previously been indentified superior to the sacral promontory are usually readily identified (Fig. 19.19).

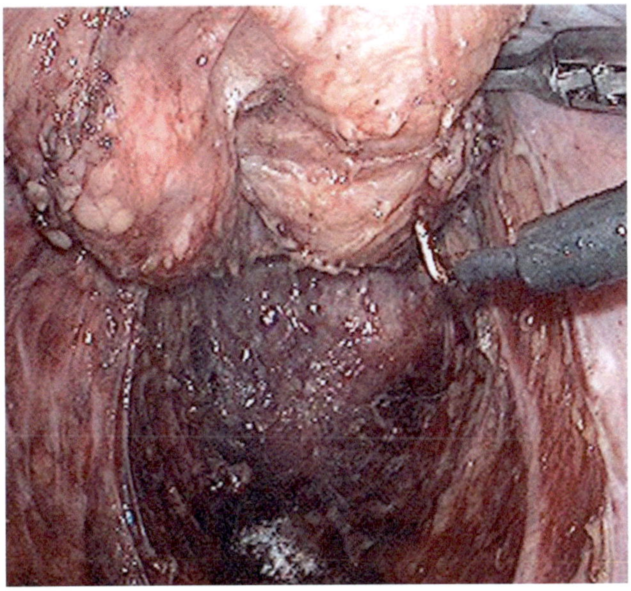

**Fig. 19.19** Hypogastric nerves seen in the pelvis

As these structures are mobilized laterally, the lateral peritoneal attachments of the rectum can then be divided with monopolar cautery down to the lateral rectal stalks. As the dissection begins, the rectum is retracted anteriorly toward the abdominal wall. This pulls the retroperitoneal structures up with the mesorectum, and as a result, the correct plane of dissection is higher than generally appreciated. As a result, if the dissection is started too low, the hypogastric trunks can be injured or divided while trying to access the presacral plane.

The nervi erigentes are encountered just below the anterior peritoneal reflection at the 10 and 2 o'clock positions. The key to good exposure in the pelvis is creating tension that is perpendicular to the energy source so the vectors of force are anterior to posterior and medial to lateral. Avoiding pulling the rectum out of the pelvis will facilitate better exposure. This is most evident when performing the anterior and lateral dissections. After the anterior reflection is incised, the rectum is retracted posteriorly and the reflection is retracted anteriorly. This tension will expose the avascular plane anteriorly. This plane is divided sharply, and the rectum can be rolled to the right to expose the left side and then rolled left to expose the right side. As mobility is created, the rectum is grasped further down in the pelvis. The correct plane is just on the shiny surface of the rectum—too lateral, the risk of injuring the parasympathetic nerves is higher and too medial, the risk of injuring the mesorectum increases. Creating adequate tension will greatly facilitate the visualization and dissection deep in the pelvis.

## Lateral and Anterior Mobilization of the Rectum

The video laparoscope can be angled to the left to mobilize the right aspect of the rectum and to the right for the left aspect of the rectum to ensure adequate working space for the surgeon. At this point, it is advantageous to incise the anterior peritoneal reflection and dissect the rectum posteriorly away from the genitourinary structures. In females, the uterus can fall down, filling much of the pelvis and making exposure difficult. The uterus can be suspended to the anterior abdominal wall with a trans-fascial fixation suture. A heavy suture on a straight needle is passed transabdominally and can be passed through the fundus of the uterus or from broad ligament to broad ligament. It is then passed back through the abdominal wall and cinched down with a clamp to suspend the uterus out of the way.

Just as described above, the vector of retraction should be with the rectum directed posteriorly and the cervix/vagina or prostate anteriorly. By gently rotating the rectum to the right and left, the lateral aspects of the dissection are facilitated. As each layer is divided, the rectum should be grasped more distally. There is limited space in the pelvic so the rectum should be grasped as close to the point of dissection as possible to maximize tension. Angling the video laparoscope superiorly (upward) facilitates this exposure.

## Dealing with the Genitourinary Structures

The genitourinary structures are reflected anteriorly to expose this plane. This can typically be accomplished with manual retraction via the suprapubic 5-mm port. In the female pelvis, gaining exposure in the setting of a bulky uterus can be facilitated by transcutaneous suture fixation to the anterior abdominal wall. Additionally, placing a vaginal manipulator can aid in identification of the proper plane and provide countertraction to aid in dissection. In the male pelvis, the seminal vesicles are first encountered laterally as the peritoneal reflection is incised, and it is important to carry this dissection just inferior to these structures to their lateral extent to avoid nuisance bleeding and for preservation of the parasympathetic nerve supply (nervi erigentes). The dissection is then carried caudally indentifying Denonvillier's fascia and again conducting the dissection just inferior to this structure to preserve periprostatic structures. Once the anterior dissection is commenced, it allows exposure and division of the lateral rectal stalks and bringing the lateral dissection plane anteriorly to complete the rectal mobilization.

## Dividing the Rectum

Once mobilization of the bowel is complete, attention is turned to division of the bowel and anastomosis creation. This can be accomplished intracorporeally with endoscopic staplers or more typically extracorporeally with open stapling techniques. The limitations in the size of the pelvis and the length and angulation of the laparoscopic staplers can make dividing the rectum difficult. The current endoscopic stapling technology is lacking particularly in distal rectal division limiting its utility. Having an assistant providing perineal pressure can bring the distal rectum further up into the pelvic to facilitate division. Also, utilizing the suprapubic port can facilitate division as close to a right angle as possible. Division of the rectum should be limited to no more than 2 firings of an endoscopic stapler as more firings are associated with an increased risk of anastomotic complications. It is imperative to ensure an adequate distal margin, which is more difficult with distal tumors. Finally, in women the posterior wall of the vagina needs to be inspected to ensure it is free from the stapler prior to firing it. Strict adherence to the principles of anastomosis creation (adequate mobilization and bloody supply, healthy bowel, and technically perfect technique) is required regardless of technical approach.

## Pelvic Bleeding

Pelvic bleeding can range from a nuisance to massive hemodynamically compromising hemorrhage. For nuisance bleeding that obscures visualization, a small sponge can be passed via a 10-mm port and used to soak up bleeding. If this does not provide adequate clearance of blood and improve visualization, a suction-irrigation device can be used. The most common areas of bleeding are deep in the pelvic along the lateral sidewalls and anterior around the seminal vesicles or posterior wall of the vagina. It is of utmost importance to have adequate visualization, prior to attempting to control active bleeding. Often bleeding results from partial injury to a vessel, so completely dividing the vessel will facilitate visualization and hemostasis. Once the bleeding is isolated, it can often be controlled with monopolar electrocautery or an alternative energy source. Presacral bleeding from a sacral vessel can often be difficult to control. These vessels often retract into the sacrum, and angle of the sacrum relative to the port sites contributes to challenges of gaining hemostasis. If bleeding is significant and cannot be controlled, packs should be placed in the pelvis to tamponade the bleeding prior to conversion to an open approach.

## Pearls and Pitfalls

- Find the ureter prior to dividing the IMA at its base. Although you may be "sure" that it is out of the way, if you haven't seen it, take the time to find it.
- In the pelvis, often another grasper may help hold the small bowel out of the way and the uterus up or provide improved traction-countertraction. It may make all the difference between struggling and having things go much easier.
- In thin male patients, when you open the anterior peritoneal reflection, the seminal vesicles may be right there.
- Provide perineal pressure when performing a low pelvic transection at the pelvic floor. It often will help the stapling and allows you to get lower.

## Conclusion

Minimally invasive techniques are available to manage a wide range of pelvic pathologic conditions. Whether the condition is approached in an open or laparoscopic fashion, the same principles of exposure, anatomic identification, and traction-countertraction to facilitate dissection are consistent. Technical considerations discussed in this chapter will allow for consistent and successful laparoscopic approaches to pelvic surgery.

## References

1. Greenblatt DY, Rajamanickam V, Pugely AJ, Heise CP, Foley EF, Kennedy GD. Short term outcomes after laparoscopic-assisted proctectomy for rectal cancer: results from the ACS NSQIP. J Am Coll Surg. 2011;212(5):844–54.
2. Lee SH, Lakhtaria P, Canedo J, Lee YS, Wexner SD. Outcome of laparoscopic rectopexy versus perineal rectosigmoidectomy for full thickness rectal prolapse in elderly patients. Surg Endosc. 2011; 25(8):2699–702.
3. Kiran RP, El-Gazzaz GH, Vogel JD, Remzi FH. Laparoscopic approach significantly reduces surgical site infections after colorectal surgery: data from national surgical quality improvement program. J Am Coll Surg. 2010;211(2):232–8.
4. Nivatvongs S, Gordon PH. Surgical anatomy, principles and practice of surgery of the colon, rectum and anus. 3rd ed. 2007;Ch 1. p. 3–38.
5. Jorge JMN, Habr-Gama A. Anatomy and embryology, The ASCRS textbook of colon and rectal surgery. 2nd ed, 2011;Ch 1. p. 1–22.

# Overcoming Technical Challenges: Reoperative Surgery

# 20

Brian R. Englum, M. Benjamin Hopkins, and John Migaly

**Key Points**

- Proper patient selection and timing of surgery are key in reoperative minimally invasive colorectal surgery.
- Distorted anatomy, adhesions, and the need for prolonged adhesiolysis and dissection are the key differences in reoperative surgery.
- Gaining entry to the abdominal cavity is the most common cause of abdominal organ injury in laparoscopic surgery.
- Most injuries during laparoscopic entry occur due to adhesions or previous abdominal surgery.
- Electrocautery is the second most common cause of injury during laparoscopy, and extreme care must be taken during reoperative lysis of adhesions.
- Understanding your limitations, especially when approaching a reoperative case laparoscopically, is a necessary component to success.

**Electronic supplementary material:** Supplementary material is available in the online version of this chapter at 10.1007/978-1-4939-1581-1_20. Videos can also be accessed at http://www.springerimages.com/videos/978-1-4939-1580-4.

B.R. Englum, M.D.
Department of Surgery, Duke University Medical Center, DUMC Box #3443, Durham, NC 27710, USA
e-mail: brian.englum@duke.edu

M.B. Hopkins, M.D.
Department of Surgery, Duke Raleigh Hospital, 3404 Wake Forest Rd., Suite 202, Raleigh, NC 27612, USA
e-mail: ben.hopkins@duke.edu

J. Migaly, M.D., F.A.C.S., F.A.S.C.R.S. (✉)
Department of Surgery, Duke University Medical Center, 7674 HAFS Building, DN, Erwin Rd., Durham, NC 27710, USA
e-mail: john.migaly@duke.edu

## Introduction

Minimally invasive surgery for colorectal disease, including cancer and inflammatory bowel disease (IBD), has become well accepted due to equivalent or improved long-term outcomes [1–3] and better short-term outcomes related to faster recovery, lower complications [4–7], and improved quality of life [8]. However, most trials examining the use of minimally invasive surgery have excluded patients with previous surgery or significant adhesive disease, questioning the degree of applicability of these benefits to this patient population. As patients live longer, the global population ages, and as surgical outcomes continue to improve, the likelihood of patients returning for second or third major abdominal operations inevitably increases. With more surgeons becoming comfortable with laparoscopic techniques and more patients expecting the associated improved cosmetic and short-term outcomes, the use of minimally invasive surgery for reoperative colorectal cases has become an important clinical and technical challenge.

Yet, this does not necessarily translate to easier surgical procedures. Distorted or altered anatomy and adhesive disease make reoperative cases challenging, whether using an open or laparoscopic approach. The potential complications are not different from more typical surgery; however, the risks of these complications may be elevated. Although some studies have indicated that prior abdominal surgery makes little difference in intraoperative or postoperative complications during laparoscopic colorectal cases [9, 10], reoperation is often cited as a risk factor for worse outcomes in these patients. In an analysis of 1,000 consecutive laparoscopic colon resections for cancer, Franko and colleagues [11] found a conversion rate of 19 % for prior abdominal surgery cases compared to 11 % for virgin abdomens. This difference appeared to be driven by a history of prior pelvic surgery, where conversion rates were 23 % (Fig. 20.1). Other complications that were elevated among laparoscopic reoperations included enterotomy (1.4 % vs. 0.2 %), ileus (6.6 % vs. 3 %),

H.M. Ross et al. (eds.), *Minimally Invasive Approaches to Colon and Rectal Disease: Technique and Best Practices*, DOI 10.1007/978-1-4939-1581-1_20, © Springer Science+Business Media New York 2015

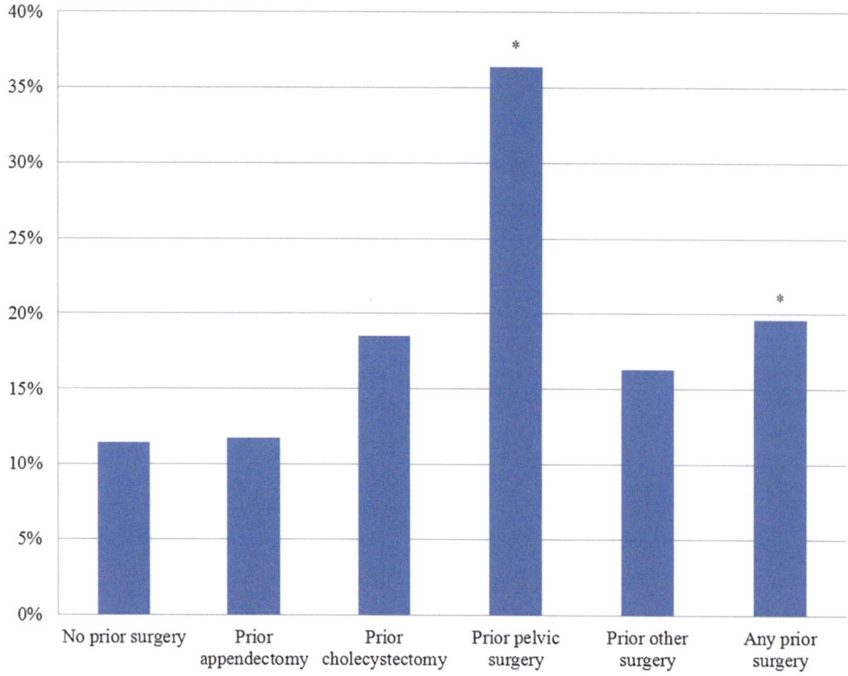


**Fig. 20.1** Conversion rate of laparoscopic colorectal surgery by type of previous operation. Figure represents data from Franko et al. [11]; 820 patients were evaluated. * represents conversion rates that were significantly different from patients without prior surgery by Pearson's chi-squared test. *With permission from Franko J, O'Connell BG, Mehall JR, Harper SG, Nejman JH, Zebley DM, et al. The influence of prior abdominal operations on conversion and complication rates in laparoscopic colorectal surgery. JSLS: Journal of the Society of Laparoendoscopic Surgeons 2006;10(2):169-75 © Society of Laparoendoscopic Surgeons* 2006 [11]

and the need for reoperation (2.3 % vs. 0.2 %). Of note, mortality, wound infection, ureteral injury, and anastomotic leak rates were similar between groups.

When considering specific metrics, the rate of enterotomy varies between studies, with Binenbaum et al. [12] reporting a rate of nearly 0.6 %. A systematic review by van der Voort and colleagues [13] found a smaller incidence of intestinal injury during laparoscopy (0.13 %); however, nearly 70 % of intestinal injuries were associated with adhesions or prior abdominal surgery. In laparoscopic cases dedicated exclusively to lysis of adhesions, enterotomy rates have been reported between 3 % and 17 % [14]. Although a rare complication in most studies, accidental enterotomy can have disastrous consequences, with mortality rates of greater than 3.5 % in these cases [13]. Mortality rates increase to between 20 % and 50 % if the enterotomy is not recognized at the time of surgery [15, 16].

Adhesions are thought to occur almost universally after transperitoneal surgery. The density of adhesions and the clinical ramifications appear to worsen with the number of previous surgeries [17] and other inflammatory processes, such as bowel injury, intra-abdominal abscess, locally advanced cancer, or IBD. While the potential for dense adhesive disease in reoperative patients poses an additional challenge for the minimally invasive surgeon, it increases the degree of difficulty rather than creating a unique set of problems. We feel that laparoscopic surgery can be performed safely and efficiently when adequately trained surgeons follow basic steps (Table 20.1) and maintain a low threshold for conversion to an open approach in especially complex cases.

**Table 20.1** Steps in the reoperative minimally invasive colorectal case

| |
|---|
| 1. Abdominal entry |
| • Initial transperitoneal entry |
| • Insufflation and inspection |
| • Safe placement of ports for Step 2 |
| 2. Anterior abdominal wall clearance |
| • Adhesiolysis of abdominal wall |
| • Optimal placement of ports for Step 3 |
| 3. Dissection and isolation |
| • Adhesiolysis, mobilization, and isolation of structures for Step 4 |
| 4. Resection and reconstruction |

When thinking about the reoperative laparoscopic case, it helps to break the procedure down into steps. These smaller components help to concentrate the surgeon on immediate goals, and each step is focused on setting the surgeon up for success in the following step. Gaining safe entry into the abdominal cavity is the first step. The goal of this step is the safe placement of adequate ports to continue adhesiolysis of the anterior abdominal wall. The first step involves initial port placement, insufflation, visual examination, and finally the safe placement of additional ports. The second step is a focused adhesiolysis. The goal of the second step is not a complete takedown of all intra-abdominal adhesions. Rather, this is an abdominal wall adhesiolysis for optimal placement of ports in order to continue the dissection and isolation of the structures of interest. Once ideal port placement has been achieved, the surgeon can begin the third step—dissecting out the structures needed to complete the case. Mobilization and isolation of these structures is key in setting up the resection and reconstruction, the final step of the procedure. Having a clear understanding of the anatomy prior to commencing a difficult dissection is critical as this will help frame the procedure and increase one's understanding of the anatomy as the dissection progresses.

In this chapter, we will examine the challenges involved in minimally invasive colorectal surgery for reoperative patients and focus on preoperative, operative, and postoperative strategies to minimize complications and achieve optimal outcomes despite the added difficulty posed by these cases.

## General Considerations

As with any surgery, appropriate patient selection is the key to achieving optimal outcomes. While most of the considerations for laparoscopic surgery in the reoperative patient are identical to those for any patient undergoing laparoscopic surgery, the reoperative patient may require additional attention centered around the potential for adhesions. In patients with a significant amount of expected adhesions, two differences between them and typical patients should be considered. First, the risk of injury during entry into the abdominal cavity may be increased compared to typical patients. This additional level of risk may alter the risk-benefit ratio of a given case and tip the scales in favor of nonoperative management (when appropriate) or open surgery.

In addition, laparoscopic adhesiolysis may be a significant portion or even the majority of a complex reoperation. Studies of open surgery have indicated that abdominal entry and time for adhesiolysis in reoperative surgery can extend the range of operative times by 20 min to several hours [18]. Although data examining operative time for abdominal entry and adhesiolysis in laparoscopic reoperation is lacking, the potential for extended times in laparoscopy is likely even greater than in open surgery. The additional time involved for this aspect of the case should be considered, and cases should be scheduled for extended blocks to avoid time constraints in the operating room (OR). Patients potentially unable to tolerate the increased fluid shifts and stress of prolonged anesthesia due to added length of surgery should be considered for an open procedure or nonoperative management.

While the emergent status of an operation is generally a contraindication for laparoscopic surgery, urgent operations are often performed laparoscopically. Even in cases considered to have a low likelihood of laparoscopic completion, practitioners feeling comfortable with laparoscopic entry find little disadvantage to starting an operation with a diagnostic laparoscopy. With a low threshold for conversion to an open procedure in the urgent setting, diagnostic laparoscopy adds little time to the procedure and may provide important visualization for diagnosis or surgical planning. In some cases, a procedure may be completed with the minimally invasive technique, sparing the patient the larger incision and associated complications. The reader is referred to Dr. Haas' excellent review of the use of a laparoscopic approach for colorectal disease in the emergent setting in Chap. 27.

## Preoperative Evaluation

Preoperative evaluation in the reoperative patient differs from the evaluation of other patients preparing for surgery due to the focus on the past surgical history. While considerations of the patient's disease and indicated procedure are important, the patient's surgery may be dominated by aspects related to his previous surgeries. The patient's surgical history should be thoroughly reviewed, with attention paid to the number and types of previous operations and resultant anatomy. Furthermore, especially in Crohn's patients, consideration should be given to determining the length of residual bowel to avoid a short bowel syndrome. Abdominal complications such as mesh placement, intra-abdominal abscesses, fistulas, bowel injuries, and other inflammatory processes that may lead to increased abdominal adhesions should be directly questioned.

A visual inspection of the abdomen may reveal scars from previous surgeries that the patient forgot or considered unimportant (Fig. 20.2). They can also be more significant and should cause reconsideration regarding whether or not you should undertake a minimally invasive approach (Fig. 20.3). These scars may also provide a road map of locations to avoid during entry, as adhesions to previous incisions or trocar sites will increase the risk of bowel injury. If possible, previous operative notes should be reviewed to help identify potential areas of dense adhesive disease to be avoided during laparoscopic entry. Areas of potential adhesion may also determine port placement, as lysis of adhesions may be the most difficult portion of the case, requiring the addition of dedicated ports.

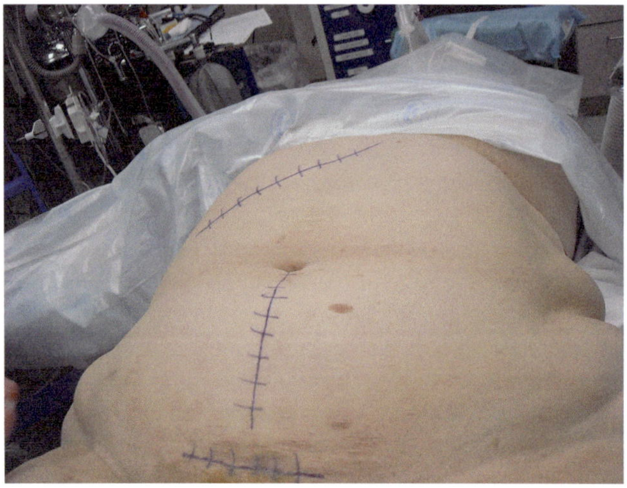

**Fig. 20.2** Abdomen demonstrating subtle previous scars throughout

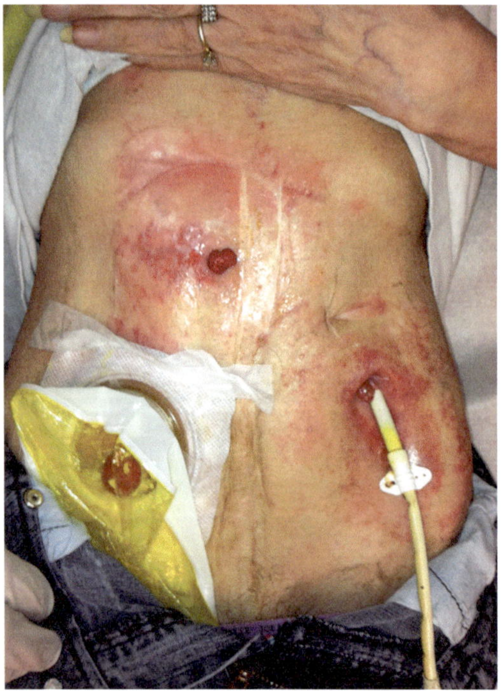

**Fig. 20.3** "Hostile" abdomen suggesting that a minimally invasive approach may be contraindicated. *Courtesy of Brad Davis, MD, with permission*

Indicated imaging, such as a barium enema to establish anastomotic patency or colonic anatomy for stoma reversal, should be performed in accordance with usual practice for any surgery. A computed tomography (CT) scan may be of additional aid in determining the potential site of adhesion in obstructive disease, and areas of the abdomen with especially dilated loops may be avoided during laparoscopic entry. In general, however, dilated loops of the bowel are not static, and minimal reliance can be placed on preoperative imaging in this regard.

Although not regularly practiced at our institution, several reports in the literature have indicated the utility of preoperative ultrasonic or cine-MRI evaluation of abdominal wall adhesions to minimize injury during laparoscopic entry into the abdominal cavity (Fig. 20.4) [19–21]. These techniques use spontaneous and induced visceral slide to detect loops of bowel or other organs adhered to the anterior abdominal wall. While these techniques have shown excellent correlation to intraoperative findings, they have not been tested for improvement in clinical outcomes and their widespread application in the non-research setting is unclear. Finally, determining both the date and results of a previous colonoscopy can be useful to avoid missing pathology or making intraoperative decisions such as the need for an en bloc resection, diversion, or intraoperative endoscopy.

## Timing of Surgery

While the timing of certain operations is out of the surgeon's control (i.e., perforation, complete obstruction, sepsis), most cases can be performed electively and provide an early opportunity to optimize the chances of success after previous operation. As with any surgery, patient nutrition and cardiopulmonary status should be optimized before undergoing a complex procedure. In the case of previous operation in the distant past, timing may make little difference to the surgery performed. However, in cases of a recent operation, the difficulty of adhesiolysis can be dramatically altered by the appropriate timing of surgery.

Adhesions form within 5–8 days of surgery [22, 23]. These initial adhesions are more vascular and diffuse, making adhesiolysis significantly more difficult and dangerous. The ability to delay surgery by 3 months beyond the previous operation (such as an ileostomy closure) will allow time for these adhesions to become better defined, with less density and vascularity [24, 25]. This delay may decrease complications, blood loss, and operative time.

For cases where delay is not possible, the surgery should be undertaken with extreme caution. In conjunction with anesthesia, a brief risk assessment can still be easily performed. In addition, consideration for the potential need for diversion is crucial, and patients should be appropriately marked in the preoperative holding area. Extended operative times and increased blood loss should be expected and planned for accordingly. Managing expectations for the patient, family, and surgical team is important, as these cases are often complicated. Blunt dissection may be less appropriate in this setting, as vascular adhesions will bleed more often, obscuring the operative field and causing increased blood loss. While laparoscopy still holds the potential for fewer postoperative complications, the risk-benefit ratio may be dramatically different in these patients and should be considered carefully.

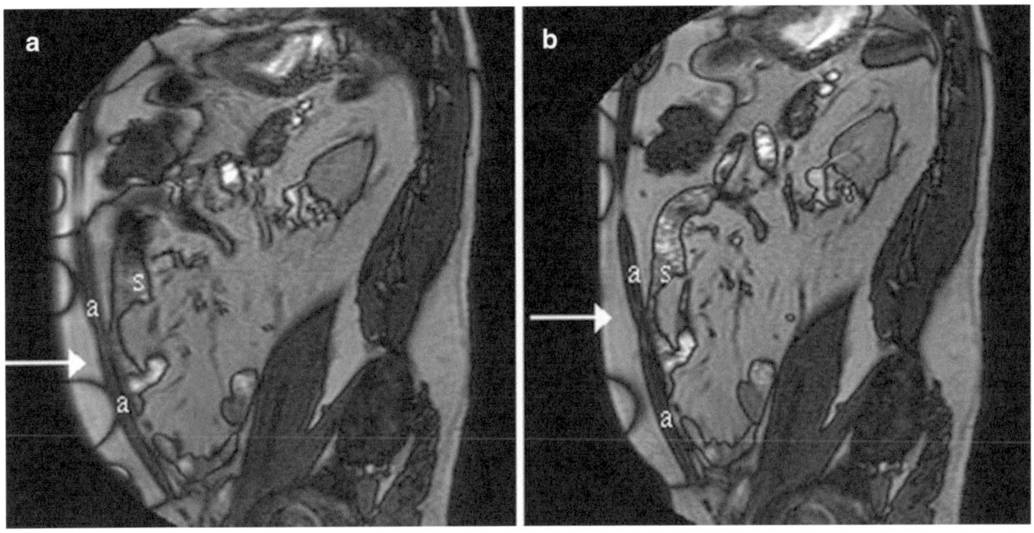


**Fig. 20.4** Midsagittal MRI showing adhesion (*arrow*) between abdominal wall (**a**) and small bowel(s) during inspiration (**a**) and expiration (**b**). *With permission from Zinther NB, Zeuten A, Marinovskij E, Haislund M, Friis-Andersen H. Detection of abdominal wall adhesions using visceral slide. Surg Endosc. 2010;24(12):3161-6 © Springer in 2010* [21]

## Gaining Access

The first step in any minimally invasive abdominal procedure is entry into the abdominal cavity, and safe performance of this step is critical in reoperative colorectal surgery. In a review of the reasons for enterotomy during laparoscopic surgery, nearly 42 % of injuries were caused by Veress needle or trocar placement, making entry into the abdominal cavity the most treacherous period of laparoscopic surgery [13]. While the incidence of these injuries is low (0.18 %), more than half of these injuries occur in patients with a previous operation [26], demonstrating the importance of caution during abdominal entry and the need for careful choice of entry technique. Large meta-analyses of laparoscopic entry have shown no difference in major complication rates between open and closed techniques [27]. The Hasson technique, which allows direct visualization as the abdominal cavity is entered, has generally provided the safest results, particularly when used away from previous surgical sites [28, 29].

The Veress needle technique is often preferred by surgeons due to speed and prevention of gas leakage at the trocar site. For reoperations in patients without a previously violated left upper quadrant (LUQ), Veress needle entry into this area may be a reasonable alternative and has demonstrated comparable outcomes in reoperative surgery with an intestinal injury rate of 0.4 % [30]. Veress needle entry into the LUQ has become our preferred method of abdominal entry, as most prior surgeries are performed in the lower quadrants or right upper quadrant (Fig. 20.5) [11]; however, prior LUQ surgeries, such as splenectomy or gastric resection, must first be excluded. Optical trocars (Fig. 20.6; Video 20.1) have been suggested as another possible alternative, allowing visualization with rapid abdominal access even in reoperative cases [31]; however, reports have indicated that optical trocars cannot prevent injury during abdominal entry [15, 32].

The "peek-port" technique [33] has been promoted as a rapid and less costly method for evaluating the potential for laparoscopic completion of a reoperative case. In this method, a small midline incision is made and used to evaluate the intra-abdominal cavity for the appropriateness of laparoscopy. In patients with a previous midline incision, an off-midline incision should be used for entry to avoid adhesions. If the patient is considered an appropriate candidate, then a hand-assist port is placed and the laparoscopic equipment is opened for a hand-assisted, laparoscopic case. If the abdomen is considered unfavorable for laparoscopy, then the midline incision is lengthened to continue the case as a laparotomy. Results from a single-institution series using this technique demonstrated 32 % rate of immediate conversion to laparotomy and a 5 % rate of late conversion after attempted laparoscopy. In cases where the peek-port technique was not used, the conversion rate to laparotomy was 2 %, potentially due to patient selection [33].

## Identifying Important Anatomy

Due to dense adhesions and distorted anatomy from previous resection, finding critical landmarks to guide surgery and avoid serious injury can be difficult in reoperative cases. Attempting to perform an extensive lysis of adhesions in an unfamiliar operative field can be a dangerous and unnerving

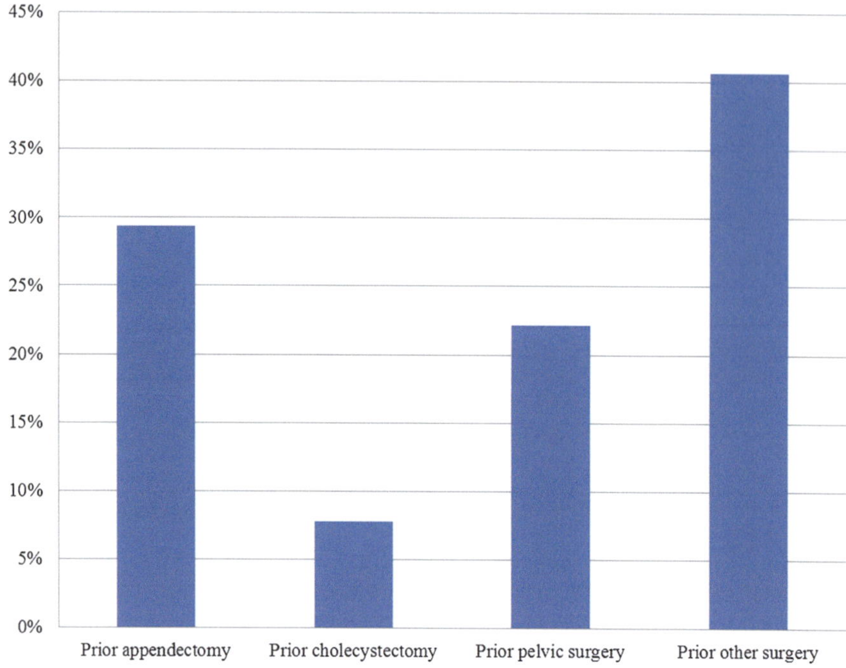


**Fig. 20.5** Rates of previous surgery type in reoperative laparoscopic colorectal surgery. Figure represents data from Franko et al. [11]; 347 patients undergoing laparoscopic colorectal surgery were identified with prior operations. *With permission from Franko J, O'Connell BG, Mehall JR, Harper SG, Nejman JH, Zebley DM, et al. The influence of prior abdominal operations on conversion and complication rates in laparoscopic colorectal surgery. JSLS : Journal of the Society of Laparoendoscopic Surgeons 2006;10(2):169-75 © Society of Laparoendoscopic Surgeons 2006* [11]

experience; therefore, the use of aids or alternate techniques may provide assistance in orienting the surgeon and decreasing the risk of injury.

## Ureters

Although identifying and preserving the ureters is always a concern during colorectal surgery, special consideration needs to be given to this topic for reoperative cases with a laparoscopic approach. Although studies have not demonstrated increased rates of ureteral injury during reoperative colorectal surgery [11], adhesive disease, distorted anatomy, and increased dissection make the safety of the ureters a special concern during these cases. In general, the ureters tend to be more medially located than normal, especially in the pelvis, following prior surgery. However, this may not always be the case, and it is important to have several options to find them if you cannot do it via standard medial and lateral approaches. One method is to start at the splenic flexure (assuming this is relatively undisturbed anatomy) and locate the ureter as it courses from the kidney along the retroperitoneum and track it caudally into the pelvis.

Another method for identification is ureteral stenting, which has a well-established history in colorectal surgery. Although studies have not demonstrated decreased rates of ureteral injuries during typical or complex surgery [34, 35], many surgeons advocate the utility of intraoperative injury recognition with stenting. With the advent of laparoscopic colorectal surgery, the tactile feedback provided by ureteral stents was replaced with lighted stents that could be visualized during surgery (Video 20.2). While no significant improvements in outcomes have been detected, rates of ureteral visualization greater than 80 % have demonstrated the potential utility of this technique [36]. Prophylactic bilateral stenting of the ureters before complex reoperative colorectal cases that involve pelvic dissection may improve ureter identification and recognition of intraoperative injuries. We strongly advocate the routine placement of lighted stents in purely laparoscopic cases due to the loss of tactile feedback.

## Bladder

Bladder catheters should be placed in all complex colorectal cases involving the pelvis to decompress the bladder, improve exposure, and decrease the chance of a bladder injury. The catheter can also allow for monitoring of urine output and an assessment of intraoperative fluid status, an important consideration in reoperative cases that may be prolonged due to extensive adhesiolysis. Finally, the catheter balloon can provide a landmark in the lower pelvis for the location of the bladder to help orient the surgeon and safeguard against bladder injury.

## Major Blood Vessels

Colorectal surgery is often performed in close proximity to several large vessels in the pelvis; however, the most commonly injured are the epigastric vessels during trocar placement in the anterior abdominal wall. Avoidance of these vessels

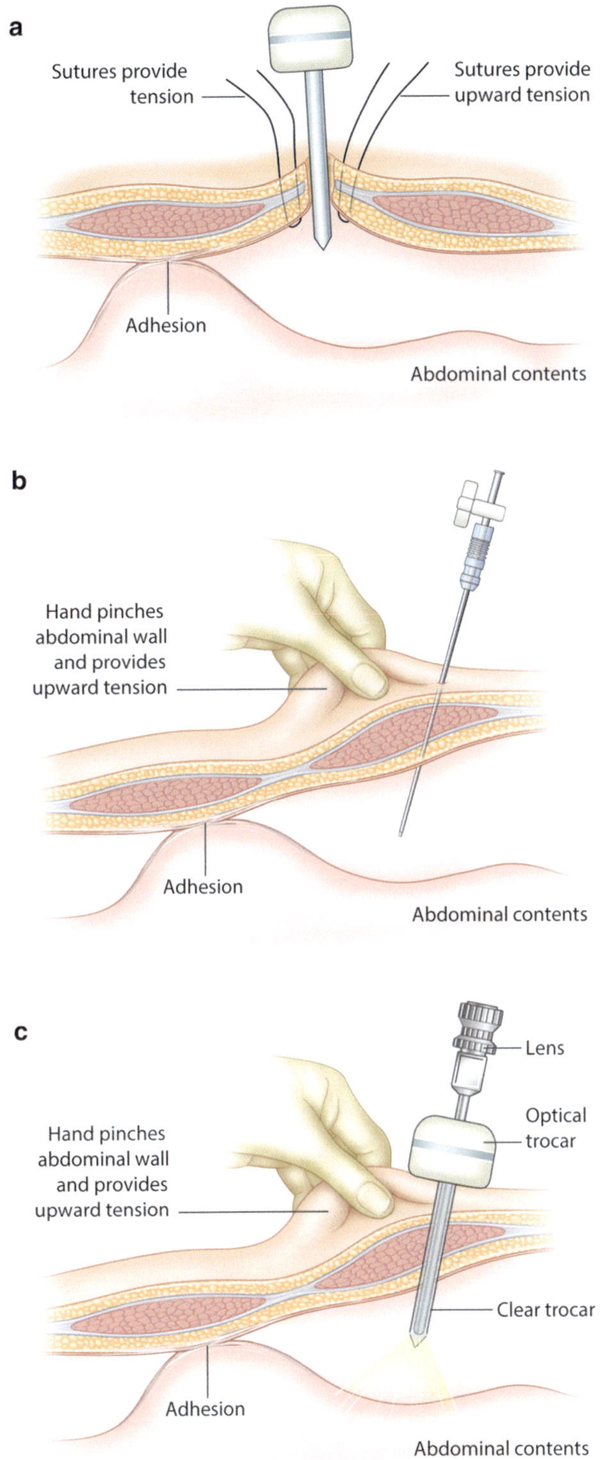


**Fig. 20.6** Abdominal entry techniques. (**a**) Trocar through upper midline abdominal entry point using Hasson technique. (**b**) Veress needle in left upper quadrant. (**c**) Optical trocar in left upper quadrant. Clear trocar tip allows light to pass from camera lens for visualization

can be managed in several ways. Initial entry in a midline position may allow for intra-abdominal examination for vessel identification. Transillumination of the anterior abdominal wall using the laparoscopic light source can help to identify the location of the epigastric vessels. In the case of dense adhesions or an obese patient, the surgeon can avoid the epigastric artery by remaining close to the midline or well lateral to the midclavicular line for port placement. Inserting the working trocars lateral to the rectus muscle will also minimize the risk of injuring these vessels. Finally, the visual inspection of the port sites both at the time of placement and removal will insure that any injury will be promptly recognized and treated.

Although damage to other major vessels such as the iliac arteries is rare, these injuries can be catastrophic. Extreme care must be exercised during a redo pelvic dissection, as normal anatomic landmarks may be missing or difficult to identify. The surgeon must be cognizant of energy sources used in dissection because the optics for these cases may be altered, leading to missed identification of normally seen pulsating structures.

## Rectum

Whether for ostomy reversal, cancer, diverticular disease, or IBD, rectal cases can be particularly difficult due to their location deep in the pelvis. To aid in identification of the rectum during dissection, the proximal aspect of the rectal stump near the staple line can be tattooed during preoperative colonoscopy. An additional technique that we have found useful intraoperatively is manipulation of the rectal stump using an EEA sizer or proctoscope to aid in visual or tactile identification of the rectum. Beyond simply orienting the surgeon, manipulation can be used to create tension, help identify tissue planes, or adjust the rectal position during dissection. If the sacral promontory can be accurately identified, an incision anterior to this point should facilitate entry into the presacral plane. The wider the incision, the more easily the plane will be visualized. The extent of the original dissection around the rectum directly impacts the difficulty of accessing this plane.

## Lysis of Adhesions (Videos 20.3, 20.4, and 20.5)

As has been previously described, lysis of adhesions can be a major part of a reoperative case, extending operative times and becoming an important consideration for abdominal entry, port placement, and patient positioning. The ability to achieve adequate exposure for visualization and instrument placement will often determine whether a surgery can be completed laparoscopically. As previously mentioned, the goals of adhesiolysis are to gain adequate access for the working ports and to clearly identify and understand the anatomy associated with the planned procedure. While adequate adhesiolysis is an important determinant of being able to complete a case, safe adhesiolysis is critical to patient outcomes. Avoiding organ injury during adhesiolysis is important for preventing prolonged procedures requiring additional resection or reconstruction as well as avoiding the added morbidity and mortality brought by these injuries. In the case of injury made during lysis of adhesions, early recognition and treatment are critical to achieving optimal patient outcomes.

Adhesions can be taken down using monopolar or bipolar electrocautery, ultrasonic shears, or blunt or sharp dissection. Electrocautery is the second most common cause of bowel injury during laparoscopic surgery after Veress needle or trocar placement [13]; therefore, we recommend the use of electrocautery only when a clear plane can be established between bowel and adhesive tissue. In addition, adequate space must separate any hollow viscus from the site of electrocautery in order to assure that thermal spread does not inadvertently damage the wall of the bowel or other organ. While bipolar electrocautery poses a lesser risk of injury due to thermal spread and capacitance, the need to grasp tissue between the forceps of the instrument make it of limited utility in a case with dense adhesions and minimal space between important organs and the tissue to be cut. Although studies have not demonstrated decreased rates of organ injury [37], animal models have suggested that ultrasonic shears have reduced thermal spread and injury than electrocautery. Unfortunately, these instruments have the same limitations as the bipolar electrocautery.

Gentle, blunt dissection using the camera, endoscopic kittner, suction irrigator, or other blunt instrument may quickly and safely release filmy adhesions and create space for further port placement. Most cases, however, require the use of nontraumatic graspers to develop tension between organs adhered to each other and the abdominal wall. Once this tension is developed, the surgeon can use sharp dissection with a laparoscopic scissors to release adhesions. Working from areas of good visualization toward areas of less exposure, the surgeon can remain confident in the difference between scar tissue and bowel or other organ. In addition, the surgeon should come back to areas of difficult dissection and lysis after attacking easier areas that will improve exposure. This technique maximizes the safety and efficiency of the difficult dissection. Moving the camera to different ports to achieve more optimal views and allow instrumentation from better angles can also be a key maneuver in making steady progress in a difficult case.

Ventral hernias from previous abdominal operations can pose a significant challenge to structure identification and surgical dissection. One technique that has proven useful to aid in orientation and safe lysis of adhesions in these cases is the external manipulation of the hernia contents to improve visualization and tension for dissection. The simple application of downward abdominal pressure on the hernia contents can create angles and visualization that may be useful during a difficult dissection. With external manipulation, multiple ports for camera view changes and instrumentation placement, and careful dissection adhering to the principles above, these hernias can usually be fully reduced, or adequate lysis can be achieved to allow for continuation of the case without full reduction.

If adequate time has passed since the prior operation (at least 3 months), adhesions should be avascular; therefore, blunt or sharp dissection should not result in significant bleeding and allow for safe and efficient adhesiolysis. When vasculature is identified in the adhesions, care should be taken to assure the proper identity of the structure and consideration given to the use of a hemostatic device, such as electrocautery, ultrasonic shears, or a clip. If structures cannot be confidently identified or the difference between bowel and scar cannot be assured despite application of several different techniques, strong consideration of conversion to an open procedure should be considered. Proceeding laparoscopically, especially with blunt dissection, runs the increased risk of either a full- or partial-thickness iatrogenic injury to the bowel and its associated increase risk of potential morbidity. If a bowel injury is created and identified, the decision to repair this laparoscopically or to exteriorize it and perform an open repair must be made. For exteriorization, the injured segment must be clearly marked so it can be identified later. Also, proper documentation of clear or suspected injuries must be included in the operative report because lack of documentation increases the risk of successful litigation if a complication occurs.

## Hand-Assist Port

Many surgeons use a hand-assist port for colorectal surgery, particularly in patients with increased BMI, cases that involve deep pelvic dissection, or for a total abdominal colectomy. For surgeons comfortable with this technique, it can provide improved ability to dissect bluntly and palpate vessels, ureters, ureteral stents, or catheter balloons. Studies have indicated no difference in short-term outcomes between hand-assisted and fully laparoscopic cases while showing a significant decrease in operative time (30 min for sigmoid colectomy and nearly 1 h for total colectomy) [38, 39]. While data is limited in the setting of reoperative cases, a surgeon may find the hand-assist port to be a good compromise, allowing for shorter surgery and better blunt dissection, mobilization, and retraction without putting the patient at increased risk for the complications of open laparotomy.

Several systems are available, including the GelPort® (Applied Medical, Rancho Santa Margarita, CA; Fig. 20.7) and HandPort® (Smith & Nephew, Inc., Endoscopy Division, Andover, MA) system and DEXTRUS device (Ethicon, Inc., Cincinnati, OH), all of which utilize a 7–9 cm lower midline or transverse (Pfannenstiel) incision. In cases of previous

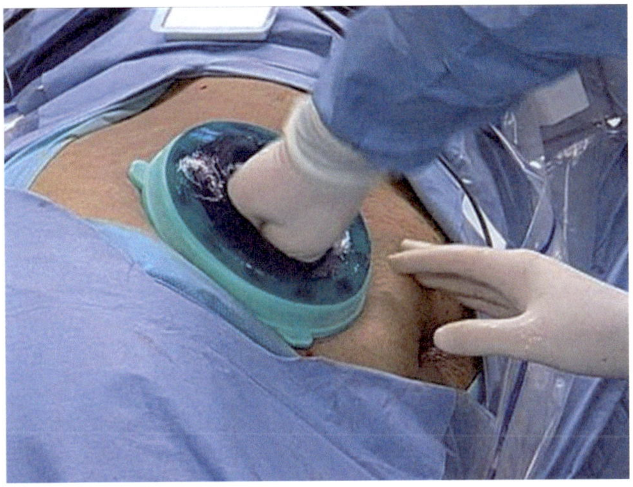

**Fig. 20.7** GelPort® (Applied Medical, Rancho Santa Margarita, CA) for hand-assisted laparoscopic surgery. *With permission from Applied Medical*

incision or potential adhesions, this location can be altered. This site can either be opened as the initial entry point into the abdomen or after laparoscopic adhesiolysis of the anterior abdominal wall. The hand-assist port is placed in the incision and the abdomen is insufflated. The surgeon's hand can then be used for blunt dissection, retraction, palpation, or hemostasis.

In especially complex cases where the surgeon continues to struggle despite placing a hand-assist port, the abdomen can be desufflated, and the port removed. The dissection can then be continued in an open fashion through the hand-assist port incision. After difficult adhesions have been lysed, the hand-assist port can be replaced, the abdomen re-insufflated, and the procedure continued laparoscopically. If, after using these methods, the surgeon still does not feel comfortable with the safety of his dissection, the hand port incision can easily be incorporated into the midline laparotomy incision, and the case can be completed using an open approach.

## Conversion to Open Procedure

Conversion to an open procedure has a known association with increased blood loss, operative time, time of return of bowel function, anastomotic insufficiency, and reoperation [40]; however, these results are likely confounded by the difficult anatomy of these patients and not necessarily related to the decision to convert. Limited data exists on the impact of early versus late conversion or the impact of starting laparoscopically in a difficult case that is eventually converted to an open procedure. However, it is clear that the outcomes are better if the conversion is preemptive rather than reactive to an intraoperative complication.

With a lack of evidence in this area, we fall back on classic surgical teaching, which would suggest that an early decision to convert to an open procedure when a lack of visualization or exposure make a laparoscopic approach hazardous is important to avoid prolonged operative times and elevated potential for abdominal organ injury. Although there are no clear guidelines about when to convert to an open procedure, factors such as operative time, blood loss, visualization, safety of future port placement, progress and difficulty of adhesiolysis, cardiopulmonary status of the patient, and the ability to perform an oncologically sound operation should all be frequently reevaluated during a complex surgery that is progressing slowly.

Although early conversion to an open procedure is recommended when the risks of laparoscopic abdominal entry or adhesiolysis are considered excessive, the conversion to an open approach will not necessarily solve the problems of a difficult procedure. Specific advantages of an open procedure, such as increased exposure and the ability to palpate structures and use fingers for blunt dissection, should be considered when contemplating a conversion to a laparotomy. If the open approach does not offer specific advantages to improve dissection in the case, then it may be prudent to continue cautiously with laparoscopic mobilization where the enhanced visualization of the camera can be advantageous. Especially in the morbidly obese patient, conversion to an open laparotomy does not necessarily translate to improved exposure, easier dissection, or improved outcomes, though HALS may provide specific advantages compared to straight laparoscopy in this select population [41].

## Specific Cases

### Ostomy Reversal

Ostomy reversals are obligatory reoperative cases. The advantages of laparoscopic approach have been well documented and include decreased blood loss, hospital stay, and rates of complications [42]. The complications of ostomy reversals are also well described. While laparoscopy may mitigate these complications, it does not eliminate them. With rates of morbidity that range from 10 % to 25 %, careful expectations must be set [42–44].

The visualization provided by the laparoscope can be helpful for all aspects of an ostomy reversal, from identifying blind ends of the bowel from a previous Hartmann's procedure to performing efficient, well-visualized takedown of the stoma. Once adhesions have been lysed and the bowel mobilized, the anastomosis can be performed in an intracorporeal fashion using a stapled or hand-sewn technique. Alternatively, if the anastomosis reaches the stoma site, the stoma can be taken down and the anastomosis performed

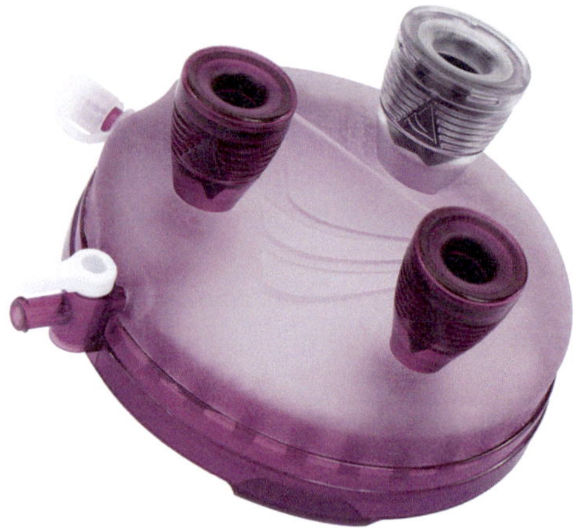

**Fig. 20.8** GelPOINT® access port (Applied Medical, Rancho Santa Margarita, CA) seals the abdominal wall for insufflation and allows introduction of laparoscopic instruments, converting an open case to a minimally invasive technique. *With permission from Applied Medical*

in an extracorporeal manner. As previously described, we recommend liberal use of ureteral stents for these cases, due to the common need for extensive dissection and mobilization.

Alternatively, the surgeon can begin the case by taking down the stoma in the standard, open fashion. Using the stoma site as a safe port of entry, the practitioner can lyse adhesion to the anterior abdominal wall around the site. Once adequate exposure has been achieved, the GelPOINT® Advanced Access Platform (Applied Medical, Rancho Santa Margarita, CA; Fig. 20.8) or similar device can be introduced to allow a seal for insufflation. Its ports allow for the introduction of laparoscopic instruments, and the case can be completed through the single incision. Additional trocars can also be placed as needed, and the stoma site converted to a hand-assist port for surgeons who feel more comfortable completing the case with a hand for dissection and retraction. The anastomosis can be performed laparoscopically or after simple exteriorization of the specimen through the ostomy site.

Even in cases of prior anastomosis and loop ostomy, some practitioners advocate the use of a laparoscopic approach to visualize the adhesions around the stoma for safer adhesiolysis, citing decreased wound infection and bowel obstruction rates, although similar overall complication rates [45]. In these cases, the bowel can be anastomosed in an extracorporeal fashion after the bowel is freed from the abdominal wall using direct visualization with the laparoscope. For more on the use of laparoscopy for stoma reversal, Dr. Gorgun provides a complete overview in Chap. 16.

## Colorectal Cancer

Because colorectal cancer cases are usually done in the absence of significant adhesive disease, substantial adhesiolysis during a cancer resection in reoperative cases can be a foreign experience for surgeons. In cases of previous non-colorectal surgery (i.e., low anterior resection after remote hysterectomy), the main complicating factor is the presence of adhesions and the way these adhesions alter the normal anatomy. As described above, great care must be taken in abdominal entry and adhesiolysis. Once adhesions have been taken down and the operative field has been appropriately exposed, mobilization of the specimen can remain challenging, due to the distortion of normal landmarks that allow identification of structures such as the ureters. Increased scarring may also make lymph node dissection more difficult. In addition, the reliability of using tattooing performed during colonoscopy to identify a lesion may be diminished if adhesions are dense in the area.

Another surgical challenge in colorectal cancer is the re-resection of a previously removed area of the colon or rectum. In the case of removing an area of positive margins or local cancer recurrence, all the previously mentioned challenges are present. In these cases, however, the anatomy is not just distorted but also is dramatically altered. Particularly if the surgeon who performed the original operation is no longer involved, orientation can be very challenging. Identification of prior resection and anastomosis sites may be a lengthy process, and mobilization of these areas particularly time-consuming. Additional mobilization may be required to allow for a tension-free anastomosis after resection, and this factor should be taken into consideration when planning the mobilization. Once the site has been identified and mobilized, surgery can proceed in the normal laparoscopic fashion.

## Diverticular Disease

Due to often repeated and sometimes prolonged episodes of inflammation associated with diverticular disease, these cases often involve considerable adhesions even without previous operation. While reoperative cases can pose the typical challenges associated with laparoscopic entry, adhesions, and anatomic distortions, literature supporting the use of minimally invasive techniques for this disease process is substantial, even in complicated cases such as stricture, abscess, or fistula [46–49]. Again, we strongly advocate the routine use of ureteral stents, particularly lighted stents for purely laparoscopic cases, in order to aid in ureter identification and injury recognition.

## IBD

In Crohn's disease, the presence of adhesions, even in the absence of prior surgery, makes the original and subsequent operations more alike. Numerous studies, including some with significant numbers of reoperative patients, have demonstrated the advantages of laparoscopic resection of

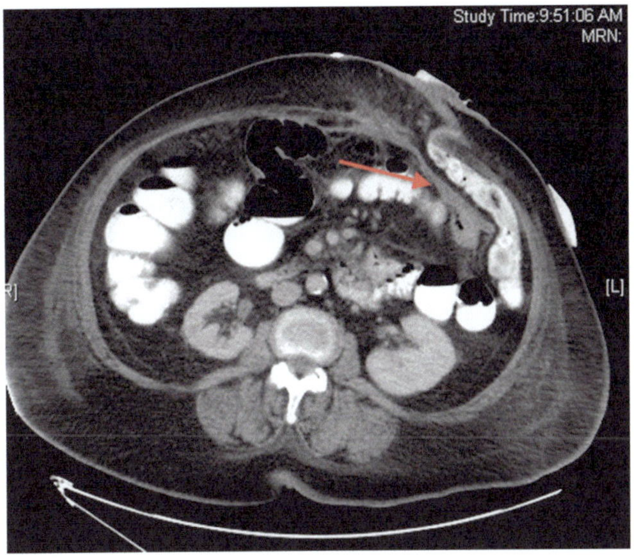


**Fig. 20.9** CT of a Sugarbaker colostomy repair demonstrating mesh (*arrow*) to the anterior abdominal wall

Crohn's complications, with shorter hospital stays and faster resumption of bowel function [6, 50–53]. Precautions for reoperative, minimally invasive surgery in these patients include those taken for any Crohn's patient, any reoperative patient, and any laparoscopic case.

In ulcerative colitis (UC), many patients will undergo an expected reoperation to establish bowel continuity after total proctocolectomy. Reports of laparoscopic ileoanal pouch anastomoses (IPAA), often performed in 2- or 3-stage procedures, have shown equivalent or improved outcomes, including improved rates of fertility [2, 5, 54]. Consideration of previous factors increasing the likelihood or density of adhesions, such as previous anastomotic leak or intra-abdominal abscess, is important for cases of reoperative laparoscopic IPAA or ostomy reversal to prove it is feasible and safe.

## Prior Hernia Repair

Prior ventral hernia repairs pose three challenges, the potential for dense adhesions to the mesh, difficult entry into the abdominal cavity, and possible contamination of incorporated mesh. While there is little data in the medical literature to guide decision-making in this patient population, it is preferable to avoid exposure of permanent mesh in these cases, due the possibility of contamination leading to infection and requiring subsequent excision. Unfortunately, cases with large sheets of mesh covering much of the anterior abdominal wall usually necessitate port placement (and sometimes specimen removal) through incorporated mesh (Fig. 20.9). Limited institutional experience would suggest that these cases can be accomplished successfully without the need for subsequent mesh excision due to contamination; however, the possibility of contamination should be discussed with the patient and form part of the risk-benefit analysis for surgery. As previously described, the abdomen should be inspected and the previous operative note reviewed in order to understand the size, position, and type of mesh previously used. Biologic or absorbable mesh placed remotely should have little impact on operative planning other than the increased potential for adhesions to the anterior abdominal wall. While it is preferable for laparoscopic port entry to be made away from the site of mesh placement, the surgeon should not perform any operation with suboptimal ports that puts the patient at increased risk for operative complications.

## Summary

Once considered a contraindication to minimally invasive surgery, reoperative cases in colorectal surgery now commonly enjoy the shorter hospital stays and reduced pain and complications from laparoscopic surgery. As laparoscopic skills and technology continue to improve, the need for conversion to an open approach will diminish. The use of laparoscopy in challenging reoperative cases can be performed safely and efficiently when the surgeon (1) selects patients and surgical plans with the aid of a careful history and physical examination, (2) breaks up the procedure into small steps with defined goals, (3) uses caution in planning and executing safe abdominal entry, (4) performs adhesiolysis with constant reassessment of potential structures in danger, (5) avoids the use of energy except on clearly defined structures, and (6) employs a variety of techniques to safely get through difficult parts of the procedure.

## References

1. Fleshman J, Sargent DJ, Green E, Anvari M, Stryker SJ, Beart Jr RW, et al. Laparoscopic colectomy for cancer is not inferior to open surgery based on 5-year data from the COST Study Group trial. Ann Surg. 2007;246(4):655–62. discussion 62-4. Epub 2007/09/26.
2. Bartels SA, D'Hoore A, Cuesta MA, Bensdorp AJ, Lucas C, Bemelman WA. Significantly increased pregnancy rates after laparoscopic restorative proctocolectomy: a cross-sectional study. Ann Surg. 2012;256(6):1045–8. Epub 2012/05/23.
3. Indar AA, Efron JE, Young-Fadok TM. Laparoscopic ileal pouch-anal anastomosis reduces abdominal and pelvic adhesions. Surg Endosc. 2009;23(1):174–7. Epub 2008/10/16.
4. Abraham NS, Young JM, Solomon MJ. Meta-analysis of short-term outcomes after laparoscopic resection for colorectal cancer. Br J Surg. 2004;91(9):1111–24. Epub 2004/09/28.
5. Dunker MS, Bemelman WA, Slors JF, van Duijvendijk P, Gouma DJ. Functional outcome, quality of life, body image, and cosmesis in patients after laparoscopic-assisted and conventional restorative proctocolectomy: a comparative study. Dis Colon Rectum. 2001; 44(12):1800–7. Epub 2001/12/14.

6. Wu JS, Birnbaum EH, Kodner IJ, Fry RD, Read TE, Fleshman JW. Laparoscopic-assisted ileocolic resections in patients with Crohn's disease: are abscesses, phlegmons, or recurrent disease contraindications? Surgery. 1997;122(4):682–8. discussion 8-9. Epub 1997/11/05.
7. Veldkamp R, Kuhry E, Hop WC, Jeekel J, Kazemier G, Bonjer HJ, et al. Laparoscopic surgery versus open surgery for colon cancer: short-term outcomes of a randomised trial. The lancet oncology. 2005;6(7):477–84. Epub 2005/07/05.
8. Weeks JC, Nelson H, Gelber S, Sargent D, Schroeder G. Short-term quality-of-life outcomes following laparoscopic-assisted colectomy vs open colectomy for colon cancer: a randomized trial. JAMA. 2002;287(3):321–8. Epub 2002/01/16.
9. Law WL, Lee YM, Chu KW. Previous abdominal operations do not affect the outcomes of laparoscopic colorectal surgery. Surg Endosc. 2005;19(3):326–30. Epub 2004/12/30.
10. Maggiori L, Cook MC, Bretagnol F, Ferron M, Alves A, Panis Y. Prior abdominal open surgery does not impair outcomes of laparoscopic colorectal surgery: a case-control study in 367 patients. Colorectal Dis. 2013;15(2):236–43. Epub 2012/06/29.
11. Franko J, O'Connell BG, Mehall JR, Harper SG, Nejman JH, Zebley DM, et al. The influence of prior abdominal operations on conversion and complication rates in laparoscopic colorectal surgery. JSLS. 2006;10(2):169–75. Epub 2006/08/03.
12. Binenbaum SJ, Goldfarb MA. Inadvertent enterotomy in minimally invasive abdominal surgery. JSLS. 2006;10(3):336–40. Epub 2007/01/11.
13. van der Voort M, Heijnsdijk EA, Gouma DJ. Bowel injury as a complication of laparoscopy. Br J Surg. 2004;91(10):1253–8. Epub 2004/09/18.
14. Szomstein S, Lo Menzo E, Simpfendorfer C, Zundel N, Rosenthal RJ. Laparoscopic lysis of adhesions. World J Surg. 2006;30(4): 535–40. Epub 2006/03/24.
15. Bhoyrul S, Vierra MA, Nezhat CR, Krummel TM, Way LW. Trocar injuries in Laparoscopic surgery. J Am Coll Surg. 2001;192(6): 677–83. Epub 2001/06/13.
16. Perrone JM, Soper NJ, Eagon JC, Klingensmith ME, Aft RL, Frisella MM, et al. Perioperative outcomes and complications of laparoscopic ventral hernia repair. Surgery. 2005;138(4):708–15. discussion 15-6. Epub 2005/11/05.
17. Van Der Krabben AA, Dijkstra FR, Nieuwenhuijzen M, Reijnen MM, Schaapveld M, Van Goor H. Morbidity and mortality of inadvertent enterotomy during adhesiotomy. Br J Surg. 2000; 87(4):467–71. Epub 2000/04/12.
18. van Goor H. Consequences and complications of peritoneal adhesions. Colorectal Dis. 2007;9 Suppl 2:25–34. Epub 2007/10/27.
19. Caprini JA, Arcelus JA, Swanson J, Coats R, Hoffman K, Brosnan JJ, et al. The ultrasonic localization of abdominal wall adhesions. Surg Endosc. 1995;9(3):283–5. Epub 1995/03/01.
20. Lang RA, Buhmann S, Hopman A, Steitz HO, Lienemann A, Reiser MF, et al. Cine-MRI detection of intraabdominal adhesions: correlation with intraoperative findings in 89 consecutive cases. Surg Endosc. 2008;22(11):2455–61. Epub 2008/03/07.
21. Zinther NB, Zeuten A, Marinovskij E, Haislund M, Friis-Andersen H. Detection of abdominal wall adhesions using visceral slide. Surg Endosc. 2010;24(12):3161–6. Epub 2010/05/22.
22. DeCherney AH. diZerega GS. Clinical problem of intraperitoneal postsurgical adhesion formation following general surgery and the use of adhesion prevention barriers. Surg Clin North Am. 1997; 77(3):671–88.
23. diZerega GS. Biochemical events in peritoneal tissue repair. Eur J Surg Suppl. 1997;577:10–6. Epub 1997/01/01.
24. Fabri PJ, Rosemurgy A. Reoperation for small intestinal obstruction. Surg Clin North Am. 1991;71(1):131–46. Epub 1991/02/01.
25. Jobanputra S, Wexner SD. Systematic guide to complex cases from adhesive disease. Colorectal Dis. 2007;9 Suppl 2:54–9. Epub 2007/10/27.
26. Schafer M, Lauper M, Krahenbuhl L. Trocar and Veress needle injuries during laparoscopy. Surg Endosc. 2001;15(3):275–80. Epub 2001/05/19.
27. Ahmad G, O'Flynn H, Duffy JM, Phillips K, Watson A. Laparoscopic entry techniques. Cochrane Database Syst Rev. 2012;2, CD006583. Epub 2012/02/18.
28. Bonjer HJ, Hazebroek EJ, Kazemier G, Giuffrida MC, Meijer WS, Lange JF. Open versus closed establishment of pneumoperitoneum in laparoscopic surgery. Br J Surg. 1997;84(5):599–602. Epub 1997/05/01.
29. Gersin KS, Heniford BT, Arca MJ, Ponsky JL. Alternative site entry for laparoscopy in patients with previous abdominal surgery. Journal Laparoendosc Adv Surg Tech Part A. 1998;8(3):125–30. Epub 1998/07/29.
30. Agarwala N, Liu CY. Safe entry techniques during laparoscopy: left upper quadrant entry using the ninth intercostal space–a review of 918 procedures. J Minim Invasive Gynecol. 2005;12(1):55–61. Epub 2005/05/21.
31. Rabl C, Palazzo F, Aoki H, Campos GM. Initial laparoscopic access using an optical trocar without pneumoperitoneum is safe and effective in the morbidly obese. Surg Innov. 2008;15(2):126–31. Epub 2008/05/16.
32. Fuller J, Ashar BS, Carey-Corrado J. Trocar-associated injuries and fatalities: an analysis of 1399 reports to the FDA. J Minim Invasive Gynecol. 2005;12(4):302–7. Epub 2005/07/23.
33. Read TE, Salgado J, Ferraro D, Fortunato R, Caushaj PF. "Peek port": a novel approach for avoiding conversion in laparoscopic colectomy. Surg Endosc. 2009;23(3):477–81. Epub 2008/07/16.
34. Bothwell WN, Bleicher RJ, Dent TL. Prophylactic ureteral catheterization in colon surgery. A five-year review. Dis Colon Rectum. 1994;37(4):330–4. Epub 1994/04/01.
35. Tsujinaka S, Wexner SD, DaSilva G, Sands DR, Weiss EG, Nogueras JJ, et al. Prophylactic ureteric catheters in laparoscopic colorectal surgery. Tech Coloproctol. 2008;12(1):45–50. Epub 2008/05/31.
36. Senagore AJ, Luchtefeld M. An initial experience with lighted ureteral catheters during laparoscopic colectomy. J Laparoendosc Surg. 1994;4(6):399–403. Epub 1994/12/01.
37. Tou S, Malik AI, Wexner SD, Nelson RL. Energy source instruments for laparoscopic colectomy. Cochrane Database Syst Rev. 2011;5, CD007886. Epub 2011/05/13.
38. HALS Study Group. Hand-assisted laparoscopic surgery vs standard laparoscopic surgery for colorectal disease: a prospective randomized trial. Surg Endosc. 2000;14(10):896–901. Epub 2000/11/18.
39. Marcello PW, Fleshman JW, Milsom JW, Read TE, Arnell TD, Birnbaum EH, et al. Hand-assisted laparoscopic vs. laparoscopic colorectal surgery: a multicenter, prospective, randomized trial. Dis Colon Rectum. 2008;51(6):818–26.
40. Scheidbach H, Garlipp B, Oberlander H, Adolf D, Kockerling F, Lippert H. Conversion in laparoscopic colorectal cancer surgery: impact on short- and long-term outcome. J Laparoendosc Adv Surg Tech Part A. 2011;21(10):923–7. Epub 2011/10/21.
41. Heneghan HM, Martin ST, Kiran RP, Khoury W, Stocchi L, Remzi FH, et al. Laparoscopic colorectal surgery for obese patients: decreased conversions with the hand-assisted technique. J Gastrointest Surg. 2013;17(3):548–54. Epub 2012/11/29.
42. Siddiqui MR, Sajid MS, Baig MK. Open vs laparoscopic approach for reversal of Hartmann's procedure: a systematic review. Colorectal Dis. 2010;12(8):733–41. Epub 2010/07/24.
43. Kaiser AM, Israelit S, Klaristenfeld D, Selvindoss P, Vukasin P, Ault G, et al. Morbidity of ostomy takedown. J Gastrointest Surg. 2008;12(3):437–41. Epub 2007/12/21.
44. Rosen MJ, Cobb WS, Kercher KW, Sing RF, Heniford BT. Laparoscopic restoration of intestinal continuity after Hartmann's procedure. Am J Surg. 2005;189(6):670–4. Epub 2005/05/25.

45. Russek K, George JM, Zafar N, Cuevas-Estandia P, Franklin M. Laparoscopic loop ileostomy reversal: reducing morbidity while improving functional outcomes. JSLS. 2011;15(4):475–9. Epub 2012/05/31.
46. O'Sullivan GC, Murphy D, O'Brien MG, Ireland A. Laparoscopic management of generalized peritonitis due to perforated colonic diverticula. Am J Surg. 1996;171(4):432–4.
47. Sher ME, Agachan F, Bortul M, Nogueras JJ, Weiss EG, Wexner SD. Laparoscopic surgery for diverticulitis. Surg Endosc. 1997;11(3):264–7. Epub 1997/03/01.
48. Siddiqui MR, Sajid MS, Khatri K, Cheek E, Baig MK. Elective open versus laparoscopic sigmoid colectomy for diverticular disease: a meta-analysis with the Sigma trial. World J Surg. 2010; 34(12):2883–901. Epub 2010/08/18.
49. Kockerling F, Schneider C, Reymond MA, Scheidbach H, Scheuerlein H, Konradt J, et al. Laparoscopic resection of sigmoid diverticulitis. Results of a multicenter study. Laparoscopic Colorectal Surgery Study Group. Surg Endosc. 1999;13(6):567–71. Epub 1999/05/29.
50. Schmidt CM, Talamini MA, Kaufman HS, Lilliemoe KD, Learn P, Bayless T. Laparoscopic surgery for Crohn's disease: reasons for conversion. Ann Surg. 2001;233(6):733–9. Epub 2001/05/24.
51. Soop M, Larson DW, Malireddy K, Cima RR, Young-Fadok TM, Dozois EJ. Safety, feasibility, and short-term outcomes of laparoscopically assisted primary ileocolic resection for Crohn's disease. Surg Endosc. 2009;23(8):1876–81. Epub 2009/02/03.
52. Tilney HS, Constantinides VA, Heriot AG, Nicolaou M, Athanasiou T, Ziprin P, et al. Comparison of laparoscopic and open ileocecal resection for Crohn's disease: a metaanalysis. Surg Endosc. 2006;20(7):1036–44. Epub 2006/05/23.
53. Vangeenberghe N, De Vogelaere K, Haentjens P, Delvaux G. Laparoscopically assisted ileocolectomy in patients with Crohn's disease: a study of 50 consecutive patients. Surg Endosc. 2009; 23(8):1797–801. Epub 2008/12/11.
54. Ouaissi M, Alves A, Bouhnik Y, Valleur P, Panis Y. Three-step ileal pouch-anal anastomosis under total laparoscopic approach for acute or severe colitis complicating inflammatory bowel disease. J Am Coll Surg. 2006;202(4):637–42. Epub 2006/03/31.

# 21 Overcoming Technical Challenges: Prevention and Managing Complications

Bradley R. Davis

**Key Points**

- The insertion of the initial trocar offers the biggest potential for injury, and reliance on only one technique has potential for harm. Knowledge of an open technique and a percutaneous technique will allow the surgeon the most versatility in accessing the abdomen.
- Enterotomy, serosal, and thermal injuries are a part of complex laparoscopy and a strategy must exist to deal with them. For enterotomies, the decision should be made immediately if the procedure needs to be converted to minimize contamination. Serosal and thermal injuries should be dealt with as soon as they are recognized, as they may not be able to be found later in the case.
- While several anastomotic techniques are utilized, adhering to the traditional principles of proper tissue handling, ensuring adequate blood supply, and avoiding tension remain essential to optimizing outcomes.
- Methods for creating adequate length for a technically sound left-sided bowel anastomosis include proper mobilization of the splenic flexure and mesentery, division of the inferior mesenteric vein near the ligament of Treitz, ligation of the inferior mesenteric artery, and rectal mobilization (when applicable).
- You should have a stepwise and thorough algorithm for troubleshooting the difficult anastomosis.
- With more operations being performed through minimally invasive approaches, laparoscopic techniques for mobilizing the colon and maintaining optimal visualization are vital to minimizing complications.
- Leak testing is a critical component to left-sided anastomoses, and you should understand what to do with a positive leak test or incomplete doughnuts.

**Electronic supplementary material:** Supplementary material is available in the online version of this chapter at 10.1007/978-1-4939-1581-1_21. Videos can also be accessed at http://www.springerimages.com/videos/978-1-4939-1580-4.

B.R. Davis, M.D. (✉)
Department of Surgery, University of Cincinnati Medical Center, 231 Albert Sabin Way, ML 0058, Cincinnati, OH 45267, USA
e-mail: davisbd@ucmail.uc.edu; bradley.davis@uc.edu

## Introduction

The practice of surgery requires a broad skill set with ever-increasing demands on our technical abilities. The application of advanced laparoscopic procedures in the management of colorectal disease has provided significant opportunities for our patients while at the same time ongoing challenges in the operating room. The development of new technology is constant and pushes the surgeon to learn new things regularly and perform procedures that may not have been part of initial surgical training. As a result, there are going to be instances when complications and technical misadventures occur, but insight into prevention of these complications remains the most effective strategy.

## Trocar Insertion

***Key Concept: The risk of injury is greatest with the initial trocar insertion, and the operator should be an expert with several different techniques for introduction of the initial trocar into the abdomen.***

One of the earliest opportunities for injury occurs during trocar insertion into the abdomen. The initial trocar insertion will provide the greatest opportunity for a bad outcome, and as such several different techniques have been described [1]. These include an open technique, a blind technique using the Veress needle, and an optical technique using specialized trocars that allow visualization of the layers of the abdominal wall using the laparoscope (Video 21.1). Mastery of one of these techniques is essential for safe access to the abdomen, and knowledge of more than one is essential to keep the operating surgeon and the patient out of trouble; however, no one technique has been shown to be superior with potential

H.M. Ross et al. (eds.), *Minimally Invasive Approaches to Colon and Rectal Disease: Technique and Best Practices*, DOI 10.1007/978-1-4939-1581-1_21, © Springer Science+Business Media New York 2015

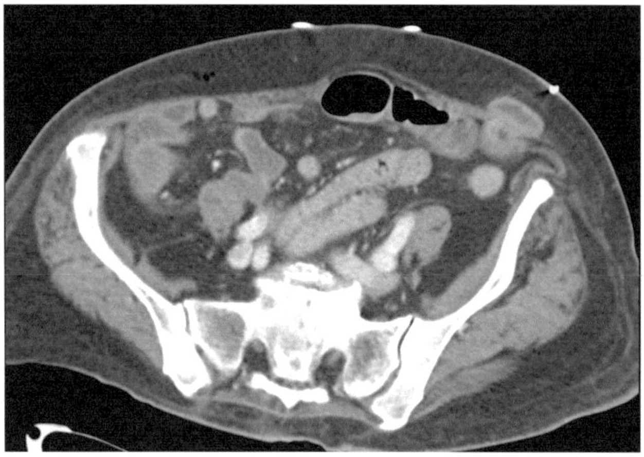

**Fig. 21.1** CT scan demonstrating a port-site hernia

pros and cons of each [2, 3]. A recent review including 28 randomized controlled trials with 4,860 individuals undergoing laparoscopy demonstrated no advantage using any single technique in terms of preventing major vascular or visceral complications. Using an open-entry technique compared to a Veress needle demonstrated a reduction in the incidence of failed entry (OR = 0.12; 95 % CI 0.02 to 0.92). There were three advantages with direct trocar entry when compared with Veress needle entry, in terms of lower rates of failed entry (OR = 0.21; 95 % CI 0.14 to 0.31), extra-peritoneal insufflation (OR = 0.18; 95 % CI 0.13 to 0.26), and omental injury (OR = 0.28; 95 % CI 0.14 to 0.55).

Advocates of the open technique regard this as the safest and most effective means to place the initial trocar [4], although there are some limitations. It is very difficult to keep the skin incisions smaller than 1 cm, and larger trocars (11 or 12 mm) are generally needed to prevent loss of pneumoperitoneum during the case. It is not always desirable or necessary to have a 12 mm trocar, particularly in the midline, and placing a trocar using an open technique off midline is difficult in all but the thinnest patients. Additionally, while acute and chronic herniation can occur through trocars as small as 5 mm [5], it is generally acceptable to close the fascial defect of trocars larger than 12 mm [6, 7] resulting in longer overall time using an open technique. Complications associated with the open technique include enterotomy, vascular and solid organ injury, as well as acute and chronic herniation, which in the immediate postoperative period can result in bowel obstruction (Fig. 21.1) and need for emergent repair. In the obese patient, it can be very difficult to visualize the fascia through a small skin incision, and if necessary, it should be enlarged to ensure an adequate closure. It's probably best to avoid this technique altogether in the significantly obese patients as the abdominal wall thickness will preclude adequate fascial visualization without a generous skin incision.

The Veress needle is an alternative to the open technique and can be used alone or in conjunction with an optical view technique. Traditionally, Veress needles are 14 gauge in size and are spring-loaded so that when resistance is met, the blunt end retracts into the needlepoint and tissues such as fascia and peritoneum can be traversed without significant trauma. The operator must feel the needle insert into the peritoneal cavity and discontinue advancing once the requisite number of "pops" is felt and no further resistance is encountered. When centered on the midline, the operator will experience two points of resistance (the midline fascia and the peritoneum), with the latter causing the spring mechanism to "pop" as resistance is encountered and the needle abruptly discontinued (corresponding to the needle traversing the peritoneum and entering the peritoneal cavity). Confirmation of safe access is determined by water drop test in which saline is introduced into the end of the Veress needle, which if correctly placed will passively flow into the abdomen due to the lower intraperitoneal pressure relative to the atmosphere. I find this test to be finicky and prefer to simply connect the insufflation tubing set on a flow rate of 3 L/m and assess my opening pressures as determined by the insufflator. The initial opening pressure should be low single digit or zero mmHg but will correlate with the patient's body mass index [8]. Anything higher in a patient who is not morbidly obese indicates that the needle is not in the correct location and insufflation should be terminated immediately and the needle repositioned or an alternative method of initial access should be pursued. Veress needles can be used in the midline, but for re-operative surgery (in which the midline has been used), an off-midline technique can be employed. Proponents of this technique recommend the left upper quadrant (Palmer's point) as the preferred site [9] as there is relatively little that can be injured here. In contrast, the liver edge often obscures the right upper quadrant, while the lower quadrants risk bowel and vascular injury and are less desirable locations. Many surgeons will want to elevate the abdominal wall when using this technique, but this may make it more difficult by pulling up on the skin and creating a long distance between the underlying fascia and the skin entry site. Many bariatric surgeons recommend not elevating the skin and simply inserting the needle. The same haptic feedback is achieved irrespective of skin elevation, and it won't be necessary to insert the full length of the needle to gain access into the peritoneum in someone with a lot of subcutaneous fat.

Injuries associated with the Veress needle entry encompass the entire spectrum of bad things that can occur with initial trocar injury—vascular, bowel, bladder, solid organ, and air embolism have all been described [2]. The key to success in using a Veress needle is experience and discipline. Multiple passes should never be needed to gain access, and the entire length of the needle (usually 12–15 cm) should rarely be needed to reach the peritoneal cavity.

The optical view technique or direct trocar insertion is newer than either the Veress or open Hasson techniques and relies on the clear plastic material of most modern trocars. A zero-degree laparoscope should always be used inside the trocar and the focus should be adjusted so that it is just beyond the tip of the trocar. Elevating the abdominal wall is not necessary and can be detrimental in an obese patient, as the trocar length will not traverse the abdominal fat. The layers of the abdominal wall can be visualized as the bladeless obturator passes through (Video 21.1). When used in conjunction with the Veress needle, the operator will have no difficulty identifying the peritoneal cavity as it will be insufflated with gas (Video 21.1). If the optical view technique is to be used without establishing pneumoperitoneum beforehand, the surgeon must be experienced in identifying the layers of the abdominal wall as seen through the trocar [10]. Otherwise, even experienced surgeons who do not routinely use this technique can find themselves below the omentum or pre-peritoneal (Video 21.2).

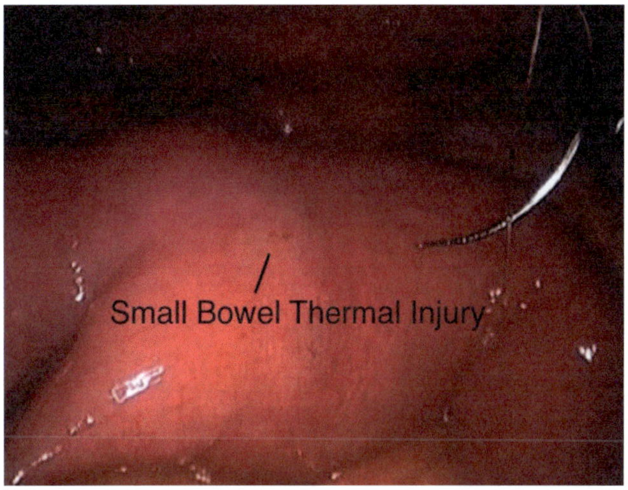


**Fig. 21.2** A thermal injury is identified on the small bowel antimesenteric surface. Notice that there is a degree of blanching with some very small visible burn formation. This may not have created any problems but it is safer to be proactive when dealing with these types of injuries

## Enterotomy, Serosal, and Thermal Injuries

***Key Concept: Enterotomies can and will occur during laparoscopy. Initial trocar entry is a risk as is lysing adhesions in a re-operative abdomen. Immediate control and repair or resection is necessary to limit contamination.***

Enterotomies can and will occur during the conduct of laparoscopic abdominal surgery. There is a risk of bowel injury associated with the initial trocar access which has been estimated between 0.5 and 0.7 % [11, 12]. Re-operative surgery also increases the risk of an enterotomy, and during re-operative colectomies, the risk is estimated to be less than 1 %; however, this is still significantly higher than the incidence when operating on a virgin abdomen [13]. When dealing with inter-loop small bowel and pelvic adhesions, the use of sharp dissection technique is preferred to avoid injury resulting from energy and heat (Video 21.3). Inadvertent bowel or serosal injuries can often be repaired if a result of sharp dissection when the true extent of the injury can be determined. It is imperative that once an enterotomy is made, it is identified and repaired immediately (Video 21.4). This will avoid any unnecessary contamination and spillage as well as the risk of not being able to find it later in the procedure. If the surgeon is not comfortable evaluating and closing the enterotomy laparoscopically, a small abdominal incision can be made and it can be repaired extracorporeally. Prior to exteriorization, the bowel should be tagged to facilitate identification of the injury.

Intestinal injury can also occur off-camera, and great care should be taken to avoid forcing an instrument into the operative field as it may be caught up in the small bowel. This is particularly true when the patient is positioned in either extremes of Trendelenburg or airplaned in either direction. In addition, when using energy sources, heat is generated on the blade of the instrument that can cause small bowel injury both on and off the camera as the instrument is withdrawn. Care should be taken when removing any instrument that is potentially hot, and it is good practice to allow the instrument to cool prior to removing.

A relatively common scenario during laparoscopy is an inadvertent serosal or thermal injury. It is our practice to repair serosal injuries irrespective of laparoscopy using a 3-0 Vicryl Lembert suture. It is important that this be done as soon as they are recognized, as they can be difficult to relocate after even a few minutes (Video 21.4). This is particularly true during a laparoscopic case where inspecting the entire bowel can be much more labor intensive than in open surgery. The utility of oversewing serosal injuries is not well studied, but animal models have failed to identify any benefit [14]. It is likely that very superficial injuries occur frequently and go unrepaired without detriment to the patient, but in the absence of demonstrable harm, we suggest repairing recognized serosal injuries for fear of delayed intestinal perforation and leaks. It is also important to recognize thermal injuries (Fig. 21.2), which can occur during use of electrosurgical devices and bipolar and ultrasonic energy devices. It is estimated that such injuries occur between 0.6 and 3 times per 1,000 cases [15]. Electrothermal injury may result from direct application, insulation failure, direct coupling, and capacitive coupling. Direct application is probably the most common and easiest to recognize. Once again, it is important to immediately evaluate the injury and decide if it necessitates repair. Finding the injury at a later time will prove difficult irrespective of laparoscopy. The decision to oversew these injuries will depend on the operator's judgment as to whether the bowel wall integrity has been compromised. Coagulation burns are deeper than those caused by a blended or cutting current [16], and injuries that blanch white have usually gotten hot enough to cause protein denaturation, but may not result in full-thickness injury. As a rule, if the injury is a result of a very short burst of energy and there is minimal tissue change, no further intervention is required.

## Bleeding: Intra-abdominal and Pelvic

***Key Concept: There are a variety of options for ligating blood vessels intracorporeally, and the surgeon should master one of these instruments and then have a plan for when they fail. All methods for ligating blood vessels are capable of failing.***

The development of reliable energy sources to ligate major vascular pedicles has been a critical step in moving laparoscopic colorectal surgery toward the mainstream. Surgeons now have a reliable method of dividing large (up to 7 mm) vessels and with this the opportunity to encounter major bleeding, both during and following surgery which may challenge the laparoscopist more so than during open surgery. When major bleeding occurs, the laparoscopic surgeon must rely not only on their skill but also those of a talented assistant. Certainly, silk and Vicryl ties can fall off of major arteries and veins, but controlling bleeding during an open surgery is generally less difficult when compared to laparoscopy, and the operator will need to have a skill set and a plan of action when major bleeding occurs during the conduct of a laparoscopic case.

The current choices for vascular ligation include laparoscopic staplers, clip appliers, bipolar energy, and radiofrequency (ultrasonic) shears or some variation of these themes. In general, the bipolar products have similar performance characteristics and are approved for 7 mm vessel ligation [17]. Many authors have favorably compared ultrasonic devices with bipolar energy, although the vessel indication is smaller (5 mm) and may result in longer operative time and greater blood loss when compared to bipolar devices [18–20].

The use of monopolar electrocautery is appropriate for dissecting in the avascular anatomic planes, but will not be effective in dealing with any vessel of significant size. The use of clips on mesentery and vascular pedicles has largely been abandoned, as they are inferior to the other readily available options [19, 21, 22].

It is preferable to be facile with one technology, as repetitive use will result in less bleeding from erroneous application. The cost-effectiveness of staplers vs. energy devices has been evaluated [20], and it is my practice to use staplers to divide the pedicle only if I plan to divide the bowel intracorporeally—a situation in which I would not open any energy device. All energy devices generate heat and have some degree of thermal spread. It is important to be mindful of this when exchanging instruments or when dividing tissue near important structures that are being preserved. It is also critical to avoid tension when ligating major vessels, as this can result in inadequate tissue sealing and bleeding. Arteries that are heavily calcified may not seal with energy due to the inability of the proteins to coagulate and an alternate approach may be preferable in this situation. Fortunately when energy devices fail, they tend to do so immediately and delayed bleeding and take backs for vessels that were clearly sealed at the initial operation are rare [23].

When bleeding does occur, the most important initial step is to gain proximal control—an attempt to clip or ligate a bleeding mesenteric or named arterial vessel without first controlling the source will be unlikely to work and can result in injury to important structures (Video 21.5). A Maryland grasper works well for this purpose and it is a good instrument to have on the Mayo stand at all times. It is good practice to abandon the technique that resulted in the bleeding and to proceed directly to an ENDOLOOP® (3-0 PDS™ II works well in this situation, Ethicon Endo-Surgery, Cincinnati, OH). Reattempting to seal a vessel that is bleeding using energy may work, but if the proximal side is short and near the mesenteric root, the stakes for failure can be very high. This is particularly true when dealing with bleeding venous structures, as they can be very unforgiving. It is my practice to always divide the inferior mesenteric vein a few centimeters distal from the duodenum in the event that if it does bleed, it can be controlled. If it is ligated very short, it may retract behind the pancreas and can rarely be salvaged laparoscopically.

When bleeding is somewhat diffuse and the source is difficult to identify, the operator has a few options—the laparoscopic suction irrigator can be difficult to use for this purpose, as it will often become occluded with tissue. Vaginal packing works well in this situation—cut to 15–20 cm strips, it can be introduced through a 12 mm trocar and act as a sponge and can be used in concert with the suction irrigator (Video 21.6). Additionally, nasal packing strips are a similar size and can be easily placed down a standard size trocar. Care should be taken to remove either right away. A sponge can also be used but will be more likely to fray and may not retain its radiopaque strip when cut. A laparotomy pad can be introduced through a hand port without much difficulty and is also a nice way to clear the field. It is imperative to remain calm during bleeding that is difficult to control. It is appropriate to attempt laparoscopic control because the time required to turn the lights on, get the nursing staff oriented, open the patient, and isolate the bleeding will typically result in more blood loss. Therefore, compress the site of bleeding with a sponge, and if it is not possible to isolate, then maintain the pressure to stem the bleeding during conversion.

Pelvic bleeding can be a source of considerable hemorrhage in both open and laparoscopic surgery. Control of presacral bleeding can be accomplished laparoscopically [24] through a variety of techniques (Video 21.7) including a welding technique using the rectus muscle of epiploic fat. The use of bovine pericardium has also been described applied to the bleeding site with a spiral tacker. The best strategy is to stay in the correct planes posteriorly and use an energy device laterally to divide the lateral stalks and peritoneum. This will keep the field dry and maintain the critical exposure, which can be difficult in a narrow pelvis.

On rare occasions when pulsatile bleeding strikes the camera, the operative field will be totally obscured—creating a situation that is particularly unnerving. It is important to determine the significance of the bleeding (omental vessel vs. IMA) and to deal with it as quickly as possible. Typically the camera operator is the least experienced surgeon or student involved in the case, and the senior surgeon must quickly take control of the situation. There is no point in proceeding until the visualization of the field can be restored; therefore, the first priority is to clear the lens by removing the laparoscope. Blood in the trocar will frustrate any attempts at good visualization, and if it cannot be cleared quickly, therefore, an alternate trocar should be chosen for the camera as long as it provides good exposure to the bleeding vessel. Alternatively, a 5 mm trocar can be upsized to accommodate a 10 mm laparoscope, which will be less temperamental in the face of blood and debris. Once the operative view has been restored, an assessment of the bleeding can be made and dealt with appropriately. When necessary, an additional 5 mm trocar can be inserted to provide a point of entry for additional instruments or an ENDOLOOP®. Never allow the lack of an additional 5 mm or 10 mm trocar to result in a conversion, advice that is often lost in the stress of the situation.

## Anastomotic Leak

***Key Concept: The most important intraoperative predictors of a healthy anastomosis are adequate blood supply and absence of tension. In the event that either of these is not achieved, the laparoscopic surgeon will need to decide if converting the case will offer a better chance of success. A technically perfect anastomosis requires intimate knowledge of the tools being used.***

There are innumerable studies looking at the risk factors and strategies to prevent anastomotic complications with some general themes that are consistent. Prevention of leak starts with a meticulous surgical technique, and surgeons can have the biggest impact on prevention of anastomotic complications by ensuring that the blood supply to the anastomosis is intact and that there is no tension across the anastomosis. While there is little in the way of data to support the latter assertion, there is a host of newer data correlating the oxygen tension in the mucosa of the bowel with rates of anastomotic leak. Testing the effect of tension across anastomosis has been done in animal models with demonstration of decrease of mucosal blood flow in the face of increasing tension. The presence of mechanical forces attempting to disrupt anastomosis does not require a study to demonstrate poor outcomes. The surgeon should do whatever is necessary to make sure that the bowel that is being joined together does so easily and without tension. The risk of leak for a right colon anastomosis should be very low, as blood supply and tension should never be an issue. Care should be taken to avoid the "180-degree twist" that is unfortunately easier to do than believed with side-to-side anastomosis and can result in kinking in the blood supply. For a left colectomy, both blood supply and tension can be problematic. The surgeon's decision to ligate the inferior mesenteric artery at its origin will have an impact on the blood supply to the subsequent conduit. If the descending colon or transverse colon is to be used as the conduit, the impact is mitigated. With the sigmoid colon, the marginal blood supply off of the middle colic may not be adequate to perfuse such a long conduit [25, 26]. If it is necessary to use the sigmoid colon as part of the colorectal or coloanal anastomosis, the left colic artery should be preserved [27, 28]. Length can be achieved by completely mobilizing the attachments of the left colon to the retroperitoneum and flexure. The other critical aspect to obtaining adequate bowel length is mobilizing the mesentery, which will tether the left colon into the abdomen unless it is freed. To gain additional length, the inferior mesenteric vein (IMV) must be ligated adjacent to the IMA and a second time at the inferior border of the pancreas just lateral to the ligament of Treitz (Fig. 21.3). Ligating the vein twice while carefully preserving the marginal artery at the splenic flexure will add several centimeters to the length of the conduit while preserving arterial blood supply. A common error in an effort to gain length is to divide the colonic mesentery up toward the splenic flexure of the colon, with the end result cutting off the blood supply to the distal conduit, which is now based on the middle colic artery. If the marginal blood supply is compromised due to inadvertent injury while mobilizing the flexure or wandering too close the mesenteric border during ligation of the mesentery, the conduit will become ischemic and very likely unusable. As a general rule, if the cut edge of the mesentery traversing the pelvic brim is too tight to allow a finger (or a laparoscopic 5 mm grasper) to easily slip underneath (Fig. 21.4), the anastomosis is at risk since the blood supply is under tension—even if the bowel ends appear to approximate easily without tension. Every effort should then be made to lengthen the mesentery, even if this has already been attempted, as often reassessment will identify a small adhesion to release. In general, if the mesentery is lax, there

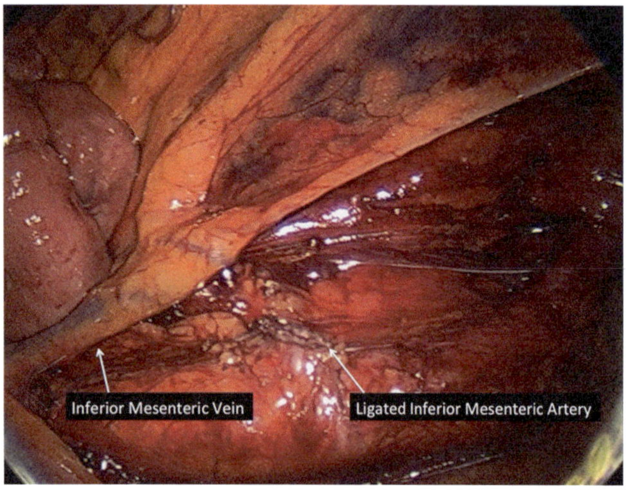


**Fig. 21.3** The inferior mesenteric vein terminate in the splenic vein and will not be paired with the artery close to this location which can tether the conduit making it difficult for the anastomosis to be created without tension. The vein can be located in this location near the ligament of Treitz and ligated with clips, staplers, or energy

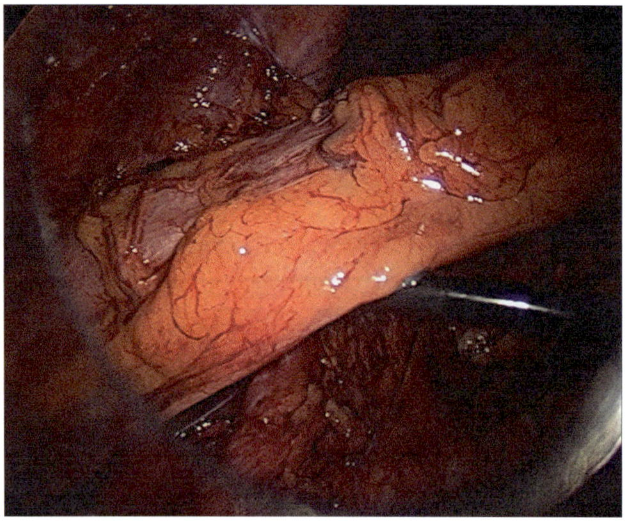

**Fig. 21.4** In this figure the conduit can be seen traversing the pelvic inlet and a grasper can easily slip below without tension

is likely no tension at the anastomosis. In those cases where only a few centimeters would allow less tension on the anastomosis, distal mobilization of the rectum to elevate it out of the pelvic hollow can also be a useful maneuver.

There are unfortunately times when despite fully mobilizing both the mesentery and the left colon, the conduit simply won't reach the pelvis. This can be due to a number of factors but is usually associated with a short fatty mesentery. You then find yourself in a situation where gaining length means dividing more mesentery (often the transverse mesocolon), which can result in further ischemia to the conduit and need for more length. There are limited options when this occurs—perform a total colectomy and an ileorectal anastomosis or rotate the right colon 180 degrees around the ileocolic pedicle in an effort to preserve the ileocecal valve. The latter option referred to as the Deloyers procedure [29] has proven successful, although a comparison to an ileorectal anastomosis has not been reported (Fig. 21.5a,b). Presumably the simplicity of an ileorectal anastomosis in cases where the entire rectum is preserved would outweigh the benefits of preserving the right colon. However, if part of the rectum has been resected, then the functional results of an ileorectal anastomosis are likely to be poor, and the Deloyers procedure would obviate the need for a permanent ostomy. The blood supply for this procedure is dependent on the ileocolic artery, and all mesenteric attachments of the ascending colon should be divided, being careful to preserve the marginal vessel adjacent to the right colon. The colonic segment is then rotated clockwise and anastomosed to the rectum. A window in the ileal mesentery has also been described, but is not necessary, as the colon will be situated anterior to the small bowel with this maneuver. Manceau et al. described their experience with this procedure in 48 consecutive cases [30] with a median follow-up of 26 months. There were no anastomotic leaks in this series, although 65 % of the patients had a temporary diverting ileostomy.

An immediate test of an anastomosis to assess for an air leak is easily performed for colorectal and left-sided resections and may help prevent or identify anastomotic leaks [31–33]. Some authors advocate endoscopic evaluation as bleeding from the staple line can also be identified [34], although the clinical significance of this intervention is less clear than an air leak test [35]. The advantage of the endoscopic evaluation of the anastomosis during laparoscopy is the confirmation that the bowel is in fact distended—this can be more difficult when occluding the bowel with a laparoscopic grasper as the haptic feedback will be missing and it is not always evident that the bowel is distended under pressure. If an air leak is identified or some other problem with the anastomosis (serosal separation, bleeding), then a laparoscopic repair is feasible [34, 35] if the surgeon has the skill sets (Video 21.8). Intracorporeal suturing can be accomplished more easily if the anastomosis is in the upper rectum and can be attempted before converting to an open or hand-assisted case. In addition to the air leak test, the anastomotic doughnuts should be inspected for completeness. Although the correlation between incomplete doughnuts and anastomotic integrity is uncertain, it will help the surgeon in the decision-making process when an air leak does occur. Regardless of the manufacturer, all of the staplers have a failure rate, and more importantly, when device failure occurs, the surgeon must have a plan to salvage the anastomosis. The exact incidence of failure is difficult to establish, but in 2007 Mardestein et al. reported on 1,188 stapler misfires reported to the FDA during a 12-month period [36]. Of the misfires, 588 occurred during colorectal procedures with failure to form staples and an inability to remove the

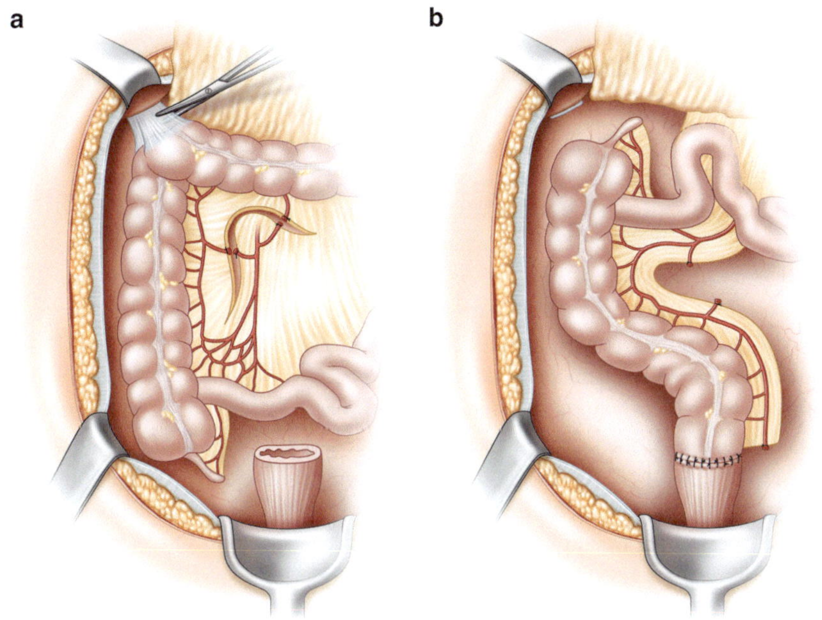


**Fig. 21.5** Deloyers procedure. (**a**) The attachments to the right colon are taken down and the vessels are divided as shown. (**b**) The right colon is rotated 180 degrees around the ileocolic pedicle in an effort to preserve the ileocecal valve, and anastomosis is performed

stapler as the most common problem. From these adverse events, 266 occurred during rectal resections and 80 were considered major, resulting in 23 unplanned permanent ostomies. Stapler misfire during a laparoscopic procedure was associated with a 43 % conversion rate. This high rate of conversion to open surgery following stapler misfire was confirmed by Pandya et al. in their analysis of 200 consecutive laparoscopic colectomies [37].

It is unknown how many of these failures were surgeon-related, but it is imperative that everyone involved in the case has intimate familiarity with the proper use of the device. The primary surgeon may not be the person deploying the stapler, and errors can occur when there is an assumption that a co-surgeon or assistant knows how to properly deploy a given stapler. In our operating room, the surgery resident is often responsible for deploying the stapler, and it is not unusual for him or her to be doing so for the first time. We have avoided this situation by focused education on the proper use of the various staplers prior to the operating room for trainees. This information can also be included into the time-out or preoperative briefing procedure so that proper orientation can occur.

## Strictures

***Key Concept: Strictures usually result from an ischemic conduit following an anastomosis; however, the use of improperly sized staplers can also contribute to their development. Recurrence of IBD can also result in stricturing and may be mitigated by a stapled anastomosis.***

Anastomotic stricture following a colon anastomosis is a well-known, but poorly defined, complication. What may be a "small" narrowing to some is a tight stricture or even "wide open" to others. Furthermore, outside of symptoms or scheduled endoscopic follow-up, the anastomosis may not be evaluated for months or years. As such, it is difficult to determine the actual rate of stricture formation for colorectal anastomoses. In 2012, Neutzling and colleagues updated their Cochrane review that consisted of 9 randomized controlled trials with 1,233 patients (622 stapled, 611 handsewn) undergoing a colorectal anastomosis [38]. While there were no other significant differences in evaluated metrics between the two methods, the authors did find stricture was more common in a stapled anastomosis [risk difference (random-effects model) 4.6 %, 95 % CI; 1.2–8.1 %)].

While little evidence exists to support one staple diameter over another, it is our practice to use the largest stapler that will safely fit into the conduit and negotiate the rectal stump. For most adults this is usually 29 mm, and we rarely use the 33 mm or 25 mm diameter stapler. There is some evidence to suggest that when stapling an ileal pouch to the anus, symptomatic strictures occur more frequently when a 29 mm stapler is used compared to a 33 mm [39]. Others have suggested that stenosis is a function of mechanical circular stapling regardless of the diameter [40]. We have not seen this in our practice and maintain like others that symptomatic stenosis is rare following stapled end-to-end anastomoses [41, 42] or side-to-end anastomosis, especially when careful attention to preservation of blood supply is maintained.

## Converting: How and When

***Key Concept: Conversions are a part of every laparoscopic case and surgeons should understand their personal rate of conversion and their outcomes. Converting proactively is***

***always the best strategy to preserve better patient outcomes. A hand port can often be used to bridge a straight laparoscopic case and a laparotomy.***

Conversions are a part of every practice and will occur for different reasons including equipment malfunction, bleeding, obscure anatomy, advanced malignancy, and intra-abdominal adhesions. The overall experience of the operator also influences the incidence of conversion with a learning curve estimated between 30 and 50 cases [43]. The decision to convert is always difficult but should be made as expeditiously as possible as a proactive conversion made early in the procedure will minimally affect the outcome when compared to the patient who underwent an open procedure [44]. It is when the surgeon struggles for prolonged periods of time creating injury and bleeding that the patient will have an adverse outcome which will be worse than if the procedure had just been done open [45]. Converting from laparoscopy to open is usually accomplished through a midline laparotomy; however, for surgeons with experience using hand-assist techniques, alternatives to performing a midline laparotomy do exist. For many left-sided and pelvic procedures, a Pfannenstiel incision can provide adequate to excellent exposure when used in combination with hand-assisted laparoscopic techniques. However, the surgeon should be certain that the lower transverse incision will adequately accomplish what needs to be addressed. For instance, it would be risky to attempt to control bleeding from the inferior mesenteric artery pedicle or upper abdominal sources using this approach. There will be times when a hand port placed in this location will require a midline extension, and based on very limited experience, it is advisable to maintain at least a 2 cm skin bridge between the Pfannenstiel and the midline incision to prevent total breakdown of the wound. When faced with a situation in which previous surgery increases the risk of conversion, the procedure should progress with minimal disposable equipment opened, and then a single trocar can be inserted to evaluate for suitability so that the amount of time and money spent for the laparoscopic procedure is minimized. An alternate approach would be a hand port placed in the midline to assess adhesions, again done with care to avoid opening a lot of disposables and avoiding unnecessary cost. The so-called "peek" port has been reported in the literature and was found to significantly limit the number of unnecessary conversions to a totally open approach [46].

## Pearls and Pitfalls: The Fatty Omentum, Small Bowel, and Maintaining Pneumoperitoneum

***Key Concepts: Performance of colorectal laparoscopy requires unobstructed views of some very important structures. The establishment and maintenance of pneumoperitoneum, displacing the omentum and small bowel, and proper patient positioning are all critical to achieve this level of visualization.***

### Omentum

The omentum can be problematic when performing laparoscopy due to its penchant to adhere to anything that has been inflamed or previously operated on as well as its capacity to store fat [47, 48]. It should be expected that when accessing the abdomen on a re-operative case, the omentum will adhere to any previous incision and can be broadly attached to the abdominal wall. This can result in the initial trocar insertion being through the omentum and will confuse the novice when the camera is inserted. Withdrawing the trocar and attempting to establish a plane between the abdominal wall and the omentum either through an open technique or an alternate trocar insertion can usually manage this (Video 21.2).

Obese patients can have very thick and stiff omentum making it difficult to get the perfect exposure. Given the increasing obesity problem in North America, surgeons will need to be able to deal with these obstacles if a laparoscopic approach is to be pursued. The basic problem is the competition for space within the insufflated abdomen with a fatty omentum occupying much more of the space that a surgeon needs to adequately visualize important structures. As an example, many surgeons approach a right colon by placing the patient in Trendelenburg with the intention of using gravity to allow the small bowel to occupy the upper abdomen while the ileocolic pedicle is being exposed and ligated. However, with a fatty omentum the upper abdomen becomes congested and space is limited. The small bowel has nowhere to go and the visualization is impaired. My approach to the obese patient for a right colectomy is to take advantage of gravity and the cephalad location of the ileocolic pedicle. The patient is placed in steep reverse Trendelenburg and the small bowel passively hangs into the lower abdomen and pelvis. To allow visualization of the bare area of the right colon and the vascular pedicle, the omentum is literally stuffed into the upper abdomen and held there by the assistant (on the patient's right side). This is accomplished by lifting directly up on the transverse colon toward the abdominal wall which then acts as a gate to keep the omentum tucked upward. An additional trocar may be necessary which is generally a good advice when dealing with difficult anatomy or obese patients.

It is generally less of a problem when dealing with left-sided anatomy. However, the omentum can become problematic in attempting to mobilize the splenic flexure, especially if attempting to do so by first entering the lesser sac between the colon and the omentum. The same problem of limited space seen on the right will come into play when trying to lift the omentum out of the left upper quadrant.

An alternate approach, which again relies on gravity, is to leave the omentum on the colon by dividing it along the greater curve of the stomach and letting it hang down in the lower abdomen.

While it is generally desirable to preserve the omentum during a total colectomy, there are times when its size will become such a liability in terms of completing the procedure safely without converting to open surgery, that it is necessary to remove it. This can be done easily in the era of effective laparoscopic energy devices. This will likely prove to be necessary in a very limited number of cases usually involving obese men who carry their weight centrally. These patients also tend to be shorter, which can significantly limit the amount of space available to safely visualize the mesentery, the major vascular pedicles, and the at-risk retroperitoneal structures such as the duodenum and left ureter.

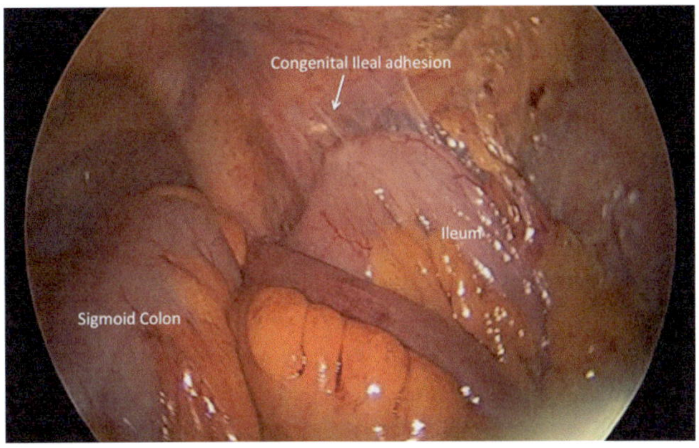


**Fig. 21.6** When the small bowel will not passively fall into the upper abdomen, the operator must assess whether there are any adhesions from the ileum to the right pelvic sidewall that may be tethering the bowel into the lower abdomen. Dividing these adhesions should free up the ileum enough to fall away passively with gravity

## Small Bowel

Like the omentum, the small bowel can also be problematic when performing a laparoscopic colectomy and can be the difference in terms of being able to complete the procedure without converting to either hand-assist or open. It is often the obese patient that poses the biggest difficulty in terms of the small bowel obscuring the operative fields due to the short nature of their mesentery. This is usually worse in men due to their tendency to deposit fat stores intra-abdominally.

For right-sided procedures, the small bowel can be directed toward the pelvis by placing the patient in steep reverse Trendelenburg, and this is usually not a problem. The lateral-to-medial approach will also be easier in cases when the small bowel is problematic, but my preferred approach for dealing with this particular issue is a hepatic flexure down approach. The omentum can either be left on the colon or dissected off (it usually can be done even with the patient in this position) and the hepatic flexure attachments can be divided using a bipolar or other energy device from the patient's left side. The duodenum will be quickly identified, and the remaining ascending colon can be mobilized from top down. It is not until the appendix and ileal attachments need to be mobilized that the patient will need to be tilted into Trendelenburg. Once the right colon is completely mobilized off the retroperitoneum, the decision can be made to take the vascular pedicle intra- or extracorporeal as it will be somewhat easier to identify once the colon can be lifted to the abdominal wall.

For left colectomies, the small bowel will need to go cephalad and the only good way to make this happen is steep Trendelenburg. It is often the distal ileum that obscures the visualization of the window below the inferior mesenteric artery. If this is a problem, take a moment to assess whether there are any adhesions that can be divided of the ileum and the right pelvic sidewall. Often patients have congenital adhesions of the ileum into the pelvis that will hinder your ability to completely displace the small bowel into the upper abdomen (Fig. 21.6). If the view remains compromised despite these maneuvers, then the operator has limited choices. My approach is to proceed with a lateral-to-medial approach and work the colon and flexure in this way. The small bowel will rarely hamper your ability to mobilize the splenic flexure. Alternatively, a hand-assisted left colectomy can be attempted as the proper use of the operator's hand can significantly increase the ability to retract the small bowel. In addition, a sponge can be brought in through the hand port and used to shield the small bowel from potential injury from cautery or energy.

## Airway Problems

One unique situation that can be very difficult to deal with is that of an inadvertent esophageal intubation. Just a few squeezes of an Ambu bag in the esophagus can completely fill the small bowel with air and little can be done to dissipate it. If a difficult airway is anticipated, a discussion with the anesthetist is warranted to minimize the chances of this complication. With modern tools such as the glide scope, this type of complication should be minimal.

## Pneumoperitoneum

Pneumoperitoneum is an essential part of every laparoscopic procedure, and while physiologic derangements occur in every patient subjected to positive intra-abdominal pressure, the clinical consequences are generally limited. These effects may be exacerbated by the use of steep head-down positioning [49, 50] and obesity [50, 51]. Decreasing the insufflation pressure may alleviate some of these changes, but short of gasless laparoscopy, there is little a surgeon can do to prevent these changes. Therefore, communication between the anesthesia team and the surgeons is critical to prevent untoward outcomes. Limiting the time spent in extreme positions and with pneumoperitoneum is an important consideration during laparoscopy on patients with hemodynamic and respiratory compromise. The maintenance of pneumoperitoneum relies on an adequate seal between the trocars or hand port and the abdominal wall. In instances where pneumoperitoneum cannot be maintained, the operative surgeon should assess for ongoing $CO_2$ losses through any of the incisions. Increasing the flow rate on the insufflator and selecting the largest trocar for gas delivery will help mitigate this problem. When attempts to seal a leaking trocar fail, sutures can be placed in the fascia or skin, or alternatively the trocar can be upsized. The use of trocars with a balloon tip that inflate below the fascia (Kii Advanced Fixation, Applied Medical, Rancho Santa Margarita, CA) can prove beneficial as a means to create a better seal.

## Summary

Knowledge of the pitfalls and technical challenges that await surgeons attempting to perform laparoscopic colorectal procedures will allow for better success and fewer conversions throughout the learning curve. Trocar insertions can be made more difficult by thick abdominal walls and previous surgery, and a variety of safe methods are available to establish the initial port. Bowel injury either from excessive traction or dissection will happen, and it will be an advantage for you to have laparoscopic suturing skills. This will also facilitate the management of serosal and thermal injuries. Bleeding is an expected problem, and a decision will need to be made quickly as to the best method of management. An ENDOLOOP® will generally be successful if the proximal side can be controlled. Anastomotic leaks are generally related to tension and ischemia, and techniques to assess the blood supply and to lengthen the conduit will mitigate some of these factors. Exposure is a critical component to success which can be threatened in the obese patient or when adhesions prevent the free movement of the small bowel and omentum.

## References


1. Varma R, Gupta JK. Laparoscopic entry techniques: clinical guideline, national survey, and medicolegal ramifications. Surg Endosc. 2008;22(12):2686–97. Epub 2008/04/11.
2. Ahmad G, O'Flynn H, Duffy JM, Phillips K, Watson A. Laparoscopic entry techniques. Cochrane Database Syst Rev. 2012;2, CD006583. Epub 2012/02/18.
3. Deffieux X, Ballester M, Collinet P, Fauconnier A, Pierre F. Risks associated with laparoscopic entry: guidelines for clinical practice from the French College of Gynaecologists and Obstetricians. Eur J Obstet Gynecol Reprod Biol. 2011;158(2):159–66. Epub 2011/05/31.
4. McKernan JB, Champion JK. Access techniques: Veress needle–initial blind trocar insertion versus open laparoscopy with the Hasson trocar. Endosc Surg Allied Technol. 1995;3(1):35–8. Epub 1995/02/01.
5. Moreaux G, Estrade-Huchon S, Bader G, Guyot B, Heitz D, Fauconnier A, et al. Five-millimeter trocar site small bowel eviscerations after gynecologic laparoscopic surgery. J Minim Invasive Gynecol. 2009;16(5):643–5. Epub 2009/10/20.
6. Chiong E, Hegarty PK, Davis JW, Kamat AM, Pisters LL, Matin SF. Port-site hernias occurring after the use of bladeless radially expanding trocars. Urology. 2010;75(3):574–80. Epub 2009/10/27.
7. Yamamoto M, Minikel L, Zaritsky E. Laparoscopic 5-mm trocar site herniation and literature review. JSLS. 2011;15(1):122–6. Epub 2011/09/10.
8. Vilos GA, Vilos AG, Abu-Rafea B, Hollett-Caines J, Nikkhah-Abyaneh Z, Edris F. Three simple steps during closed laparoscopic entry may minimize major injuries. Surg Endosc. 2009;23(4):758–64. Epub 2008/07/16.
9. Vilos GA, Ternamian A, Dempster J, Laberge PY. The Society of O, Gynaecologists of C. Laparoscopic entry: a review of techniques, technologies, and complications. J Obstet Gynaecol Can. 2007;29(5):433–65.
10. Agresta F, Mazzarolo G, Bedin N. Direct trocar insertion for laparoscopy. JSLS. 2012;16(2):255–9. Epub 2013/03/13.
11. Larobina M, Nottle P. Complete evidence regarding major vascular injuries during laparoscopic access. Surg Laparosc, Endosc Percutan Tech. 2005;15(3):119–23. Epub 2005/06/16.
12. Ten Broek RP, Van Goor H. Laparoscopic reintervention in colorectal surgery. Minerva Chir. 2008;63(2):161–8. Epub 2008/04/23.
13. Yamamoto M, Okuda J, Tanaka K, Kondo K, Asai K, Kayano H, et al. Effect of previous abdominal surgery on outcomes following laparoscopic colorectal surgery. Dis Colon Rectum. 2013;56(3):336–42. Epub 2013/02/09.
14. Binnebosel M, Klink CD, Grommes J, Jansen M, Neumann UP, Junge K. Influence of small intestinal serosal defect closure on leakage rate and adhesion formation: a pilot study using rabbit models. Langenbeck's Arch Surg. 2011;396(1):133–7. Epub 2010/07/09.
15. Wu MP, Ou CS, Chen SL, Yen EY, Rowbotham R. Complications and recommended practices for electrosurgery in laparoscopy. Am J Surg. 2000;179(1):67–73. Epub 2000/03/29.
16. Chino A, Karasawa T, Uragami N, Endo Y, Takahashi H, Fujita R. A comparison of depth of tissue injury caused by different modes of electrosurgical current in a pig colon model. Gastrointest Endosc. 2004;59(3):374–9. Epub 2004/03/05.
17. Tou S, Malik AI, Wexner SD, Nelson RL. Energy source instruments for laparoscopic colectomy. Cochrane Database Syst Rev. 2011;5, CD007886. Epub 2011/05/13.
18. Di Lorenzo N, Franceschilli L, Allaix ME, Asimakopoulos AD, Sileri P, Gaspari AL. Radiofrequency versus ultrasonic energy in laparoscopic colorectal surgery: a metaanalysis of operative time and blood loss. Surg Endosc. 2012;26(10):2917–24. Epub 2012/05/15.
19. Targarona EM, Balague C, Marin J, Neto RB, Martinez C, Garriga J, et al. Energy sources for laparoscopic colectomy: a prospective randomized comparison of conventional electrosurgery, bipolar computer-controlled electrosurgery and ultrasonic dissection. Operative outcome and costs analysis. Surg Innov. 2005;12(4):339–44. Epub 2006/01/21.
20. Campagnacci R, de Sanctis A, Baldarelli M, Rimini M, Lezoche G, Guerrieri M. Electrothermal bipolar vessel sealing device vs ultrasonic

coagulating shears in laparoscopic colectomies: a comparative study. Surg Endosc. 2007;21(9):1526–31. Epub 2007/02/09.
21. Hubner M, Demartines N, Muller S, Dindo D, Clavien PA, Hahnloser D. Prospective randomized study of monopolar scissors, bipolar vessel sealer and ultrasonic shears in laparoscopic colorectal surgery. Br J Surg. 2008;95(9):1098–104. Epub 2008/08/12.
22. Marcello PW, Roberts PL, Rusin LC, Holubkov R, Schoetz DJ. Vascular pedicle ligation techniques during laparoscopic colectomy. A prospective randomized trial. Surg Endosc. 2006;20(2): 263–9. Epub 2005/12/20.
23. Abarca F, Saclarides TJ, Brand MI. Laparoscopic colectomy: complications causing reoperation or emergency room/hospital readmissions. Am Surg. 2011;77(1):65–9. Epub 2011/03/15.
24. D'Ambra L, Berti S, Bonfante P, Bianchi C, Gianquinto D, Falco E. Hemostatic step-by-step procedure to control presacral bleeding during laparoscopic total mesorectal excision. World J Surg. 2009;33(4):812 5. Epub 2008/12/19.
25. Rutegard M, Hemmingsson O, Matthiessen P, Rutegard J. High tie in anterior resection for rectal cancer confers no increased risk of anastomotic leakage. Br J Surg. 2012;99(1):127–32. Epub 2011/11/01.
26. Karanjia ND, Corder AP, Bearn P, Heald RJ. Leakage from stapled low anastomosis after total mesorectal excision for carcinoma of the rectum. Br J Surg. 1994;81(8):1224–6. Epub 1994/08/01.
27. Lange MM, Buunen M, van de Velde CJ, Lange JF. Level of arterial ligation in rectal cancer surgery: low tie preferred over high tie. A review. Dis Colon Rectum. 2008;51(7):1139–45. Epub 2008/05/17.
28. Buunen M, Lange MM, Ditzel M, Kleinrensink GJ, van de Velde CJ, Lange JF. Level of arterial ligation in total mesorectal excision (TME): an anatomical study. Int J Color Dis. 2009;24(11):1317–20. Epub 2009/07/18.
29. Deloyers L. Suspension of the right colon permits without exception preservation of the anal sphincter after extensive colectomy of the transverse and left colon (including rectum). technic -indications- immediate and late results. Lyon Chir. 1964;60:404–13. Epub 1964/05/01. La bascule du c olon droit permet sans exception de conserver le sphincter anal apr'es les colectomies etendues du transverse et du c olon gauche (rectum y compris). technique -indications- r'esultats imm'ediats et tardifs.
30. Manceau G, Karoui M, Breton S, Blanchet AS, Rousseau G, Savier E, et al. Right colon to rectal anastomosis (Deloyers procedure) as a salvage technique for low colorectal or coloanal anastomosis: postoperative and long-term outcomes. Dis Colon Rectum. 2012; 55(3):363–8. Epub 2012/04/04.
31. Beard JD, Nicholson ML, Sayers RD, Lloyd D, Everson NW. Intraoperative air testing of colorectal anastomoses: a prospective, randomized trial. Br J Surg. 1990;77(10):1095–7. Epub 1990/10/01.
32. Yalin R, Aktan AO, Yegen C, Dosluoglu H, Okboy N. Importance of testing stapled rectal anastomoses with air. Eur J Surg. 1993; 159(1):49–51.
33. Ricciardi R, Roberts PL, Marcello PW, Hall JF, Read TE, Schoetz DJ. Anastomotic leak testing after colorectal resection: what are the data? Arch Surg. 2009;144(5):407–11. discussion 11-2. Epub 2009/05/20.
34. Li VK, Wexner SD, Pulido N, Wang H, Jin HY, Weiss EG, et al. Use of routine intraoperative endoscopy in elective laparoscopic colorectal surgery: can it further avoid anastomotic failure? Surg Endosc. 2009;23(11):2459–65. Epub 2009/03/21.
35. Shamiyeh A, Szabo K, Ulf Wayand W, Zehetner J. Intraoperative endoscopy for the assessment of circular-stapled anastomosis in laparoscopic colon surgery. Surg Laparosc, Endosc Percutan Tech. 2012;22(1):65–7. Epub 2012/02/10.
36. Marderstein E TJ, Stulberg J, Champagne B, Reynolds H, Delaney CP. Analysis of stapler misfire during colorectal surgical procedures using a national event report database. 2007; Available from: http://www.casesurgery.com/research/Abstract08WEB.pdf.
37. Pandya S, Murray JJ, Coller JA, Rusin LC. Laparoscopic colectomy: indications for conversion to laparotomy. Arch Surg. 1999;134(5):471–5. Epub 1999/05/14.
38. Neutzling CB, Lustosa SA, Proenca IM, da Silva EM, Matos D. Stapled versus handsewn methods for colorectal anastomosis surgery. Cochrane database Syst Rev (Online). 2012;2:CD003144. Epub 2012/02/18.
39. Kirat HT, Kiran RP, Lian L, Remzi FH, Fazio VW. Influence of stapler size used at ileal pouch-anal anastomosis on anastomotic leak, stricture, long-term functional outcomes, and quality of life. Am J Surg. 2010;200(1):68 72. Epub 2010/07/20.
40. Polese L, Vecchiato M, Frigo AC, Sarzo G, Cadrobbi R, Rizzato R, et al. Risk factors for colorectal anastomotic stenoses and their impact on quality of life: what are the lessons to learn? Colorectal Dis. 2012;14(3):e124–8. Epub 2011/09/14.
41. Kyzer S, Gordon PH. Experience with the use of the circular stapler in rectal surgery. Dis Colon Rectum. 1992;35(7):696–706. Epub 1992/07/01.
42. Detry RJ, Kartheuser A, Delriviere L, Saba J, Kestens PJ. Use of the circular stapler in 1000 consecutive colorectal anastomoses: experience of one surgical team. Surgery. 1995;117(2):140–5. Epub 1995/02/01.
43. Tekkis PP, Senagore AJ, Delaney CP. Conversion rates in laparoscopic colorectal surgery: a predictive model with, 1253 patients. Surg Endosc. 2005;19(1):47–54. Epub 2004/11/19.
44. Casillas S, Delaney CP, Senagore AJ, Brady K, Fazio VW. Does conversion of a laparoscopic colectomy adversely affect patient outcome? Dis Colon Rectum. 2004;47(10):1680–5. Epub 2004/11/13.
45. Guillou PJ, Quirke P, Thorpe H, Walker J, Jayne DG, Smith AM, et al. Short-term endpoints of conventional versus laparoscopic-assisted surgery in patients with colorectal cancer (MRC CLASICC trial): multicentre, randomised controlled trial. Lancet. 2005; 365(9472):1718–26. Epub 2005/05/17.
46. Read TE, Salgado J, Ferraro D, Fortunato R, Caushaj PF. "Peek port": a novel approach for avoiding conversion in laparoscopic colectomy. Surg Endosc. 2009;23(3):477–81. Epub 2008/07/16.
47. Ngu SF, Cheung VY, Pun TC. Left upper quadrant approach in gynecologic laparoscopic surgery. Acta Obstet Gynecol Scand. 2011;90(12):1406–9. Epub 2011/08/23.
48. Levrant SG, Bieber E, Barnes R. Risk of anterior abdominal wall adhesions increases with number and type of previous laparotomy. J Am Assoc Gynecol Laparosc. 1994;1 (4, Part 2)(4):S19. Epub 1994/08/01.
49. Kadono Y, Yaegashi H, Machioka K, Ueno S, Miwa S, Maeda Y, et al. Cardiovascular and respiratory effects of the degree of head-down angle during robot-assisted laparoscopic radical prostatectomy. Int J Med Robotics. 2013;9(1):17–22. Epub 2013/01/26.
50. Meininger D, Westphal K, Bremerich DH, Runkel H, Probst M, Zwissler B, et al. Effects of posture and prolonged pneumoperitoneum on hemodynamic parameters during laparoscopy. World J Surg. 2008;32(7):1400–5. Epub 2008/01/29.
51. Nguyen NT, Wolfe BM. The physiologic effects of pneumoperitoneum in the morbidly obese. Ann Surg. 2005;241(2):219–26. Epub 2005/01/15.

# Part IV

# New Horizons

# Single-Incision Laparoscopic Approaches to Colorectal Disease

# 22

Virgilio George

**Key Points**

- Single-incision laparoscopy is safe and feasible in major colorectal surgery.
- The learning curve is quite short and almost nonexistent for those already skilled in conventional laparoscopic surgery and, more specifically, right hemicolectomy.
- Using different length instruments and a 30-degree 5-mm camera will aid in avoiding extracorporeal instrumentation collisions.
- A right-angled light cord adapter is a must.
- Do not sacrifice safety and adequacy of an operation for a limited approach.

## Introduction

New surgical techniques are constantly being developed around the world. Yet, some interventions never gain traction, while others become an important part of a surgeon's skill set. Single-port laparoscopy is one approach that has steadily gained popularity across various surgical disciplines, including colorectal surgery, and is a frequent topic of discussion and investigation. It would appear that single-port laparoscopy will remain a part of surgical therapy for some time.

As the field of single-port laparoscopy grows, the trend in publications changes with it. To date, there have been a number of studies within the general, urologic, and gynecologic surgery literature looking at the feasibility and safety of the single-port laparoscopic approach to various operations [1–7]. Although the technique may vary, it would appear that nearly any surgery that can be done laparoscopically can also be done using a single-port approach [8].

Colon and rectal surgery is no stranger to this trend and in recent years has seen a vast increase in publications about the use of single-port laparoscopy [9, 10]. Our group has published the largest series of single-port laparoscopic right hemicolectomies to date and has since had a growing experience with more complex procedures using a single-port approach [11].

It is important to keep in mind that when learning any new procedure, there is a learning curve that each person must complete in order to become proficient. Single-port surgery is no different. Although the steps of a colectomy may be well engrained and the point of achieving competency using a laparoscopic approach is long past, bringing in the single-port dimension adds a degree of difficulty to the mix. There has been some data addressing the learning curve for single-port laparoscopy [12–14]. However, there have been no specific studies examining the learning curve for performing single-port laparoscopic colorectal procedures, specifically. In this chapter we will address the technical aspects of single-port surgery for various colorectal operations and highlight tips to hopefully make this approach much easier, no matter where you are on your learning curve.

## Indications

Laparoscopic surgery has been shown to have multiple advantages when compared to open surgery: decreased morbidity, decreased pain, faster recovery, and shorter hospital stay [15, 16], as well as equivalent oncological results seen in the COST and MRC CLASICC trial [17–20]. Single-incision laparoscopic surgery (SILS) uses only one incision in the abdominal wall, allowing all operative work to be done in the same opening, but this does not change the fundamental tenants of laparoscopic surgery: proper exposure, triangulation, and the use of instruments and devices tailored for in-line viewing.

---

**Electronic supplementary material:** Supplementary material is available in the online version of this chapter at 10.1007/978-1-4939-1581-1_22. Videos can also be accessed at http://www.springerimages.com/videos/978-1-4939-1580-4.

V. George, M.D. (✉)
Associate Professor of Surgery, Indiana University School of Medicine, Department of Surgery, Richard L. Roudebush VA Medical, Center, 545 Barnhill Dr., #500, Indianapolis, IN 46202, USA
e-mail: vigeorge@iupui.edu

H.M. Ross et al. (eds.), *Minimally Invasive Approaches to Colon and Rectal Disease: Technique and Best Practices*, DOI 10.1007/978-1-4939-1581-1_22, © Springer Science+Business Media New York 2015

During the past years, numerous reports of SILS procedures have been published showing the feasibility of this approach for even complex colon and rectal procedures [10]. To date, all types of colorectal procedures have been performed through single-port laparoscopy, from a minimally invasive stoma to a total proctocolectomy and ileoanal pouch. It is not a result of a "landmark" randomized, prospective study but rather through experience that single-site outcomes have been shown to be equivalent to multiple-site laparoscopy and open laparotomy from all perspectives. In many cases, this approach has become the preferred technique for surgeons.

The most common single-site procedures will be reviewed here, including right colectomy, sigmoid colectomy, and total abdominal proctocolectomy with J pouch.

## Preoperative Planning

Whether you are performing a procedure through an open, laparoscopic or single-incision laparoscopic approach, a good history and physical examination is mandatory. In addition, appropriate patients should have a complete blood count, chemistry, and carcinoembryonic antigen (CEA) levels as indicated by their comorbidities and disease process. Additional assessment for staging and localization of a tumor includes CT scan and colonoscopy to confirm the exact location and mark the lesion with India ink. While still controversial, a bowel preparation typically follows the preference of the individual institution and surgeon. In my institution, we do not routinely prescribe bowel prep for right colectomies and use oral laxative for the other colectomies. Also, intravenous antibiotics are used perioperatively for all patients.

Appropriate patient selection cannot be overemphasized. During my initial experience, I selected patients with a low body mass index (BMI). In addition, I avoided patients with previous surgeries, due to the time-consuming lysis of adhesions, as well as patients with large tumors that can be difficult to handle.

As my experience has grown, I now use single-incision laparoscopy for all my right colectomies as well as those undergoing a total abdominal colectomy with J pouch. Regarding BMI or previous surgery, I perform single-site laparoscopic resection in selective cases for sigmoid and left colectomy when the cosmetic results are important to the patient.

## Single-Incision Port Types and Port Placement

Multiple access devices have been developed and are constantly changing in an attempt to improve this developing technique of minimally invasive single-port surgery. Among them is the recent addition of a robotic single-port platform. At present, the most popular are the following six systems including:

1. The platform most commonly used is the SILS port (Covidien, Inc. Norwalk, CT), which is made from an elastic polymer. It is hourglass-shaped and can be deployed through a 2-cm fascial incision. It contains four openings: one for insufflation via a right-angled tube and three that can accommodate trocars 5–15 mm in size.
2. The GelPOINT® (Applied Medical, Rancho Santa Margarita, CA) port uses a wound protector that is also very helpful for retraction, accommodating multiple trocars 5–12 mm. This platform allows for laparoscopic surgery by providing a flexible, airtight position for multiple trocars and multiple positions that allows an easy triangulation and less collision. It's large enough to allow bowel exteriorization for extracorporeal resection and anastomosis using standard instrumentation. By offering an increased range of motion and maximum retraction and exposure, the GelPOINT platform provides the utmost versatility and access for a wide range of abdominal and transanal procedures.
3. The TriPort® (Advanced Surgical, Co. Wicklow, Ireland) has three channels, allowing up to one 12-mm and two 5-mm instruments.
4. The QuadPort (Advanced Surgical) has four lumens, permitting up to one 15-mm, two 10-mm, and one 5-mm instruments.
5. The Uni-X single-port laparoscopic device (Pnavel Systems Morganville, NJ) is a system designed to allow the simultaneous use of three 5-mm laparoscopic instruments through a single fascial incision. It requires fascial fixation sutures and curved laparoscopic instruments. The Uni-X system seems to be used primarily in urology procedures [4, 21–23]. Initial technical notes are provided by Remzi et al. [10].
6. Ethicon Endo-Surgery SSL Access System (Ethicon, Cincinnati, OH) consists of two 5-mm seals and a larger 15-mm seal in a low-profile design. Unique to the device is the 360-degree rotation of the seal cap that enables quick reorientation of instruments during procedures and reduces the need for instrument exchanges.

## Right Hemicolectomy (Video 22.1)

### Operative Technique

After anesthesia is induced, a Foley catheter and orogastric tube are placed. Then the patient is positioned supine on the table; the left arm is padded and tucked. Some kind of restraint device (beanbag or chest and leg straps) needs to be used to prevent the patient from falling from the table during position manipulation.

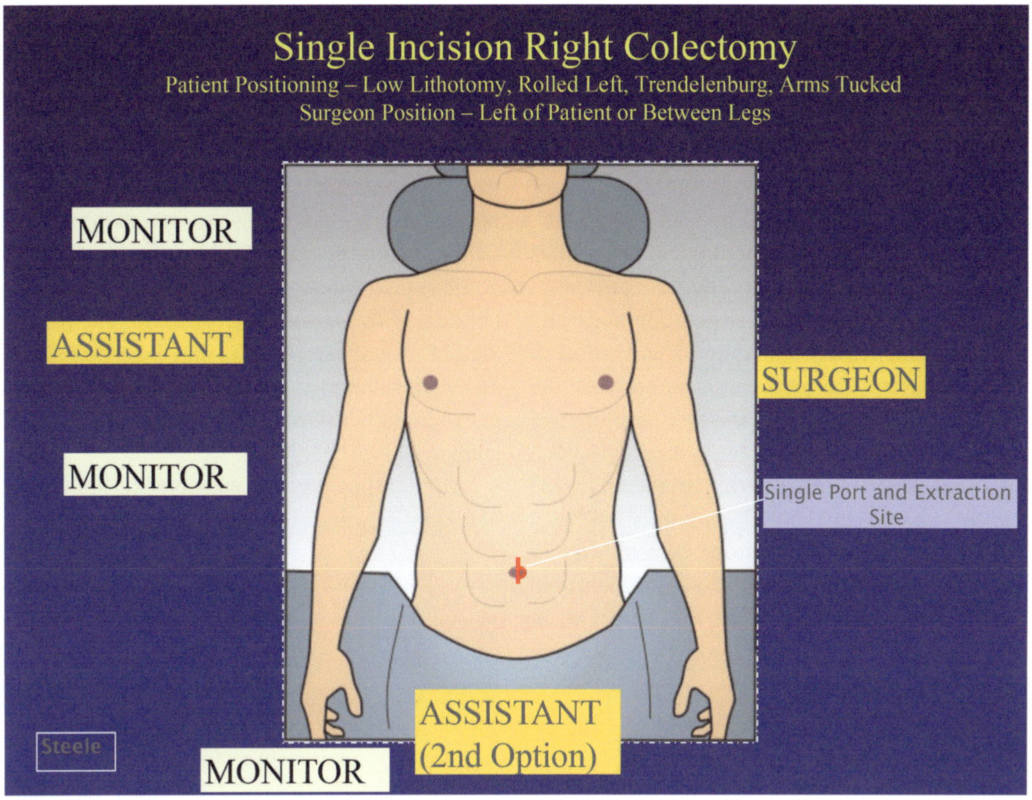


**Fig. 22.1** Port placement for single-incision right colectomy. Note the left colectomy can be in the umbilicus or in the Pfannenstiel position

The patient is prepped and draped in standard fashion. The surgeon and assistants are located on the left side of the patient. Visual monitors, as many as are needed, are positioned on the opposite side of the surgeon, which allows comfort and good visualization (Fig. 22.1).

The operative technique starts with placement of the SILS™ port device placed in the umbilicus using an open technique. This provides an added degree of safety against inadvertent intra-abdominal injury [24], as well as a cosmetic benefit by hiding the future scar. A vertical incision is made in the fascia large enough to accommodate the single-port trocar (~2 to 3 cm; Fig. 22.2). A fascial opening bigger than the device will cause loss of insufflation during extreme movement of the instrumentation and can add time and frustration to the procedure and the surgeon.

Our preference is to use standard laparoscopic instrumentation (i.e., straight) including the scope. This decreases the learning curve and allows the surgeon to perform the procedure with tools to which they are accustomed (Video 22.2). A standard 5-mm 30° laparoscope of bariatric length is then inserted (or rarely a 30° 10-mm laparoscope), followed by two 5-mm working ports with non-articulating instruments: (1) atraumatic bowel grasper and (2) an energy device with multifunctional capability such as the ENSEAL® (Ethicon Endo-Surgery, Inc, Cincinnati, OH) (Fig. 22.3).

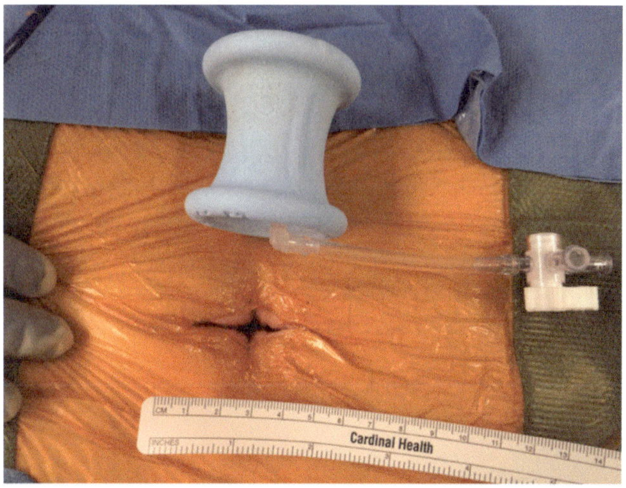


**Fig. 22.2** Single-port and umbilical incision. Notice the small incision to accommodate the port to reduce air leaks

I prefer to orient the trocar with the gas port aimed toward the patient's feet, helping to keep triangulation on the 5-mm port, as well as using the top of the triangle for the camera port (Fig. 22.4).

The abdominal cavity is explored for adhesions, and most importantly when performing the surgery for colon cancer, the peritoneum and liver must be inspected for metastatic disease. The patient is then positioned in Trendelenburg position and left side down. The omentum is grasped and placed on top of the transverse colon. My common approach is to begin medial-to-lateral dissection where the vascular pedicle is ligated before the mobilization of the colon or the tumor. I prefer to maintain the "no touch" technique and adhere to standard oncological principles [25] with gentle traction on the cecum. The ileocolic pedicle is then elevated; the small bowel is positioned on the left side of the abdominal cavity, allowing visualization of the base of the mesentery. The peritoneum underlying the ileocolic pedicle and the base of the mesentery are opened (Fig. 22.5) using laparoscopic scissors or an energy device of the surgeon's preference in order to dissect the colon off its retroperitoneal attachments and the duodenum in a medial-to-lateral fashion. Careful retroperitoneal dissection continues until the duodenum is completely identified and the head of the pancreas is seen. Once this is complete, a mesenteric window is created and the ileocolic vessels are divided using an energy device.

After the division of the vascular pedicle, this space is developed in cephalad direction, above the duodenum, between the first portion of the duodenum and the transverse mesocolon. Identification of the right branch of the middle colic vein and artery must happen while dissecting at the origin (Fig. 22.6). Then this can be ligated using an energy device. The mesenteric of the transverse colon is then divided to encircle a distal portion of the colon for the creation of the ileocolic anastomosis. The patient is then positioned into reverse Trendelenburg; the omentum is grasped and divided to be included in the en bloc resection from its attachments to the transverse colon. Next, the hepatic flexure and the lateral attachments are taken down from superior to inferior (Fig. 22.7). Careful dissection should be used when approaching the lateral attachment in the right lower quadrant to minimize the risk of ureteral injury. After confirming the completed mobilization and division of the mesentery of the terminal ileum, the cecum is grasped with a locking instrument to help during extraction (Fig. 22.8). The fascial incisions are enlarged as necessary to exteriorize the specimen for division and anastomosis. The use of a wound protector is recommended to prevent contamination of the wound, tumor seeding, and helping with the exposure. The colon is then exteriorized, ensuring you maintain proper orientation of the specimen (Fig. 22.9). The previously selected area of the transverse colon and the terminal ileum is divided and the anastomosis is created according to surgeon's preference in either side-to-side or end-to-side fashion with staplers.

After inspecting the anastomosis intracorporeally, I do not routinely close the mesenteric defect. Then the fascia is

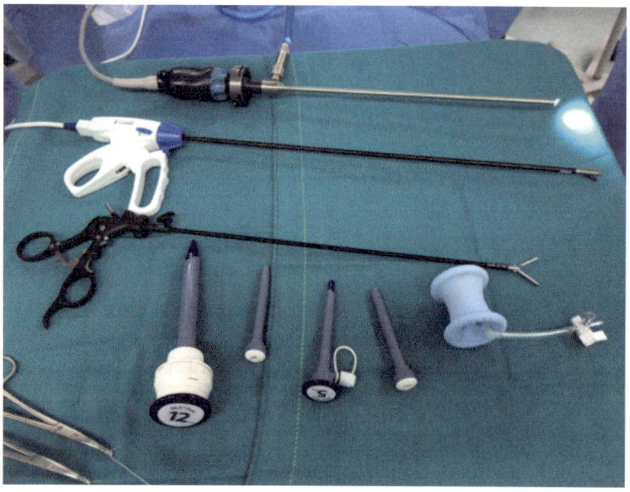

**Fig. 22.3** Instruments: 30-degree camera, energy device, bariatric length, and atraumatic bowel grasper. Different lengths will help decrease the extracorporeal collision

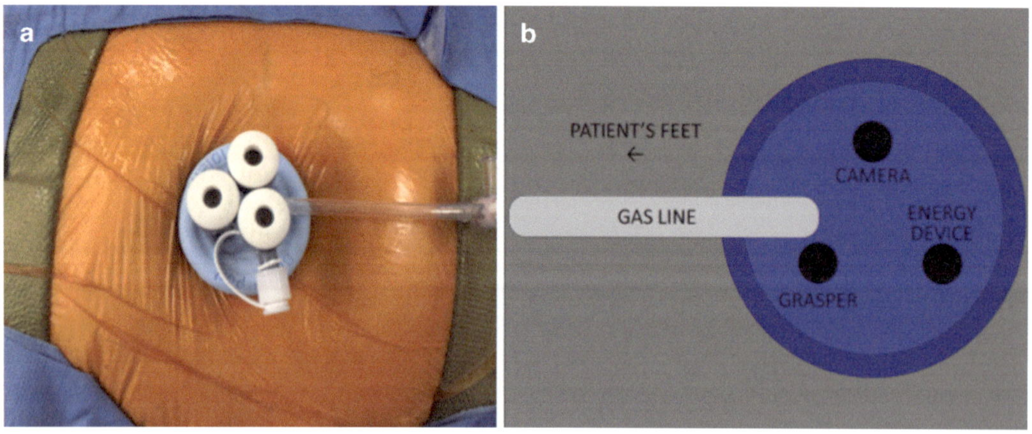


**Fig. 22.4** (**a**) A vertical incision is made in the fascia large enough to accommodate the single-port trocar even in obese patients. (**b**) Diagram indicating the orientation of the port to allow triangulation of the instruments with the gas line port toward the patient's feet

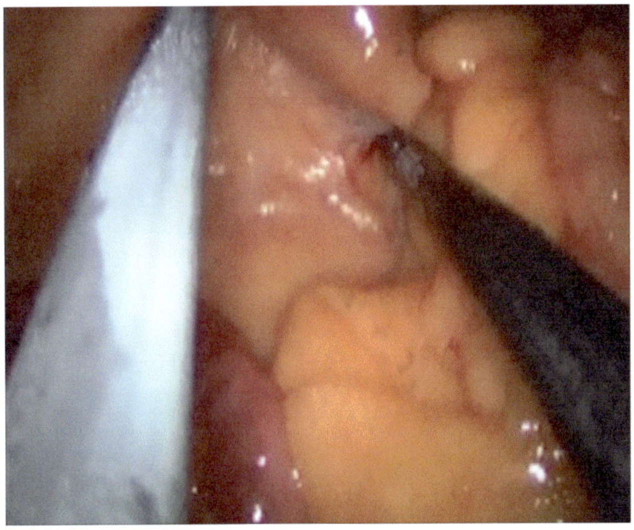

**Fig. 22.5** The ileocolic pedicle is elevated to allow tension to help open the peritoneum underlying the ileocolic pedicle. This is extended to the base of the mesentery

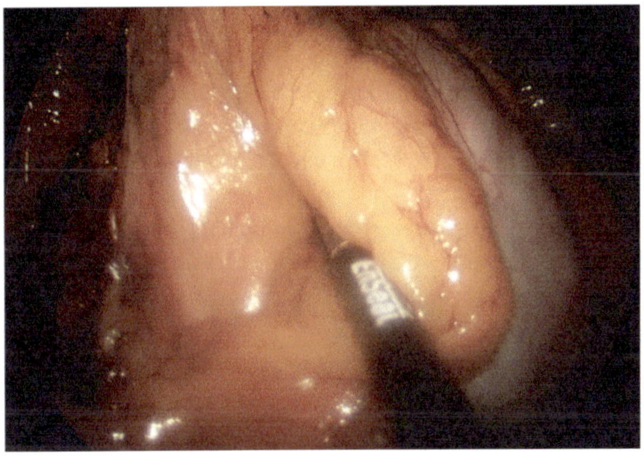

**Fig. 22.6** Right branch of the middle colic artery and vein. Notice that division of the ileocolic pedicle decreases the visualization of the duodenum

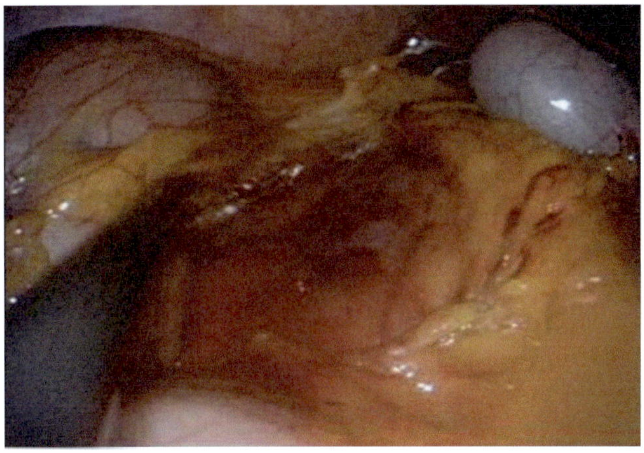

**Fig. 22.7** Takedown of hepatic flexure and the lateral attachments in a superior-to-inferior fashion

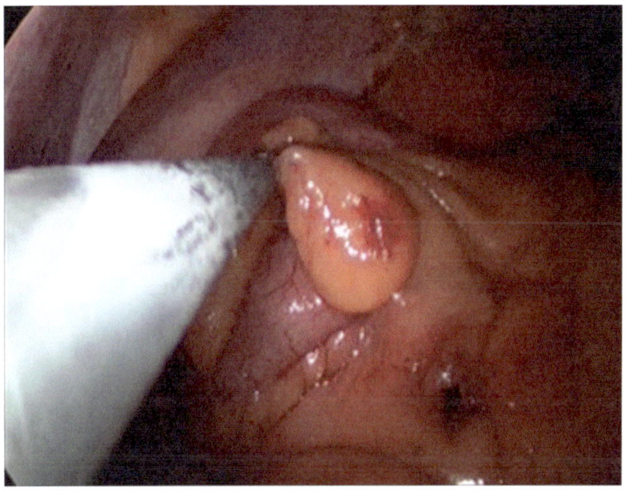

**Fig. 22.8** After complete mobilization and division of the mesentery of the ileum, the cecum is grasped with a locking instrument to help during extraction

closed in either a running or figure-of-eight fashion (Fig. 22.10).

## Single-Port Left Colectomy

The indications for the SILS left colectomy are the same as the open colectomy or laparoscopy. Advantages of the SILS approach depend on the surgeon's experience and the search for alternative operative techniques as well as better cosmetic and highest patient satisfaction results [26–28]. Similar to a right colectomy, there is not an absolute contraindication for the use of single-port laparoscopy, as long as procedure meets the safe surgery criteria. Also, if needed, an additional trocar can be added for camera access or retraction.

### Surgical Procedure

The patient's preoperative evaluation is the same as previously described in this chapter including mechanical bowel preparation and intravenous pre-op antibiotics. After induction of the anesthesia, the patient is placed in lithotomy position with arms tucked to the sides and protected. Special attention is focused to secure the patient to the anesthesia table to prevent falling or moving during extreme table position changes. The routine use of the left ureteral stent for left colectomy may prevent any injury [29], though more likely may allow recognition of any intraoperative injury, as well as early identification of the ureter itself to help expedite the procedure.

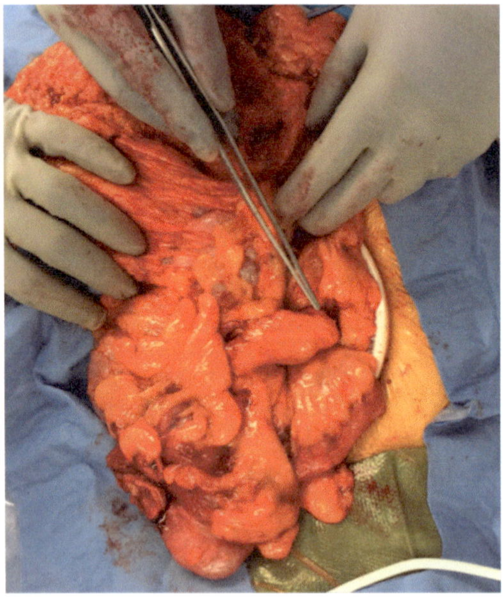

Fig. 22.9 Extraction of the colon with a cecal tumor through the wound protector. Notice the ileocolic pedicle seen at the tip of the instrument

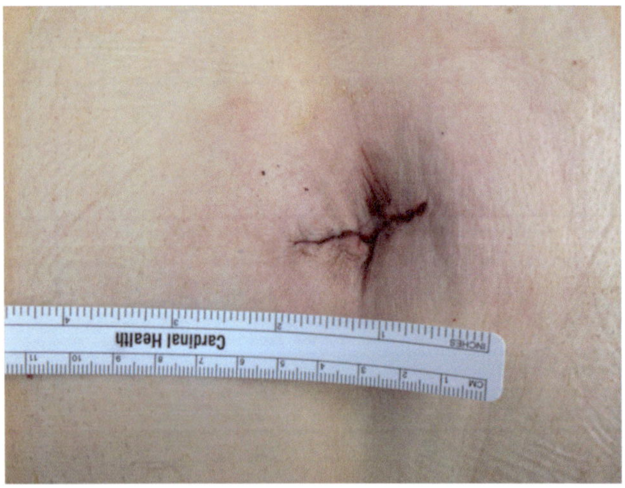



Fig. 22.10 Final incision after single-incision right colectomy

## Port at the Umbilicus

The surgeon and the operative assistant are positioned on the right side of the patient if the single-port trocar is placed in the umbilicus. The surgeon may also need to stand between the legs of the patient and the assistant on the right of the patient when the alternative port placement of a suprapubic location is used. This suprapubic port site hides the scar and can also be used for colon specimen extraction. The suprapubic location is also over the rectal-sigmoid junction, allowing for direct vision, division of the rectum, and performing the anastomosis.

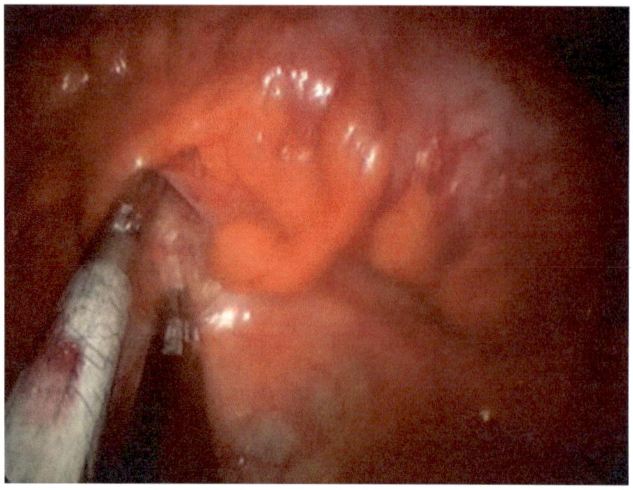

Fig. 22.11 The peritoneum is opened between the inferior mesenteric vein and inferior mesenteric artery; the longer the incision, the better the exposure of the retroperitoneum will be

An open technique is used to make a 3-cm abdominal wall incision to accommodate the SILS port. After entering the peritoneal cavity and achieving adequate insufflation, exploration of the abdominal cavity for adhesions and metastatic disease should be performed if colon cancer is a preoperative diagnosis. If the indication is cancer, then specific identification of the location of the tumor should be the next step. Ideally a previous, preoperative colonoscopy with intraluminal colon marking with ink identifies anatomic location or, if necessary, intraoperative colonoscopy with $CO_2$ to ensure the location. Both colonoscopy techniques are superior to intraoperative manual palpation with instruments.

The patient is positioned in Trendelenburg, and the right side of table is lower than the left. This uses gravity retraction to position the bowel on the right side of the abdomen. Placement of the omentum on top/caudal to the transverse colon allows for identification of the transverse colon and localization of the middle colic vessels and the inferior mesenteric vein (IMV) at the level of the ligament of Treitz. After scoring the mesentery along the medial aspect of the left colon from the inferior mesenteric artery (IMA) to the IMV, the surgeon may use a medial-to-lateral dissection approach with ureteral stents in place.

Surgeons may alternate between the next two steps. First, with the SILS trocar in the umbilicus, the area between the IMV and IMA can be easily accessed using a monopolar scissor. The peritoneum is opened; the longer the incision, the better the exposure of the retroperitoneum (Fig. 22.11). The retroperitoneal dissection is started under the descending mesocolon, which helps retraction by elevating the mesocolon with a sweeping movement up and down. This allows the embryological plane to be identified and bluntly separated. This dissection should be bloodless (Fig. 22.12 a,b).

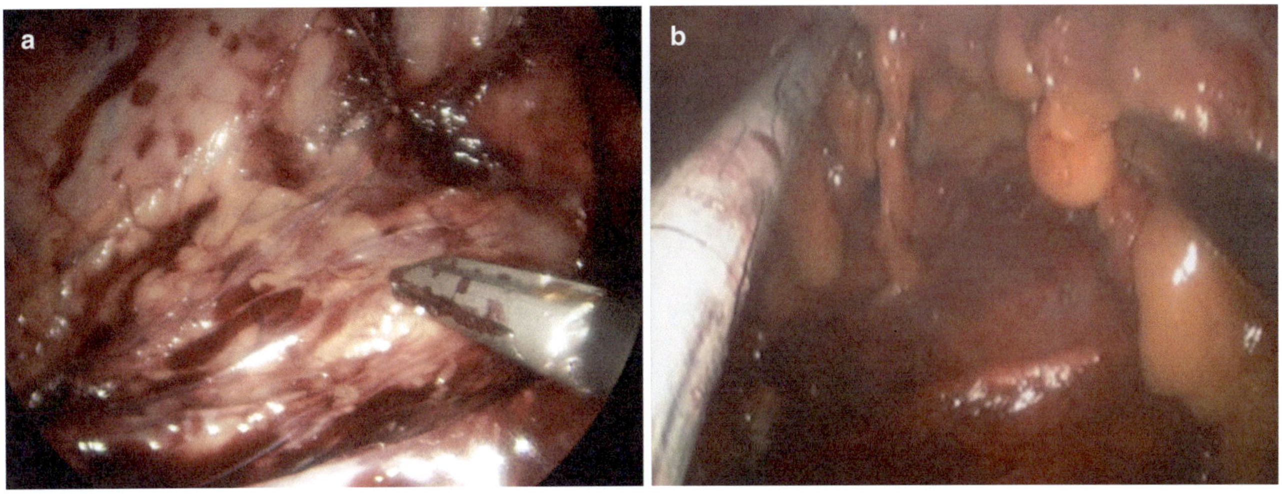


**Fig. 22.12** Retroperitoneal dissection. Notice the elevation of the mesocolon with left arm and bloodless plane (**a**) before IMA division and (**b**) after IMA division

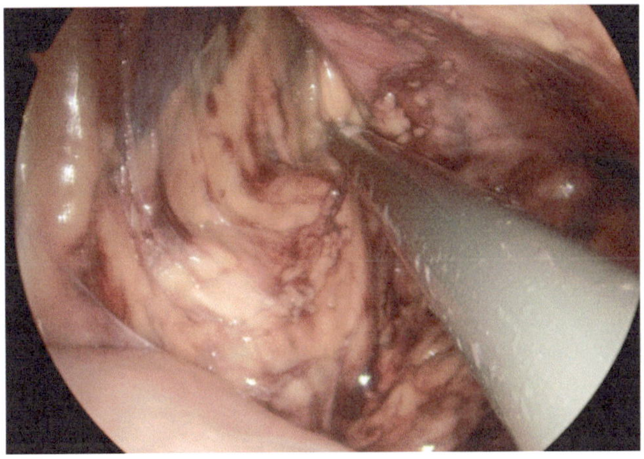

**Fig. 22.13** Retroperitoneal dissection without division of the inferior mesenteric vein. This dissection is lateral and superior, with identification of the inferior border of the pancreas

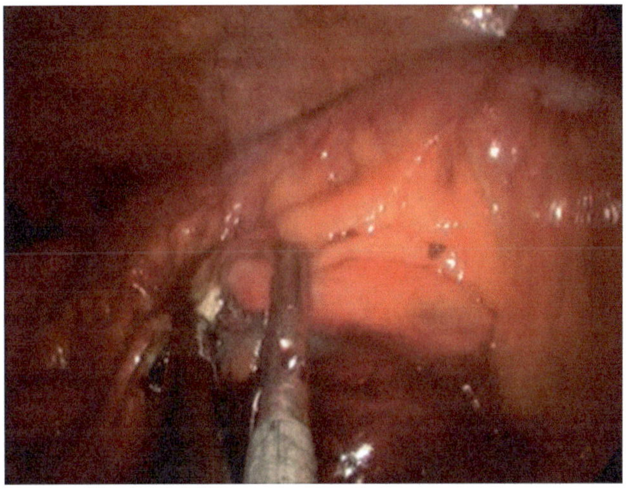

**Fig. 22.14** Division of the IMA using an energy device. Notice the in-line view and the triangulation with the crossover instruments

With elevation of the IMV and continued dissection of the retroperitoneum above Gerota's fascia, you need to identify the inferior border of the pancreas. Dissection continues all the way to the lateral colon attachments with hand-over-hand instrument exchanges (Fig. 22.13).

Caudal dissection is continued to visually encircle the IMA and identify the left ureter. Once this is performed, the dissection space around the IMA exposes the origin of the artery and sweeps the nerves around the IMA-aorta junction to prevent injury to the sympathetic and parasympathetic nerve plexus. Division of the IMA can be done according to the surgeon's preference using an energy device, stapler, or clip ligation (Fig. 22.14). Dissecting the IMV without division facilitates the medial dissection of the splenic flexure and the lesser sac. Early division of the IMV will allow the heavy, floppy mesentery to fall on top of the camera and often create the need for an extra instrument to retract the mesentery. The extended dissection of the retroperitoneum will make the dissection on the lateral left colon attachments easier.

The next step involves opening the avascular area on top of the pancreas to enter the lesser sac. Identification of the posterior wall of the stomach helps confirm the correct location (Fig. 22.15). Continued use of the energy device helps to divide the colon mesenteric attachments to the inferior border of the pancreas until the left lateral attachment to the abdominal wall is reached.

Attention is now turned to the lateral attachments of the colon, starting with gentle retraction of the sigmoid medially. This will expose the lateral attachments at the level of the pelvic brim (Fig. 22.16a,b). Using the monopolar scissors will facilitate this step. After an opening is created in the lateral attachment, visual identification of the left ureter is easy. The left-hand instrument is used to keep the lateral attachment window open, and continued division of the attachments in a cephalad (toward the splenic flexure) direction will mobilize the entire left colon (Fig. 22.17). The left lateral dissection meets the previous medial dissection at the splenic flexure.

## Suprapubic Location of the Port

With the single access port in the suprapubic area, through a Pfannenstiel incision, the initial exploration is the same as described earlier, even with the view somewhat different from caudal to cephalic. The patient is rotated right side down to allow the small bowel to be placed in the right upper quadrant. The sigmoid colon or the descending colon is elevated with the left-hand instrument, an atraumatic grasper (bariatric length), exposing the superior hemorrhoidal artery at the level of the sacrum promontory. A long incision is made in the peritoneum, medial and below the artery exposing the retroperitoneum. The sigmoid mesentery is elevated and the dissection in the retroperitoneum is carried caudal to cephalic. The left ureter is recognized and dissection continues on top to the ureter and lateral as long as possible without division of the IMA.

After identification of the left ureter, the IMA is encircled around the junction with the aorta. Exposure is created by elevating the sigmoid mesentery and dissection is continued to the medial aspect between the IMA and IMV. The artery can be ligated according to the surgeon's preference: energy device, ligation, or stapler.

After ligation of the IMA, grasping the artery pedicle helps in the retroperitoneal dissection by continuing cephalad until identification of the inferior border of the pancreas and the IMV. Lateral dissection is carried as much as possible to facilitate the lateral mobilization later. Careful attention should be made to keep the ureter down in the retroperitoneum and the dissection kept between Gerota's fascia and the mesentery of the descending colon.

After identification of the inferior border of the pancreas, the IMV should be isolated. This can be accomplished with traction at the level of the ligament of Treitz. The division of the IMV with an energy device should be accomplished to avoid tension. Recognize that it can become a source of quick and massive bleeding and difficult to control during single-port surgery. Do not hesitate to place an additional port if needed to control this.

The medial dissection should be completed by this point. Attention is now turned to the lateral attachments starting with gentle medial retraction of the sigmoid colon. This will expose the lateral attachments at the level of the pelvic brim (Fig. 22.16). Using the monopolar scissors facilitates this

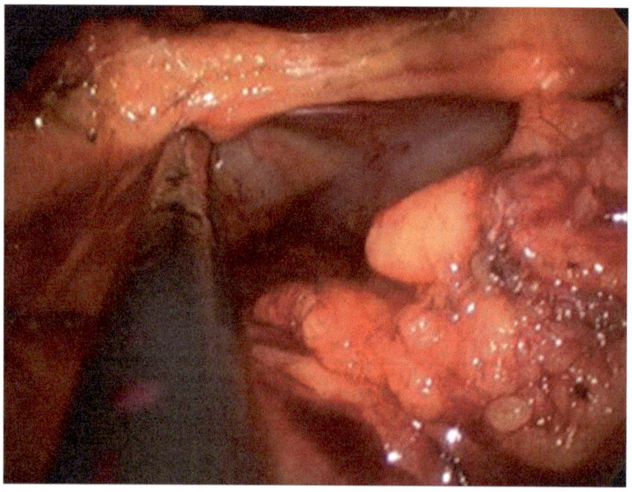

**Fig. 22.15** Opening the avascular area on top of the pancreas to enter the lesser sac. Identification of the posterior wall of the stomach helps confirm the location

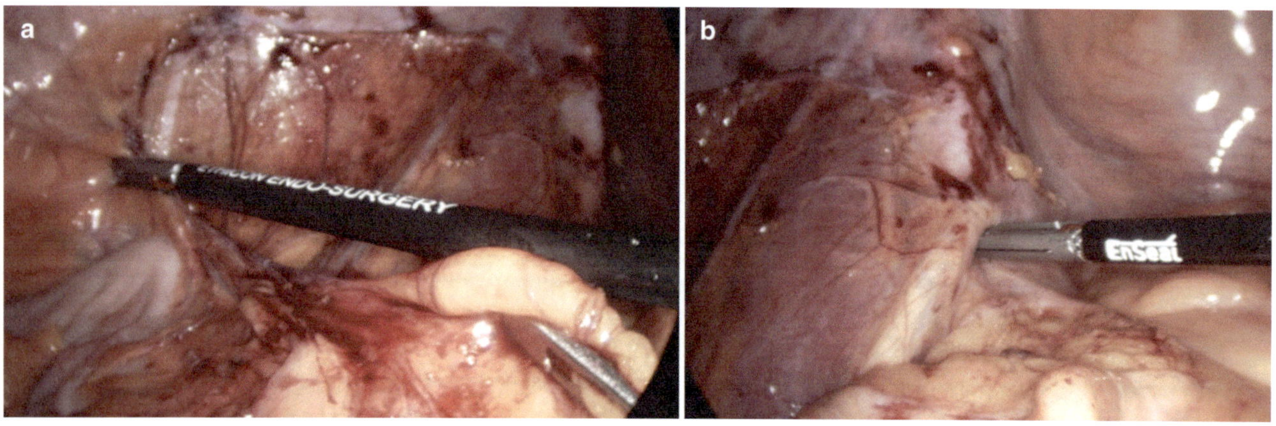


**Fig. 22.16** Takedown of the lateral attachments starting at the pelvic brim. Notice the in-line instruments. (**a**) The retroperitoneum with gonadal vein. (**b**) Tip of the instrument points at the left ureter

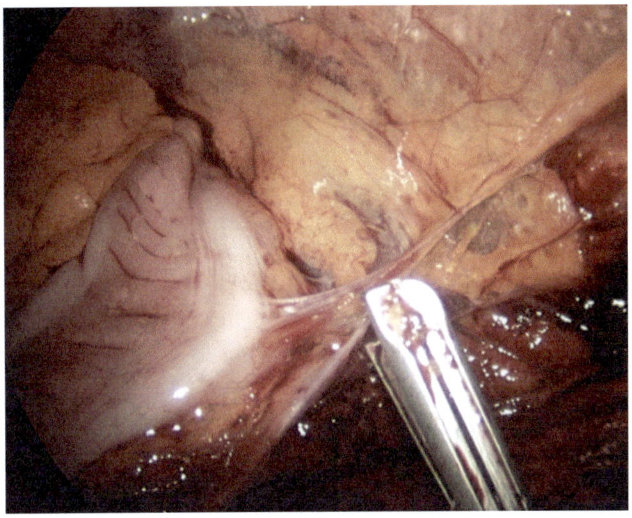

**Fig. 22.17** Division of the left lateral colonic attachments (white line of Toldt)

step. After an opening is created in the lateral attachments, visual identification of the left ureter is easy. The left-hand instrument is used to keep the lateral attachment window open, and the right instrument continues division of the remaining lateral attachments along the white line of Toldt cephalad until the entire left colon is mobilized (Fig. 22.17) at the splenic flexure.

My preference is to take down the colonic splenic ligament using the ENSEAL® energy device. The lesser sac is entered laterally and the inferior border of the pancreas is identified. The patient is now placed in reverse Trendelenburg to allow better exposure of the omental attachments to the transverse colon. Elevation of the omentum with the left-hand instrument provides traction, and by using the energy device, the gravity will keep the colon away (i.e., countertraction).

You should continue to separate the omentum until the middle transverse colon or the falciform ligament is reached. At this point, all of the colon should be retracted to the right side of the abdomen to complete exposure and allow dissection of the retroperitoneum. Dividing the peritoneal attachments at the splenic flexure will allow entry to the lesser sac. With continued dissection from the left side, all attachments between the transverse colon and the inferior border of the pancreas are serially divided until the midline and the stump of the IMV are visualized.

The colon is then returned to normal anatomical position, and the patient is returned to deep Trendelenburg. A 12-mm trocar is placed through the SILS trocar to be able to place an endostapler, and the distal colon rectal juncture is divided. Alternatively, this can be done through the wound when in the suprapubic incision (although exposure through a small fascial opening is limited). The colon is exteriorized through the incision after careful placement of a wound retractor Alexis® wound protector, which will facilitate the extraction. The proximal area of the colon then is selected, and the mesentery of the colon is divided between clamps or using the energy device.

The colorectal intracorporeal anastomosis is created by first securing the circular anvil in the proximal colon and then returning the bowel into the abdomen. The single-port trocar is replaced in the incision. If the incision was enlarged to accommodate the specimen, the fascia can be approximated with a simple suture in each corner or as many as are needed to ensure an appropriate seal. If the wound protector is kept in place, a wet lap can be used to keep the airtight seal. Insufflation is obtained and the circular stapler is placed through the anal canal after dilatation of the anal sphincter. The spike is opened just inferior to the previous rectal stapler line, which will help if any anastomotic defect or air leak occurs, as the defect will potentially be anterior and is easier to visualize and repair. After the anvil and the spike of the stapler meet, the stapler is closed, inspected, and fired. The stapler is removed and the anastomosis doughnuts are checked. An air-leak test is performed using a flexible sigmoidoscopy. Compression of the proximal colon is performed while the pelvis is filled with fluid, submerging the anastomosis, and the sigmoidoscope is advanced to the anastomosis. This final inspection is performed to ensure that the anastomosis is airtight. The abdomen is aspirated dry, and the small bowel is evaluated and should be on top to the cutting edge of the colon mesentery to prevent internal hernias; then the trocar is removed, and the incision is closed.

## Single-Port Laparoscopic Total Proctocolectomy with Ileal Pouch Anal Anastomosis Reconstruction Using Standard Laparoscopic Instrumentation (Video 22.3)

Single-port laparoscopic operations have recently gained attention and may extend and expand beyond the benefits of conventional multiport laparoscopy [26–28]. The cosmetic benefit has been fairly straightforward to appreciate; however, any additional benefits, such as decreased hospital stay, morbidity, or cost, to the patient have yet to be confirmed in large randomized studies. In the meantime, patients with ulcerative colitis and familial adenomatous polyposis that present in early stages of life who are often very concerned about cosmetic results may seek surgeons with a desire to improve patient outcomes and satisfaction and press on to explore the potential of single-port laparoscopy in smaller series. I will describe the steps of a multi-quadrant surgery performed through a single-port laparoscopy—the total proctocolectomy with J pouch—one of the most complex operations a colon and rectal surgeon performs.

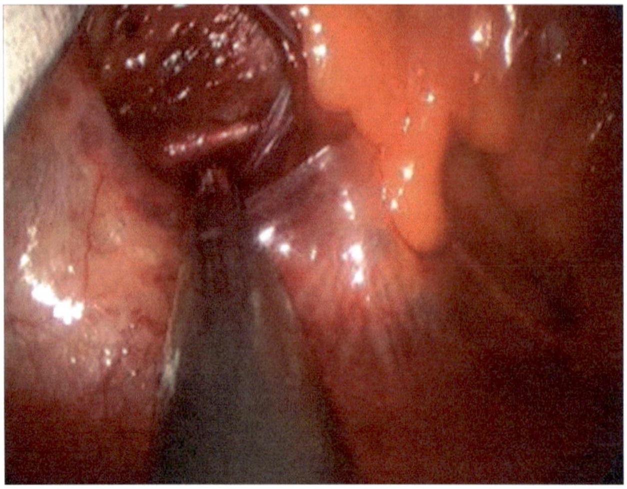

**Fig. 22.18** The left ureter is recognized at the tip of the instrument

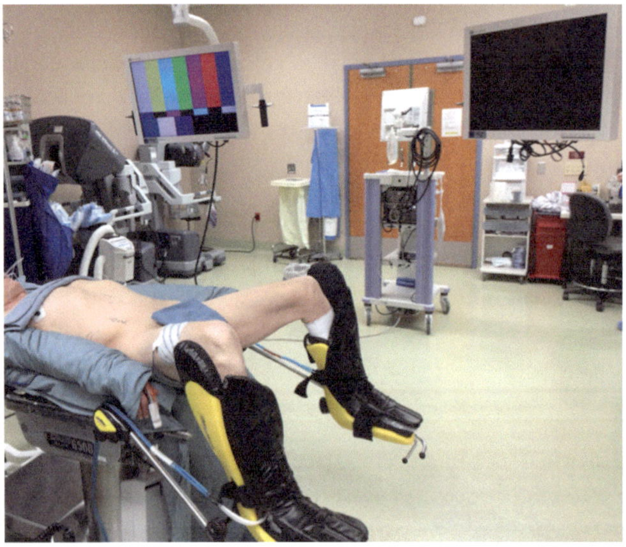

**Fig. 22.19** The patient secured to the table with a 3-inch tape, in a modified lithotomy position

## Preparation and Positioning

The patient should be marked appropriately by an enterostomal therapist for ileostomy placement in the right lower quadrant prior to proceeding to the operating room. Once on the operating table, the patient should be placed in a low lithotomy position using the Allen stirrups and both arms are tucked close to the patient with pads to protect for ulnar and radial nerve injuries and allow the operative team to rotate freely around the patient during the evolution of the procedure (Fig. 22.18). The patient is strapped securely using a 3-inch silk tape around the chest in order to facilitate frequent and pronounced bed movement throughout the case (Fig. 22.19). Ureteral stents are beneficial and may be placed at this time [29]. As with other colon and rectal procedures, mechanical bowel preparation before the surgery and appropriate intravenous antibiotics are given prior to the initial skin incision.

Single-port total colectomy can be accomplished by an experienced single surgeon. An assistant of any level may assist during most of the cases. The participation of the assistant can vary throughout the procedure, but at a minimum, they be facile at operating the laparoscopic camera.

The operation is performed through a SILS™ port. I use a standard laparoscopic scope, 5-mm 30-degree angle, for the duration of the case. Many surgeons find that a flexible scope is useful in some portions of the procedure, allowing the camera holder to establish a farther distance away from the surgeon; however, at the same time, it adds a level of difficulty and requires experience in the use of the device. Instrumentation includes atraumatic bowel grasper; energy device with multifunctional capability, ENSEAL® (Ethicon Endo-Surgery, Inc); endostapler 60 mm with blue reloads for bowel resection and creation of the pouch; 25- or 26-mm circular stapler for end-to-end ileoanal pouch anastomosis; and Alexis® wound retractor (Applied Medical).

## Position of the Patient and Single-Port Multi-trocar Access System Placement (SILS ™)

For the right-side part of the procedure, the patient will be in reverse Trendelenburg with the left side down to allow gravity to locate the small bowel in the left side of the abdomen and facilitate in the identification of the ileocolic artery. During the transverse colon mobilization, the patient is in Trendelenburg but leveling the table; then for the left side and rectal dissection, the table will go to Trendelenburg with right side down.

The surgeon should start by making a circular incision at the ileostomy site. After dissecting down to the level of the fascia, the rectus muscle is separated and the posterior fascia is opened; an incision is made in order to accommodate the single-port access system of the surgeon's choice.

## Colonic Dissection

Starting with the right colon, a window is made into the retroperitoneal space just below the ileocolic pedicle similar to the right colectomy earlier. Prior to ligating the vessels, mobilization of the colon proceeds in a medial-to-lateral fashion. Next, the lateral attachments of the right colon are taken down from superior to inferior. When mobilizing and ligating the vessels to the transverse colon, the omentum is left in place. Once ready to take down the left and sigmoid colon, the inferior

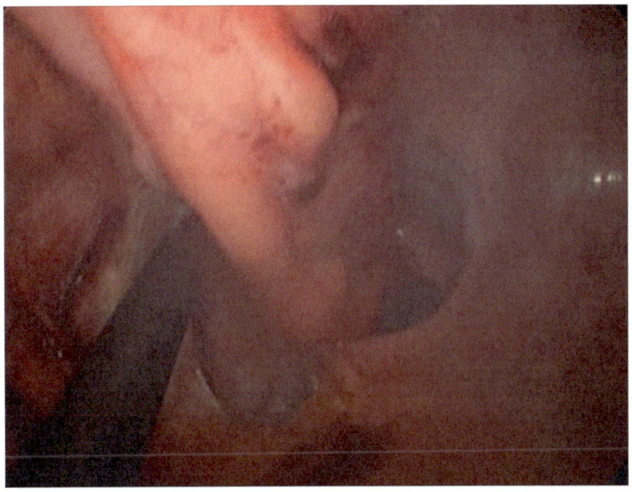

**Fig. 22.20** The dissection of the rectum is carried out by staying in the planes between the layers of the fascia propria of the mesorectum and the presacral fascia

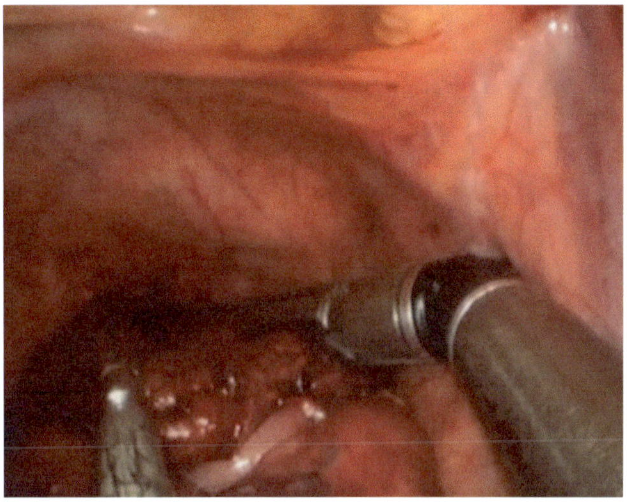

**Fig. 22.21** The laparoscopic stapler is placed from the right side to the left, anterior to posterior. The key is to have good traction and using the stapler with both articulation and rotation

mesenteric artery can be ligated early to allow medial-to-lateral dissection to proceed. In this case, the lateral attachments of the left colon are easier to remove working from inferior to superior (pedal to cephalic).

## Proctectomy

The rectum is often better dissected using monopolar cautery. We use endoscissors, as these are bloodless and expeditious in dissection. It is important to identify the ureters at the pelvic brim and avoid injury to the nervi erigentes. The dissection of the rectum is carried out by staying in the correct planes between the layers of the fascia propria of the mesorectum and the presacral fascia (Fig. 22.20). The posterior dissection is continued down in the midline between the rectal fascia and Waldeyer's fascia to the level of the levator ani. It's important to stay in this plane to prevent injury to the sacral venous plexus, which will result in major bleeding. One of the 5-mm ports must then be swapped out for a 12-mm port in order to accommodate a large laparoscopic articulating GIA stapler. With a laparoscopic Allis clamp, traction is performed to the left side of the rectum, and the stapler is placed in the right side of the pelvis with a maximum articulation from right to left and up to down (Fig. 22.21). The key is to have good traction and use the stapler with a rotational component. Also, the previous dissection should be all the way to the anal canal to eliminate the extra fat of the mesorectum that can make the placement of the stapler more difficult. The rectal division is completed with the fewest number of staple loads as possible—usually two. On occasion, an extra trocar in the left quadrant can be placed and used as a drain site.

## Specimen Extraction

A wound protector is placed at the ileostomy site and the excised specimen is brought out. The terminal ileum can now be divided extracorporeally. The most important step in making an ileoanal pouch is to create a tension-free anastomosis. These can be difficult to evaluate during the extracorporeal formation of the pouch. To create a tension-free anastomosis, we assess the potential for the pouch to reach the anus before the pouch is created. This is done by ensuring the pouch reaches the symphysis pubis externally, and then a standard 12- to 15-cm J pouch is created using the same Endo GIA stapler. The anvil of a circular stapler is secured to the distal aspect of the pouch and then returned to the abdomen.

## Ileoanal Anastomosis

We perform a double-stapled anastomosis technique. After reestablishing pneumoperitoneum, we ensure that there is no tension or torsion of the pouch. Then place the circular stapler through the anus and secure the anvil to the spike of the stapler. After firing, the anastomosis should be air-leak tested and the doughnuts checked for two complete intact rings of tissue (Fig. 22.22a–c).

## Ostomy

After inspecting the abdomen a final time, a loop of ileum is selected approximately 15–20 cm proximal to the pouch in order to form a temporary loop ileostomy.

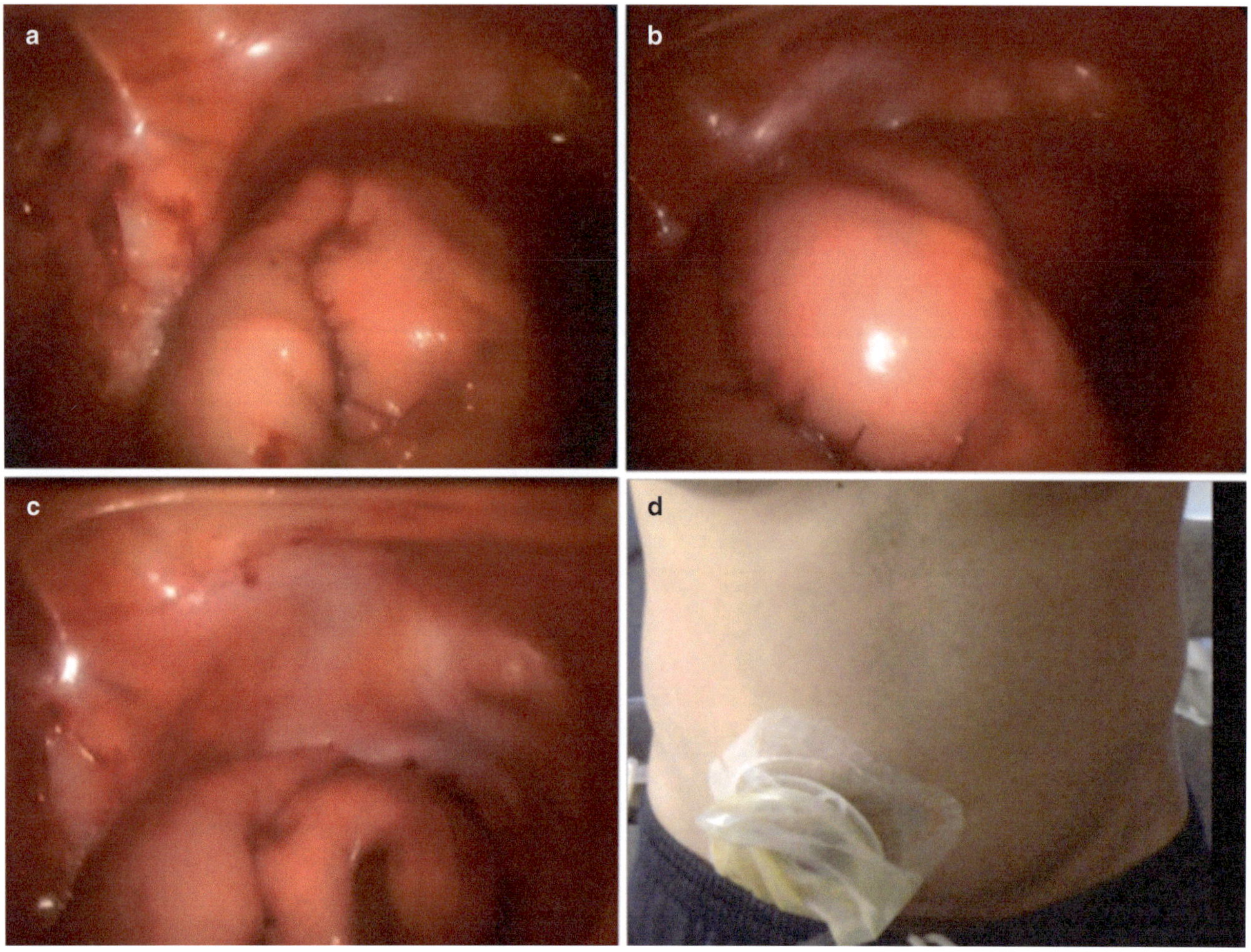

**Fig. 22.22** (**a–d**) Pouch leak test (**a**) pouch anastomosis in place, (**b**) air in the anal canal with proctoscopy anastomosis underwater, (**c**) pouch desufflated, (**d**) postoperative day one with only the ostomy visible

This ostomy is matured in the standard fashion. No drains are placed, and the patient is left with a visible ileostomy-only incision (Fig. 22.22d).

## Postoperative Care

All the patients get regional anesthesia with a transversus abdominal plane (TAP) block using bupivacaine liposome injectable suspension for postoperative pain control as well as intravenous acetaminophen. The patients are allowed to drink a clear liquid diet with a nutritional supplementation. If liquid diet is tolerated, the intravenous fluid is discontinued and they are advanced to regular diet. The Foley catheter is removed on postoperative day one in almost all the patients. When the patient is tolerating a regular diet, they are changed to oral pain medication. Once they are comfortable with the stoma, taking enough calories and liquids, and passing flatus, they may be discharged home.

## Complications

In my experience, single-incision laparoscopic colectomy can be used as a safe and efficacious approach to colorectal resections in patients eligible for traditional laparoscopy with minimal additional equipment. Single-incision laparoscopy was undertaken without an increase in morbidity or mortality. All of the standard complications ranging from wound infections to abscesses may occur. Intraoperative bleeding is more difficult to control during a single-incision operation due to the lack of triangulation and space to place the additional instrument or suction. In this case, you can use clips, Endoloops™ (Ethicon, Cincinnati, OH), or an energy device or place another trocar.

## Outcomes

Among the potential advantages of single-incision laparoscopic colectomy compared with the standard laparoscopic colectomy, cosmesis is an important factor. The perspective of body image is often very important in young patients, and single-incision approaches facilitate this trait.

Postoperative pain and recovery typically show to be improved by this approach. The patients typically demonstrate a significantly lower postoperative analgesic requirement, early ambulation, and early discharge.

## Pearls and Pitfalls

- Single-port laparoscopic surgery allows common laparoscopic procedures to be performed entirely through the umbilicus and permits the surgeon to convert the procedure to multiport laparoscopic surgery at any point during the operation.
- Modification of the operative technique can allow a colectomy to be performed without any additional access sites and without any minilaparotomy using the single-port access as extraction site.
- Operative time is probably longer in the single-incision laparoscopy in the beginning but will continue to decrease as additional cases are performed.
- The single-incision laparoscopic colectomy, as opposed to laparoscopic colectomy, can be harder to teach. Only one person can work at a time during a single-port laparoscopy case. It is an ergonomic challenge to get the cameraperson and the surgeon positioned so that the case can proceed.
- The division of the vessel during single incision should be accomplished with minimal tension. Recognize that it can become a source of quick and massive bleeding and difficult to control during single-port surgery.

## Conclusion

Single-port laparoscopy is becoming a popular option in the field of colorectal surgery. However, because it is a relatively new approach, many surgeons do not have any formal training in performing the operations with the new instruments. Those who are taking it upon themselves to learn this new technique do not yet know the number of cases it takes to become proficient in safely performing this operation. Many surgeons have found that the learning curve is quite short and almost nonexistent for those already skilled in conventional laparoscopic surgery and, more specifically, right hemicolectomy.

## References


1. Brunner W, Schirnhofer J, Waldstein-Wartenberg N, Frass R, Weiss H. Single incision laparoscopic sigmoid colon resections without visible scar: a novel technique. Color Dis. 2010;12:66–70.
2. Romanelli JR. Single-port laparoscopic surgery: an overview. Surg Endosc. 2009;23:1419–27.
3. Rane A, Rao P, Rao P. Single-port-access nephrectomy and other laparoscopic urologic procedures using a novel laparoscopic port (R-port). Urology. 2008;72:260–3.
4. Kaouk JH, Goel RK, Haber GP, Crouzet S, Desai MM, Gill IS. Single-port laparoscopic radical prostatectomy. Urology. 2008;72:1190–3.
5. Nguyen NT, Hinojosa MW, Smith BR, Reavis KM. Single laparoscopic incision transabdominal (SLIT) surgery-adjustable gastric banding: a novel minimally invasive surgical approach. Obes Surg. 2008;18(12):1628–31.
6. Gumbs AA, Milone L, Sinha P, Bessler M. Totally transumbilical laparoscopic cholecystectomy. J Gastrointest Surg. 2009;13(3):533–4.
7. Esposito C. One-trocar appendectomy in pediatric surgery. Surg Endosc. 1998;12:588–94.
8. Pfluke JM, Parker M, Stauffer JA, Paetau AA, Bowers SP, Asbun HJ, Smith CD. Laparoscopic Surgery Performed Through a Single Incision: A Systematic Review of the Current Literature. J Am Coll Surg. 2010 Oct;28.
9. Bucher P, Pugin F, Morel P. Single port access laparoscopic right hemicolectomy. Int J Colorectal Dis. 2008;23:1013–6.
10. Remzi FH, Kirat HT, Kaouk JH, Geisler DP. Single-port laparoscopy in colorectal surgery. Colorectal Dis. 2008;10(8):823–6.
11. Waters JA, Rapp BM, Guzman MJ, Jester AL, Selzer DJ, Robb BW, Johansen BJ, Tsai BM, Maun DC, George VV. Single-port laparoscopic right hemicolectomy: the first 100 resections. Dis Colon Rectum. 2012;55:134–9.
12. Gawart M, Dupitron S, Lutfi R. Laparoendoscopic single-site gastric bands versus standard multiport gastric bands: a comparison of technical learning curve measured by surgical time. Am J Surg. 2012;203:327–9. discussion 30.
13. Hernandez J, Ross S, Morton C, McFarlin K, Dahal S, Golkar F, Albrink M, Rosemurgy A. The learning curve of laparoendoscopic single-site (LESS) cholecystectomy: definable, short, and safe. J Am Coll Surg. 2010;211:652–7.
14. Wang L, Liu B, Wu Z, Yang Q, Hehir M, Chen W, Xu Z, Xiao L, Wang F, Sun Y. Transumbilical laparoendoscopic single-site surgery: more than 1-year experience in radical nephrectomy and its learning curve study. J Endourol. 2011;25:1859–65.
15. Lacy A. Colon cancer; laparoscopic resection. Ann Oncol. 2005;16:88–92.
16. Curet MJ. Laparoscopic-assisted resection of colorectal carcinoma. Lancet. 2005;365:1666–8.
17. The Clinical Outcomes of Surgical Therapy (COST) Study Group. A comparison of laparoscopically assisted and open colectomy for colon cancer. N Engl J Med. 2004;350:2050–9.
18. Fleshman J, Sargent DJ, Green E. for The Clinical Outcomes of Surgical Therapy Study Group. Laparoscopic colectomy for cancer is not inferior to open surgery based on 5-year data from the COST Study Group trial. Ann Surg. 2007;246:655–62.

19. Leung KL, Kwok SP, Lam SC, Lee JF, Yiu RY, Ng SS, et al. Laparoscopic resection of rectosigmoid carcinoma: prospective randomized trial. Lancet. 2004;363:1187–92.
20. Jayne DG, Guillou PJ, Thorpe H, Quirke P, Copeland J, Smith AM, et al. UK MRC CLASICC Trial Group. Randomized trial of laparoscopic-assisted resection of colorectal carcinoma: 3-year results of the UK MRC CLASICC Trial Group. J Clin Oncol. 2007; 25:3061–8.
21. Kaouk JH, Haber GP, Goel RK, Desai MM, Aron M, Rackley RR, Moore C, Gill IS. Single-port laparoscopic surgery in urology: initial experience. Urology. 2008;71:3–6.
22. Goel RK, Kaouk JH. Single-port-access renal cryoablation (SPARC): a new approach. Eur Urol. 2008;53:1204–9.
23. Kaouk JH, Palmer JS. Single-port laparoscopic surgery: initial experience in children for varicocelectomy. BJU Int. 2008;102:97–9.
24. Opilka M, Starzewski J, Lorenc Z, Tarnowski A, Zawada Z. Open versus closed laparoscopy entry–which are the evidences? Hepatogastroenterology. 2009;56(89):75–9.
25. Turnbull RB, Kyle K, Watson FR, Spratt J. cancer of the colon: the influence of no-touch isolation technic on survival rates. Ann Surg. 1967;166:420–5.
26. Gandhi DP, Ragupathi M, Patel CB, Ramos-Valadez DI, Pickron TB, Haas EM. Single incision versus hand-assisted laparoscopic colectomy: a case-matched series. J Gastrointest Surg. 2010;14: 1875–80.
27. Cahill RA, Lindsey I, Jones O, Guy R, Mortensen N, Cunningham C. Single-port laparoscopic total colectomy for medically uncontrolled colitis. Dis Colon Rectum. 2010;53:1143–7.
28. Adair J, Gromski MA, Lim RB, Nagle D. Single-incision laparoscopic right colectomy: experience with 17 consecutive cases and comparison with multiport laparoscopic right colectomy. Dis Colon Rectum. 2010;53:1549–54.
29. da Silva G, Boutros M, Wexner SD. Role of prophylactic ureteric stents in colorectal surgery. Asian J Endosc Surg. 2012;5(3): 105–10.

# Natural Orifice Surgery (NOTES)

# 23

Mark H. Whiteford

## Key Points

- Natural orifice translumenal endoscopic surgery (NOTES) involves passing instruments through a natural orifice (mouth, anus, vagina) then through a surgically created hole in a hollow viscous into the peritoneal cavity.
- NOTES surgery has several different categories: pure NOTES procedures, hybrid NOTES procedures, and natural orifice specimen extraction (NOSE).
- Colorectal surgeons possess the fundamental skill sets to perform NOTES surgery.
- NOSE of the sigmoid colon during laparoscopic sigmoid resection can safely be performed in experienced hands.
- Transanal NOTES surgery is currently in an investigational phase of development.
- Transanal total mesorectal excision is a favorable candidate for NOTES transanal surgery.

## Introduction

Abdominal wall surgical skin incisions, purposely created through a highly sensate and mechanically important normal body part, provide no true benefit to the patient, only harm. This impairment, however, has always been considered a necessary evil required to carry out the steps of the prescribed intra-abdominal operation. The transition to laparoscopic, minimally invasive surgery, however, has realized significant short-term patient benefit by minimizing surgical access trauma—all the while maintaining the established principles of open surgery. This dramatic avoidance of pain and morbidity associated with large abdominal wall wounds led to the quick acceptance of laparoscopic surgical techniques in general surgery.

In 2004, work from Kalloo et al. heralded a new chapter for minimal access surgery. An intra-abdominal operation was wholly completed via instruments passed through a natural orifice (per oral) by means of a surgically created hole through the stomach into the peritoneal cavity of a swine [1]. This was soon followed by the first human case reported by Rao and Reddy of an appendectomy performed transgastrically utilizing an upper endoscope [2]. Such approaches heralded the prospect of surgery with no abdominal wall access trauma and the morbidity thereby associated. This new surgical paradigm has been coined natural orifice translumenal endoscopic surgery (NOTES®).

Immediately apparent to the early innovators of NOTES was that this represented a major paradigm shift, harboring many areas of real and potential concerns regarding patient safety and methods of clinical introduction of these novel techniques. A unique collaborative effort involving leadership from the American Society of Gastrointestinal Endoscopy (ASGE) and the Society of American Gastrointestinal and Endoscopic Surgery (SAGES) convened a working group to formulate a plan for the safe adoption, research, and clinical introduction of NOTES. This group chose the name NOSCAR®, Natural Orifice Surgery Consortium for Assessment and Research. Their discussions and recommendations for early research and clinical work have been laid out in the NOTES White Paper [2], created to promote a tempered, thoughtful, safe, and collaborative development of this new surgical paradigm. Parallel collaborative groups were quickly developed in Europe (EURO-NOTES, European Association for Translumenal Surgery, D-NOTES), South America (Natural Orifice Surgery Latin America, NOTES Research Group Brazil), and Asia

**Electronic supplementary material:** Supplementary material is available in the online version of this chapter at 10.1007/978-1-4939-1581-1_23. Videos can also be accessed at http://www.springerimages.com/videos/978-1-4939-1580-4.

M.H. Whiteford, M.D., F.A.C.S., F.A.S.C.R.S. (✉)
Gastrointestinal and Minimally Invasive Surgery Division, The Oregon Clinic, Portland, OR, USA

Providence Cancer Center, 4805 NE Glisan, Suite 6N60, Portland, OR 97213, USA

Oregon Health & Science University, Portland, OR, USA
e-mail: mwhiteford@orclinic.com

H.M. Ross et al. (eds.), *Minimally Invasive Approaches to Colon and Rectal Disease: Technique and Best Practices*, DOI 10.1007/978-1-4939-1581-1_23, 

**Table 23.1** Taxonomy and abbreviations

| |
|---|
| *Hybrid NOTES*: A primarily NOTES procedure assisted by addition of a secondary modality such as laparoscopy |
| *NOSE*: Natural orifice specimen extraction. The use of a natural orifice through which to extract a surgical specimen |
| *NOTES*: Natural orifice translumenal endoscopic surgery |
| *Pure NOTES*: Surgical procedure completed wholly via a natural orifice without assistance provided through skin incisions |
| *taTME*: Transanal total mesorectal excision. Total mesorectal excision performed via a combined abdominal (open or laparoscopic) and transanal endoscopic approach |
| *Viscotomy*: A full-thickness surgical opening through a hollow viscous into the peritoneal (retroperitoneal, thoracic, mediastinal) space used to perform a diagnostic or therapeutic procedure in the peritoneal (retroperitoneal, thoracic, mediastinal) space |

(India NOTES, Japan NOTES). Nomenclature has also been developed to assist in accurate and uniform reporting (Table 23.1).

Following a few years of initial excitement and hype of NOTES, a more critical phase of grounded scientific investigation ensued. Benchtop and clinical research confirmed the safety and feasibility of a few focused procedures and dispelled some early NOTES concerns, particularly in regard to the risk of peritoneal contamination, safe viscotomy creation and closure, and the technical steps. Hence, clinical efforts in NOTES have become increasingly focused on a few targeted applications based on the route of access, each in varying stages of development and clinical application. The most common transvaginal procedures are cholecystectomy, appendectomy, and hybrid laparoscopic colon resections with transvaginal specimen extraction [3, 4]. Per-oral and transgastric procedures have focused on per-oral endoscopic myotomy (POEM) for the treatment of achalasia and transgastric resection of small gastric tumors. The least common NOTES access route, transanal, has (to date) been limited mostly to laparoscopic rectosigmoid resections with transanal specimen extraction (NOSE) and hybrid transanal-laparoscopic rectosigmoid resection for benign and malignant diseases. The most mature of these procedures is a hybrid transanal and laparoscopic total mesorectal (taTME) excision for the treatment of rectal cancer.

## GI NOTES

During GI NOTES surgery, the natural orifice can be utilized in three different ways. First, the orifice is utilized as a site of specimen extraction following a standard laparoscopic resection. This technique is called natural orifice specimen extraction (NOSE). An example would be a laparoscopic sigmoid colectomy with transanal specimen extraction instead of extracting the specimen through an abdominal wall extraction site. A second method is utilizing the natural orifice as a route of access to the peritoneal cavity in order to perform a diagnostic or therapeutic operation on a separate body part. An example of this is a transvaginal cholecystectomy. The third method involves natural orifice access to perform an operation on the access organ. Examples of this include a transgastric tumor resection or transanal total mesorectal excision. As current clinical applications in the transanal NOTES realm do not yet include transanal access for operations on non-colorectal organs, this chapter will focus on NOSE and taTME.

## Natural Orifice Specimen Extraction (NOSE)

Laparoscopic rectosigmoid resection has become the preferred treatment for rectosigmoid cancer and diverticulitis. The key steps of the procedure—complete left colon and splenic flexure mobilization, mesenteric vascular ligation, and intracorporeal anastomosis—can be safely completed exclusively through 5 and 10 mm trocars. Removal of the intact specimen, however, requires creation of a 5–10 cm abdominal wall incision. Several surgeons, in an effort to realize the greatest benefits of minimally invasive surgery, omitted this large abdominal extraction incision by using the open rectum through which to remove the colonic specimen (Video 23.1). This technique has come to be termed natural orifice specimen extraction (NOSE). Both transanal and transvaginal specimen (Videos 23.2 and 23.3) extraction have been described [5], but this section will focus on transanal specimen extraction following laparoscopic rectosigmoid resection. Interest in NOSE has significantly increased over the past 10 years.

Franklin was the first to report a large case series of NOSE during laparoscopic rectal and sigmoid resections dating back to 1991. He described delivering "the resected specimen out of the peritoneal cavity through an anatomic passage rather than through an abdominal incision" [6, 7]. This technique has subsequently been utilized and modified by others [8, 9]. The key steps of the technique are listed in Table 23.2. A standardized laparoscopic low anterior resection and mobilization is completed utilizing a total mesorectal excision technique. Intraoperative colonoscopy or proctoscopy is performed to confirm location of the pathology. Prior to rectal division, the rectum is copiously cleansed with 5 % Betadine solution irrigation. The bowel is divided intracorporeally either sharply or with endoscopic

**Table 23.2** Steps of a laparoscopic sigmoid colectomy with natural orifice specimen extraction (NOSE)

| |
|---|
| 1. Laparoscopic mobilization of the left/sigmoid/rectum |
| 2. Confirm location of the pathology (i.e., intraoperative endoscopy) |
| 3. Rectal washout with 5 % povidone-iodine solution |
| 4. Resection completed with intracorporeal division (i.e., energy, scissors) |
| 5. Bag the specimen |
| 6. Transanal specimen extraction (following gentle dilation of the anus) |
| 7. End-to-end anastomosis |
| 8. Leak test |

linear stapling devices, ensuring adequate oncologic margins. The specimen is then placed in a retrieval bag and passed to a ring forceps placed through the gently dilated anus. The specimen is extracted through the open rectum. The anvil of the circular stapler is then passed into the abdomen transrectally and secured in the proximal bowel. The upper rectum is then closed with a laparoscopic linear stapling device. End-to-end or side-to-end colorectal anastomosis is fashioned using a transanally delivered circular stapler. Finally, confirmatory air leak test is then performed.

Franklin has reported remarkably good results in 277 patients undergoing transanal specimen removal [7]. The anastomotic leak rate was 1.1 %, with a major complication rate of 3.6 %. Hospital length of stay, however, remained comparable to standard specimen extraction at 6.9 days. Some complaints of minor fecal soiling were reported, but significant fecal incontinence has only occurred in three patients (1 %) [6]. They also do not report on what their specimen size cutoff was, as attempting to remove a large specimen transanally might damage the rectum or sphincter. Other groups have limited transanal specimen size to 4–5 cm, and larger specimens would then be delivered via an abdominal extraction incision.

Yet, in order to successfully utilize this approach, morbidity (including infectious complications and anastomotic leak) must be kept to a minimum. A prospective study of peritoneal fluid contamination following laparoscopic left-sided resections with and without NOSE demonstrated positive peritoneal cultures in 100 % and 89 % of patients, respectively. Only one of 17 patients in the NOSE group developed an anastomotic leak, and there was no difference in infectious complications between the two groups [10].

Despite the success in using natural orifice specimen extraction at these selected institutions, this technique has not yet caught on in most centers due to the additional time and technical skills required to perform these increasingly complex operations. In addition, there are ongoing concerns regarding potential damage to the rectum and sphincter complex, as well as fecal contamination of the peritoneum. As with the other complex laparoscopic procedures, more surgeons will likely adopt this technique over time as clinical experience and confidence increase.

## NOTES Transanal Rectosigmoid Resection, Transanal TME (taTME)

### Development of NOTES Transanal Rectosigmoid Resection

Early NOTES procedures that made headlines involved operations performed transorally or transvaginally. Further development of transoral procedures, however, has been markedly hindered because of their exclusive reliance on flexible instrumentation. To date, flexible endoscopic platforms fail to provide consistent and reliable traction and countertraction, visibility, hemostasis, and viscotomy closure capabilities compared to the laparoscopic corollary. In addition, the small diameter of the esophagus and pharynx limits specimen extraction size. Transvaginal access therefore became the most common NOTES access site as it overcomes much of these limitations. Using this platform, flexible instruments are replaced by the more familiar long laparoscopic instruments. Entry and closure of the viscotomy (i.e., colpotomy) is relatively simple and safe, and the vagina permits large specimen extraction with a low risk of complications.

Transanal NOTES was initially eschewed by many because of the obvious concerns over fecal contamination of the peritoneal cavity and the risk of a leak at the viscotomy site. These real concerns aside, the key components of NOTES are conceptually grounded in the training and practice of colorectal surgery. Colorectal surgeons regularly operate through the natural orifice (i.e., the anus) and are trained in the recognition and management of associated complications. Most colorectal surgeons are also adept at both advanced therapeutic endoscopy and advanced laparoscopic surgery. Lastly, intraperitoneal entry and closure via the anus occurs not infrequently during already established colorectal procedures such as an Altemeier perineal rectosigmoidectomy for rectal prolapse [11] and transanal endoscopic surgery [12]. Anatomically, the rectum and anus share the potential benefits of vaginal access, including a viscotomy site located close to the natural orifice (15 cm or less) and a compliant organ that allows for insertion of larger surgical instruments and permit extraction of large specimens. This collection of key skills and clinical experience provide the foundation from which the development of transanal NOTES surgery has occurred.

It is well known that total mesorectal excision (TME) remains the gold standard for rectal cancer surgery. The principle behind a proper TME is sharp dissection, under direct vision, in the embryonic fusion planes between the mesorectum and the surrounding parietal tissues continued down to the pelvic floor [13]. The TME plane of dissection also affords identification and avoidance of the parasympathetic and sympathetic nerves innervating the urogenital regions. Despite its wide acceptance, TME does have its technical challenges related to exposure and dissection of the proper planes in the confines of the deep bony pelvis. The pelvic curvature makes visualization of the anterior structures difficult, particularly in the obese or in males with an enlarged prostate. Long lighted retractors and/or headlights are required to gain visualization in the deep pelvis. Identification of the distal oncologic margin is estimated by techniques of external palpation, digital rectal examination, or visualization of a diffused tattoo—and this critical step is relegated to the end of the procedure. Even following successful pelvic dissection, current laparoscopic stapling devices utilized for rectal division have limited angulations, making a perpendicular rectal division and seal with a single cartridge application the exception rather than the rule. Hence, distal rectal division often necessitates several overlapping staple lines to complete the distal rectal transection, which may lead to increased risk of anastomotic leak [14, 15].

While NOTES surgery is being performed in very select cases in specialized centers, in reality, it is proceeding through three overlapping phases of clinical development. The first (and still ongoing) phase involves preclinical work identifying safety and efficacy, appropriate procedures, technical factors, and instrument development. A second phase will be early adoption of hybridized procedures that are a combination of established laparoscopic and transanal procedures. This phase is also starting to gain traction, though still remains somewhat of a niche. With increasing experience and new instrument development, the laparoscopic components can be phased out, and the third phase of fully transanal NOTES procedures will transcend.

## Phase 1: Preclinical NOTES Developments

Based on the tenets laid fourth by the NOTES White Paper [2] calling for preclinical laboratory investigations prior to clinical introduction, several investigators began laying the groundwork for transanal NOTES procedures. Radical transanal sigmoid colectomy with intracorporeal anastomosis was initially performed in the cadaver model using off the shelf transanal endoscopic surgery instrumentation, demonstrating the feasibility and fundamental steps of this procedure [16]. This and other studies confirmed the reproducibility of this technique for pelvic rectal dissection [17–19]. From these experiences, it seems that the primary technical limitation of a pure NOTES rectosigmoid resection was not the pelvic dissection, but rather the sacral curvature and sacral promontory that limited current rigid and flexible instruments access and safe dissection higher in the abdomen. Key portions of the rectosigmoid resection such as high ligation of the inferior mesenteric artery and vein and left colon and splenic flexure mobilization could not reliably be accomplished with either currently available rigid or flexible instruments [17, 19, 20]. To overcome these obstacles, a hybrid transanal proctectomy with laparoscopic assistance for the abdominal portions of the procedure was the initial transanal NOTES procedure to break into the human clinical realm.

The potential benefit of a hybrid transanal TME realized during these studies was that it allowed surgeons to overcome some of the challenges of operating in the deep pelvis by performing the deep pelvic dissection from the bottom up. This includes better visualization of the mesorectal envelope with easier retraction and dissection, as well as a more precise determination of the oncologic distal margin. The potential disadvantages include the learning curve in adopting this new point of view, the remaining underlying technical difficulty of the procedure, and the potential risk of bacterial or tumoral peritoneal contamination.

Due to these limitations and obvious concerns over patient safety, the initial foray into transanal total mesorectal excision was performed in a hybrid fashion whereby the deep pelvic portion of the surgery was performed transanally, and the left colon mobilization, vascular ligation, upper pelvic dissection, and air leak test were all performed via standard laparoscopic techniques. What seems apparent is that for the foreseeable future, laparoscopic assistance will be required until technological advancements in surgical instrumentation permit reproducible facile performance of the abdominal steps of the operation in a safe, reliable, and cost-effective fashion.

## Phase 2: Initial Clinical NOTES Developments, Hybrid Laparoscopic and Transanal Rectosigmoid Resection (Transanal Total Mesorectal Excision (taTME))

The first hybrid transanal total mesorectal excision was performed by the team of Sylla and Lacy in 2009 [20]. This patient was a 76-year-old woman with node-positive rectal cancer treated with preoperative chemoradiotherapy. They performed a combined transanal, transvaginal, and laparoscopic total mesorectal excision. Since then, the number of case reports detailing various modifications of taTME is approaching 100 patients [3, 21]. The collective early experience for transanal total mesorectal excision in cancer patients has shown feasibility by demonstrating intact mesorectal specimens, negative circumferential radial margins, adequate lymph node harvest rate, and acceptable complication rates in properly selected patients [21]. Unfortunately, to date, the long-term oncologic results have yet to be reported, and future implementation of this method depends largely on these outcomes.

*Patient selection*: Most clinical studies included patients preoperatively staged at T1-3, N0-1, M0, and with a negative predicted circumferential margin based on preoperative clinical examination and imaging. One study varied from this theme and included particularly high-risk patients with T4 tumors, recurrent cancers, and cancers with less than 1 mm circumferential radial margin [22]. Not surprisingly, they report an increased positive circumferential margin rate of 13 % and higher cancer recurrence rates. At present, these high-risk patients should be excluded from early investigations.

## Transanal TME (taTME) Procedural Steps (Table 23.3)

The patient receives a mechanical bowel preparation, perioperative antibiotics, and pharmacologic thromboembolic prophylaxis. Preferred positioning in the operating room is lithotomy prepped for synchronous abdominal laparoscopy and transanal endoscopic surgery (Fig. 23.1). The operation commences with placement of an anoscope to visualize the rectal lumen and the tumor. A suture purse string is then secured 1–2 cm distal to the tumor to mechanically occlude the proximal bowel from stool spillage during the case (Fig. 23.2). A circumferential, full-thickness, hemostatic incision is then created to transect the rectum just distal to the purse string. This step can be performed via traditional anoscope or via a transanal endoscopic surgery (TES) platform. Several platforms have been described including TEM (transanal endoscopic microsurgery, Richard Wolf GmbH, Knittlingen, Germany), TEO (transanal endoscopic operations, Karl Storz GmbH, Tuttlingen, Germany), or TAMIS (transanal endoscopic minimally invasive surgery) disposable platforms: SILS™ Port, (Covidien, Mansfield, MA) or GelPOINT Path (Applied Medical, Rancho Santa Margarita, CA) (Fig. 23.3). The remaining of the pelvic dissection is performed via the TES platform of choice.

**Table 23.3** Procedural steps of transanal total mesorectal excision

| | |
|---|---|
| 1. | Transanal identification of the distal margin and purse-string occlusion of the lumen |
| 2. | Use of a rigid reusable transanal endoscopic surgical or disposable TAMIS platforms to perform transanal mesorectal excision |
| 3. | Monopolar and bipolar energy utilized for transanal pelvic dissection |
| 4. | Identification and avoidance of the pelvic nerves |
| 5. | Laparoscopic left colon, high vascular ligation, and (when needed) splenic flexure mobilization. Usually performed synchronously with the transanal portion |
| 6. | Transanal specimen extraction |
| 7. | Coloanal hand-sewn or circular-stapled anastomosis |
| 8. | Diverting-loop ileostomy (performed in majority of cases) |

Dissection is initiated in a cephalad direction along the TME plane around the fascia propria of the mesorectum and along the levator muscles. The carbon dioxide pneumodistention aids in identifying the proper planes. Dissection is initially established posterolaterally followed by following the plane around anteriorly. Digital vaginal examination can also facilitate anterior dissection in women. A dry dissection plane is maintained through the use of both monopolar and bipolar cautery devices and small gauze swabs. The parasympathetic nerve roots at S3–5 are swept laterally during the mid-pelvic dissection. The curvature of the sacrum is followed posteriorly along the TME plane. Anteriorly, dissection continues between the rectum and Denonvilliers fascia. As pneumodistention is instrumental in maintaining adequate visualization and retraction during transanal endoscopic surgery, intraperitoneal entry, typically accomplished anteriorly, should be avoided until the majority of the pelvic dissection is completed (Fig. 23.4). Once connection to the peritoneum occurs, pneumodistention of the TME plane collapses and visibility is markedly hampered.

Several potential challenges exist during the transanal TME dissection. Particular care is required at the start of the pelvic dissection to correctly identify the TME plane on the surface of the mesorectal envelope. A plane too lateral or radial will risk injury to the pelvic nerves, sidewall structures, presacral vessels, urethra, prostate, or vagina. A plane too medial or central will risk violating the rectal wall and mesorectum. However, once the correct mesorectal plane is established, it has the same appearance of the plane when dissected from above in the standard fashion.

The abdominal portion of the procedure can be performed laparoscopically by a simultaneous team working from above (Fig. 23.5). Left colon and splenic flexure mobilization,

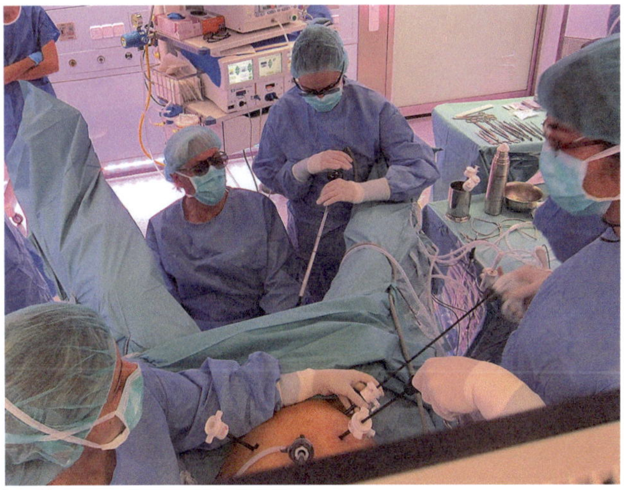

**Fig. 23.1** Transanal total mesorectal excision (taTME) positioning in modified lithotomy allowing perineal and abdominal access simultaneously. *Courtesy of Mark Whiteford, MD and Antonio Lacy, MD*

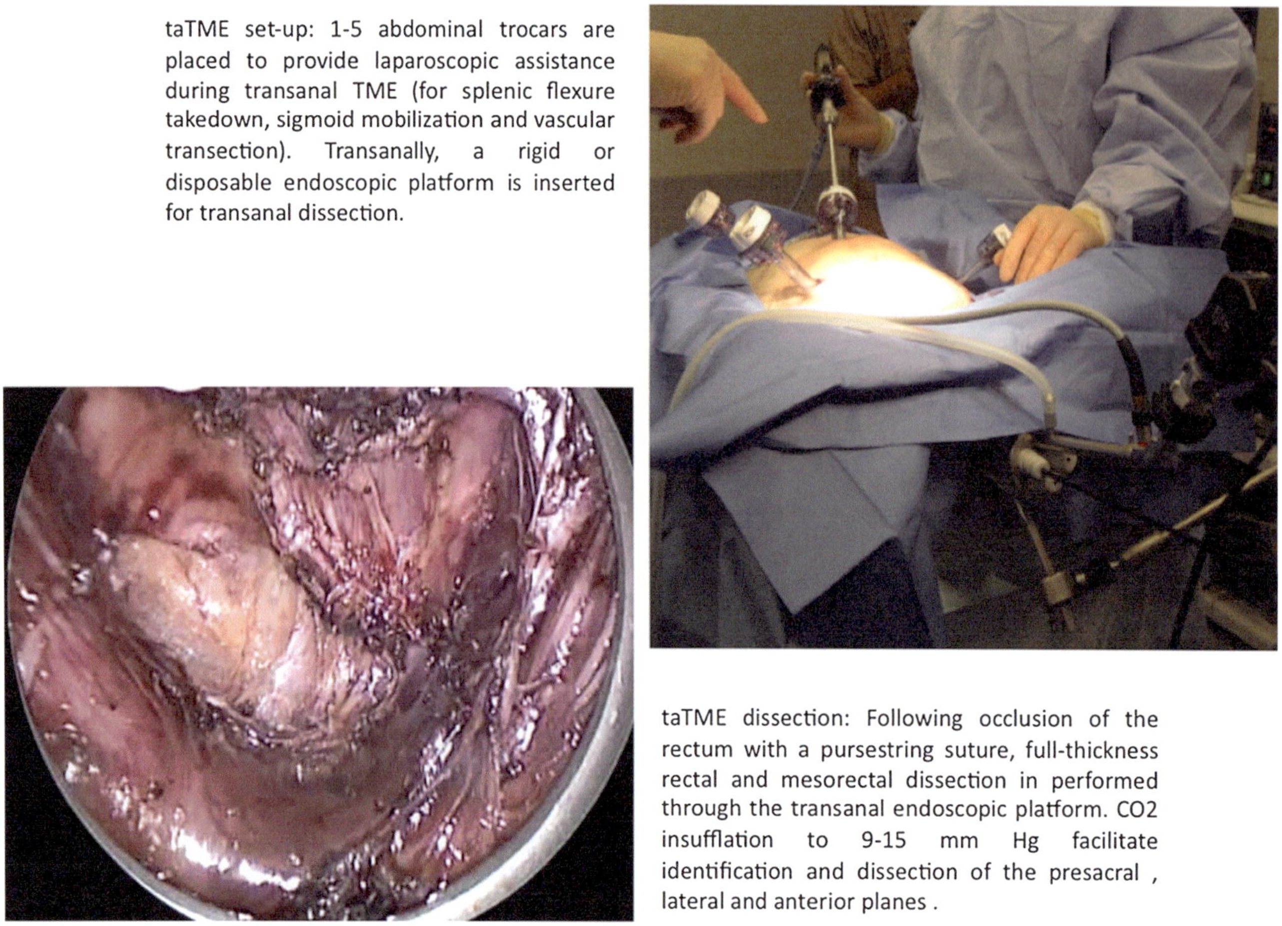


**Fig. 23.2** taTME setup and initial dissection. *Courtesy of Patricia Sylla, MD, with permission*

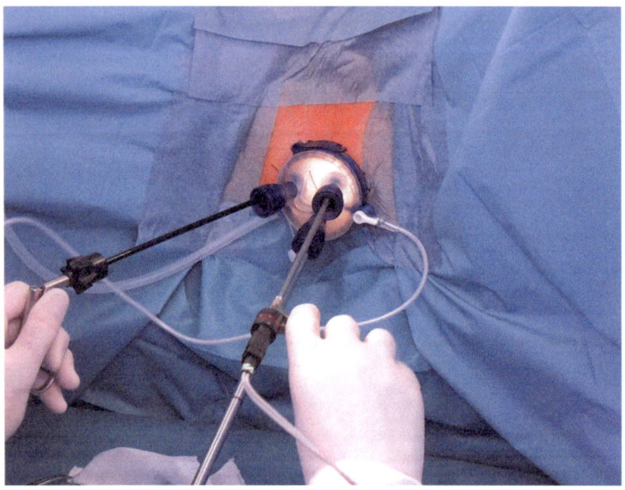

**Fig. 23.3** taTME perineal setup. *Courtesy of Mark Whiteford, MD and Antonio Lacy, MD*

mesenteric vascular ligation, ureteric identification, and the proximal mesorectal dissection are all completed in the conventional fashion. The laparoscopic and transanal surgeons typically join up anteriorly under direct vision, usually at or just below the peritoneal reflection. Working together, they circumferentially complete the remaining TME mobilization. The mesentery proximal to the resection margin is then divided with a laparoscopic vessel-sealing device.

The specimen is properly oriented then delivered and divided transanally. If the specimen is too bulky, then an abdominal extraction should be performed to avoid anorectal damage and tumor exfoliation. The specimen is then inspected for mesorectal grading and confirmation of adequate margins. The anastomosis can either be created as a hand-sewn coloanal or with a circular stapler. The latter involves securing the stapler anvil in the proximal bowel segment, placing a purse string on the open distal rectum, and completing the double purse-string circular-stapled anastomosis. Leak test can then be performed followed by proximal fecal diversion in most cases.

*Outcomes*: A review of the first 72 cases of taTME has demonstrated encouraging results [21]. What stands out is that the average BMI was less than or equal to 26 in all series. Most tumors were located in the mid and low rectum. Most patients underwent stage-appropriate neoadjuvant

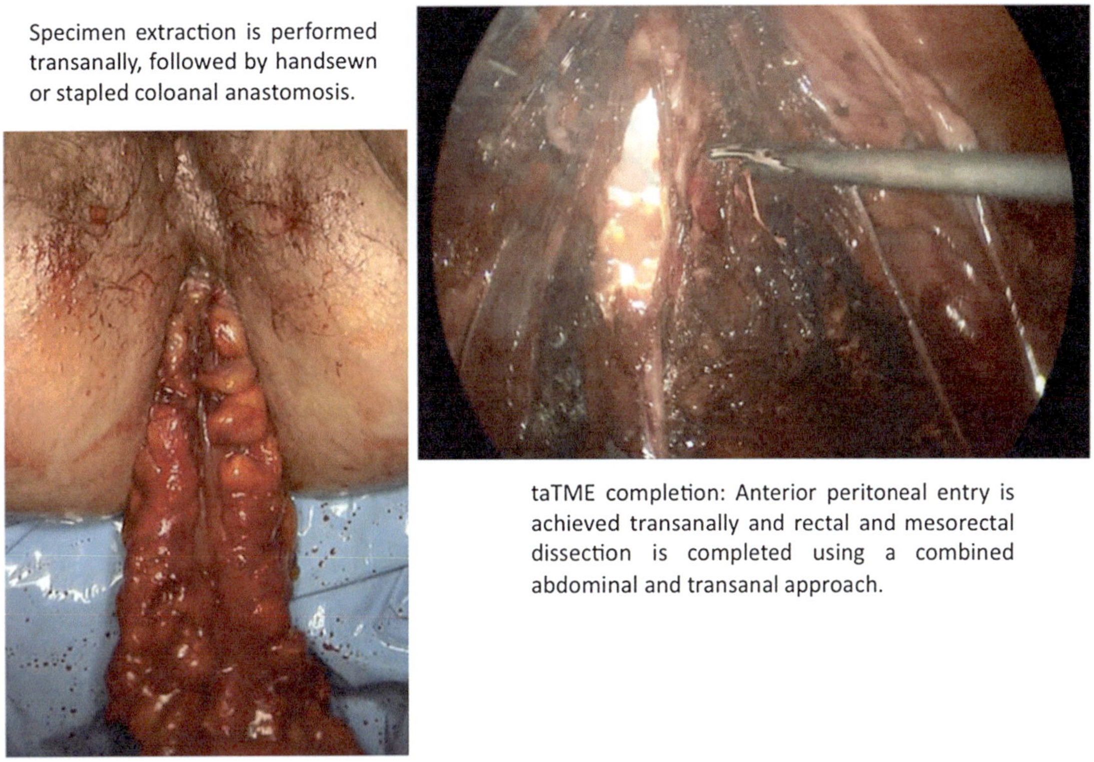


**Fig. 23.4** taTME anterior dissection with peritoneal entry and specimen extraction. *Courtesy of Patricia Sylla, MD, with permission*

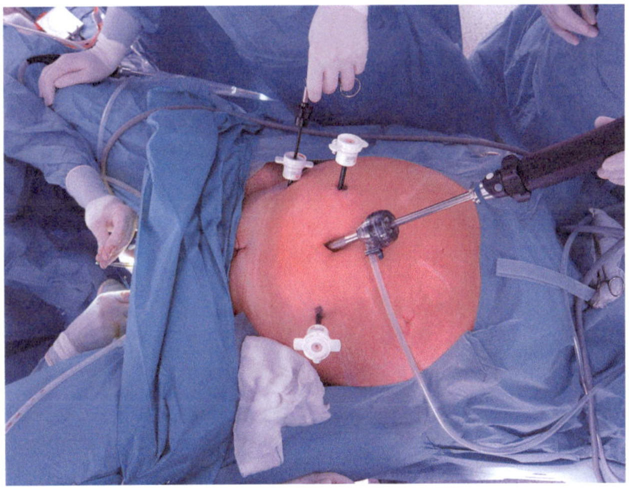

**Fig. 23.5** Aerial view of port placement for taTME. *Courtesy of Mark Whiteford, MD and Antonio Lacy, MD*

chemoradiotherapy. Overall, operative times ranged from 125 to 460 min, with most cases lasting 4–5 h. Nearly all of the intraoperative complications occurred in patients with locally advanced or recurrent tumors. These included two urethral injuries and two patients converted to open surgery. One study reported that two of five patients experienced post-operative urinary retention, thought to be secondary to transient parasympathetic nerve injury [22]. Short-term oncologic outcomes were also adequate. The quality of the mesorectal specimen was complete in all patients, and resection margins were negative in all patients preoperatively staged as having T3 or less disease. Lymph node harvest rates were likewise comparable to historical TME patients. As expected, long-term oncologic data have yet to be reported.

## Phase 3: Initial Clinical Pure NOTES Transanal Resection

At present, two cases of transanal total mesorectal excision without the assistance of laparoscopy have been reported in the literature [23–25]. Both were performed using either a rigid or flexible transanal platform, and primary anastomoses were performed in each case. Mesorectal excisions were graded as complete and lymph node harvest was adequate. Neither patient was diverted and the short-term outcomes were good. One patient had a postoperative hematoma requiring drainage. These cases did not require splenic flexure mobilization. Obviously, further experience is needed to determine the ultimate role of this approach in the surgeon's armamentarium.

## Pearls and Pitfalls

- While NOSE and NOTES offer certain theoretical advantages, they should be performed by experienced teams or special monitored circumstances.
- Patients deemed high risk for increased recurrence or inability to gain margins should be avoided until further experience is gained.
- Although the NOTES approach is unique and technically demanding, the principles of oncologic surgery and operating in the pelvis remain the same as open or standard laparoscopy.

## Summary

A considerable foundation of benchtop research and clinical progress has occurred since the NOTES White Paper was published in 2006 and called for a safe and rational introduction of this new surgical paradigm. It is likely that NOTES progress will continue in a gradual, stepwise fashion, as did laparoscopic surgery, which had its humble beginnings near the start of the twentieth century, yet did not attain widespread use as a therapeutic modality until the 1980s. The tipping point for laparoscopy was when the enabling technological advancement (the video chip) liberated the procedure from that of a one-handed, solo operator tied to monocular scope to the multiport, multimember surgical team now capable of working in a coordinated fashion to accomplish complex integrated tasks [26].

Colorectal NOTES procedures are becoming a reality. Natural orifice specimen extraction of large colonic specimens following laparoscopic resection can be performed safely in experienced hands. Early investigation and clinical experience of transanal total mesorectal excision has been met with excitement as a potentially easier method to perform the deep pelvic dissection during TME. With time and further experience, these techniques will become refined and applicable to more surgeons and situations.

Until that the elusive enabling technology declares itself, it is likely that colorectal NOTES procedures will gradually progress as modifications of hybrid laparoscopic, transanal, and natural orifice specimen extraction procedures for the foreseeable future. In the meantime, though, the dream of NOTES has inspired some secondary gains in the general surgical realm. These include single-port surgery, the increased use of transanal minimally invasive surgery, and advanced endoscopic surgical procedures such as the per-oral endoscopic myotomy (POEM) as a scarless and fully endoscopic treatment for achalasia.

## References


1. Kalloo AN, Singh VK, Jagannath SB, et al. Flexible transgastric peritoneoscopy: a novel approach to diagnostic and therapeutic interventions. Gastrointest Endosc. 2006;60:114–7.
2. Rattner D, Kalloo A, The SAGES/ASGE Working Group on Natural Orifice Translumenal Endoscopic Surgery, October 2005. ASGE/SAGES working group on natural orifice translumenal endoscopic surgery. Gastrointest Endosc. 2006;63(2):329–33.
3. Fuchs KH, Meining A, von Renteln D, et al. Euro-NOTES status paper: from the concept to clinical practice. Surg Endosc. 2013; 27:1456–67.
4. Lehmann KS, Ritz JP, Wibmer A, et al. The German registry for natural orifice translumenal endoscopic surgery: report of the first 551 patients. Ann Surg. 2010;252(2):263–70.
5. Sanchez JE, Marcet JE. Colorectal natural orifice transluminal endoscopic surgery (NOTES) and transvaginal/transrectal specimen extraction. Tech Coloproctol. 2013;17 Suppl 1:S69–73.
6. Franklin Jr ME, Liang S, Russek K. Natural orifice specimen extraction in laparoscopic colorectal surgery: transanal and transvaginal approaches. Tech Coloproctol. 2013;17 Suppl 1:S63–7.
7. Franklin Jr ME, Liang S, Russek K. Integration of transanal specimen extraction into laparoscopic anterior resection with total mesorectal excision for rectal cancer: a consecutive series of 179 patients. Surg Endosc. 2013;27(1):127–32.
8. Wang Q, Wang C, Sun D-H, Kharbuja P, Cao X-Y. Laparoscopic total mesorectal excision with natural orifice specimen extraction. World J Gastroenterol. 2013;19(5):750–4.
9. Leroy J, Costantino F, Cahill RA, et al. Laparoscopic resection with transanal specimen extraction for sigmoid diverticulitis. Br J Surg. 2011;98(9):1327–34.
10. Costantino FA, Diana M, Wall J, Leroy J, Mutter D, Marescaux J. Prospective evaluation of peritoneal fluid contamination following transabdominal vs. transanal specimen extraction in laparoscopic left-sided colorectal resections. Surg Endosc. 2012;26(6): 1495–500.
11. Altemeier WA, Culbertson WR, Schowengerdt C, Hunt J. Nineteen years' experience with the one-stage perineal repair of rectal prolapse. Ann Surg. 1971;173(6):993–1006.
12. Gavagan JA, Whiteford MH, Swanstrom LL. Full-thickness intraperitoneal excision by transanal endoscopic microsurgery does not increase short-term complications. Am J Surg. 2004;187(5): 630–4.
13. Heald RJ, Moran BJ, Ryall RDH, Sexton R, MacFarlane JK. Rectal Cancer: the basingstoke experience of total mesorectal excision, 1978–1997. Arch Surg. 1998;133:894–9.
14. Ito M, Sugito M, Kobayashi A, Nishizawa Y, Tsunoda Y, Saito N. Relationship between multiple numbers of stapler firings during rectal division and anastomotic leakage after laparoscopic rectal resection. Int J Colorectal Dis. 2008;23(7):703–7.
15. Kim JS, Cho SY, Min BS, Kim NK. Risk factors for anastomotic leakage after laparoscopic intracorporeal colorectal anastomosis with a double stapling technique. J Am Coll Surg. 2009;209(6): 694–701.
16. Whiteford MH, Denk PM, Swanstrom LL. Feasibility of radical sigmoid colectomy performed as natural orifice translumenal endoscopic surgery (NOTES) using transanal endoscopic microsurgery. Surg Endosc. 2007;21(10):1870–4.
17. Rieder E, Spaun GO, Khajanchee YS, et al. A natural orifice transrectal approach for oncologic resection of the rectosigmoid: an experimental study and comparison with conventional laparoscopy. Surg Endosc. 2011;25(10):3357–63.

18. McLemore EC, Coker AM, Devaraj B, et al. TAMIS-assisted laparoscopic low anterior resection with total mesorectal excision in a cadaveric series. Surg Endosc. 2013;27(9):3478–84.
19. Telem DA, Han KS, Kim MC, et al. Transanal rectosigmoid resection via natural orifice translumenal endoscopic surgery (NOTES) with total mesorectal excision in a large human cadaver series. Surg Endosc. 2013;27(1):74–80.
20. Sylla P, Rattner DW, Delgado S, Lacy AM. NOTES transanal rectal cancer resection using transanal endoscopic microsurgery and laparoscopic assistance. Surg Endosc. 2010;24(5):1205–10.
21. Emhoff IA, Lee GC, Sylla P. Transanal colorectal resection using natural orifice translumenal endoscopic surgery (NOTES). Dig Endosc. 2013;28.
22. Rouanet P, Mourregot A, Azar CC, et al. Transanal endoscopic proctectomy: an innovative procedure for difficult resection of rectal tumors in men with narrow pelvis. Dis Colon Rectum. 2013;56(4): 408–15.
23. Sylla P, Bordeianou LG, Berger D, et al. A pilot study of natural orifice transanal endoscopic total mesorectal excision with laparoscopic assistance for rectal cancer. Surg Endosc. 2013;27(9):3396–405.
24. Leroy J, Barry BD, Melani A, Mutter D, Marescaux J. No-scar transanal total mesorectal excision: the last step to pure NOTES for colorectal surgery. JAMA Surg. 2013;148(3):226–30.
25. Zhang H, Zhang YS, Jin XW, Li MZ, Fan JS, Yang ZH. Transanal single-port laparoscopic total mesorectal excision in the treatment of rectal cancer. Tech Coloproctol. 2013;17(1):117–23.
26. Nagy AG. History and development of laparoscopic surgery. In: Eubanks WS, Swanstrom LL, Soper NJ, editors. Mastery of endoscopic and laparoscopic surgery. Philadelphia, PA: Lippincott, Williams, and Wilkins; 2000.

# Robotic Surgery

# 24

Mehraneh Dorna Jafari, David E. Rivadeneira, and Alessio Pigazzi

**Key Points**

- The specific indications for the utilization of a robotic approach continue to evolve.
- Advantages of robotic surgery include better visualization, surgeon-controlled camera, improved ergonomics, and overall dexterity.
- At present, pelvic, more than colonic, operations allow for a more wide application of the robotic advantages.
- A robotic approach allows an intracorporeal anastomosis during a right colectomy to be much more feasible.
- Left colectomy and pelvic operations can be performed via a hybrid or totally robotic approach using a one or two docking method.
- Robotic surgeons should be proficient in advanced laparoscopic surgery.

## Introduction

Robotic surgery has been evolving since its first introduction in 1994. The FDA approved the use of the da Vinci® robotic system (Intuitive Surgical Inc., Sunnyvale, CA, USA) as the first telerobotic manipulation system for intra-abdominal surgery in 2000. An explosion of robotic surgery utilization has occurred mostly in the last decade with more than 350,000 procedures done worldwide by 2011 (Fig. 24.1). This increase in robotic procedures has been mostly brought about from our other pelvic subspecialist colleagues, namely, urology and gynecology (Fig. 24.2). Robotic colorectal surgery was first reported in 2001 [1], and the first of total mesorectal excision was reported in 2006 [2]. Although multiple case series and at least one randomized prospective study have demonstrated the feasibility and safety of robotic surgery in colorectal resections [3–12], its adoption in the colorectal surgical community has been increasing slowly. A recent study of national trends of robotic surgery in the United States showed that it is utilized in only 2.8 % of minimal invasive colorectal surgery [13].

This slow adoption is despite the many purported advantages of robotic surgery including better visualization, improved ergonomics, and overall dexterity. The robot provides a steady camera with highly magnified stereoscopic optics, which provides 3-D visualization and improved depth perception of the operative field. Furthermore, the surgeon at the console has complete control of the camera, removing any potential distraction of an assistant that normally used in traditional laparoscopic surgery. The superior surgical dexterity provided by the robotic approach is due to the instruments having seven degrees of freedom, 180° articulation, and 540° rotation—all allowing for easier manipulation within small spaces. The robot also allows for motion scaling and tremor filtering, which again facilitate technically challenging laparoscopic procedures. Moorthy et al. reported that the robot was associated with an enhanced dexterity by 65 %, reduction in skill-based errors by 93 %, and reduction in time needed to complete a task by 40 % [14]. The robot also allows for superior ergonomics [15], as the enhanced dexterity and superior visualization are especially helpful in the narrow confines of the pelvis, and is very appealing for surgical subspecialties that deal with pelvic pathology such as urologists, gynecologists, and colorectal surgeons.

**Electronic supplementary material:** Supplementary material is available in the online version of this chapter at 10.1007/978-1-4939-1581-1_24. Videos can also be accessed at http://www.springerimages.com/videos/978-1-4939-1580-4.

M.D. Jafari, M.D. (✉)
Department of Surgery, University of California, Irvine School of Medicine, 333 City Blvd. West Ste 850, Orange, CA 92868, USA
e-mail: jafarim@uci.edu; apigazzi@uci.edu

A. Pigazzi, M.D., Ph.D.
Colorectal Surgery, University of California, Irvine Medical Center, 333 City Blvd. West Ste 850, Orange, CA 92868, USA
e-mail: jafarim@uci.edu; apigazzi@uci.edu

D.E. Rivadeneira, M.D., M.B.A., F.A.C.S., F.A.S.C.R.S.
North Shore-LIJ Health System, Huntington Hospital, Hofstra University School of Medicine, Huntington, NY, USA
e-mail: drivadeneira@nshs.edu

H.M. Ross et al. (eds.), *Minimally Invasive Approaches to Colon and Rectal Disease: Technique and Best Practices*, DOI 10.1007/978-1-4939-1581-1_24, 

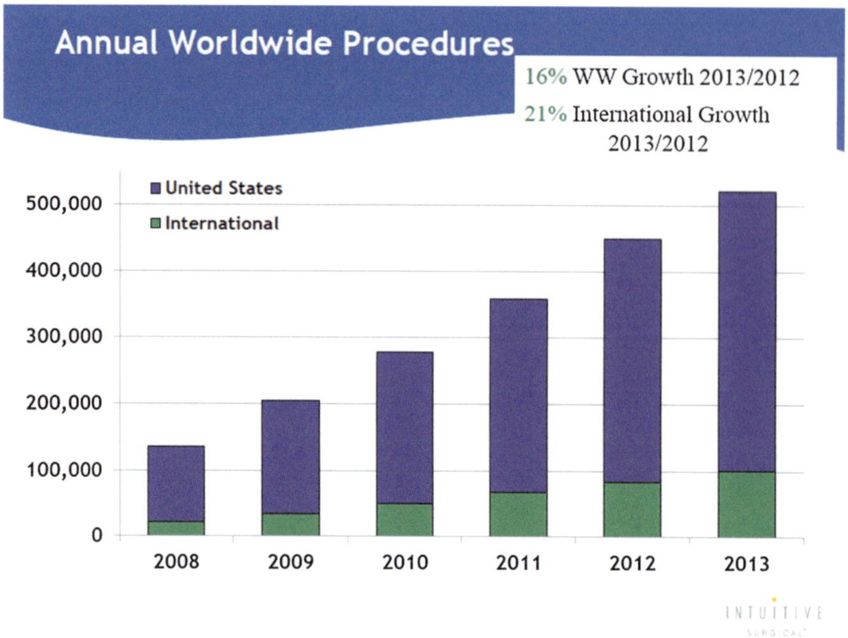


**Fig. 24.1** Total robotic procedures performed worldwide (2005–2011). *With permission from Intuitive Medical*

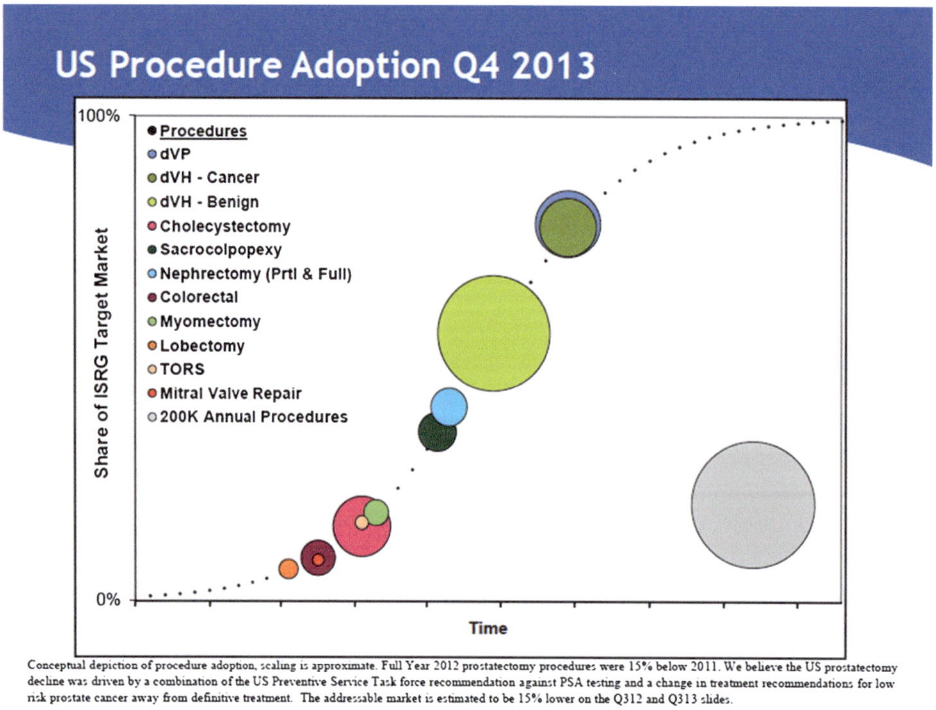


**Fig. 24.2** Robotic cases by specific procedure. *With permission from Intuitive Medical*

The disadvantages of robotic-assisted surgery can be attributed to lack of haptic feedback, longer operative time, and cost. The time-consuming aspect of robotic surgery is docking, especially in certain totally robotic colorectal approaches which can require multiple docking and/or reengaging of instruments. However, it has been shown in rectal surgery that as experience is gained, operative time will improve [16]. Recent meta-analyses have suggested that operating time for robotic rectal procedures is similar to that for a conventional laparoscopic approach [12, 17]. The authors agree that with continued experience of an assembled robotic surgical team, the operative times of robotic colorectal procedures will approach the times of similar laparoscopic procedures. While there continues to be a debate regarding the cost-effectiveness of the robot, especially given the current lack of clinical evidence demonstrating its superiority compared to the laparoscopic approach, there is no doubt it has an expanding role for colorectal surgeons. In this chapter, we will review the technical aspects of robotic use for colorectal surgery and share several tips and tricks we have found useful in our experience with robotic approaches to colorectal disease.

## Indications

The specific indications for the utilization of the robot when compared to laparoscopy continue to evolve. To date, there are no large randomized controlled studies that demonstrate the benefits of the robotic approach with regard to colorectal surgery. In fact, the majority of data detailing robotic use comes from single institution cases series. Therefore, the specific indications for colorectal surgery are evolving as new evidence comes to light. The clinical outcomes of robotic and laparoscopic colorectal procedures have overall been similar.

The utilization of robotics for colorectal resection is at the discretion of the surgeon. As mentioned above, the use of robotics can increase operative time, but once the learning curve is overcome, this is not a hindrance to the use of the robot. During segmental resections, the robot will allow for easier intracorporeal suturing, given the EndoWrist® technology. However, intracorporeal suturing has not translated into superior outcomes [18]. In short, despite the technological advantages afforded by the robot, and proven feasibility, there have been no tangible clinical improvements reported with the use of the robot for colon resections [13, 19, 20]. Rather, laparoscopic colon resection has the same clinical outcomes as robotic colon resection with a lower cost and shorter operative time.

Currently, however, there may be stronger indications for robotic rectal surgery given that studies have shown lower rate of conversion when robotic technology is used to facilitate total mesorectal excision (TME) [12, 13, 21]. The anatomical confines of the pelvis render rectal surgery more difficult compared to colon surgery, especially using a minimally invasive approach. Total mesorectal excision demands a high degree of precision, since anatomic dissection of the mesorectal envelope allows for the best oncological outcomes for rectal cancer. Moreover, the degree of difficulty for TME is directly proportional to the size of the pelvis [22]. Laparoscopic TME can be very challenging, especially in males and in those with very low tumors and obese patients [23]. Using the nonarticulating laparoscopic instrumentation and obtaining an optimal surgical view can become very challenging and lead to higher rates of conversion [24, 25]. The abovementioned advantages of the robot can overcome these challenges and, in fact, lead to lower conversion rates [12, 13].

We should point out that there are no absolute contraindications to the utilization of a robot in colorectal surgery—only the experience and expertise of the surgeon. Similar to laparoscopy, the robot is a tool or approach used to complete the same operation as in an open case. The robot can be used for diverticular disease, inflammatory bowel disease, and malignancy. The loss of haptic feedback may be more difficult in certain inflammatory conditions, and extra care must be taken when handling inflamed tissue. However, the indication should rely mostly on the underlying disease process; then consideration should be given to whether or not the patient can tolerate a pneumoperitoneum, steep Trendelenburg for pelvic cases, and perhaps longer operative times that occur with a robotic approach.

## Equipment

The equipment needed for a laparoscopic case, as described by Dr. Bafford in Chap. 1, should be available for all robotic cases, especially when using the hybrid approach. Therefore, additional towers for insufflator, electrosurgical units, and extra monitors in rooms that are used for laparoscopic and robotic cases are necessary. The operating room setup should provide adequate space for staff and large equipment and allow the surgeon to have a direct view of the patient from the surgeon's console. The room should also allow docking of the robot from several angles (Fig. 24.3).

### Robotic System

The da Vinci® exists in five models: standard, streamline (S), S-high definition (HD), and S-integrated (i) HD. At the time of this writing, the new da Vinci Xi has just been introduced into the market. This system features improved robotic arm movements and the ability to introduce the camera in any of the arms. The standard system originally was a three-arm robot. In 2006, the S-system offered numerous improvements including motorized patient cart, color-coded optic connection, easier instrument exchange, improved trocars, and increased range of motion and reach of instruments. The da Vinci® surgical system consists of three components: the surgeon's console, the cart with the four robotic arms, and the electronic/vision tower (Fig. 24.3). The HD camera was an addition for the S-HD model, while the most recent version includes the enhanced HD vision at 1080i, upgrades to surgeon console and ability for dual console.

The surgeon operates at the console (Fig. 24.4); a three-dimensional image is obtained through the stereoviewer, which can be adjusted via the pod controls. The instruments are controlled using the master controllers and foot pedals. The surgeon's instruments and console are only active when the surgeon's head is at the stereoviewer. This allows for immediate deactivation of the surgical arms when the surgeon looks away from the surgical field.

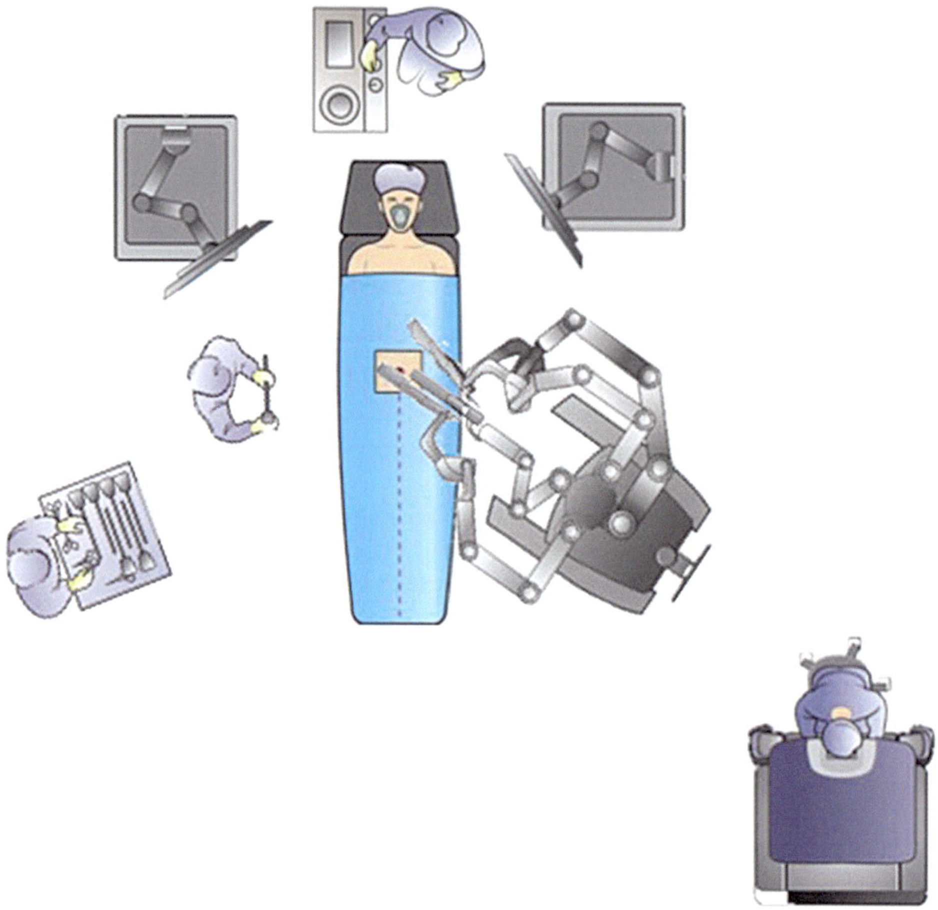

**Fig. 24.3** Operating room setup should include ample room for robotic cart and laparoscopic and robotic towers. The system includes a robotic cart, console, and tower. *With permission from Intuitive Medical*

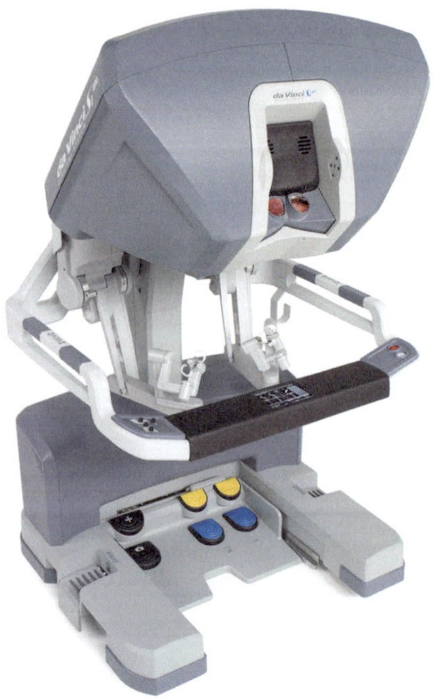

**Fig. 24.4** The da Vinci Si™ console, which includes master controls and pedals. *With permission from Intuitive Medical*

The surgeon controls the instruments via the master controllers using the index finger and thumb. The robotic technology (without delay) scales, filters, and relays the information to the instruments. The surgeon should keep in mind the ergonomics while using the controllers and should be able to sit comfortably without overreaching. The robot is dual energy capable, and both monopolar and bipolar instruments can be used simultaneously.

The patient cart has 3–4 arms, one of which is the camera. Each arm has multiple clutch buttons for gross and fine movements (Fig. 24.5).

## Camera

The endoscope is available as a 0° and 30° lens. Our preference for robotic colectomy is to use a 30° lens, while we normally use a 0° scope for robotic TME. The camera system has digital zoom and allows for magnifications by pressing the left and right arrow keys on the left-side pod controls or depressing the camera pedal and moving the masters together or apart.

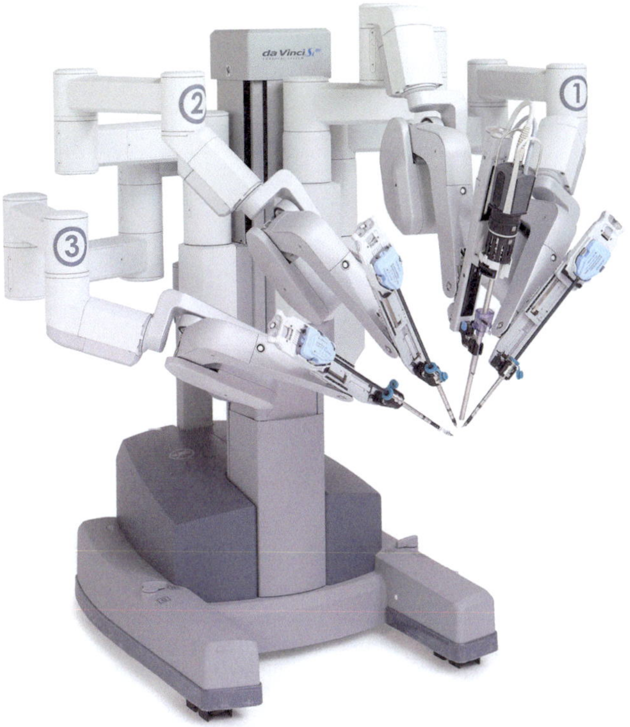


**Fig. 24.5** Four-Arm da Vinci Si™ robotic cart. *With permission from Intuitive Medical*

### Instruments

As mentioned above, the EndoWrist® instruments allow for seven degrees of freedom, 180° of articulation, and 540° of rotation. Instruments are reusable but have a fixed number of uses, and the system keeps track of the number. The S-model instruments are 57 cm in length with blue housing and are made up of release levers, instrument shaft, wrist, and tip. Instruments come in a 5 mm "snake joint" (Fig. 24.6) or an 8 mm "angle joint" (Fig. 24.7). The snake joint uses a larger radius for rotation when compared to the angle joint. Our preferred instruments for colon resection and total mesorectal excision include prograsper in Arm 3, fenestrated bipolar forceps in Arm 2, and monopolar scissors/hook in Arm 1. Given the decreased haptic feedback, caution must be used when grasping the tissue. The mesorectum should not be grasped since this may cause tearing and bleeding.

## Procedure-Specific Considerations

### Positioning

Specific precautions as to patient positioning follow the same principles discussed in Chap. 2. However, we will reiterate that patients should be secured to the table so that they may not slip during the procedures. The use of shoulder and neck restraints is strongly discouraged, as these have been reported to cause brachial plexus injuries. The authors have successfully used a variety of methods including beanbags, gel pads, and the Pink Pad™, a proprietary specialized pad specifically made for patient positing during laparoscopic and robotic cases. For rectal cases, the patient should be positioned so that the operating room table and the robotic cart do not hinder access to the anus. The docking of the robot is procedure dependent.

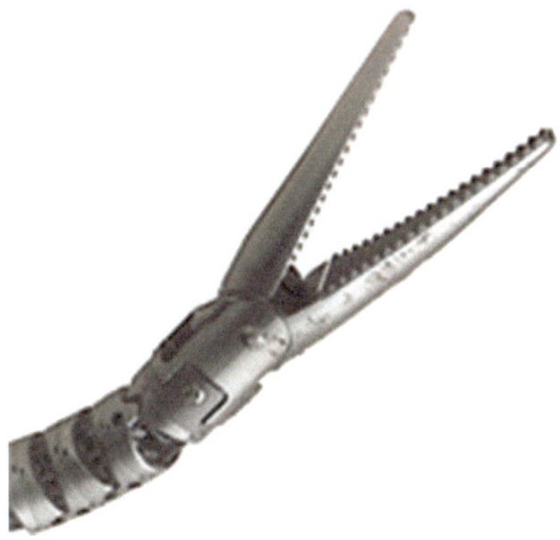

**Fig. 24.6** 5 mm snake joint Maryland dissector. *With permission from Intuitive Medical*

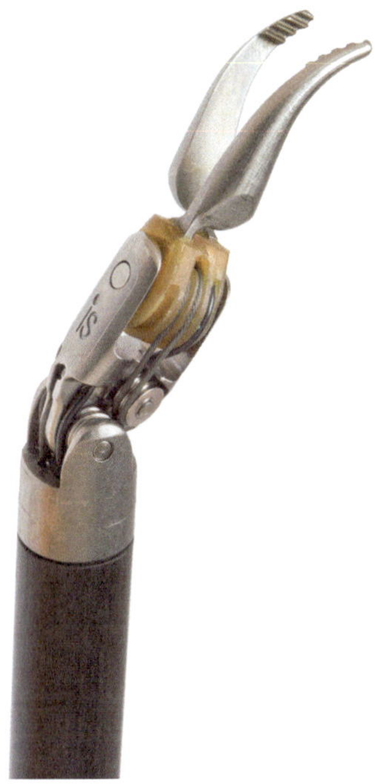

**Fig. 24.7** 8 mm angle joint bipolar dissector. *With permission from Intuitive Medical*

### Port Placement

In this chapter we will describe port placement that suits best the S/Si systems. It goes without saying that the new Xi platform will considerably change robotic approaches in a variety of operations and allow greater freedom in port placement.

The setup described in this chapter have been optimized for single and two quadrant surgery in most cases; the new Xi system will surely make multi-quadrant robotic surgery much more feasible in the near future, but the experience with this device is still too limited at the time of this writing to describe it in detail. As in laparoscopic surgery, trocars are placed as to optimize triangulation, avoid collision within the body, and in the case of robotics avoid collision of the robotic arms outside the body. The principles of triangulation are maintained by assuring that minimum distance between trocars is at least one handbreadth apart. Ports should be placed under direct vision, and the small bowel swept out of the surgical field prior to docking of the robot.

We will describe port placement for each procedure below and will designate camera port (C), the three robotic trocars as R1, R2, and R3. Unless otherwise specified, Arm 1 will be docked in R1, Arm 2 in R2, and Arm 3 in R3. Arm 1 will usually be the operating arm and will be connected to a monopolar scissors, hook cautery, and/or robotic vessel sealer. Arm 2 and Arm 3 will provide traction and counter-traction to aid in dissection. Arm 2 will often be connected to bipolar energy. A laparoscopic-assistant port can be helpful in further traction and/or suction/irrigation.

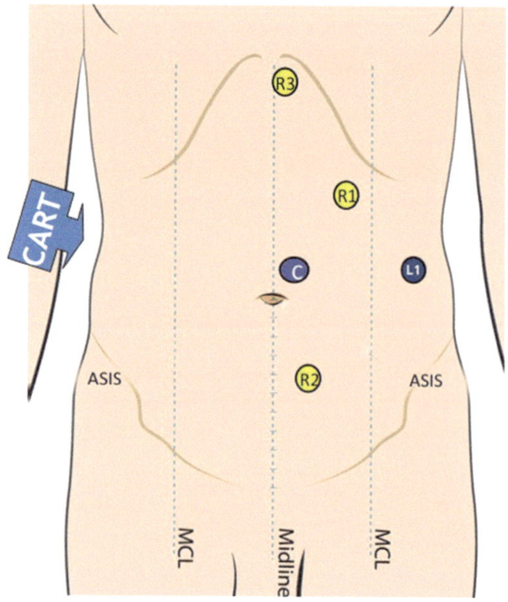


**Fig. 24.8** Right colectomy port placement: *C* indicates camera port; *L1* is a 12 mm laparoscopic assistant port. *R1*, *R2*, and *R3* are 8 mm robotic ports. *MCL* midclavicular line, *ASIS* superior iliac spine. *With permission from Intuitive Medical*

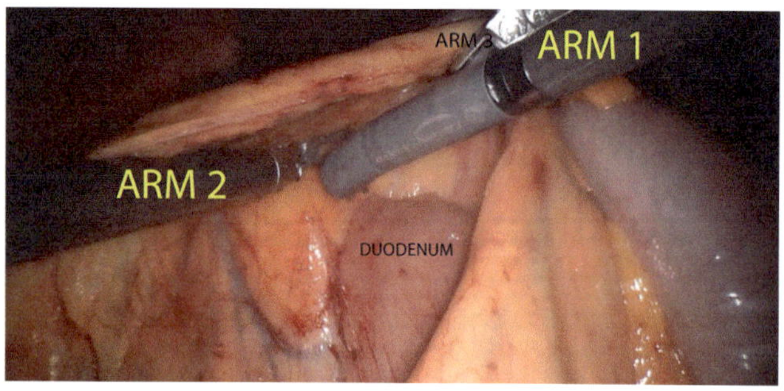


**Fig. 24.9** The retroperitoneal structures, the duodenum and the head of the pancreas, are carefully swept posteriorly using Arm 3 for anterior retraction and Arms 1 and 2 for dissection

## Right Colectomy

### Positioning

The patient can be placed supine and/or in modified lithotomy position. Both arms should be tucked to allow standing room for the assistant and the cart. Once entrance into the abdomen is gained, and a laparoscopic view deems that patient anatomy is feasible to a minimally invasive approach, the table should be rotated to the left by approximately 20–30°. The robotic cart is docked at the patient's right flank, and ports placed in the left abdomen as described below. The surgeon's assistant will stand on the left side of the patient.

### Port Placement

The camera port (C) is placed about two fingerbreadth to the left of midline, midway between the xiphoid and the pubis. R1 is an 8 mm trocar that is placed one handbreadth cephalad and lateral to C. R2 is an 8 mm trocar be placed one handbreadth inferior and medial to C. R3 is placed at a subxiphoid position. A 12 mm assistant port can be placed midway between C and the left anterior superior iliac spine (ASIS) and can be used for stapling, additional retraction, and passing sutures (Fig. 24.8).

### Procedure

Once the ports are placed and the patient is appropriately positioned, the robot is docked as described above. We prefer a medial-to-lateral approach for our colonic resection. The right colon is elevated and retracted anteriorly via Arm 3 (providing countertraction), and Arm 1 and Arm 2 are used for dissection and fine traction. The ileocolic pedicle is identified by the tenting of the mesentery and is isolated using monopolar cautery via Arm 1, while traction is provided via R2. The retroperitoneal structures, the duodenum and the head of the pancreas, are carefully swept posteriorly using Arm 1 and Arm 2 (Fig. 24.9). Once the pedicle is isolated, it is divided using the daVinci EndoWrist® One™ Vessel Sealer, clips, and/or an appropriate laparoscopic vessel sealing device or stapling devices inserted via the assistant port (Fig. 24.10). Our preferred method includes using Weck® Hem-o-lok® clips and vessel sealing device to divide the vasculature. Be sure to take the ileocolic pedicle at its origin for cancer cases. Once the ileocolic pedicle is divided, the dissection will proceed above the duodenum and head of the pancreas; the mesentery is gently stretched laterally, and the right branch of the middle colic artery is identified and divided. The terminal ileum and right colon are freed from

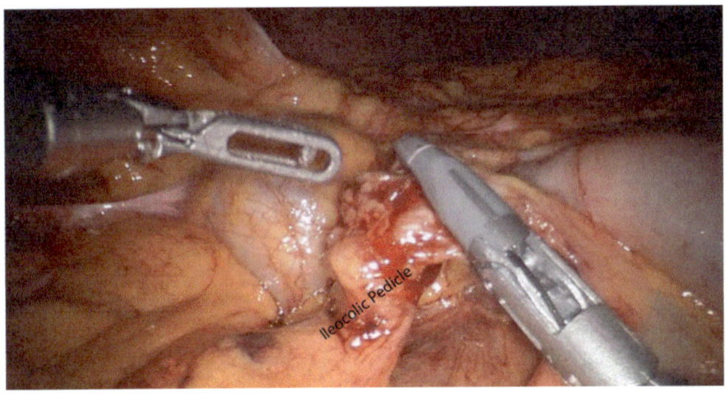


**Fig. 24.10** The robotic vessel sealer device is used to divide the ileocolic pedicle

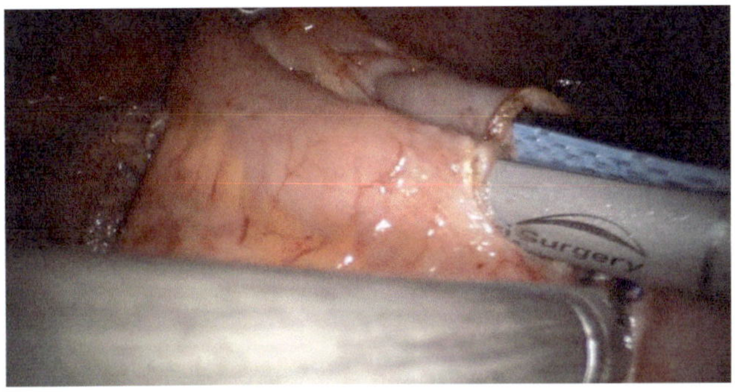

**Fig. 24.11** Intracorporeal anastomosis is created by aligning the terminal ileum and the transverse colon in an isoperistaltic fashion and firing a single 60 mm linear stapler cartridge to create the side-to-side anastomosis

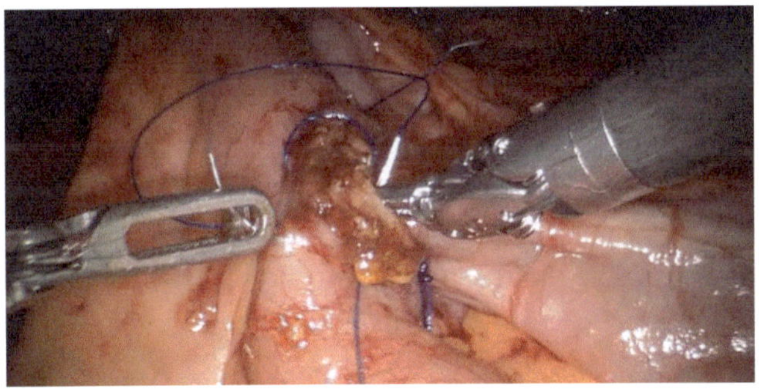

**Fig. 24.12** The enterotomies are closed using an intracorporeal suturing

their attachment to the pelvic sidewall and abdominal wall. Arm 3 will retract medially, while Arm 2 creates countertraction and Arm 1 takes down the line of Toldt via monopolar cautery. Once the bowel is fully mobilized, it can be extracted via a minilaparotomy for extracorporeal anastomosis. However, our preferred method is to create an intracorporeal anastomosis and extract via Pfannenstiel incision (Fig. 24.11). This is accomplished by aligning the terminal ileum and the transverse colon in an isoperistaltic fashion, creating an enterotomy and a colotomy, and firing a single 60 mm linear stapler cartridge to create the side-to-side anastomosis. The enterotomy can then be closed robotically in a running fashion using absorbable sutures (Fig. 24.12).

## Left Colectomy/Low Anterior Resection

### Positioning

If a totally robotic approach is planned, the robot may need to be docked twice for left/sigmoid colectomy to allow for a full splenic flexure mobilization and then re-docked for the left colon mobilization. The splenic flexure mobilization will be most effectively conducted via the left shoulder approach, and the colon can be mobilized via the left hip approach.

The robot may also have to be re-docked for a fully robotic low anterior resection to allow for optimal visualization and triangulation during the case. However, our preferred approach for a low anterior resection is via a hybrid approach, utilizing a laparoscopic medial-to-lateral colonic mobilization and vessel ligation followed by the docking of the robot for the low pelvic part of the operation. We find this be to be a less cumbersome and more efficient use of the robot.

#### Colonic Mobilization and Vessel Ligation

The patient is placed in modified lithotomy position with both arms tucked. Once entrance into the abdomen is gained and the small bowel is swept out of the pelvis and packed in the right upper quadrant, the bed is rotated with the left side elevated by approximately 20–30°. The robotic cart is docked from a left hip approach. The assistant will stand on the right side of the patient.

#### Total Mesorectal Excision (Hybrid Approach)

After the completion of the splenic flexure and colon mobilization and vessel ligation, the patient is placed in Trendelenburg. The robot is docked from a left hip approach [26]. The robot can also be docked at the pelvis [10]. The placement of robotic cart at the pelvis will limit access to the anus for digital rectal exams, transanal stapling, and endoscopy during the case. The surgeon's assistant will stand on the right side of the patient.

### Port Placement

#### Left Colectomy

The camera port (C) is placed about two fingerbreadths to the right of the midline, midway between the xiphoid and the pubis. R1 is a 12 mm trocar placed midway between C and the right ASIS. The robotic or the laparoscopic stapler will use R1. R2 is an 8 mm trocar placed one handbreadth cephalad to C. R3 is an 8 mm trocar, placed one handbreadth cephalad to R2 in the left upper abdomen. Again, this will provide traction and countertraction. The assistant port (5- or 12 mm port) is placed in the right lateral mid-abdomen (Fig. 24.13).

#### Low Anterior Resection

Camera port (C) is placed in the midline halfway between the xiphoid process and symphysis pubis. R1 is a 12 mm trocar inserted in the midclavicular line (MCL) halfway in

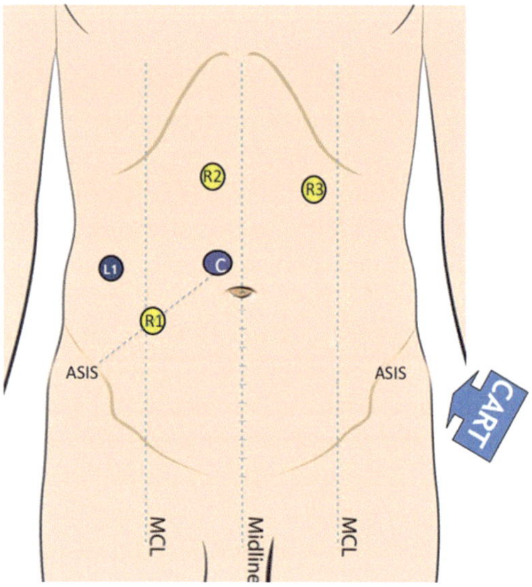


**Fig. 24.13** Left colectomy port placement: *C* indicates camera port; *L1* is a 5 mm or 12 mm laparoscopic assistant port. *R1* is a 12 mm robotic trocar. *R2* and *R3* are 8 mm robotic ports. *MCL* midclavicular line, *ASIS* superior iliac spine. *With permission from Intuitive Medical*

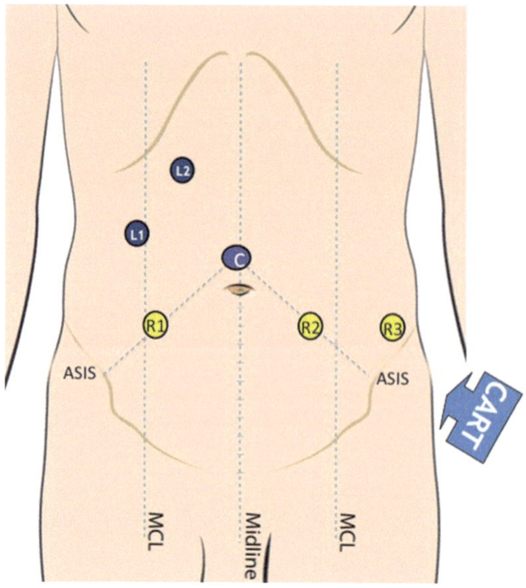


**Fig. 24.14** Robotic-assisted laparoscopic low anterior resection port placement for a hybrid approach. *C* indicates camera port; *L1* and *L2* are laparoscopic 5 mm ports. *R1* is a 12 mm robotic port, and *R2* and *R3* are robotic 8 mm ports. *MCL* midclavicular line, *ASIS* superior iliac spine. *With permission from Intuitive Medical*

between C and the right anterior superior iliac spine (ASIS). This port can be used for ileostomy placement and is used for the stapler. R2 is an 8 mm trocar inserted as a mirror image of R1. R3 is an 8 mm trocar inserted 8–10 cm lateral to R2, usually directly above the left ASIS. A first laparoscopic-assisted port (L1) is a 5 mm trocar inserted in the MCL about 12 cm superior to R1 (this port can be converted to a 12 mm trocar for stapling a very low rectum if necessary at the completion of the proctectomy). A second laparoscopic port (L2) is a 5 mm port inserted halfway between the MCL and midline about 12 cm superior to L1. R1, the two laparoscopic ports, and C are used during the laparoscopic section of the hybrid approach. The same port placement can be used for all rectal cases including pelvic mass excision, rectopexy, and abdominoperineal resection. We prefer a hybrid approach, which consists of laparoscopic medial-to-lateral dissection of the colon using R1, L1, and L2, followed by a robotic TME (Fig. 24.14).

## Procedure

### Laparoscopic Splenic Flexure Mobilization and Medial-to-Lateral Dissection of the Left Colon

For a complete resection that will need the colon to reach toward the pelvis, dissection is usually begun at the inferior mesenteric vein (IMV), which is found lateral to the ligament of Treitz. Once the IMV is clipped, the left colon is elevated and retracted anteriorly, and the inferior mesenteric artery (IMA) is now tented within the mesentery. Using blunt dissection, the retroperitoneal structures are identified and swept posteriorly. At this junction, care is taken to avoid injury to the hypogastric nerves. Once the left ureter is identified, the vessel is ligated at its origin (for cancer operations) using clips, a vessel sealing device, or a stapler (Video 24.1).

The left colon is retracted medially, and the colon is mobilized off the left abdominal sidewall. The splenic flexure is then taken down by entering the lesser sac, and the colon attachments to the spleen are completely divided together with the gastrocolic ligament. Care should be taken to avoid injury to the tail of the pancreas. Mobilization should be tailored to the procedure and the length of the colon needed to allow for a tension-free anastomosis.

### Total Mesorectal Dissection

The robot is docked as described above, and dissection is begun posteriorly. The assistant retracts the rectum cephalad and anterior using L2 and provides countertraction via L1; the surgeon at the console will use Arm 3 for retraction and Arms 1 and 2 to develop the plane of dissection within the mesorectal space between the mesorectum and the presacral fascia. Dissection is carried first posteriorly toward the coccyx as distal as possible following the areolar plane between the fascia propria and the presacral fascia, then laterally, taking care to avoid injury to the pelvic autonomic plexus that resides in this location (Video 24.2). Dissection is lastly carried anteriorly using Arm 3 to retract anteriorly and Arm 2 to push the rectum posteriorly. Ultimately, Denonvilliers' fascia/pouch of Douglas (rectovesical/rectovaginal pouch) is entered by incising the peritoneal reflection between the anterior wall of the rectum and posterior wall of the vagina or the seminal vesicles. Dissection is carried below the level of the tumor. Separation of the low rectum from its attachments to the pelvic floor musculature can be carried out very effectively secondary to the articulating robotic instruments. At the most distal end of the rectum, the mesorectum ends, and the naked surface of the rectum will become obvious. Several digital rectal examinations are necessary together with intraoperative endoscopy, if necessary, to assess the location of the tumor and ensure an adequate distal margin. Once clear distal margins are achieved, the bowel is divided via either R1 (using the robotic stapler or by the assistant using a laparoscopic approach) or R2 depending on the amount of retraction needed to expose the surface of the rectum (Video 24.3).

After undocking the robot, the bowel is extracted through a Pfannenstiel incision, and the proximal colon is divided extracorporeally. After insertion of the appropriate anvil, an anastomosis using an EEA stapler is then performed under laparoscopic vision.

Transanal extraction is also a possibility by placing a wound protector through the rectum. The specimen is delivered via the anus, and extracorporeal resection can be achieved and the specimen placed back into the abdomen. Then using a PDS suture, the rectal stump is closed in a single layer around the stapling device spike, and the anastomosis is achieved via a single stapling technique (Video 24.4).

This approach can also be applied to abdominoperineal resections (APR). We prefer, in most cases, an extra-levator APR. Once the TME is completed, the dissection is carried distally, avoiding "coning" in at the level of the levators and its associated "waist" in the specimen. Rather, a wide resection of the levators near their origin is carried out prior to continuing the dissection distally into the ischiorectal fat as far as feasible just before encountering the perineal skin. Once this is accomplished, the robot is undocked, and a circumferential incision around the anus from the perineal body to the coccyx, and laterally to the tuberosities, is made from a perineal approach until the previous dissection plane is met. The perineal incision is then closed in three layers. The use of drains is at the discretion of the surgeon.

### Hybrid Approach vs. Total Robotic Approach

The exact approach to robotic cases is again surgeon dependent. There are no studies that would dictate one approach is superior to another. However, each approach has its inherent advantages and disadvantages. A total robotic approach can be used in a right and left colectomy, as well as a low anterior and abdominoperineal resections. For a total mesorectal excision with splenic flexure mobilization, the total robotic approach can be disadvantageous in that it requires additional time for the surgeon to re-dock in order to facilitate the splenic flexure mobilization. Also multiple re-docking will require precise port placement that will avoid collision of the operative configuration of the robot as multiple quadrants are accessed.

The hybrid approach specifies that a portion of the case be performed laparoscopically. This is mainly utilized in low anterior resections. For a low anterior resection, the mobilization of the splenic flexure, left colon, and vessel ligation is performed laparoscopically as described above. The robot is docked for total mesorectal excision. This approach allows for the robot to be used for its maximal benefit, which becomes apparent in the narrow confines of the pelvis. Robotic surgeons should be proficient in advanced laparoscopic surgery, and therefore, it may be easier to perform the portions of the operation that require change in patient position via laparoscopy.

## Pearls and Pitfalls

The robotic surgeon must become proficient with the following tasks:

1. Overcoming the loss of tensile and tactile feedback by:
   (a) Recognizing visual cues with regard to tension and manipulation of the tissues.
   (b) Conceptualizing the spatial relationships of robotic instruments and reposition safely without direct visualization.
   (c) Minimizing external collision and optimizing range of motion of robotic arms by mentally visualizing the spatial relationships of the robotic arms and external clashing and optimizing maneuverability and range of motion.
2. Expert laparoscopic skills prior to the utilization of the robotic technology can facilitate the acquisition of the above tasks.

*Avoid Complications*:

1. Keep in mind that the principles of laparoscopic surgery such as triangulation and visualization continue to apply with robotic surgery:
   (a) Make sure you maintain adequate visualization of surgical field. Instruments should always be in the field of view.
   (b) Place ports at least one handbreadth or 10 cm apart to reduce the risk of arm collisions.
2. Novices should familiarize themselves extensively and train with the robot, the instruments, as well as the console in a simulator setting prior to embarking on live surgery.
3. The surgeon needs to be aware of the lack of haptic feedback:
   (a) Extra care must be taken to handle tissue gently, especially when the bowel is friable as seen in acute ulcerative colitis and Crohn's patients.
   (b) During total mesorectal excision, avoid grabbing the mesorectum; rather, gently retract the rectum via the fenestrated bipolar graspers.

4. Make sure that you are aware of all instruments:
   (a) Failure to keep activated instruments in view may cause inadvertent injury.
   (b) Be sure that the correct arms are activated and that the activated instruments are in view.
   (c) A good technique is to use the fourth robotic arm for retraction, deactivate this arm and keep in position, while using the two other active arms.
5. The fourth robotic arm should be used for every case to aid in traction/countertraction.
6. Choose the robotic cart position to best suit the operation.
7. The hybrid approach is efficient and allows for one docking.

**Disclosure** Drs. Pigazzi and Rivadeneira serve as consultants for Intuitive Surgical (Sunnyvale, CA).

## References


1. Ballantyne GHMP, Weber A, Wasielewski A. Robotic solutions to the pitfalls of laparoscopic colectomy. Osp Ital Chir. 2001; 7(405):405–12.
2. Pigazzi A, Ellenhorn JD, Ballantyne GH, Paz IB. Robotic-assisted laparoscopic low anterior resection with total mesorectal excision for rectal cancer. Surg Endosc. 2006;20(10):1521–5. PubMed PMID: 16897284.
3. Weber PA, Merola S, Wasielewski A, Ballantyne GH. Telerobotic-assisted laparoscopic right and sigmoid colectomies for benign disease. Dis Colon Rectum. 2002;45(12):1689–94. PubMed PMID: 12473897; discussion 95-6.
4. Delaney CP, Lynch AC, Senagore AJ, Fazio VW. Comparison of robotically performed and traditional laparoscopic colorectal surgery. Dis Colon Rectum. 2003;46(12):1633–9. PubMed PMID: 14668588.
5. D'Annibale A, Orsini C, Fiscon V, Trevisan P, Sovernigo G, Morpurgo E, et al. [Videolaparoscopic surgery in the treatment of colorectal disease: our experience with 200 patients]. Chirurgia italiana. 2002;54(6):777–83. PubMed PMID: 12613325. La chirurgia videolaparoscopica nel trattamento della patologia colo-rettale: nostra esperienza di 200 pazienti.
6. Braumann C, Jacobi CA, Menenakos C, Borchert U, Rueckert JC, Mueller JM. Computer-assisted laparoscopic colon resection with the Da Vinci system: our first experiences. Dis Colon Rectum. 2005;48(9):1820–7. PubMed PMID: 16142433.
7. Rawlings AL, Woodland JH, Crawford DL. Telerobotic surgery for right and sigmoid colectomies: 30 consecutive cases. Surg Endosc. 2006;20(11):1713–8. PubMed PMID: 17008953.
8. Rawlings AL, Woodland JH, Vegunta RK, Crawford DL. Robotic versus laparoscopic colectomy. Surg Endosc. 2007;21(10):1701–8. PubMed PMID: 17353988.
9. Hellan M, Anderson C, Ellenhorn JD, Paz B, Pigazzi A. Short-term outcomes after robotic-assisted total mesorectal excision for rectal cancer. Ann Surg Oncol. 2007;14(11):3168–73. PubMed PMID: 17763911.
10. Spinoglio G, Summa M, Priora F, Quarati R, Testa S. Robotic colorectal surgery: first 50 cases experience. Dis Colon Rectum. 2008;51(11):1627–32. PubMed PMID: 18484134.
11. Baik SH, Ko YT, Kang CM, Lee WJ, Kim NK, Sohn SK, et al. Robotic tumor-specific mesorectal excision of rectal cancer: short-term outcome of a pilot randomized trial. Surg Endosc. 2008; 22(7):1601–8. PubMed PMID: 18270772.
12. Trastulli S, Farinella E, Cirocchi R, Cavaliere D, Avenia N, Sciannameo F, et al. Robotic resection compared with laparoscopic rectal resection for cancer: systematic review and meta-analysis of short-term outcome. Colorectal Dis. 2012;14(4):e134–56. PubMed PMID: 22151033.
13. Halabi WJ, Kang CY, Jafari MD, Nguyen VQ, Carmichael JC, Mills S, et al. Robotic-assisted colorectal surgery in the United States: a nationwide analysis of trends and outcomes. World J Surg. 2013;6. PubMed PMID: 23564216.
14. Moorthy K, Munz Y, Dosis A, Hernandez J, Martin S, Bello F, et al. Dexterity enhancement with robotic surgery. Surg Endosc. 2004;18(5):790–5. PubMed PMID: 15216862.
15. Kenngott HG, Fischer L, Nickel F, Rom J, Rassweiler J, Muller-Stich BP. Status of robotic assistance–a less traumatic and more accurate minimally invasive surgery? Langenbecks Arch Surg. 2012;397(3):333–41. PubMed PMID: 22038293.
16. Baek SJ, Kim SH, Cho JS, Shin JW, Kim J. Robotic versus conventional laparoscopic surgery for rectal cancer: a cost analysis from a single institute in Korea. World J Surg. 2012;36(11):2722–9. PubMed PMID: 22855217.
17. Yang Y, Wang F, Zhang P, Shi C, Zou Y, Qin H, et al. Robot-assisted versus conventional laparoscopic surgery for colorectal disease, focusing on rectal cancer: a meta-analysis. Ann Surg Oncol. 2012;19(12):3727–36. PubMed PMID: 22752371.
18. Magistro C, Lernia SD, Ferrari G, Zullino A, Mazzola M, De Martini P, et al. Totally laparoscopic versus laparoscopic-assisted right colectomy for colon cancer: is there any advantage in short-term outcomes? A prospective comparative assessment in our center. Surg Endosc. 2013;9. PubMed PMID: 23397503.
19. Baik SH. Robotic colorectal surgery. Yonsei Med J. 2008;49(6):891–6. PubMed PMID: 19108010; Pubmed Central PMCID: 2628019.
20. Park JS, Choi GS, Park SY, Kim HJ, Ryuk JP. Randomized clinical trial of robot-assisted versus standard laparoscopic right colectomy. Br J Surg. 2012;99(9):1219–26. PubMed PMID: 22864881.
21. Antoniou SA, Antoniou GA, Koch OO, Pointner R, Granderath FA. Robot-assisted laparoscopic surgery of the colon and rectum. Surg Endosc. 2012;26(1):1–11. PubMed PMID: 21858568.
22. Baik SH, Kim NK, Lee KY, Sohn SK, Cho CH, Kim MJ, et al. Factors influencing pathologic results after total mesorectal excision for rectal cancer: analysis of consecutive 100 cases. Ann Surg Oncol. 2008;15(3):721–8. PubMed PMID: 18058183.
23. Champagne BJ, Makhija R. Minimally invasive surgery for rectal cancer: are we there yet? World J Gastroenterol. 2011;17(7):862–6. PubMed PMID: 21412496; Pubmed Central PMCID: 3051137.
24. Guillou PJ, Quirke P, Thorpe H, Walker J, Jayne DG, Smith AM, et al. Short-term endpoints of conventional versus laparoscopic-assisted surgery in patients with colorectal cancer (MRC CLASICC trial): multicentre, randomised controlled trial. Lancet. 2005; 365(9472):1718–26. PubMed PMID: 15894098.
25. Ng KH, Ng DC, Cheung HY, Wong JC, Yau KK, Chung CC, et al. Laparoscopic resection for rectal cancers: lessons learned from 579 cases. Ann Surg. 2009;249(1):82–6. PubMed PMID: 19106680.
26. Hellan M, Stein H, Pigazzi A. Totally robotic low anterior resection with total mesorectal excision and splenic flexure mobilization. Surg Endosc. 2009;23(2):447–51. PubMed PMID: 19057962.

# Transanal Minimally Invasive Surgery (TAMIS): Operative Technique, Pitfalls, and Tips

# 25

Francisco Quinteros, Kumaran Thiruppathy, and Matthew R. Albert

**Key Points**

- TAMIS improves vision and accessibility when performing transanal procedures resulting in superior outcomes.
- Accurate preoperative evaluation of tumors is required to ensure good outcomes.
- The authors advise pre-dissection circumferential marking of dissection area around tumor.
- Standard laparoscopic equipment can be used with the TAMIS platforms; however, advanced innovative equipment is available to simplify difficult steps, if required.
- Post-excision rectal defect closure is ideal but not essential.
- Peritoneal entry when excising high rectal lesions can be repaired simply by a combined laparoscopic and TAMIS approach.

## Introduction

There has been a recent resurgence in the interest in transanal resections due to advances in technology and techniques, along with the efforts of pioneering surgeons. Traditionally, poor visualization and access, in particular when dealing with rectal lesions further than 5 cm from the anal verge, made conventional transanal resections unfavorable. However, the introduction of transanal endoscopic microsurgery (TEMS) in the 1980s dramatically advanced transanal visibility and access, which contributed to improved postoperative outcomes [1]. TEMS offers superior quality of resections, with decreased local recurrence and improved survival when compared to conventional transanal resections.

TEMS utilizes a fixed platform with a 40 mm diameter and a varying length rigid sigmoidoscope that is attached to a fixed articulating stabilizer arm. The TEMS scope has binocular vision or a standard laparoscope and additional working instrument ports. A specialized insufflator allows constant low-pressure distension in combination with suction and irrigation. This permits a single surgeon using specialized TEMS instruments to perform rectal surgery within a visual field of 180–210°. Due to the steep learning curve, position-dependent limitations, and costs, TEMS has been largely restricted to subspecialty units and surgeons worldwide.

The recent introduction of transanal minimally invasive surgery platforms has made transanal microsurgery more accessible to colorectal surgeons and led to a resurgence of this technique. Two FDA-approved surgical platforms, the GelPOINT path (Applied Medical, Rancho Santa Margarita CT) and the SILS™ port (Covidien, Samford, CT), exist in the United States [2, 3] (Fig. 25.1). In combination with these access devices, standard insufflators and traditional laparoscopic instruments afford excellent intraluminal visualization of the rectum and proximal reach of tumors as high as 15 cm. In early studies, TAMIS has shown to confer all of the advantages of TEMS with improved excision of neoplasms when compared to traditional transanal excision [4]. Furthermore, the short learning curve compared to TEM, especially for surgeons already facile with basic laparoscopic skills, as well as the inexpensive initial cost makes TAMIS an attractive alternative [5].

Traditionally, transanal resections were reserved for treatment of benign lesions or malignant lesions in patients not otherwise suitable for classical oncologic resection.

**Electronic supplementary material:** Supplementary material is available in the online version of this chapter at 10.1007/978-1-4939-1581-1_25. Videos can also be accessed at http://www.springerimages.com/videos/978-1-4939-1580-4.

F. Quinteros, M.D. • M.R. Albert, M.D., F.A.C.S., F.A.S.C.R.S. (✉)
Department of Colorectal Surgery, Center for Colon and Rectal Surgery, Florida Hospital Orlando,
601 East Rollins St, Orlando, FL 32803, USA
e-mail: matthew.albert.md@flhosp.org

K. Thiruppathy, F.R.C.S. (Eng)., M.B.B.S., M.Phil., B.Sc.
Department of Colorectal Surgery, Center for Colon and Rectal Surgery, Florida Hospital Orlando, 601 East Rollins St, Orlando, FL 32803, USA

Department of Colorectal Surgery, Colchester General Hospital, Turner Road, Essex CO4 5JL, UK

H.M. Ross et al. (eds.), *Minimally Invasive Approaches to Colon and Rectal Disease: Technique and Best Practices*,
DOI 10.1007/978-1-4939-1581-1_25, © Springer Science+Business Media New York 2015

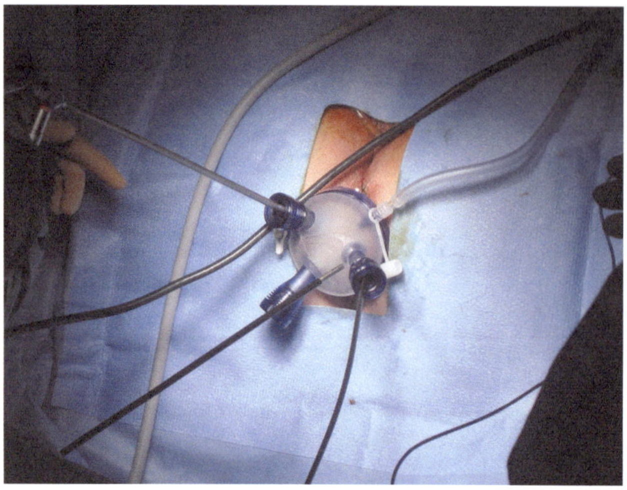

**Fig. 25.1** The port shown with instruments in the trocars

With a growing understanding of colorectal tumor biology, disease progression, and advances in medicine, selected malignant tumors are preferentially being treated by local excision transanally to negate the morbidity and mortality of a major resection [4, 6]. As skills and instrumentation evolved, there has been an increasing interest in TAMIS as a key instrument in transanal total mesorectal excision of rectum and in natural orifice tumor extraction (NOTES) procedures; however, these are currently still in the early stages of development [7]. Anecdotal evidence suggests that the transanal total mesorectal excision (ta-TME) of the rectum offers significant advantages, particularly in patients with low-lying tumors, internal sphincter involvement, and especially in the narrow, difficult pelvis typical of the obese male [8].

## Indications for TAMIS

The indications for TAMIS in the resection of tumors are the same as for TEMS. This includes benign, premalignant, and selected malignant rectal tumors that are not suitable for endoscopic resection and otherwise would require low anterior resection with or without colostomy. Traditionally, lesions should not occupy more than 30 % of the luminal diameter. However, in the experience of the authors, larger lesions and even circumferential sleeve excisions have routinely been feasible. Well-selected malignancies include tumors less than 3 cm, well-to-moderately differentiated tumors, early submucosal invasion (T1 sm1, sm2), and no evidence of lymphovascular invasion or other poor pathologic features that increase the risk of lymph node metastasis. Patients with advanced disease have also been offered TAMIS for palliation instead of a larger non-curative abdominal procedure. The maximum height of lesions that can be readily accessed and subsequently removed from the rectum varies. However, from our experience of 125 patients requiring rectal tumor resections, we are able to successfully excise all lesions that could be visualized by office proctoscopy without prohibitive patient discomfort. In the same series, several patients had rectal tumor excisions between 14 and 16 cm from the anal verge [4, 9].

The "gold standard" for rectal cancers has traditionally been the low anterior resection (LAR) or abdominoperineal resection (APR) [10, 11]. These operations carry with them significant morbidity and mortality, including anastomotic leak, urinary and sexual dysfunction, fecal incontinence, and almost universally chronic functional changes or low anterior syndrome [12, 13]. In well-selected $T_1N_0$ cancers, where the risk of nodal spread is low, TAMIS offers local rectal excision with curative intent and significantly reduced risk of morbidity and mortality. In fact, although several studies have demonstrated increased rates of locoregional recurrence, no comparison has ever demonstrated a survival advantage of radical resection over transanal excision. Ongoing randomized trials should further help delineate this controversial issue (TREC trail, Birmingham University Hospital, UK).

Current indications for TAMIS may also be broadened to include local excision of the "scar"—grossly negative lesions in patients with locally advanced rectal cancer after neoadjuvant therapy—for the purpose of confirming complete local pathological response (ypT0) [14]. Modern neoadjuvant chemoradiotherapy can offer up to 20–50 % of patients with rectal adenocarcinoma a complete pathological response [15, 16]. In this subset of patients, LAR or APR can be avoided with fairly low risk. If radical resection is ultimately required following transanal excision because of margin positivity, preoperative understaging, or adverse histological features, this can be performed with no negative long-term impact on survival or cure. Delay in surgery for 6 weeks or longer to allow the mesorectal defect to heal in order to maintain the "holy plane" is recommended.

## Preoperative Work-Up

Optimal management of rectal tumors is dependent on obtaining accurate and detailed staging information at the time of diagnosis. Therefore, all patients should undergo adequate oncologic preoperative evaluation including full assessment of the colon by colonoscopy or other radiographic means to rule out synchronous lesions. Digital rectal assessment and proctoscopy/sigmoidoscopy should also be performed in order to determine sphincter tonicity, confirm tumor height, and verify orientation. Local tumor and lymph node staging should be performed by endoanal ultrasound, MRI with endorectal endocoil, or 3-T MRI. Any of these modalities can provide detailed information about tumor depth and lymph node involvement, with MRI providing

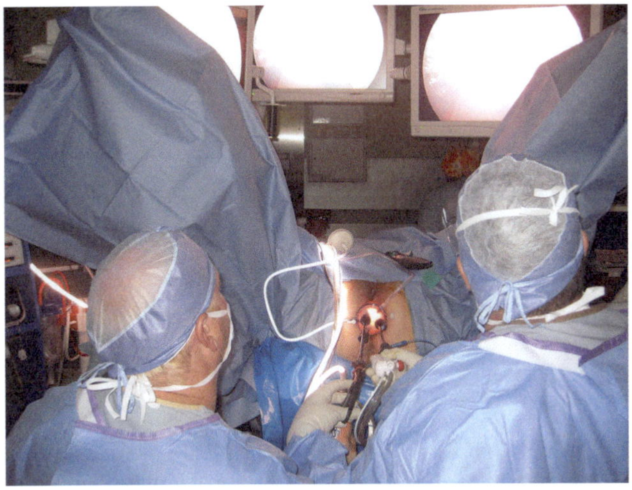

**Fig. 25.2** The patient position is shown during the operation as well as the surgeon positioning

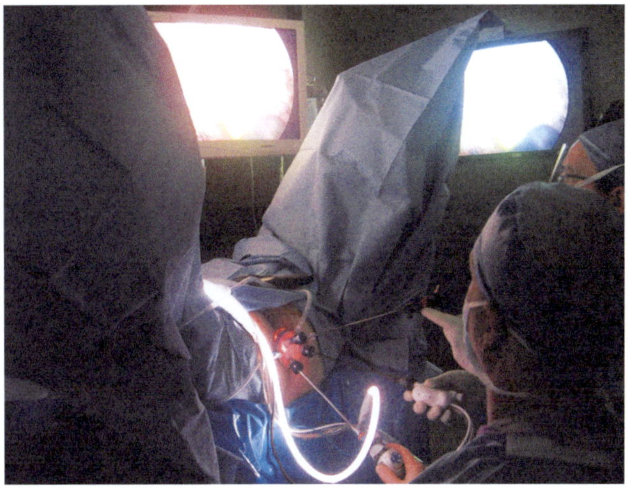

**Fig. 25.3** The monitors are placed to provide the most comfortable view

additional information regarding extramural vascular invasion (EMVI), threatened circumferential resection margin (CRM), and mucin deposits—all of which are negative prognostic markers and can influence treatment options [17–19]. For malignant lesions, metastatic workup with computed tomography of the chest, abdomen, and pelvis is performed as well as consideration of combined CT/PET scan.

## Technique (Videos 25.1 and 25.2)

Mechanical bowel preparation is recommend for all patients to maximize visualization of the rectum with minimal contamination. The authors routinely have good results using only two phosphate enemas preoperatively. For inadequate bowel preparation, transanal lavage using a proctoscope or catheter system can be performed, but this technique is not ideal. If visualization is impaired in any way after these maneuvers, the procedure should be terminated and rescheduled with a more thorough preparation. A single dose of intravenous antibiotic is given approximately 30 min before the procedure. TAMIS can be performed in any position. The authors find the high lithotomy position most advantageous for the anesthesiologist and surgeon because it permits the surgeon to perform the operation while sitting comfortably and with minimal neck strain with the viewing monitor placed between the patient's legs, while providing the anesthesiologist ready access to the airway (Figs. 25.2 and 25.3). The versatility of the TAMIS ports ensures the surgeon can gain good access to the lesion from the lithotomy position regardless the position of the tumor, unlike the TEM system. Positioning in Trendelenburg provides an advantageous view into the rectal lumen throughout the procedure, particularly for anteriorly based lesions that require challenging positioning when using traditional TEM. The authors have used lateral or prone position at times, but when using the TAMIS port, we have not found any intraoperative limitations due to the location of the lesion when using the high lithotomy. In addition, the abdominal cavity may be easily accessed if the need arises intraoperatively.

All current transanal access devices are deployed using similar techniques. Gentle two-finger dilatation is performed with or without a perianal block. The port is inserted into the rectum either by hand or ringed forcep with generous lubrication until it seats at the anorectal ring. An obturator is often used to facilitate placement when using the GelPOINT path or Endorec port (Aspide Medicale, La Talaudiere, France). Confirmation of the correct placement is followed by placement of stay sutures through the port eyelets or port itself. Although port dislodgement in a properly deployed device is a rare event, stay sutures can prevent the port from rotating during the procedure and inadvertently changing the location of the camera and working ports, thereby also minimizing trauma to the anorectal canal. Newer-designed access devices permit some variation in port placement to minimize instrument collisions; however, generally three 5 mm ports are placed in a triangular orientation.

Adequate insufflation is generally the most critical component to a successful procedure and ideally achieves a tensely distended rectum for the duration of the procedure. The insufflation port should be placed on the top of the port so that you are not insufflating through any pooled blood. Insufflation is achieved with a standard laparoscopic insufflator at 15 mmHg pressure on high flow, although the pressure may be increased as needed. Pressures as high as 25 mmHg have been attained using bariatric insufflators. To date, there have been no reports of barotrauma or other adverse events to the colon or rectum as a result of insufflation. Complete relaxation with general endotracheal anesthesia is critical to prevent collapse of the rectum or, subtler though equally distracting, bellowing during respiration, the effects of which are magnified during excision of small neoplasms. Recently, spinal anesthesia has been described to perform TAMIS without difficulty; however, any problems should prompt early conversion to a full general anesthetic [9]. Although nearly every surgeon performing TEM or TAMIS has at some point experienced difficulty with poor insufflation, a series of routine laparoscopic troubleshooting strategies will almost always resolve this sufficiently to allow completion of the procedure.

There are multiple options for instrument selection for the procedure. A 5 mm 30° camera is optimal because it provides high-definition visualization for the procedure with the ability to manipulate the angle of the scope based on tumor location. A larger camera and corresponding trocar may be used, but the smaller size is preferable in light of the already small working area and increasingly high-quality picture of smaller laparoscopes. Using a standard colonoscope to provide a wider visual field with more flexibility has been described by Mclemore [20]. Articulating cameras have also been used, but this requires an experienced camera holder and, in most cases, additional expense. The authors have not found that the articulation benefits outweigh the grainier image quality.

In general, the basic instruments should function to grasp and bluntly dissect tissue, to provide cautery, and to evacuate smoke and any blood. The majority of procedures can be performed with a Maryland dissector for fine grasping and either a needle-tip or spatula cautery attached to a suction irrigator. If needed, cautery can be connected to the Maryland dissector for coagulation of a bleeding vessel which commonly occurs in the mesorectal fat. More troublesome bleeding can often be controlled with ease using one of many bipolar energy devices or ultrasonic dissectors. This added luxury might be of significant benefit for more proximal lesions where retraction is limited and bleeding is more difficult to stop. The use of extra-long instruments may prove beneficial to some in minimizing instrument or hand collisions.

Whether using traditional TEM or newer transanal platforms, the quality of resection is paramount. The true marker of outcomes for this procedure is the quality of the specimen. Given the increased rate of resecting malignancies of the rectum with this technique, as well as the malignant potential of adenomas, an accurate, well-executed, technically correct operation with strict indications is imperative. The procedure begins by marking with cautery the intended resection margins on the mucosa 5 mm to 1 cm away from the tumor (Fig. 25.4). A mucosal or full-thickness incision is then performed at the most distal marking (Fig. 25.5). As the tension changes, retraction is frequently adjusted by grasping the tissue as close as possible to the dissection site and using short bursts of monopolar cautery. This is a very dynamic procedure that requires frequent changes in laparoscope angulation and retraction angles. Also, there may be a benefit to exchanging the instruments and camera into different ports to gain a better view or working angle as needed. Direct tumor grasping should be avoided to prevent tumor fragmentation and possible seeding. When performing a full-thickness excision in the correct plane just into the perirectal fat deep to the muscularis propria, the areolar tissue begins to pneumo-dissect from the insufflation pressure. Advancing and retracting the lesion proximally into the rectum while working "underneath" the tumor is the easiest technique. The lesion is slowly encircled while dissecting more proximal in the rectum, frequently reassessing the proximal margin (Figs. 25.6, 25.7, 25.8, 25.9, and 25.10). Finally, the proximal margin is divided and the lesion detached, again facilitated by retracting proximally into the rectum rather than pulling the lesion towards the camera and the port (Fig. 25.11).

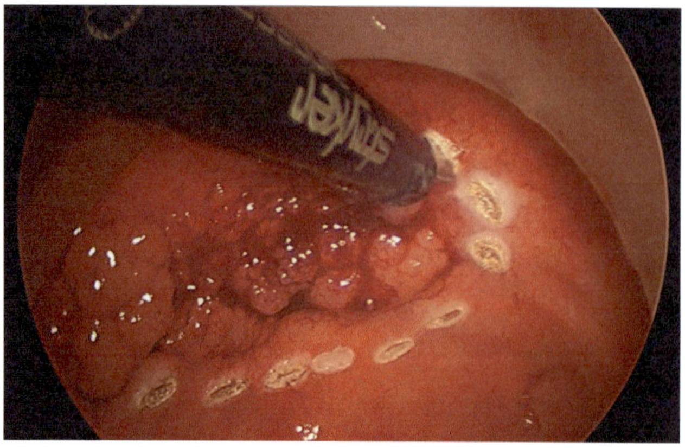

**Fig. 25.4** The tumor resection margins are outlined with cautery at the outset of the procedure. The margin of normal tissue that is included in the specimen will serve as a handle to grasp the tissue and provide traction

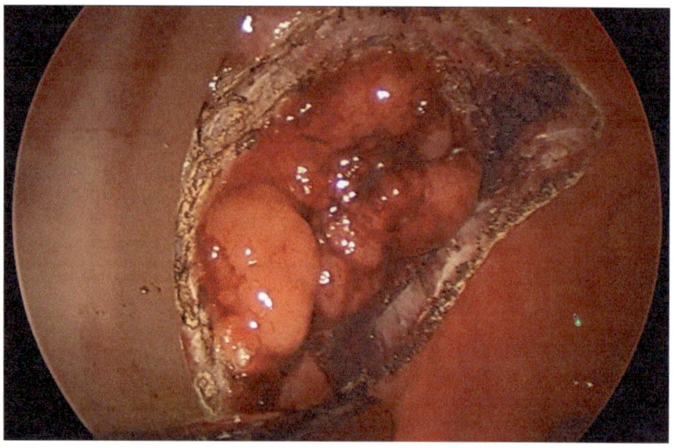

**Fig. 25.5** The tumor outline is completed. The effects of the pneumodissection and the amount of contracture of the tissue start to be noticeable at this point

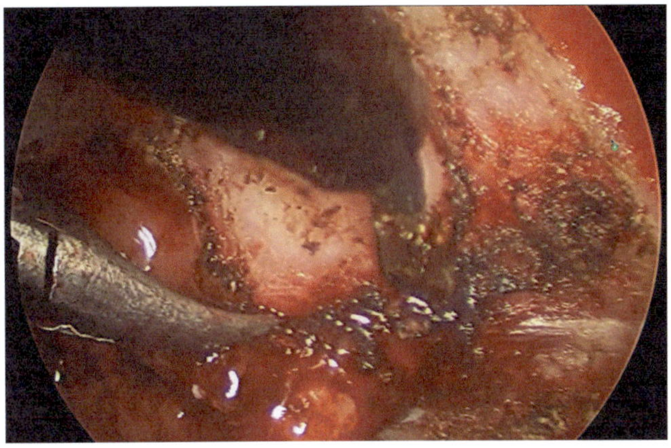

**Fig. 25.6** The tumor is cauterized in the full-thickness plane. The traction applied to allow easy cauterization of the tissue is well demonstrated

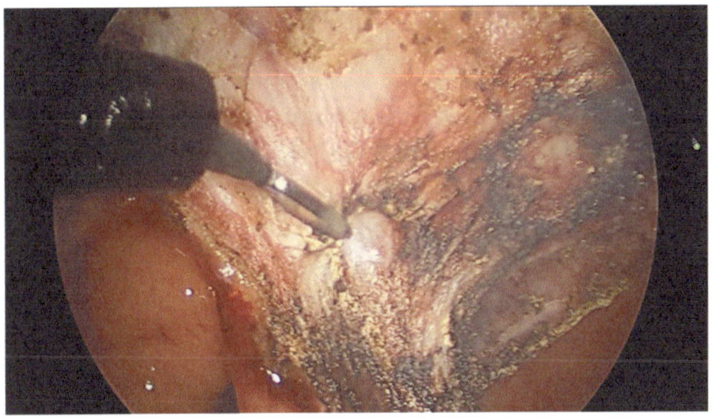

**Fig. 25.7** Dissection continues on the medial side. Notice the full-thickness dissection

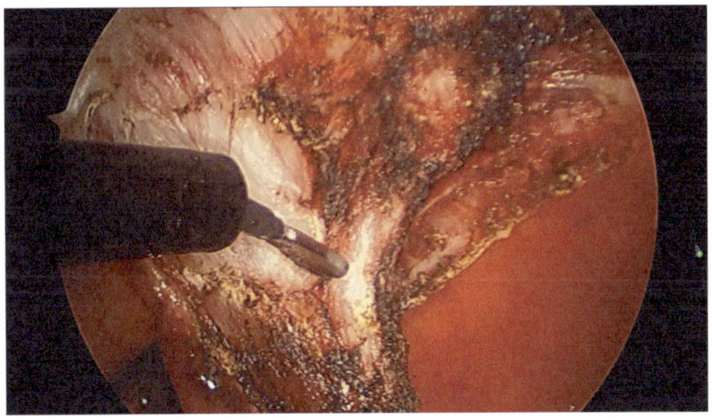

**Fig. 25.8** As the dissection continues in the full-thickness plane, traction allow excellent visualization

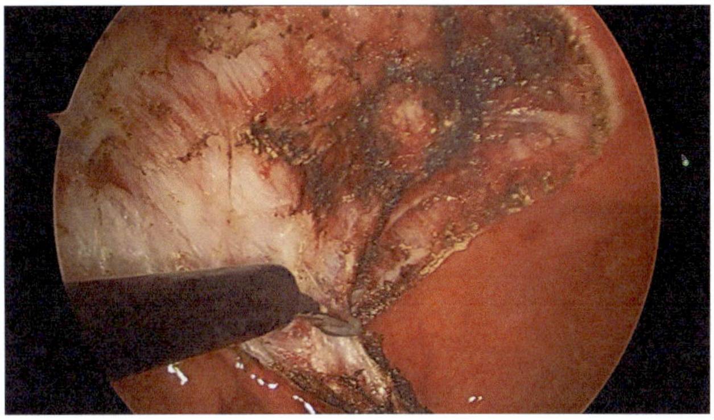

**Fig. 25.9** Continued full-thickness dissection on the inferior aspect of the lesion. Notice the excellent hemostasis

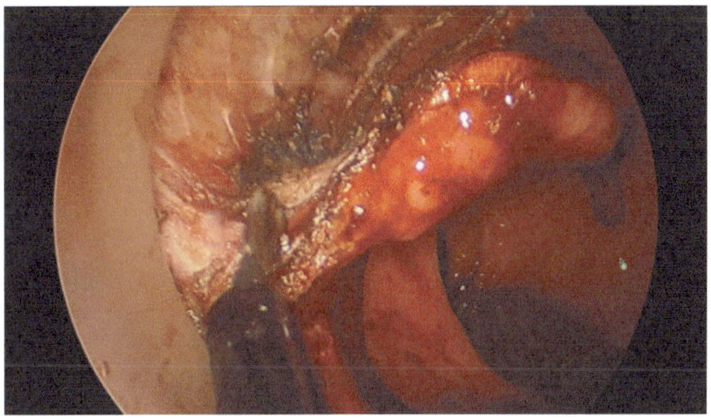

**Fig. 25.10** Dissection continues in the previously marked lateral boundary to complete the resection

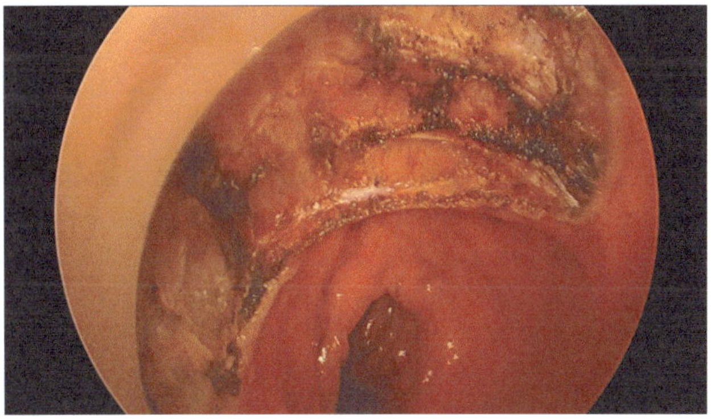

**Fig. 25.11** The size of the defect can be appreciated in this defect. It was approximately 40 % of the circumference of the rectum

Specimen extraction should be performed at completion of resection and prior to closure to maintain specimen integrity and avoid accidental proximal migration. The specimen is then pinned in place or marked per surgeon and pathologist preference (Figs. 25.12 and 25.13). The majority of platforms accommodate extraction by allowing removal of the faceplate; however, some ports require removal of the entire device with reinsertion for closure. Irrigation of the excision bed with dilute betadine, presumably for its tumoricidal and bactericidal effects, is a common practice. However, no evidence-based literature exists to support this technique.

For tumors that are extremely low, in the distal rectum and even abutting the dentate line, a hybrid technique can maintain all the benefits of TAMIS and facilitate a superior resection.

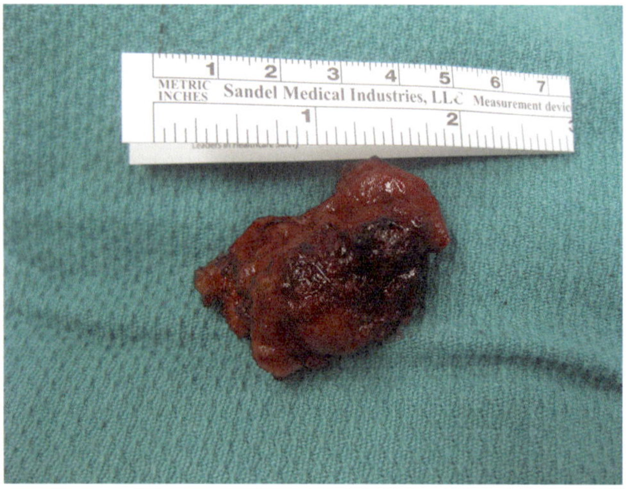


**Fig. 25.12** A full-thickness specimen after extraction. The mesorectal fat is evident on the portion of the specimen that was not anterior

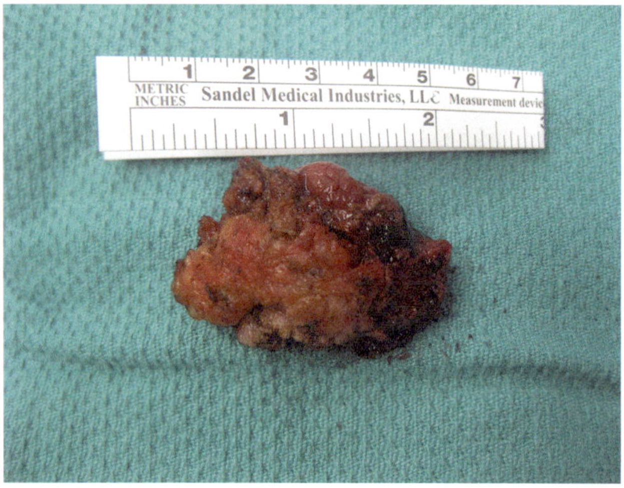


**Fig. 25.13** Notice the perirectal fat on the posterior aspect of the tumor to confirm full-thickness resection

Although these can be performed with traditional anorectal retractors to avoid additional expense, we believe that use of a transanal port is extremely advantageous in bulky friable villous tumors, circumferential or near circumferential tumors, or lesions that extend more proximally into the rectum. The distal incision is made prior to port insertion with dissection carried proximally a short distance. This is followed by port deployment and standard excision once the mass is above the anorectal ring, where the port will be seated.

Closure is performed by placing a suture for traction at the midportion of the proximal rectal wall followed by port removal and replacement with an anorectal retractor. Easy closure is permitted with perfect alignment of the rectal wall. There is no consensus as to whether it is necessary to close the remaining mural defect in the rectal wall. Certainly, this can be the most difficult component of the operation.

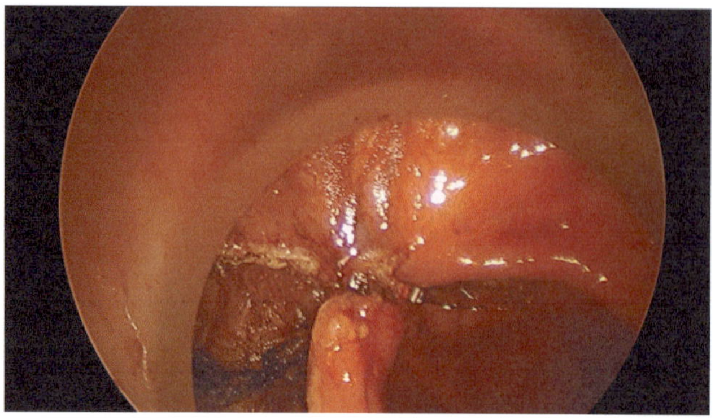

**Fig. 25.14** The defect is first re-approximated at the midportion using an absorbable stitch

Extraperitoneal full-thickness resections can be left to heal without closure of the defect. This technique almost certainly arose from the amount of difficulty and time it took to close a defect with conventional transanal surgery, as well as the common belief that wound dehiscence and abscess are a regular occurrence. Aside from the aesthetic pleasure, the authors recommend closure of all defects with a 2-0 or 3-0 absorbable sutures for postoperative hemostasis. In addition to minimizing bleeding complications, the wound usually remains closed at postoperative office proctoscopy, and this facilitates quicker healing.

Laparoscopic suturing with traditional laparoscopic needle holders is challenging due to the ergonomic difficulties of suturing within a confined space. Wound closure can be performed using interrupted, figure-of-eight, or running sutures. Initially, decreasing the insufflator pressure by 3–5 mmHg can "shrink" a seemingly daunting defect to one that is more manageable. Defects should be closed from proximal to distal and not side to side to avoid narrowing of the lumen. Given the compliance of the rectal wall, it is uncommon to have to mobilize the proximal rectum to oppose the wound. Dividing the defect into two sections by re-approximating the midportion of the defect can be helpful (Fig. 25.14). Intracorporeal knot tying is time consuming and difficult and can be avoided using a standard 25 cm laparoscopic knot pusher or an automated suture tying device. Alternatively, performing a continuous sutured closure with a barbed suture avoids the need to tie altogether. The use of modern laparoscopic suture devices endoluminally to close defects can dramatically shorten the learning curve and improve precision of closure, but requires increased procedural costs (Endostitch, Ethicon, Cincinnati, OH; LSI, Covidien, CT). With practice, given the minimal increase in operative time and technical difficulty, the authors feel that closure is warranted to minimize any complications (Fig. 25.15).

Entry into the peritoneal cavity is not an uncommon occurrence with anterior-based tumors, especially in women where the peritoneal reflection is lower and is surrounded by

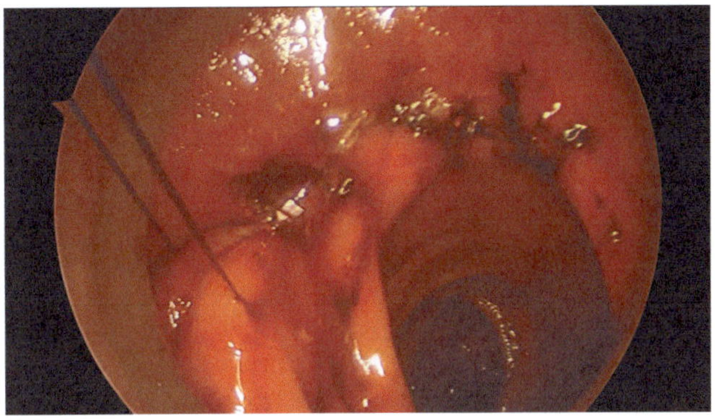

**Fig. 25.15** The wound is shown nearly closed, with only the last suture requiring a tie. The lumen is clearly visible and is not narrowed with the closure

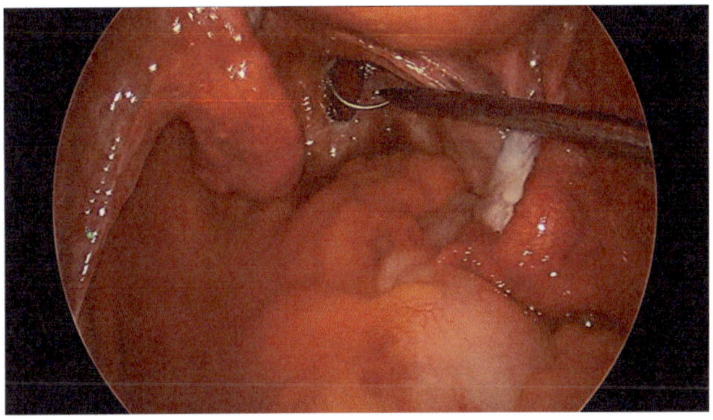

**Fig. 25.16** An anterior rectal mass leading to entry into the peritoneal cavity is shown from an abdominal perspective. The loss of pneumorectum made closure not possible transanally and required placement of laparoscopic trocars. The peritoneal wound was closed with interrupted sutures, and the rectum was then re-insufflated and closed with interrupted sutures as well

less perirectal fat (Fig. 25.16). This should be anticipated by tumor localization on preoperative proctoscopic evaluation and appropriate precautions and discussion with the patient. During the early history of TEM, this commonly necessitated conversion to laparotomy with the need for resection and frequently colostomy. In addition, the potential for transperitoneal seeding in the setting of malignancy was a common concern. More recently, Gavagan demonstrated this to be a low-risk event, which does not mandate conversion [21]. Obviously, a secure closure becomes mandatory. A two-layer closure of outer peritoneum first followed by full-thickness closure of the rectal wall is recommended. In this scenario, some surgeons have suggested a water-soluble contrast study the following morning prior to discharge. In our experience with peritoneal entry during TAMIS, we have had two cases where insufflation failed to maintain distention of the rectum to permit adequate closure. In both of these instances, laparoscopy with suture closure of the peritoneal defect from the abdominal side allowed reestablishment of the pneumorectum with completion of the closure endoluminally. These patients were discharged the following day without further studies.

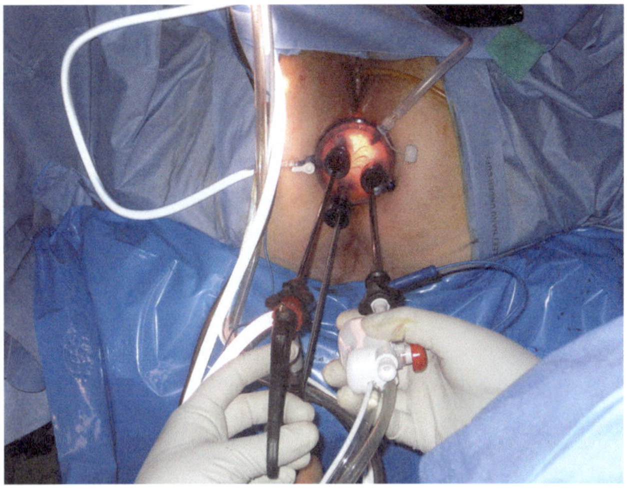

**Fig. 25.17** The instruments are positioned at a comfortable height

Minimal postoperative care with same-day discharge can be accomplished in most patients, except those with excessive comorbidities. No postoperative antibiotics are required and patients may resume normal diet and activity immediately. Postoperative surveillance of adenomas over the initial postoperative year can be performed with proctoscopy at regular intervals. Small recurrences can often be removed with endoscopic techniques. Patients with malignancy should be followed by standard NCCN or locoregional guidelines with quarterly follow-up and CEA levels. Serial MRI or endoscopic ultrasound has been advocated for early detection of mural and mesorectal recurrences that tend to occur following local excision; however, no standard guidelines currently exist. If "salvage" operation is required for patients with more advanced lesions than suspected preoperatively or with later findings of nodal disease, no negative prognosis has thus far been associated with the initial TAMIS approach followed by abdominal surgical resection in our experience.

## Pearls and Pitfalls

- Select your patients wisely, especially at the beginning. Posterior, <3 cm, mid-rectal lesions are often the best candidates. Even if they can be performed by traditional transanal methods, use TAMIS for increased visualization and better instrumentation.
- Position the patient and set up the room to maximize ergonomics. These are complex operations, but will only become harder if you are uncomfortable with the instrumentation and straining (Figs. 25.17, 25.18, and 25.19).

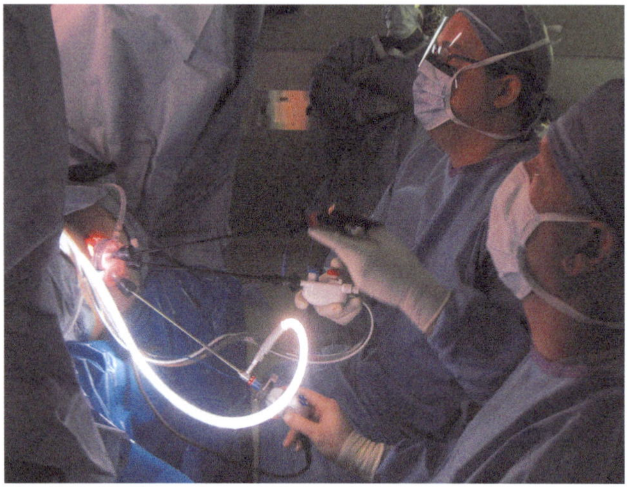

**Fig. 25.18** An experienced assistant or surgeon is invaluable

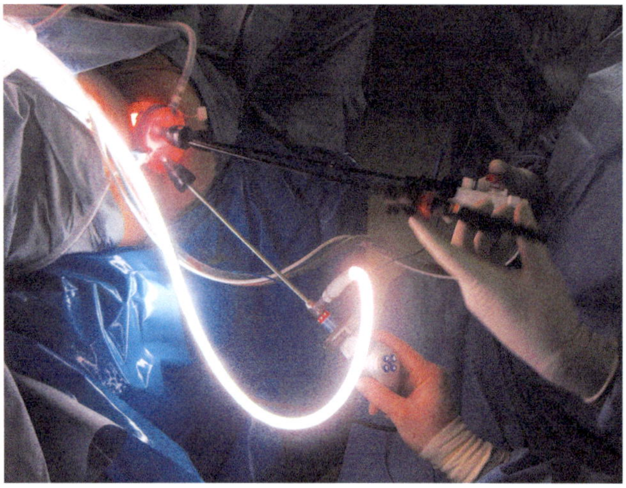

**Fig. 25.19** Creating space between the different instrumentations provides clear visualization while avoiding collisions

- Ensure you have adequate margins. Marking your boundaries of resection closer to 1 cm at the onset of the case, especially in your early experience, and ensuring you have a full-thickness excision are imperative. Although the defect will be slightly larger, it is better than the alternative of positive margins.
- It is imperative that your anesthesiology team has completely paralyzed the patient and continues to re-dose during the procedure as needed. Failure to ensure this is done will compromise your visualization.
- Take care of the troublesome bleeding right away. Don't let small nuisance bleeding obstruct your visualization.
- Although the lesion is fixed, be active in changing angles of the camera and of changing which ports your instruments and cameras use. Impossible angles typically become very easy when the perspectives are changed.
- Immediately prior to transecting the final attachments on the specimen, ensure you have proper orientation prior to removal to assist in marking the boundaries for pathology. A grasper placed on the anterior (i.e., distal) midline facilitates this process.
- Attempt intracorporeal suturing in easy cases, but don't waste time, effort, and frustration—use one of the described methods above to make things much easier.
- Preoperatively discuss with your patient the potential for an inability to complete the case purely via TAMIS and the possibility of abdominal exploration if peritoneal entry occurs.

## Conclusion

Transanal minimally invasive surgery is a feasible technique that has maximized the advantages introduced by minimally invasive techniques and evolving laparoscopic instrumentation. The improved access to the rectum enhances visualization, improves resection, and extends the upper limits of resection in comparison to traditional transanal excision. TAMIS should be a part of every colorectal specialist's armamentarium.

**Disclosures** Dr. Quinteros and Dr. Thiruppathy have no disclosures. Dr. Albert is a paid speaker, program director, and consultant for Applied Medical and is a speaker for Lifecell.

## References

1. Buess G, Theiss R, Gunther M, Hutterer F, Pichlmaier H. [Transanal endoscopic microsurgery]. Leber Magen Darm. 1985;15(6):271–9.
2. Atallah S, Albert M, Larach S. Transanal minimally invasive surgery: a giant leap forward. Surg Endosc. 2010;24(9):2200–5.
3. Matz J, Matz A. Use of a SILS port in transanal endoscopic microsurgery in the setting of a community hospital. J Laparoendosc Adv Surg Tech A. 2012;22(1):93–6.
4. Albert MR, Atallah SB, deBeche-Adams TC, Izfar S, Larach SW. Transanal minimally invasive surgery (TAMIS) for local excision of benign neoplasms and early-stage rectal cancer: efficacy and outcomes in the first 50 patients. Dis Colon Rectum. 2013;56(3):301–7.
5. Atallah SB, Albert MR. Transanal minimally invasive surgery (TAMIS) versus transanal endoscopic microsurgery (TEM): Is one better than the other? Surg Endosc. 2013;27(12):4750–1.
6. Allaix ME, Arezzo A, Caldart M, Festa F, Morino M. Transanal endoscopic microsurgery for rectal neoplasms: experience of 300 consecutive cases. Dis Colon Rectum. 2009;52(11):1831–6.
7. de Lacy AM, Rattner DW, Adelsdorfer C, Tasende MM, Fernandez M, Delgado S, et al. Transanal natural orifice transluminal endoscopic surgery (NOTES) rectal resection: "down-to-up" total mesorectal excision (TME)-short-term outcomes in the first 20 cases. Surg Endosc. 2013;27(9):3165–72.
8. Marks J, Nassif G, Schoonyoung H, Denittis A, Zeger E, Mohiuddin M, et al. Sphincter-sparing surgery for adenocarcinoma of the distal

3 cm of the true rectum: results after neoadjuvant therapy and minimally invasive radical surgery or local excision. Surg Endosc. 2013;27(12):4469–77.
9. Lee TG, Lee SJ. Transanal single-port microsurgery for rectal tumors: minimal invasive surgery under spinal anesthesia. Surg Endosc. 2013;28(1):271–80.
10. Heald RJ, Moran BJ, Ryall RD, Sexton R, MacFarlane JK. Rectal cancer: the Basingstoke experience of total mesorectal excision, 1978-1997. Arch Surg. 1998;133(8):894–9.
11. MacFarlane JK, Ryall RD, Heald RJ. Mesorectal excision for rectal cancer. Lancet. 1993;341(8843):457–60.
12. Morino M, Parini U, Giraudo G, Salval M, Brachet CR, Garrone C. Laparoscopic total mesorectal excision: a consecutive series of 100 patients. Ann Surg. 2003;237(3):335–42.
13. Hendren SK, O'Connor BI, Liu M, Asano T, Cohen Z, Swallow CJ, et al. Prevalence of male and female sexual dysfunction is high following surgery for rectal cancer. Ann Surg. 2005;242(2).212–23.
14. Morino M, Arezzo A, Allaix ME. Transanal endoscopic microsurgery. Tech Coloproctol. 2013;17 Suppl 1:S55–61.
15. Habr-Gama A, Perez RO, Nadalin W, Sabbaga J, Ribeiro Jr U, Silva E, et al. Operative versus nonoperative treatment for stage 0 distal rectal cancer following chemoradiation therapy: long-term results. Ann Surg. 2004;240(4):711–7.
16. Zmora O, Dasilva GM, Gurland B, Pfeffer R, Koller M, Nogueras JJ, et al. Does rectal wall tumor eradication with preoperative chemoradiation permit a change in the operative strategy? Dis Colon Rectum. 2004;47(10):1607–12.
17. Salerno GV, Daniels IR, Moran BJ, Heald RJ, Thomas K, Brown G. Magnetic resonance imaging prediction of an involved surgical resection margin in low rectal cancer. Dis Colon Rectum. 2009; 52(4):632–9.
18. Shihab OC, Moran BJ, Heald RJ, Quirke P, Brown G. MRI staging of low rectal cancer. Eur Radiol. 2009;19(3):643–50.
19. Brown G. Thin section MRI in multidisciplinary pre-operative decision making for patients with rectal cancer. Br J Radiol. 2005;78(Spec No. 2):S117–27.
20. McLemore EC, Coker A, Jacobsen G, Talamini MA, Horgan S. cTAMIS: endoscopic visualization for transanal minimally invasive surgery. Surg Endosc. 2013;27(5):1842–5.
21. Gavagan JA, Whiteford MH, Swanstrom LL. Full-thickness intraperitoneal excision by transanal endoscopic microsurgery does not increase short-term complications. Am J Surg. 2004;187(5):630–4.

# 26 Combined Endo-Laparoscopic Surgery (CELS)

Kelly A. Garrett and Sang W. Lee

**Key Points**

- The technique of combined endo-laparoscopic surgery is for patients with benign colon polyps that cannot be removed endoscopically.
- Colonoscopy report and pathology results should be reviewed at initial consultation.
- $CO_2$ colonoscopy should be employed in order for this technique to be more often successful.
- The polyp should be localized first endoscopically and its location marked using dilute indigo carmine solution.
- The colon wall adjacent to the polyp can be manipulated laparoscopically to facilitate snare polypectomy.
- If a repair of the colon wall is performed, repair should be leak-tested with the colonoscope.
- Endoscopic-assisted laparoscopic wall excision may be necessary in some locations.
- If there are features of malignancy, the procedure can be converted to laparoscopic colectomy.
- If CELS is successful, but final pathology reveals malignancy, patients may go on to require colectomy in the postoperative period.

**Electronic supplementary material:** Supplementary material is available in the online version of this chapter at 10.1007/978-1-4939-1581-1_26. Videos can also be accessed at http://www.springerimages.com/videos/978-1-4939-1580-4.

K.A. Garrett, M.D., F.A.C.S., F.A.S.C.R.S
Division of Colorectal Surgery, Department of Surgery, NY Presbyterian Hospital, Weill Cornell Medical College, 525 East 68th Street, Box 172, New York, NY 10065, USA

S.W. Lee, M.D., F.A.C.S., F.A.S.C.R.S. (✉)
Division of Colon and Rectal Surgery, Department of Surgery, Weill-Cornell Medical College, New York Presbyterian Hospital, New York, NY, USA
e-mail: sal2013@med.cornell.edu

## Background

Large colon polyps and those on or behind a haustral fold can be very challenging to remove endoscopically. Although endoscopic mucosal resection (EMR) and submucosal dissection (ESD) have been performed for these polyps, this technique is not widely available and does not provide a solution for certain polyps [1, 2]. For this reason, the most common recommendation for these patients who cannot have their polyps removed through endoscopic means has traditionally been segmental colectomy. There are many studies that demonstrate that laparoscopic colectomy has quicker recovery rates, faster return of bowel function, and earlier return to normal activities in comparison with open colectomy. However, while the laparoscopic approach can minimize the morbidity associated with colectomy, only a minority of the colon resections performed in the United States are being performed laparoscopically [3]. Furthermore, even if a minimally invasive approach is employed, it still entails a major abdominal operation with the potential for associated morbidities. In place of resection, combined endo-laparoscopic surgery (CELS) removal of the polyps has been described as an alternative in select patients [3–10].

The technique of laparoscopic-assisted polypectomy was first described in 1993 as a means to avoid the morbidities associated with a major bowel resection [4]. Larger retrospective studies have since been published indicating that the technique is safe and effective [3, 6, 7, 10–12]. The benefits of CELS include mobilization of the colon to make the polyp easier to resect with the colonoscope, the ability to directly observe the wall of the colon laparoscopically to ensure there is not a full-thickness defect, the capacity to repair an injury if there is one, and the option of converting directly to a laparoscopic resection if the polyp cannot be resected endoscopically or there are findings suspicious for malignancy (Fig. 26.1). Many different techniques and approaches have been described including laparoscopic-assisted colonoscopic resection, endoscopic-assisted

H.M. Ross et al. (eds.), *Minimally Invasive Approaches to Colon and Rectal Disease: Technique and Best Practices*, DOI 10.1007/978-1-4939-1581-1_26, © Springer Science+Business Media New York 2015

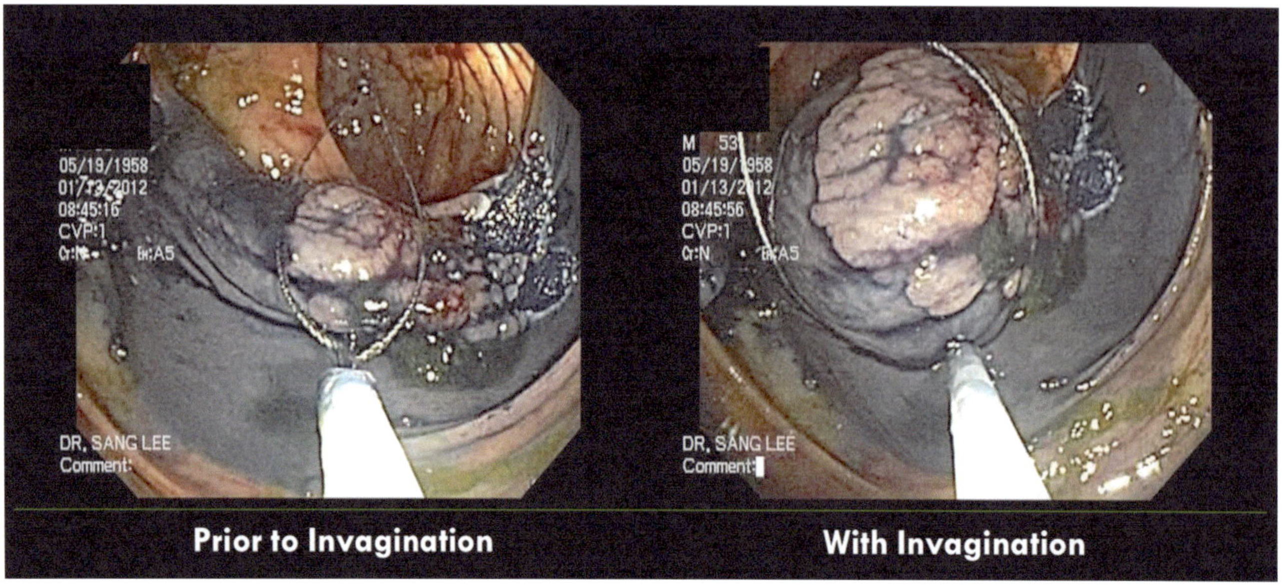


**Fig. 26.1** Combined endo-laparoscopic polypectomy. Laparoscopic manipulation of the bowel wall allows invagination of the bowel wall (*right*) facilitating polypectomy

laparoscopic wedge resection, and endoscopic-assisted laparoscopic resection [13–15]. The largest study to date was performed by Franklin et al., which included long-term follow-up of 160 patients with 209 polyps. At a median follow-up of 65 months (range 6–196 months), there were no recurrences of completely resected polyps [16].

## Indications

Current indications for CELS include large benign colon polyps or polyps in a difficult anatomic location that are unable to be removed by colonoscopic snare polypectomy. In addition, a similar polyp that has been incompletely removed via traditional endoscopic techniques may be considered for CELS. Patients should have a preoperative colonoscopic biopsy that is benign, although polyps with high-grade dysplasia can be included. If patients have other polyps, they should be able to be removed colonoscopically or with CELS technique. CELS should not be performed on patients with a known polyposis syndrome. Finally, relative contraindications for CELS would include a history of multiple previous abdominal surgeries or polyps that are too close to the ileocecal valve.

## Preoperative Planning

A complete history and physical examination should be done including past medical and surgical history. If the patient has a history of multiple abdominal operations, then CELS may not be feasible. Generally, if the colonoscopy has been done elsewhere, it is important to obtain both the colonoscopy and pathology report, and frequently the pathology slides themselves for internal review. If the polyp is on the left side, it is often useful to evaluate the area in the office with a flexible sigmoidoscope to determine the exact location, polyp characteristics, and feasibility of CELS.

Patients should undergo a preoperative workup as they would for any other abdominal procedure including blood work, electrocardiogram, and chest X-ray. Patients should receive a full mechanical bowel preparation the day prior to the procedure in order to aid in visualization of the polyp. When discussing the procedure, the patient should be informed that colonoscopic polypectomy would be attempted; however, if the polyp cannot be resected endoscopically or if there are findings suspicious for malignancy, then laparoscopic colectomy will need to be performed. In addition, patients should be made aware that even if CELS is successful in completely removing the polyp, it is possible that the final pathology may reveal a malignancy and that they may require a bowel resection at a later date.

## Procedure (Video 26.1)

### Setup

After the induction of general anesthesia, Venodyne boots, a nasogastric tube, and a Foley catheter are placed. The patient is positioned in modified lithotomy, ensuring the legs are abducted and placed in padded yellow fin stirrups to facilitate the insertion and manipulation of the colonoscope during the operation. Both arms are tucked at the sides, and the hands

**Table 26.1** Equipment needed for CELS

| |
|---|
| Adult or pediatric colonoscope with monitor ($CO_2$ insufflation if available) |
| Indigo carmine diluted 50 % with injectable saline |
| Endoscopic injector needle |
| Endoscopic snare |
| Endoscopic Roth net® (US Endoscopy, Mentor, OH) |
| Suction trap |
| Bovie cautery |
| Laparoscopic monitors |
| High-definition, flexible-tip laparoscope |
| Trocars: 5 mm × 4, 10 mm × 1, and 12 mm × 1 |
| Laparoscopic bowel graspers and scissors |
| Laparoscopic needle driver |
| Laparoscopic energy device (surgeon preference) |
| Micro-laparoscopic (3 mm) instruments if available |
| Laparoscopic linear stapler (with appropriate loads) |
| Endo Catch bag (Covidien, Norwalk, CT) |
| Wound protector |
| Polysorb or vicryl sutures |

*CELS* combined endo-laparoscopic surgery

and wrists are padded. All equipment should be available to perform colonoscopic polypectomy as well as laparoscopic and open colectomy (though only opened as needed) (Table 26.1). Subcutaneous heparin and intravenous antibiotics are given prior to incision.

Laparoscopic monitors will be placed depending on the location of the lesion. For right colon polyps, monitors are placed on the patient's right side and toward the head of the bed (Fig. 26.2). For left colon lesions, the monitors are placed at the patient's left and toward the foot of the bed. For transverse colon or flexure lesions, the monitors are placed at the head of the bed as the surgeon may stand between the patient's legs (as will the endoscopist).

Endoscopic equipment may vary. Surgeons may prefer to use pediatric versus an adult colonoscope. In addition, we feel it is a prerequisite to have $CO_2$ colonoscopy available in the operating room. Simultaneous performance of laparoscopy and colonoscopy with room air can present technical challenges. Insufflation using room air can significantly obscure the laparoscopic view and compromise exposure. For institutions where this is not possible, a technique of laparoscopically clamping the terminal ileum to minimize bowel distention during laparoscopy has been described, but we have found that colonic distention alone still is a major impediment to this method [3, 4]. Since 2003, our group has been performing colonoscopy with the use of $CO_2$ insufflation during laparoscopy. Because the bowel absorbs $CO_2$ gas approximately 150 times faster than room air, there is minimal unwanted dilation of the colon and excellent simultaneous endoscopic and laparoscopic visualization. We have previously demonstrated that intraoperative $CO_2$ colonoscopy is safe during laparoscopy and can be used to avoid excessive bowel dilation during CELS procedures [9, 17]. Therefore, if available, it is preferred to have $CO_2$ for insufflation during colonoscopy.

## Procedure Steps

### Endoscopy

- After the abdomen is prepped and draped in a sterile fashion, $CO_2$ colonoscopy is performed to locate the lesion (Fig. 26.3). We then use dilute indigo carmine solution (50 % dilution of indigo carmine with injectable saline solution) to mark the area directly under and surrounding the polyp.

### Port Placement

- *Initial access*: A periumbilical incision is made and the fascia is entered sharply. A 5 mm port is placed and pneumoperitoneum is established. A 5 mm, high-definition, flexible-tip laparoscope is preferred for better visualization. The abdomen is explored and the site that was previously marked is located.
- *Secondary trocars*: Depending on the location of the lesion, typically two 5 mm trocars may be placed. For right colon lesions, trocars can be placed in the left lower quadrant and suprapubically. For left colon lesions, trocars can be placed in the right lower quadrant and suprapubically. For transverse colon lesions, trocars can be placed on both sides in both the lower and upper quadrants. If available, micro-laparoscopic (3 mm) instruments are used.
- *Optional trocars*: A 5–12 mm port may be needed for a stapler if a colonoscopic-assisted laparoscopic wall excision is anticipated.
- *GelPort*: For CELS, a hand port is not necessary. However, if converting to a segmental or formal colectomy, then some may elect to place a GelPort™ for hand-assisted laparoscopy.

### Mobilization

- For laparoscopic-assisted colonoscopic polypectomy, the lesion is located by the endoscopist, and its position is confirmed by laparoscopic visualization with the use of transillumination and/or by endoscopic visualization during laparoscopic manipulation of the colon (Fig. 26.4). This maneuver can also expose areas that were not previously visualized because of mucosal folds or segmental kinks of the colon. The location of the polyp in relation to the peritoneum is important. Polyps that are located on the retroperitoneal side or mesenteric side require lateral mobilization of the colon for adequate exposure.
- If the polyp is in a difficult location (i.e., at a flexure or near the mesenteric border of the colon) and this area cannot be manipulated, the colon will need to be mobilized. This is done as in any laparoscopic procedure. We prefer to use an energy device along the line of Toldt and carried in the native planes. Once the colon is mobilized adequately, the polyp can then be manipulated.

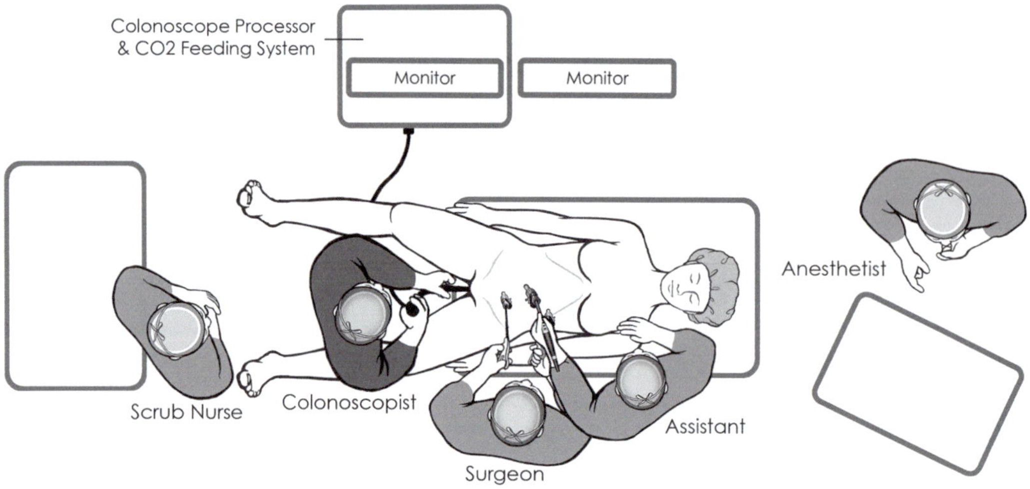


**Fig. 26.2** Patient positioning and room setup for a right-sided CELS procedure

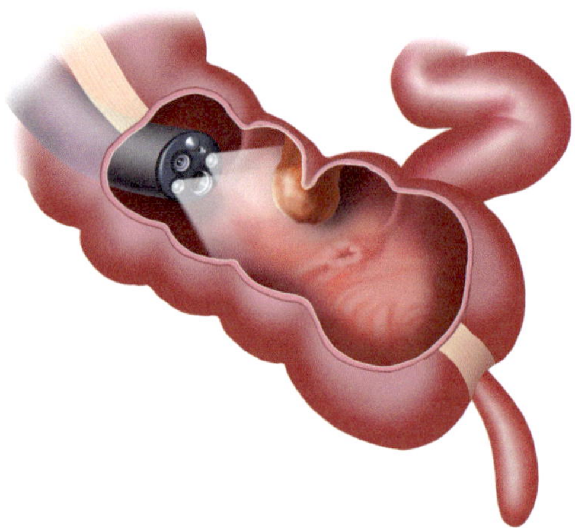

**Fig. 26.3** $CO_2$ colonoscopy to determine lesion location. *With permission from Yuko Tonohira*

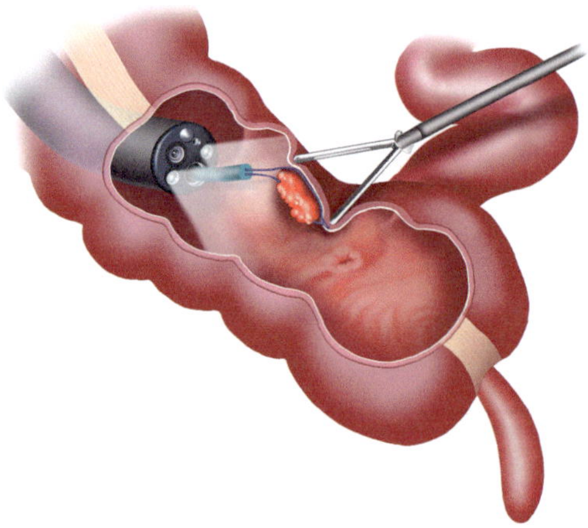

**Fig. 26.5** Endoscopic snare is placed around the polyp while the wall is invaginated laparoscopically. *With permission from Yuko Tonohira*

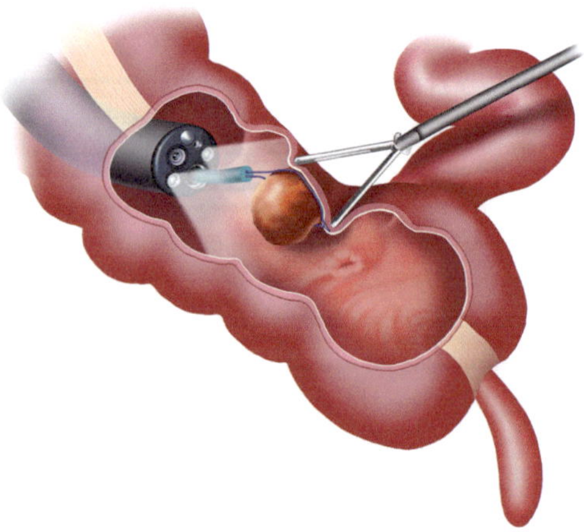

**Fig. 26.4** Laparoscopic manipulation of the bowel wall helps to put the polyp in ideal position for endoscopic removal. *With permission from Yuko Tonohira*

## Polypectomy

- As stated previously, the polyp is lifted with dilute indigo carmine solution. This aids in visualizing the polyp in comparison to the normal surrounding mucosa and also aids in seeing the location of the polyp laparoscopically. It also provides a "buffer" zone to facilitate endoscopic resection without causing a full-thickness injury.
- Polypectomy is performed using an electrosurgical snare. This can be done using a single attempt or in a piecemeal fashion. For polyps that are either flat or situated in tough location, laparoscopic manipulation of the polyp during snare polypectomy can facilitate delivery of the polyp into the snare (Fig. 26.5).
- During polypectomy, the serosal aspect of the colon should be monitored closely. If there is any subtle change to the area, this can be immediately recognized and then

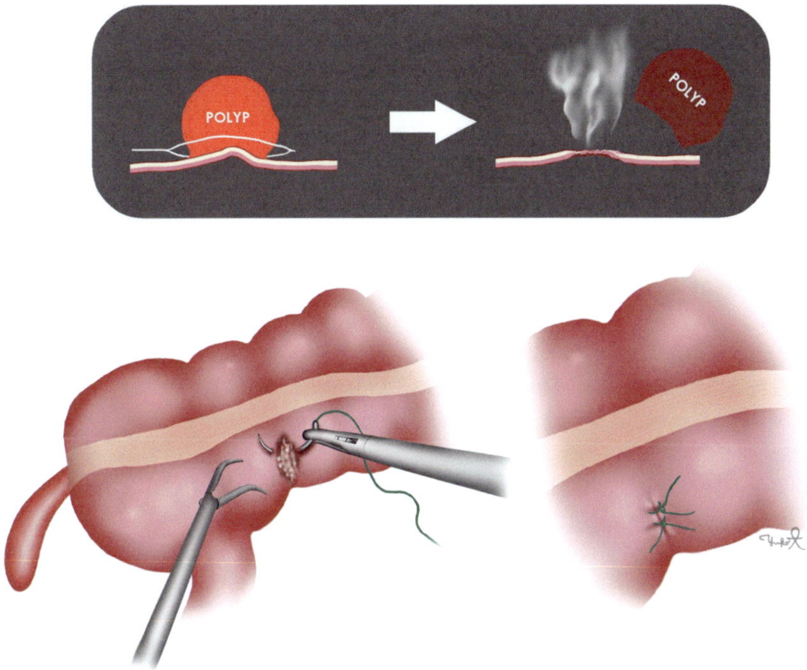


**Fig. 26.6** Laparoscopic closure of the bowel wall. *With permission from Yuko Tonohira*

oversewn if needed (Fig. 26.6). Typically, seromuscular sutures are placed if a full-thickness thermal injury or perforation is noted. If there is some evidence of blanching or deterioration of muscle layers, the area can also be reinforced to avoid the evolution of partial-thickness to full-thickness injuries in the postoperative period. The ability to laparoscopically repair potential damage allows for a more aggressive polypectomy.

## Colonoscopic-Assisted Laparoscopic Wall Excision

- For polyps that are located in the cecum where the wall of the colon is the thinnest, one may elect for a laparoscopic sleeve excision of the polyp.
- Colonoscopy is used to locate the lesion and monitor adequate surgical margins. It should be noted if polyps are located very close to the ileocecal valve in order to avoid injury to this structure. This can be monitored with the colonoscope.
- Sleeve resection is performed using a laparoscopic linear stapler through a 12 mm port (Fig. 26.7). Once the specimen is removed, it can be placed within an Endo Catch bag (Covidien, Norwalk, CT) and brought out through the 12 mm port site. The specimen can be opened in the operating room to make sure there is a clear margin.
- Oversewing of the staple line can be performed laparoscopically as needed.

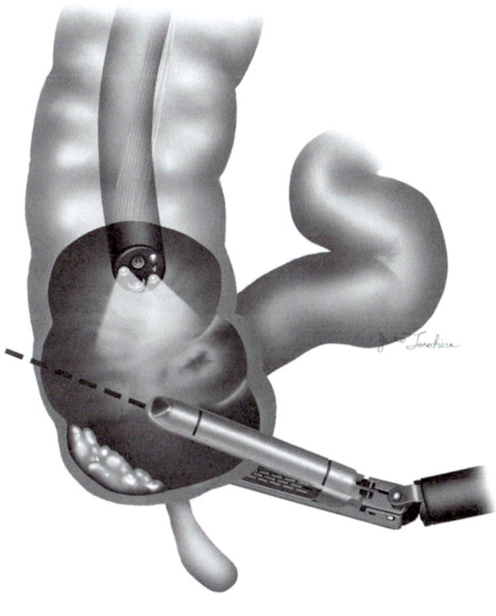

**Fig. 26.7** Sleeve resection of a polyp using CELS. *With permission from Yuko Tonohira*

## Leak Test

- A leak test using $CO_2$ insufflation with the colonoscope and immersion of the bowel segment under saline (using gravity to make the correct area dependent) should be performed.

### Polyp Retrieval

- For polyp retrieval, an endoscopic Roth net® (US Endoscopy, Mentor, OH) can be used if the polyp is resected en bloc. For polyps that are resected piecemeal, a trap can be added to the suction device, and the polyp can be suctioned through the scope.

## Postoperative Care

For patients that undergo standard snare polypectomy and there are no concerns intraoperatively, these patients may have a very short hospital stay and may even go home the same day as the procedure. Most groups report length of stay between 1 and 2 days, although other large studies report a mean length of stay of 4–8 days [9, 12, 16]. Patients that have a partial- or full-thickness injury or undergo colonoscopic-assisted laparoscopic wall excision should be monitored in the hospital for observation and to await return of bowel function. These patients should be admitted to the hospital and treated like any patient that has had a laparoscopic abdominal procedure. Patients are encouraged to ambulate early and frequently and use incentive spirometry to avoid postoperative morbidity. Venous thromboembolism (VTE) prophylaxis is used consisting of subcutaneous heparin and sequential compression devices. Diet is advanced as tolerated, and once patients have return of bowel function, intravenous fluids and pain medications are discontinued. Patients will usually follow up within 2 weeks after discharge for review of the final pathology and determination if additional treatment is needed.

## Complications

Intraoperative complications can be related to the endoscopic portion of the procedure or to laparoscopic port placement and mobilization.

In a large retrospective study, the risk of colonoscopic perforation for all comers was less than 1 % [18]. The benefit of the laparoscopic and endoscopic combined approach is that any full-thickness injury to the colon from electrocautery, barotrauma, or scope trauma can be immediately recognized and repaired. Franklin et al. reported a 10 % rate of serosal suture placement [16]. Our group reported a higher rate of 43 %. However, in all of these patients, there was no evidence of a full-thickness injury, but rather concern that the wall appeared to have a partial-thickness compromise that could easily be prepared at the time [9]. The other benefit of doing a concomitant colonoscopy is that a leak test can be performed to assess the site of injury and repair.

The risk of laparoscopic complications should be similar to any other laparoscopic abdominal procedure and potentially even less if no mobilization of the colon is required. There is risk of abdominal wall and intra-abdominal injury with port placement, bowel injury related to grasper trauma, or the use of an energy device and injury to surrounding viscera such as the bowel, the ureter, or the gonadal or iliac vessels.

For patients that undergo a successful CELS procedure, postoperative morbidity is low as reported in the literature. Franklin reported a 9 % postoperative complication rate, with all complications being minor and mostly consisting of ileus, atelectasis, and seroma [16]. Our group reported an overall rate of 4.2 %, with postoperative complications including urinary retention and wound hematoma [7].

## Outcomes

There are few large studies that report on the combined approach of laparoscopy and colonoscopy for polyp removal. The longest follow-up for these patients is a median of 65 months, which is reported by both our group and Franklin's group [7, 16]. Overall, the long-term outcome of patients undergoing CELS is excellent. For patients with benign polyps that are successfully resected with a CELS technique, there are variable recurrence rates in the literature. Our group reports a recurrence in five patients (10 %). Four of these patients underwent a repeat colonoscopic polypectomy, and one patient had a subsequent laparoscopic segmental colectomy, and all patients had benign pathologies [7]. Franklin's group reports no recurrences over a median follow-up of 65 months, but three patients were reoperated on for polyps in different locations [16].

There is concern that with patients that ultimately are diagnosed with a cancer on final pathology that there are potential risks associated with a potential perforated cancer. However, although follow-up is limited in patients that have had evidence of cancer on final pathology and have then gone on to have formal resection, there are no reports of tumor recurrence [16].

## Pearls and Pitfalls

In the preoperative workup of these patients with benign polyps, there should be awareness that there can be discrepancy in pathology. It is important to have pathology slides reviewed by pathologists at your own institution to make sure there is consensus. In addition, the colonoscopy report should be reviewed, as well as pictures of the polyp, to ensure that the polyp seems to be acceptable for CELS.

It is important to perform colonoscopy first in the operating room prior to laparoscopic port placement. Intermittently, the polyp, which may have previously been deemed unresectable by a referring gastroenterologist, may actually be amenable to traditional colonoscopic polypectomy alone.

This combined technique can be technically demanding, and the surgeon must be proficient in both laparoscopic and endoscopic techniques. For the first several cases, it is useful to have an assistant that is proficient in both of these techniques in order to be successful.

During the CELS procedure, it is important to try and recognize the signs of a potential malignancy. Many times, polyps that have been biopsied or previously had attempts at snaring may be scarred and difficult to lift with submucosal injection. These findings must be contrasted with findings of a possible cancerous polyp. These findings include central umbilication, ulceration, vascular pattern on narrow band imaging, and firmness. If these findings are present, options are to continue with CELS and perform an intraoperative frozen section or to proceed to formal colectomy. We do not feel that it is necessary to perform frozen section on all polyps resected as this can add to the operative time and cost of the case. In our experience, the rate of cancer on polyps that were thought to be benign was only 2 % (1/48). Therefore, frozen section should only be done on patients with suspicion of malignancy. In our experience, 12 patients underwent colectomy instead of CELS for suspected malignancy, and only 4 (33 %) of these patients actually had cancer.[7] Although this is a low sensitivity, this may reflect our overly cautious attempts to avoid performing CELS for potential malignancy.

## Conclusion

Combined endo-laparoscopic surgery (CELS) appears to be a safe and effective for the treatment of benign colon polyps and may help to avoid laparoscopic colectomy in most cases.

## References


1. Fujishiro M, Goto O, Kakushima N, Kodashima S, Muraki Y, Omata M. Endoscopic submucosal dissection of stomach neoplasms after unsuccessful endoscopic resection. Dig Liver Dis. 2007;39(6):566–71.
2. Zhou PH, Yao LQ, Qin XY. Endoscopic submucosal dissection for colorectal epithelial neoplasm. Surg Endosc. 2009;23(7):1546–51.
3. Franklin Jr ME, Diaz-E JA, Abrego D, Parra-Davila E, Glass JL. Laparoscopic-assisted colonoscopic polypectomy: the Texas Endosurgery Institute experience. Dis Colon Rectum. 2000;43(9):1246–9.
4. Beck DE, Karulf RE. Laparoscopic-assisted full-thickness endoscopic polypectomy. Dis Colon Rectum. 1993;36(7):693–5.
5. Guller U, Jain N, Hervey S, Purves H, Pietrobon R. Laparoscopic vs open colectomy: outcomes comparison based on large nationwide databases. Arch Surg. 2003;138(11):1179–86.
6. Ommer A, Limmer J, Mollenberg H, Peitgen K, Albrecht KH, Walz MK. Laparoscopic-assisted colonoscopic polypectomy—indications and results. Zentralbl Chir. 2003;128(3):195–8.
7. Lee SW, Garrett KA, Shin JH, Trencheva K, Sonoda T, Milsom JW. Dynamic article: long-term outcomes of patients undergoing combined endolaparoscopic surgery for benign colon polyps. Dis Colon Rectum. 2013;56(7):869–73.
8. Lee MK, Chen F, Esrailian E, et al. Combined endoscopic and laparoscopic surgery may be an alternative to bowel resection for the management of colon polyps not removable by standard colonoscopy. Surg Endosc. 2013;27(6):2082–6.
9. Yan J, Trencheva K, Lee SW, Sonoda T, Shukla P, Milsom JW. Treatment for right colon polyps not removable using standard colonoscopy: combined laparoscopic-colonoscopic approach. Dis Colon Rectum. 2011;54(6):753–8.
10. Wilhelm D, von Delius S, Weber L, et al. Combined laparoscopic-endoscopic resections of colorectal polyps: 10-year experience and follow-up. Surg Endosc. 2009;23(4):688–93.
11. Franklin Jr ME, Leyva-Alvizo A, Abrego-Medina D, et al. Laparoscopically monitored colonoscopic polypectomy: an established form of endoluminal therapy for colorectal polyps. Surg Endosc. 2007;21(9):1650–3.
12. Winter H, Lang RA, Spelsberg FW, Jauch KW, Huttl TP. Laparoscopic colonoscopic rendezvous procedures for the treatment of polyps and early stage carcinomas of the colon. Int J Colorectal Dis. 2007;22(11):1377–81.
13. Feussner H, Wilhelm D, Dotzel V, Papagoras D, Frimberger E. Combined endoluminal and endocavitary approaches to colonic lesions. Surg Technol Int. 2003;11:97–101.
14. Mal F, Perniceni T, Levard H, Boudet MJ, Levy P, Gayet B. Colonic polyps considered unresectable by endoscopy. removal by combinations of laparoscopy and endoscopy in 65 patients. Gastroenterol Clin Biol. 1998;22(4):425–30.
15. Le Picard P, Vacher B, Pouliquen X. Laparoscopy-assisted colonic polypectomy or how to be helped by laparoscopy to prevent colectomy in benign colonic polyps considered to be unresectable by colonoscopy. Ann Chir. 1997;51(9):986–9.
16. Franklin Jr ME, Portillo G. Laparoscopic monitored colonoscopic polypectomy: long-term follow-up. World J Surg. 2009;33(6):1306–9.
17. Nakajima K, Lee SW, Sonoda T, Milsom JW. Intraoperative carbon dioxide colonoscopy: a safe insufflation alternative for locating colonic lesions during laparoscopic surgery. Surg Endosc. 2005;19(3):321–5.
18. Hamdani U, Naeem R, Haider F, et al. Risk factors for colonoscopic perforation: a population-based study of 80118 cases. World J Gastroenterol. 2013;19(23):3596–601.

# Part V

# Special Situations

# 27 Emergent Laparoscopic Colorectal Surgery

Rodrigo Pedraza and Eric M. Haas

**Key Points**

- Laparoscopic colorectal surgery is both safe and feasible in many emergent cases. Proper patient selection is crucial to for optimal outcomes.
- Port placement is challenging, as the left upper quadrant is typically used for access however, if there is any question of safety, the right upper quadrant may be used as the first point of access, taking care to avoid liver injury.
- Optical trocars are preferred to gain abdominal access.
- For colonoscopic perforations, laparoscopic procedures range from primary single-layer repair to segmental resection—with or without ostomy creation.
- For perforated diverticulitis, emergent interventions range from laparoscopic lavage to resection with diversion, depending on the case.
- Small bowel obstruction are ideal emergent laparoscopic cases, since the majority require only a lysis of adhesions with no bowel resection.
- Managing malignant obstructions laparoscopically, can be fraught with major morbidity and intraoperative complications intervention is often limited to proximal diversion and distal decompression.

**Electronic supplementary material:** Supplementary material is available in the online version of this chapter at 10.1007/978-1-4939-1581-1_27. Videos can also be accessed at http://www.springerimages.com/videos/978-1-4939-1580-4.

R. Pedraza, M.D. • E.M. Haas, M.D., F.A.C.S., F.A.S.C.R.S. (✉)
Division of Minimally Invasive Colon and Rectal Surgery,
Department of Surgery, The University of Texas Medical School
at Houston, 7900 Fannin Street, Suite 2700,
Houston, TX 77030, USA
e-mail: ehaas@houstoncolon.com

## Introduction

Over the past two decades, laparoscopic colorectal surgery has gained acceptance and rates of adoption are increasing with proven clinical advantages. Recent reports demonstrate nearly 45 % of elective colectomies are performed laparoscopically [1–3]; however, emergent laparoscopic colorectal surgery is less common. Current use in the emergent setting is be than 10 %, reflecting the complexity and challenges even in expert hands.

The ability to use laparoscopy for colorectal emergencies depends on both patient and surgeon factors. The most common utilizations include acute diverticulitis and malignant obstruction. In addition, emergent laparoscopy for colonoscopic perforations has also been advocated [4]. However, each case is individualized to determine the safety, risk, and benefits for laparoscopy compared with open laparotomy. The ultimate success lies in proper patient selection.

In this chapter, we address the trends in utilization, indications, technical considerations, and pitfalls of emergent laparoscopic colorectal resection. The descriptions are based on generalities in the urgent setting; specific presentations may require alternative approaches.

## Advantages and Disadvantages of Emergent Laparoscopic Colorectal Surgery

The principles of laparoscopic colorectal surgery can be employed in the emergency setting. The absolute contraindications for laparoscopy include an unstable patient who cannot tolerate pneumoperitoneum, inability to safely access the abdomen, and insufficient laparoscopic experience.

Despite its challenges, laparoscopic colorectal surgery has many advantages in the emergent context. With initial laparoscopic intervention, the surgeon is able to thoroughly evaluate the peritoneal cavity and establish the most appropriate intervention without committing the patient to a large

H.M. Ross et al. (eds.), *Minimally Invasive Approaches to Colon and Rectal Disease: Technique and Best Practices*,
DOI 10.1007/978-1-4939-1581-1_27, 

incision. Often the pathology can be addressed maintaining a laparoscopic approach. Even if the condition requires an open incision, the laparoscopic exploration affords accurate identification of the pathology, leading to a better localization, smaller incisions, less subsequent pain, less postoperative complications, and faster recovery. In some cases, the benefits of a minimally invasive approach can be salvaged when conversion is required by utilizing hand-assisted laparoscopic surgery.

In the emergent setting, avoiding open laparotomy has many advantages. First, large incisions may be difficult to close, with a risk of abdominal compartment syndrome. The small incision size also has advantages in this patient population, where immunosuppression, sepsis, or shock are common and can jeopardizing healing and wound integrity. Laparoscopy lowers the risk of wound complications (e.g., dehiscence, evisceration, and infection), q major source of postoperative morbidity and mortality. Moreover, wound complications may result in hernia formation, which ultimately require further surgery. Consequently, wound complications result in significant increases in hospital resource utilization and cost.

Despite the advantages of laparoscopic emergent colorectal intervention, there are several limitations. Safe abdominal entry may be compromised, risking injury to bowel, solid organs, and vascular structures. This may turn an already difficult scenario into a disastrous one. We recommend extensive experience with various laparoscopic entry techniques, especially direct visualization with optical trocars, such as with the OptiView® (Ethicon Endo-Surgery, Cincinnati, OH) and Visiport™ Plus (Covidien, Mansfield, MA, USA).

Another important consideration is the hemodynamic instability that can result from decreased venous return and increased peripheral vascular resistance after establishing pneumoperitoneum. The surgeon and anesthesiologist must communicate about the patient's condition; release of pneumoperitoneum facilitates prompt recovery of hemodynamic parameters and may allow finishing with through a the minimally invasive approach.

Additional factors hampering the utilization of laparoscopy in emergent colorectal surgery include the relative inability to place the patient in extreme positions as well as the lack of available instrumentation and trained staff during non-elective procedure times.

## Approach and Abdominal Entry

Consideration to the minimally invasive technique to gain safe entry is crucial. Emergency patients often present with extreme abdominal distension and rigid abdomens, and caution must be taken during entry. Such presentations may deter from considering laparoscopic intervention; however, after anesthesia induction and ensuing relaxation of the abdominal wall muscles, laparoscopic approach may be very reasonable. Once abdominal entry is accomplished, the placement of the remaining laparoscopic ports may remain challenging, since in severe inflammatory cases, the omentum is friable and tends to adhere to the peritoneum (Video 27.1). We typically utilize either conventional multiport laparoscopy or hand-assisted laparoscopic surgery. The abdominal entry is commonly safely achieved through a port placed in the left upper quadrant along the costal margin (Fig. 27.1). Alternatively, when access to the left upper quadrant is unsafe, access through the right upper quadrant may be accomplished inferior to the costal margin to avoid liver injury. We favor direct visualization with an optical trocar for abdominal entry, as it provides a safer approach when compared with blind access. This approach is also advantageous for patients with prior abdominal surgery or when the source or extent of pathology is unknown. An alternative is hand-assisted or single-incision laparoscopic surgery, though the abdominal laparotomy entry may still be difficult. These are most appropriate when it is safer to enter the abdomen through a direct *mini-laparotomy* incision.

## Indications

### Colorectal Perforation

#### Acute Colonoscopic Perforation

Laparoscopic intervention can be a suitable approach for both acute and delayed colonoscopic perforations. The procedure depends on the degree and cause of perforation, timing following the event, degree of peritoneal contamination, and overall clinical condition of the patient. Nearly all cases can be managed laparoscopically, whether primarily repairing the perforation or resecting with or without ostomy creation.

##### Procedure Steps

- Abdominal entry: left upper quadrant port placement under direct visualization.
- Exploration: the abdominal and pelvic cavities are explored to assess the location, extent of injury, and presence of fluid or fecal contamination. If fecal contamination is encountered, conversion to hand-assisted laparoscopic surgery or laparotomy for lavage, bowel resection, and fecal diversion is recommended. Fecal washout cannot often be adequately performed with pure laparoscopic techniques. However, if minimal contamination is recognized, the bowel injury can often be primarily repaired. The entirety of the large bowel is examined to identify the perforation. Intraoperative colonoscopic assistance utilizing carbon dioxide may be required to aid visualization of the perforation. Once identified, proximal bowel clamping is performed to avoid further contamination.

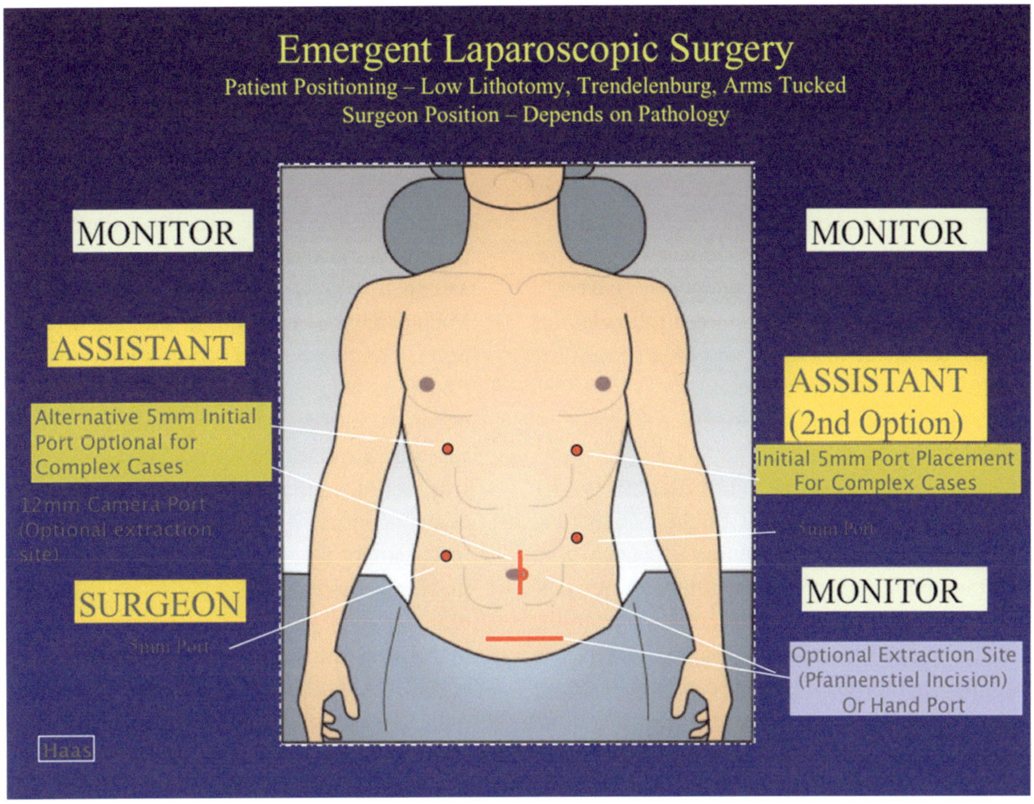


**Fig. 27.1** Port placement alternatives for emergent colorectal surgery

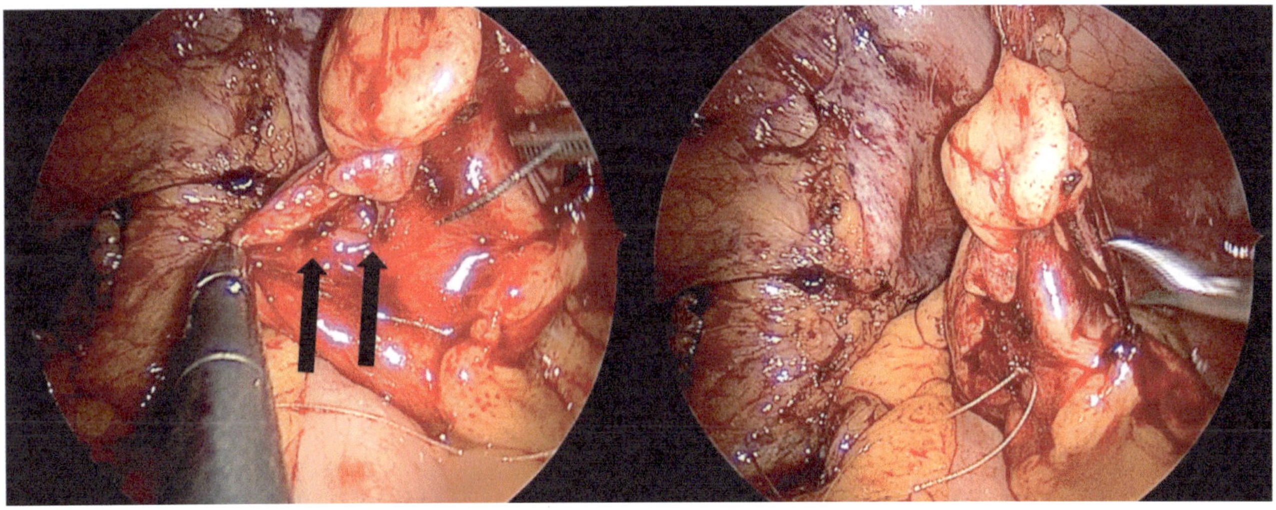

**Fig. 27.2** Intraoperative view of a colonic perforation following colonoscopy (*arrows*). The perforation was successfully repaired with single-layer primary colorrhaphy

- Laparoscopic management alternatives:
  (a) Laparoscopic colorrhaphy (Video 27.2): the perforation borders are defined and debrided if devitalized tissue is encountered. The repair is achieved with a one-layer colorrhaphy with absorbable suture (Fig. 27.2). The use of multiple layer colorrhaphy may potentially result in lumen narrowing, especially in the sigmoid colon. Following the repair, an air insufflation test and direct intraluminal visualization of the perforation site should be performed to confirm the integrity of the repair. Injuries extending into the mesentery may be more challenging to repair, and care must be taken to identify the entire extent of the perforation. The borders of the mesentery, which often bleed, may obscure the view and lead to failure to recognize and address the entire extent of the perforation.

(b) Segmental resection: after visualizing the perforation, if primary repair is not appropriate, laparoscopic segmental colectomy may be performed with or without ostomy creation. The same principles of laparoscopy in the elective setting are followed and often a medial-to-lateral approach is favored to avoid the inflamed bowel with associated adhesions and friable tissue.

(c) Bowel diversion: in extreme cases, proximal diversion with colonic lavage may be a temporary measure. Concomitant diversion is also considered following (a) or (b) above, under the discretion and judgment of the surgeon at the time of the operation.

## Acute Perforated Diverticulitis

The management of acute perforated diverticulitis varies depending on the clinical presentation of the patient and must be approached on an individual basis. Those who require emergent intervention typically present with free perforation, with an intra-abdominal abscess and/or peritonitis. Laparoscopic surgery in this setting can be both diagnostic and therapeutic. The therapeutic measures can include drainage of abscesses, lavage, primary closure of perforation, resection, and/or diversion. Although, it has been generally agreed that the presence of fecal peritonitis requires an open lavage, we have been successful using hand-assisted technique to effectively evacuate the contamination while maintaining a minimally invasive platform.

### Procedure Steps

- Abdominal entry: left upper quadrant optical trocar port placement under direct visualization.
- Abdominopelvic exploration: often, the omentum is inflamed and adhered to the peritoneal lining and pelvis requiring mobilization to explore the abdomen. The peritoneal cavity is then thoroughly examined to evaluate the nature of the contamination. For patients with Hinchey 3 (purulent peritonitis), we perform laparoscopic lavage with or without over-sewing the bowel wall with placement of drains through the port sites. It is important to evaluate for inter-loop abscesses, which may be a case for treatment failure if not identified and adequately drained during the procedure. It is also important to locate the perforation site itself, as an occult abscess may be present at or adjacent to this area, which is often shielded by inflamed tissue (Video 27.3). For those presenting with Hinchey 4 (fecal peritonitis), we typically perform hand-assisted laparoscopic technique, which allows evacuation of the fecal content as well as sigmoid resection with colostomy. A 5–7 cm umbilical or Pfannenstiel incision can be used to place the hand assist device. However, if this technique does not afford complete evacuations of the fecal contents, an open laparotomy is required.
- Lavage: it is necessary to lavage all four quadrants including perihepatic, perisplenic, right and left gutters, and pelvis (Video 27.3). Often occult fluid collections are identified and attended to in this process. Although no standard volume of irrigation has been reported, we recommend lavage until the fluid return is clear. The laparoscopic lavage is an excellent device to episode jet irrigation and allows litters of heated fluid to be utilized in an expeditious fashion.
- Management of perforation site: the diverticular perforation is typically walled off; however, gentle teasing of the tissues around the perforation should be performed, as occult abscesses may lie around the perforation. In the case that the diseased sigmoid is densely adhered, aggressive mobilization should be avoided, since this may result in an uncontained perforation. If perforation site is visualized, some advocate over-sewing the perforation or placing a tissue patch with adjacent epiploica or omentum. There is, however, no consensus and these various maneuvers all warrant consideration on an individual basis. The fallback "conservative" approach, however, typically involves resection of the diseased segment.
- Bowel diversion: if diversion is considered, laparoscopic loop ileostomy or colostomy may be performed depending on the clinical presentation of the patient. The laparoscopic technique is accomplished in a conventional fashion (Chap. 15). In either case, if diversion is performed without bowel resection, on-table lavage of the distal segment should be performed to clear the intraluminal fecal content.
- Laparoscopic resection: in some cases segmental colectomy may be warranted during the emergent presentation. In such cases, a laparoscopic sigmoid colectomy is performed utilizing a medial-to-lateral approach (Chap. 6/Chap. 7) to afford early identification and preservation of the critical vascular structures and the left ureter. Placement of ureteral stents and hand-assisted techniques should all be entertained in this scenario.

## Postoperative Anastomotic Perforation

Anastomotic perforation may manifest with peri-anastomotic abscess and purulent or fecal peritonitis. An isolated abscess can often be managed with image-guided drainage, whereas peritonitis or the presence of multiple abscesses may require laparoscopic lavage and further interventions. Although such perforations are typically approached with open surgery, laparoscopic reoperation is a safe and feasible alternative for those with technical expertise [5].

### Procedure Steps

- Abdominal entry: left upper quadrant port placement under direct visualization.
- Exploration: as with any type of perforation, the entirety of the peritoneal cavity is explored. It is common to

experience a hostile intra-abdominal environment with inflamed and adhered omentum and mesentery.

- Lavage: thorough peritoneal washout is performed to clear out the contamination.
- Anastomotic takedown and diversion: anastomotic resection should be contemplated in all cases with proximal diversion. In cases in which the anastomosis is not accessible for resection—such as those deep in the pelvis—diversion alone must be accompanied with on-table lavage.

## Bowel Obstruction

### Postoperative Small Bowel Obstruction

Small bowel obstruction is the ideal scenario for laparoscopic intervention. Since the majority of cases do not require bowel resection, a sizable incision of any length is usually not required. The general principles of management of bowel obstruction are followed including gastrointestinal decompression and fluid/electrolyte replacement before operative intervention. Patients with small bowel obstruction may seem severely distended on clinical exam, causing many surgeons to abort the laparoscopic approach; however, upon induction of anesthesia, the distention diminishes significantly, allowing safe laparoscopic entry.

#### Procedure Steps (Video 27.4)

- Abdominal entry: left upper quadrant access with an optical trocar. If the patient has prior scars in this region, right upper quadrant can be used. Once entered, a second trocar is placed at any location in which the laparoscopic visualization permits. Often, placement of the second trocar is the most difficult. Once 2 trocars are placed, lysis of adhesions can be initiated allowing for multiple ports. If one cannot safely gain entry in this fashion, a hand port can be placed through a midline infraumbilical incision. Hand-assisted laparoscopic surgery, however, is less useful in small bowel obstruction due to the loss of abdominal domain from the distended bowel.
- Exploration: Abdominal and pelvic exploration is performed to identify the etiology of the obstruction.
- Resection: if the case warrants segmental resection, such as in severe strangulation with bowel infarction, the affected segment is mobilized and extracorporealized through a wound protector (Fig. 27.3). Resection and primary anastomosis can then readily be achieved extracorporeally.

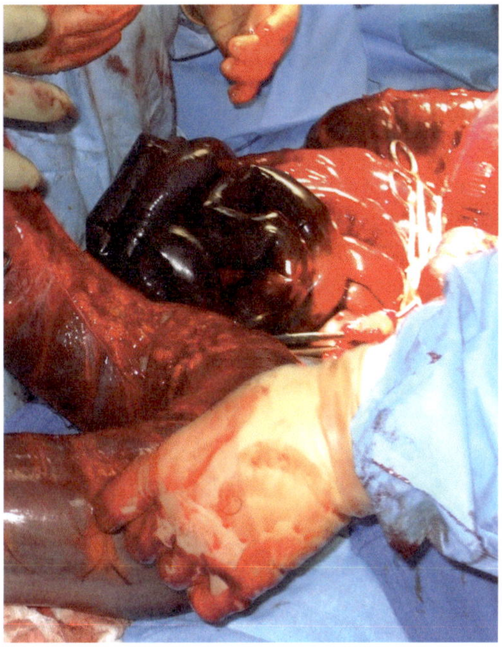

**Fig. 27.3** Gangrenous bowel from bowel obstruction

### Malignant Obstruction

Malignant obstruction encountered in the emergent setting typically involves the left colon, and the disease is usually locally advanced. It is also commonly associated with massively dilated and fragile proximal colonic dilation. In this setting, primary resection can be fraught with major morbidity and intraoperative complications. Therefore, attempts at nonoperative intervention, such as intraluminal stenting for decompression should be strongly considered before committing to surgical intervention. Laparoscopic intervention is often limited to creation of proximal diversion to decompress the obstruction and allow resuscitation and recovery. In addition, this will allow the size mismatch to resolve that frequently would prevent creation of an anastomosis in the acute setting. Therefore, distal decompression is required with either loop colostomy or end colostomy with mucus fistula.

#### Procedure Steps

- Abdominal entry: laparoscopic abdominal entry is challenging in patients with bowel obstruction secondary to abdominal distention, with the risk for perforation especially high during laparoscopic access. For multiport approach, left or right upper quadrant access is preferred, depending on the location of the disease. For cases requiring ostomy alone, a single-incision laparoscopic surgery with the single-access port placed at the proposed ostomy site is another option. In cases in which resection is contemplated, hand-assisted laparoscopic surgery is the preferred approach in our institution. This approach affords safe abdominal entry and domain allowing for adherence to the principles of an oncologic resection. The incision depends on the location of the tumor: for right-sided and mid transverse colon tumors, a midline *mini-laparotomy* incision is made, whereas for left-sided tumors, a Pfannenstiel incision is preferred.

- Bowel decompression: in cases in which there is severe distention and an ostomy is necessary, one can extracorporealize the bowel, perform an enterotomy for decompression, and utilize this segment for further ostomy creation. Once decompressed, it is often possible to perform the resection while maintaining a minimally invasive platform, typically utilizing hand-assisted laparoscopic surgery.
- Segmental resection: a conventional laparoscopic technique for segmental resection in a medial-to-lateral fashion with oncologic principles is performed (Chaps. 4–7). Even if laparotomy is required, we favor performing some portions of the procedure (e.g., splenic and hepatic flexure takedown) laparoscopically to minimize the incision length.

## Pearls and Pitfalls

- Know your limitations and choose your patients wisely. Wasting time with a minimally invasive approach in a septic patient may result in more risk and worse outcomes than open laparotomy.
- Mobilization of a perforated diverticulum may identify occult abscesses, but avoid the urge to mobilize densely adhered bowel, as this may result in additional bowel injury and the need for resection.
- Gravity is your friend to help with visualization and keeping the small bowel out of the way. However, as you may encounter inflamed bowel, dilated bowel, or intra-abdominal stool or purulence), have additional sponges on hand to keep the field of view "clean."
- The omentum is often adherent and restricts visibility; the adhesions must be released, especially those tethering the omentum to the pelvic structures. The omentum is mobilized caudally and flipped over the transverse colon for optimal exposure.
- The laparoscopic irrigator is essential, as it provides jet irrigation in an expeditious fashion. Irrigation is required in the perisplenic and perihepatic areas as well as the gutters and pelvis to help minimize risk of postoperative abscesses.

## References

1. Haas EM PR, Ragupathi M, Carman R, Nieto J. Is laparoscopic colectomy a clinically and economically favorable approach in the modern health care environment: results from a cohort of 56,000 patients. Abstract S12 The American Society of Colon and Rectal Surgeons annual meeting; 2013.
2. Delaney CP, Chang E, Senagore AJ, Broder M. Clinical outcomes and resource utilization associated with laparoscopic and open colectomy using a large national database. Ann Surg. 2008;247:819–24.
3. Fox J, Gross CP, Longo W, Reddy V. Laparoscopic colectomy for the treatment of cancer has been widely adopted in the United States. Dis Colon Rectum. 2012;55:501–8.
4. Haas EM, Pedraza R, Ragupathi M, Mahmood A, Bartley PT. Laparoscopic primary colorrhaphy for acute iatrogenic perforations during colonoscopy. Minim Invasive Surg. 2013;2013:823506.
5. Haas EM PR, Faraj C, Ragupathi M, Pickron TB. Reoperative minimally invasive surgery for the management of colorectal surgical complications. Abstract Society of American Gastrointestinal and Endoscopic Surgeons; 2013.

# Laparoscopy in the Elderly Patient

28

Joshua I.S. Bleier and Brian R. Kann

**Key Points**

- Assessment of the elderly patient is based on physiologic age rather than chronologic age.
- Preoperative assessment is based on a careful history and physical examination aimed at determination of high-risk comorbidities.
- Preoperative testing is based on functional assessment and presence of known comorbidities.
- Laparoscopic colectomy in the elderly is increasing commensurate with the overall increase in laparoscopic colorectal surgery across all ages.
- Laparoscopic colectomy in the elderly seems to yield similar benefits when using an enhanced recovery protocol as seen in younger patients.
- Pneumoperitoneum induces myriad physiologic changes that may have more significant effects in the elderly with comorbid conditions.

## Introduction

Aging is, of course, defined chronologically; however, subjectively, physiologically, and medically, it is more often a function of "how old you feel."

To a large degree, management of colorectal issues, whether benign or malignant, is pathology driven. In most instances, colon cancers that are resectable should be resected, metastatic disease is an indication for adjuvant therapy, multiple recurrent attacks of diverticulitis indicate resection, and low rectal cancers that don't involve the sphincters may be treated by sphincter-sparing operations, including colo-anal anastomoses. However, the wise surgeon knows that indications are only part of the decision process. Pathology alone may provide the *indication* for surgery, but not necessarily the *decision* for it. Patient factors must be taken into consideration. Every assessment of the potential surgical patient takes into account fitness for surgery, as well as the assessment of being able to tolerate the outcome. But where does age play into this equation? Age is a nonspecific factor that may provide predictive information about how well a patient will tolerate a procedure. In general, the older the patient, the more comorbidities, the higher the risk for healing problems, the worse the baseline continence and sphincter function, and the higher the risk for concomitant cardiovascular disease. Chronologic age is indisputable, but physiologic age is variable. Consider the unfortunate condition of progeria, in which children succumb to the physiologic maladies of advanced age such as heart attack, stroke, and atherosclerotic disease—and rarely live past the age of 13—to the 100-year-old man who completed a marathon in Toronto in 2011! The concept of physiologic age truly determines the assessment of the elderly patient. Determination of the physiologic age of the patient is an amalgam of all of the physiologic parameters that will be affected by the operation and its recovery. Prior dogma dictating age as a relative contraindication to surgery has been replaced by determination of fitness. Advances in perioperative management have demonstrated that mere chronologic age does not directly determine fitness and the ability to recover from surgery. Rather, it merely informs us of the increased possible risks, while overall fitness for intervention is determined by factors that are projected to be affected by the surgery. The use of laparoscopic surgery has further redefined risks and must be incorporated into our decision-making processes. This chapter will deal with these issues and the factors that affect them.

J.I.S. Bleier, M.D., F.A.C.S., F.A.S.C.R.S. (✉)
Division of Colon and Rectal Surgery, Pennsylvania Hospital, University of Pennsylvania, 800 Walnut St. 20th Floor, Philadelphia, PA 19106, USA
e-mail: joshua.bleier@uphs.upenn.edu

B.R. Kann, M.D., F.A.C.S., F.A.S.C.R.S.
Division of Colon and Rectal Surgery, Pennsylvania Hospital, University of Pennsylvania, 51 N. 39th St Suite W-266, Philadelphia, PA 19104, USA
e-mail: brian.kann@uphs.upenn.edu

H.M. Ross et al. (eds.), *Minimally Invasive Approaches to Colon and Rectal Disease: Technique and Best Practices*, DOI 10.1007/978-1-4939-1581-1_28, © Springer Science+Business Media New York 2015

## Evaluation for Surgery

### Determination of Cardiovascular and Physiologic Risk Stratification

The World Health Organization has broadly defined "elderly" as any patient who is eligible for pension benefits. However, given the varied standards across the world, anyone over the age of 50 may be loosely defined as "elderly." In the USA, this definition is likely inappropriate, as the retirement age is most commonly 65, and health risks do not substantially increase in the sixth decade of life. Nevertheless, most screening standards do change in the age group over 50. After 50 it is recommended that all patients receive a preoperative chest X-ray and preoperative lab work. There is no mandatory age indicating preoperative cardiovascular testing, rather this decision is the responsibility of the operating surgeon.

### Preoperative Risk Assessment

Appropriate preoperative risk assessment is the surgeon's responsibility when planning for surgery of any kind. This is more important in the elderly patient due to the increased incidence of significant comorbidities associated with age. The most recent American Heart Association guidelines [1] delineate the recommended approach to risk stratification. Not surprisingly, an appropriate history and physical examination provides most of the information that will be needed to identify risk factors.

The initial decision process should be aimed at identifying any cardiac condition that would increase the risk of an adverse cardiac event in the perioperative period. In general, any patient with active cardiac disease such as unstable coronary syndrome, decompensated or worsening CHF, significant arrhythmia, or significant valvular disease should receive cardiology evaluation and baseline cardiac testing (Table 28.1).

In the absence of serious comorbidities, a rough assessment of exercise tolerance may be all that is needed to determine if further testing is needed (Table 28.2). Age as a sole criterion defines only the need for EKG and chest X-ray for patients over 50 years. Advanced age alone is *not* an indication for further cardiac testing. In patients with good exercise tolerance (>4 METS) [2], further testing for any elective procedure is usually unnecessary. Of note, elective abdominal operations are considered intermediate-risk operations.

Other significant clinical risk factors include a history of ischemic heart disease, compensated or prior CHF, diabetes mellitus, renal insufficiency, and cerebrovascular disease, which all represent comorbidities that may require preoperative evaluation.

**Table 28.1** Active cardiac conditions for which the patient should undergo evaluation and treatment before non-cardiac surgery

| Condition | Examples |
|---|---|
| Unstable coronary syndromes | Unstable or severe angina (CCS class III or IV)[a] |
| | Recent MI[b] |
| Decompensated heart failure (NYHA functional class IV, worsening or new-onset HF) | |
| Significant arrhythmias | High-grade AV block |
| | Mobitz II AV block |
| | Third-degree AV block |
| | Symptomatic ventricular arrhythmias |
| | Supraventricular arrhythmias (including atrial fibrillation) with uncontrolled ventricular rate (HR > 100 bpm at rest) |
| | Symptomatic bradycardia |
| | Newly recognized ventricular tachycardia |
| Severe valvular disease | Severe aortic stenosis (mean pressure gradient greater than 40 mmHg, aortic valve area <1.0 cm$^2$, or symptomatic) |
| | Symptomatic mitral stenosis (progressive dyspnea on exertion, exertional presyncope, or HF) |

*CCS* Canadian Cardiovascular Society, *HF* heart failure, *HR* heart rate, *MI* myocardial infarction, *NYHA* New York Heart Association

[a]May include stable angina in patients who are unusually sedentary

[b]The American College of Cardiology National Database Library defines recent MI as more than 7 days but less than or equal to 1 month (within 30 days)

Adapted from Fleisher LA, Beckman JA, Brown KA, Calkins H, Chaikof EL, Fleischmann KE, et al. ACC/AHA 2007 Guidelines on Perioperative Cardiovascular Evaluation and Care for Noncardiac Surgery: Executive Summary: A Report of the American College of Cardiology/American Heart Association Task Force on Practice Guidelines (Writing Committee to Revise the 2002 Guidelines on Perioperative Cardiovascular Evaluation for Noncardiac Surgery) Developed in Collaboration With the American Society of Echocardiography, American Society of Nuclear Cardiology, Heart Rhythm Society, Society of Cardiovascular Anesthesiologists, Society for Cardiovascular Angiography and Interventions, Society for Vascular Medicine and Biology, and Society for Vascular Surgery. J Am Coll Cardiol 2007 Oct 23;50(17):1707–1732. [1] With permission

Exercise tolerance is an excellent overall assessment of fitness, and in the setting of good exercise tolerance, even with multiple clinical risk factors described above, often intermediate-risk surgery can be undertaken with acceptable risk. Perioperative heart rate control with beta-blockade should be considered mandatory in anyone with any of the above risk factors since this has been shown to reduce cardiac morbidity and mortality [3].

When a patient has any of these other significant comorbidities, a specific workup may be indicated as per the AHA guidelines [2]:

*Pulmonary Disease*. The presence of restrictive or obstructive pulmonary disease significantly increases the risk of

**Table 28.2** Estimated energy requirements for various activities

| Metabolic equivalent (MET) | Activity |
|---|---|
| 1 MET | Eat, dress, use the toilet |
| | Walk indoors around the house |
| | Walk a block or 2 on level ground at 2–3 mph? |
| 4 MET | Do light housework (dusting, washing dishes) |
| | Climb a flight of stairs or walk up a hill? |
| | Walk on level ground at 4 mph? |
| | Run a short distance |
| | Do heavy housework (scrubbing floors, lifting/moving furniture) |
| | Participate in moderate recreational activities (golf, bowling, dancing, double tennis, baseball or football catch) |
| >10 METS | Participate in strenuous sports (swimming, single tennis, football, basketball, skiing) |

Adapted from Fleisher LA, Beckman JA, Brown KA, Calkins H, Chaikof EL, Fleischmann KE, et al. ACC/AHA 2007 Guidelines on Perioperative Cardiovascular Evaluation and Care for Noncardiac Surgery: Executive Summary: A Report of the American College of Cardiology/American Heart Association Task Force on Practice Guidelines (Writing Committee to Revise the 2002 Guidelines on Perioperative Cardiovascular Evaluation for Noncardiac Surgery) Developed in Collaboration With the American Society of Echocardiography, American Society of Nuclear Cardiology, Heart Rhythm Society, Society of Cardiovascular Anesthesiologists, Society for Cardiovascular Angiography and Interventions, Society for Vascular Medicine and Biology, and Society for Vascular Surgery. J Am Coll Cardiol 2007 Oct 23;50(17):1707–1732. [1] With permission

perioperative pulmonary complications. In these cases, preoperative pulmonary testing to determine volume and diffusion capacity, response to bronchodilators, and a baseline blood gas will help guide postoperative therapy.

*Diabetes Mellitus*. This is the most common metabolic disease associated with advanced age and is often associated with coronary disease. The presence of insulin-dependent DM increases the risk of perioperative myocardial ischemia and heart failure. Careful attention to glucose management with insulin infusions and tight glycemic control has been found to significantly reduce postoperative wound infection in CABG pts, and this paradigm can be applied to major abdominal surgery.

*Renal Failure*. Renal failure is associated with an increased risk of perioperative cardiac morbidity. In addition, preoperative levels of creatinine >2 mg/dl are associated with an increased risk of postoperative renal failure, cardiac complications, and increased mortality.

*Hematologic Disorders*. Preoperative anemia can impose cardiac stress, worsen ischemia, and exacerbate preexisting CHF. In one study looking at patients undergoing prostate and major vascular surgery, a hematocrit <28 % was associated with an increased risk of perioperative ischemia and postoperative complications.

## Laparoscopy in the Elderly: What Are the Outcomes?

As improvements in health care and advances in medicine have led to an aging population, colorectal surgeons are now required to evaluate and operate on increasingly older patients. The use of a laparoscopic approach would seem to be an attractive alternative to traditional open approaches in this patient population in whom minimizing postoperative complications and enhancing postoperative recovery are likely to have significant benefit. A population-based study of laparoscopic colorectal cancer surgery in the United Kingdom from 2006 to 2008 showed that the use of laparoscopy for colorectal procedures increased from 10.0 % in 2006 to 28.4 % in 2008. Of 58,135 resections, 54.6 % were inpatients greater than 70 years of age. Age did not have an effect on whether laparoscopy was attempted; 18.5 % of resections in patients older than 70 years were performed laparoscopically, which was similar to the overall rate of 18.8 % in all patients [4].

### Early Studies

Early in the experience with laparoscopic colorectal surgery, initial reports sought to establish safety, in terms of equivalency or improved morbidity and mortality, compared with open procedures. In 1995, Peters and Fleshman published the results of a prospective study describing the outcomes of minimally invasive colectomy attempted in 103 patients greater than 65 years old, 78.6 % of which were able to be completed laparoscopically. Complication rates were no different in patients who underwent successful laparoscopic resection compared with those who required conversion to laparotomy. The length of stay was significantly lower in patients who underwent successful minimally invasive colectomy (5.3 vs. 8.1 days, $p<0.001$) [5].

In 1996, Reissman and Wexner published the results of a study looking at outcome in "older" patients, which they defined as age greater than 60 years. Thirty-six "older" patients (mean age 73) undergoing laparoscopic or laparoscopic-assisted colorectal procedures were compared with 36 younger patients (mean age 44). No differences were seen in rates of complications (11 % vs. 14 %), conversion (8 % vs. 11 %), length of ileus (2.8 vs. 4.2 days), or hospital stay (5.2 vs. 6.5 days) [6].

More recently, a review of data from the Nationwide Inpatient Sample (NIS) database for 2009 showed that 35.4 % of colorectal resections were performed laparoscopically [7]. Controlling for a number of factors, including age,

**Table 28.3** Comparison of outcomes for laparoscopic colectomy in younger vs. older patients

| Author | Year | Age | $N$ | Conversion rate (%) | Hospital stay (days) | Morbidity (%) | Mortality (%) |
|---|---|---|---|---|---|---|---|
| Reissman [6] | 1996 | <60 | 36 | 8 | 5.2 | 11 | 0 |
| | | >60 | 36 | 11 | 6.5 | 14 | 0 |
| Delgado [39] | 2000 | <70 | 70 | 11.4 | 5±2 | 15.6 | 0 |
| | | >70 | 59 | 16.9 | 6±2 | 21.4 | 1.6 |
| Senagore [22] | 2003 | <60 | 181 | | 3.9±5.9 | 10.5 | 0 |
| | | >70 | 50 | | 4.2±3.0 | 16 | 0 |
| Sklow [8] | 2003 | <75 | 38 | 16 | 6.1±0.4 | 29 | 0 |
| | | >75 | 39 | 8 | 6.1±0.3 | 31 | 2.6 |
| Chautard [9] | 2008 | <70 | 103 | 16 | 10±9 | 27 | 0 |
| | | >70 | 75 | 21 | 11±8 | 32 | 0 |
| Akiyoshi [11] | 2009 | <75 | 228 | 0.4 % | 15 | 13.6 | 0 |
| | | >75 | 44 | 0 | 19 | 11.8 | 0 |
| Fiscon [20] | 2010 | <75 | 50 | 4 | 9 | 8 | 0 |
| | | >75 | 50 | 6 | 10 | 24* | 0 |
| Roscio [10] | 2011 | <70 | 101 | 2 | 8.1±2.8 | 3.8 | 0 |
| | | >70 | 58 | 1.7 | 10.8±6.6* | 3.4 | 1.7 |

*$p<0.05$

multivariate analysis showed improved short-term outcomes in the laparoscopy group, as well as decreased length of stay and lower cost.

## Comparisons of Laparoscopic Outcomes in the Young vs. Elderly

A number of reports have shown equivalent short-term outcomes in older patients when compared with younger patients undergoing laparoscopic colorectal surgery. Unfortunately, most of these are small case series or case-control studies (Table 28.3).

Sklow et al. published a retrospective review of patients greater than and less than 75 years of age undergoing laparoscopic colectomy who were case-matched with controls undergoing open colectomy. Complication rates were similar between the laparoscopy and open groups, and laparoscopy was associated with a faster return of bowel function and less narcotic usage postoperatively. Interestingly, faster postoperative recovery was seen with laparoscopic left colectomies in the older group compared to the open group, while faster recovery was seen with laparoscopic right colectomies in the younger group compared with the open group [8]. In 2008, Chautard et al. described a matched case-control study comparing 75 patients greater than 70 years old with 103 patients less than 70 years old undergoing laparoscopic colorectal surgery. While the older group had more frequent cardiopulmonary preoperative comorbidities (80 % vs. 33 %, $p<0.001$), the groups had similar operative time (244±89 vs. 242±80 min), complication rates (32 % vs. 26 %), and hospital stay (11±8 vs. 10±9 days) [9].

Roscio et al. reported a series of 159 consecutive patients undergoing laparoscopic resection for colorectal cancer grouped by age less than or greater than 70 years and found no differences in terms of time to return of bowel function or postoperative complications. Older patients in this study had more comorbid conditions and had a significantly longer length of stay [10].

Looking specifically at rectal cancer, Akiyoshi et al. compared 44 elderly patients greater than 75 years of age undergoing laparoscopic rectal resection (group A) with 228 patients less than 75 years old undergoing laparoscopic proctectomy (group B) and 43 patients greater than 75 years old undergoing open rectal resection (Group C). While group A had a higher ASA classification than group B, the rate of postoperative complications did not differ between the two (13.6 % vs. 11.8 %). Complications were seen less frequently in group A than in C (13.6 % vs. 25.6 %), though this did not reach statistical significance. Group A also demonstrated faster return to flatus (1.3 vs. 3.7 days, $p<0.001$), shorter time to liquid diet (2.2 vs. 7.0 days, $p<0.001$), and a shorter hospital stay (19 vs. 22 days, $p=0.002$) [11].

## Comparisons of Laparoscopic vs. Open Outcomes in the Elderly

Similar to comparisons of laparoscopy in the young vs. the elderly, most of the published data comparing laparoscopic to open procedures in the elderly is limited to case-control series (Table 28.4). In 2000, Stocchi et al. described a series of 42 patients greater than 75 years old undergoing laparoscopic-assisted colectomies that were matched to 42 similar patients

**Table 28.4** Comparison of outcomes for laparoscopic vs. open colectomy in the elderly (*$p<0.05$)

| Author | Year | Open vs. lap | N | Conversion rate (%) | Hospital stay (days) | Morbidity (%) | Mortality (%) |
|---|---|---|---|---|---|---|---|
| Stewart [13] | 1999 | Lap | 42 | 11.9 | 9 | 16.6 | 7.1 |
| | | Open | 35 | | 17 | 42.8* | 11.4 |
| Delgado [39] | 2000 | Lap | 59 | 16.9 | 6±2 | 10.2 | 1.6 |
| | | Open | 67 | | 7±3* | 31.3 %* | 0 |
| Stocchi [12] | 2000 | Lap | 42 | 14.3 | 6.5±4.0 | 14.3 | 0 |
| | | Open | 42 | | 10.2±4.4* | 33.3* | 0 |
| Law [14] | 2002 | Lap | 65 | 12.3 | 7 | 27.7 | 1.5 |
| | | Open | 89 | | 9* | 37 | 5.6 |
| Senagore [22] | 2003 | Lap | 50 | | 4.2±3.0 | 16 | 0 |
| | | Open | 123 | | 9.3±7.6* | 37.4* | 1.6 |
| Sklow [8] | 2003 | Lap | 39 | 8 | 6.1±0.3 | 31 | 2.6 |
| | | Open | 39 | | 7.8±0.6* | 31 | 0 |
| Vignali [15] | 2005 | Lap | 61 | 6.1 | 9.8 | 21.5 | 1.6 |
| | | Open | 61 | | 12.9* | 31.1 | 2.2 |
| Feng [16] | 2006 | Lap | 51 | 3.9 | | 17.6 | 0 |
| | | Open | 102 | | | 37.3* | 1.9 |
| Frasson [17] | 2007 | Lap | 89 | 4.5 | 9.5 | 18 | 4.5 |
| | | Open | 112 | | 13* | 42* | 0.9 |
| Akiyoshi [11] | 2009 | Lap | 44 | 0 | 19 | 13.6 | 0 |
| | | Open | 43 | | 22* | 25.6 | 2.3 |
| Lian [18] | 2010 | Lap | 97 | 14.4 | 6 | 37.1 | 5.2 |
| | | Open | 97 | | 7* | 43.3 | 5.2 |

undergoing open colectomy. Despite longer operative times (190 vs. 142 min, $p<0.001$), the laparoscopic-assisted group had fewer complications (14.3 % vs. 33.3 %, $p=0.04$), less narcotic usage (2.7 vs. 4.8 days, $p<0.001$), faster return to bowel movements (3.9 vs. 5.9 days, $p<0.001$), and shorter hospital stay (6.5 vs. 10.2 days, $p<0.001$). Additionally, independent-living status was more frequently maintained postoperatively in the laparoscopic-assisted group compared with the open group (35/37 vs. 29/38, $p=0.025$)—a key factor in looking at outcome with elderly patients that many studies do not address [12].

Stewart et al., in 1999, compared patients aged 80 years or greater undergoing elective laparoscopic ($n=42$) and open ($n=35$) colorectal procedures. The open group demonstrated a higher incidence of cardiopulmonary complications, wound infections, postoperative ileus, and ICU admission; patients in the laparoscopy group had a shorter length of stay and were more likely to be discharged to home instead of to a rehabilitation facility or nursing home. At 6-month follow-up, 82 % of surviving patients in the laparoscopy group who were independent preoperatively were living independently postoperatively, compared with only 64 % of surviving patients in the open group, indicating that a fair number of elderly patients undergoing major open abdominal surgery never return to an independent lifestyle [13].

Law et al. compared laparoscopic and open colectomy in patients greater than 70 years old and found that laparoscopy was associated with less operative blood loss, earlier return of bowel function, earlier resumption of solid diet, shorter hospital stay, and less cardiopulmonary morbidity [14]. In 2005, Vignali et al. published the results of a case-matched control study comparing 61 octogenarians undergoing laparoscopic colectomy for cancer with 61 patients undergoing open colectomy, matched for gender, age, year of surgery, site of cancer, and comorbidities. Despite longer operative times in the laparoscopic group (220 vs. 171 min, $p=0.01$), postoperative morbidity rates were similar (25.5 % vs. 31.1 %, $p=0.30$), and the laparoscopy group demonstrated faster return of bowel function (4.8 vs. 5.9 days, $p=0.005$) and shorter length of stay (9.8 vs. 12.9 days, $p=0.001$). Laparoscopy also allowed better preservation of postoperative independence status compared with open surgery (98 % vs. 82 %, $p=0.02$) [15].

Feng et al., in 2006, compared 51 patients greater than 70 years old with colorectal cancer undergoing laparoscopic resection with 102 matched controls undergoing open resection. Overall morbidity was significantly reduced in the laparoscopic group (17.6 % vs. 37.3 %, $p=0.013$), suggesting a preferential benefit to laparoscopy over open surgery in elderly patients [16]. Frasson and colleagues described a cohort of 535 patients with colorectal disease randomly assigned to laparoscopic or open resection, 37.6 % of whom were greater than 70 years old. In both the younger and the older groups, complication rates and length of stay were lower in the laparoscopic resection arm compared with the open resection arm. However, in terms of reduced morbidity and length of stay, the advantages were much more pronounced in the older group of patients, again suggesting a benefit to laparoscopy in this population [17].

Lian and associates compared 97 patients more than 80 years of age (mean age 82.8 years) undergoing elective laparoscopic colectomy with similar case-matched patients undergoing open colectomy. The laparoscopy group demonstrated shorter hospital stay (6 vs. 7 days, $p=0.001$) and similar complication, readmission, and mortality rates. Contrary to other reported studies, the rate of discharge to home without assistance was not significantly different between the two groups (63.9 % vs. 62.9 %, $p=0.88$) [18].

## Is Laparoscopy *Not* Beneficial in the Elderly Population?

In contrast to the majority of published literature, there are some published series suggesting that elderly patients undergoing laparoscopic colorectal surgery may have poorer outcomes. Kirchhoff et al. found in a multivariate analysis of risk factors associated with elective laparoscopic colorectal procedures that age greater than 75 was a significant risk factor for intraoperative (OR 1.69, 95 % CI 1.09–2.62, $p=0.019$) and postoperative (OR 1.57, 95 % CI 1.15–2.13, $p=0.004$) complications [19]. Fiscon et al. reported that when a group of 50 patients greater than 75 years old (median age 79.7 years) undergoing laparoscopic colorectal resection for cancer was matched by ASA score and operation with 50 patients less than 75 years old (median age 62 years), there was a significantly higher morbidity rate seen in the older group—24 % vs. 8 % ($p=0.05$) [20].

## Laparoscopic Colorectal Surgery in the Elderly: Enhanced Recovery Protocols

A number of published studies have shown a clear benefit to the use of enhanced recovery, or "fast-track," protocols following laparoscopic colorectal surgery. More recently, these have been expanded to apply to elderly patients with similarly favorable outcomes. In fact, reports of discharge less than 24 h postoperatively following laparoscopic right colectomy for cancer in octogenarians have been described [21].

In 2003, Senagore et al. evaluated the short-term outcomes in age-matched cohorts of patients undergoing laparoscopic vs. open segmental colectomy managed with an enhanced recovery protocol. Length of stay was significantly shorter for the laparoscopy groups in each cohort. Unlike prior studies, the authors also found a significant reduction in direct hospital costs associated with laparoscopy in the older (greater than 70 years old) cohort ($3,920 vs. $6,448) but *not* the younger (less than 60 years old) cohort ($3,616 vs. $3,804). Readmission rates were similar for laparoscopic vs. open procedures in older patients (6.0 % vs. 6.5 %, $p=\text{NS}$) but significantly higher for laparoscopic procedures in the younger cohort (9.4 % vs. 4.1 %, $p<0.05$). Postoperative complication rates were also significantly reduced in the laparoscopy group for older patients (16 % vs. 37.4 %, $p<0.05$) but not in the younger group (10.5 % vs. 13.1 %, $p=\text{NS}$). The authors concluded that laparoscopic colectomy managed with an enhanced recovery program offers particular advantages to older patients [22].

In one of the few randomized controlled trials in the literature evaluating laparoscopic colorectal surgery in the elderly, Wang described the outcomes for 78 patients greater than 65 years of age (mean age 71) undergoing laparoscopic colorectal resection who were randomized to a "fast-track" protocol vs. a "conventional care" group. The fast-track group had a faster return of bowel function as measured by three separate indices, including a shorter length of stay (5.5 vs. 7.0 days, $p<0.001$), and fewer complications (5.0 % vs. 21.1 %, $p=0.045$) [23]. Pawa et al. published outcomes for 688 colorectal resections managed with an enhanced recovery protocol, 18.9 % of which were inpatients greater than 80 years old; 93.1 % of resections in the older cohort were performed laparoscopically, compared with 97.1 % in younger cohort ($p=0.036$). Both groups demonstrated similar lengths of stay and readmission rates; however, there was a higher complication rate (mainly cardiopulmonary and urinary) in the older group (26.2 % vs. 9.3 %, $p<0.0001$). The authors noted that there was more difficulty with adherence to the protocol in older group, particularly with timely discontinuation of urinary catheters and intravenous fluids [24].

## What Are the Long-Term Outcomes?

While short-term outcomes regarding outcomes for laparoscopic colorectal procedures in the elderly are well described, data regarding long-term outcomes is generally lacking. The COST trial, which proved similar oncologic outcomes in patients undergoing laparoscopic and open colectomy, did not stratify patients by age. However, keeping in mind that a number of studies define "elderly" as greater than 70 years old and that the median ages in the open and laparoscopic groups in the COST trial were 69 and 70, respectively, one might surmise from this that oncologic outcomes in elderly patients undergoing laparoscopic colectomy for cancer approximate those of patients undergoing open colectomy, at least in the setting of a strict, randomized controlled trial [25].

In the one study specifically looking at long-term outcomes, Cheung described a series of 101 octogenarians (mean age of 83 years) undergoing laparoscopic colorectal resection for cancer. At a median follow-up of 24 months, there were 22 recurrences. The overall 5-year survival rate was 51 %, and 5-year disease-free survival rate was 49 % [26]. Determination of the true long-term benefits of laparoscopic colorectal surgery would require a randomized control trial incorporating quality of life measures to definitively answer the question of whether laparoscopic colorectal surgery in the elderly population offers a true advantage over open surgery.

## Operating Room Considerations

### Physiology of Pneumoperitoneum

The common theme in terms of the elderly patient's ability to tolerate laparoscopy depends not on the chronologic age, but more so on comorbid conditions and sufficient physiologic reserve. Laparoscopy in the elderly has previously been approached with reservation because of concerns over the possible adverse hemodynamic effects of pneumoperitoneum in this population that perhaps may have a more limited cardiopulmonary reserve. With laparoscopic surgery, concerns have been raised regarding issues such as the duration of the procedure and extreme positioning which may exacerbate this limited reserve (Fig. 28.1).

Insufflation of the peritoneal cavity to create pneumoperitoneum during laparoscopy induces a number of physiologic changes (Table 28.5). In a healthy patient with normal physiologic reserve, standard insufflation to an intra-abdominal pressure of 15 mmHg produces relatively little in the way of clinically relevant changes. However, in elderly patients in whom this reserve may be limited due to underlying comorbid conditions, the physiologic changes induced by pneumoperitoneum can have profound effects [27].

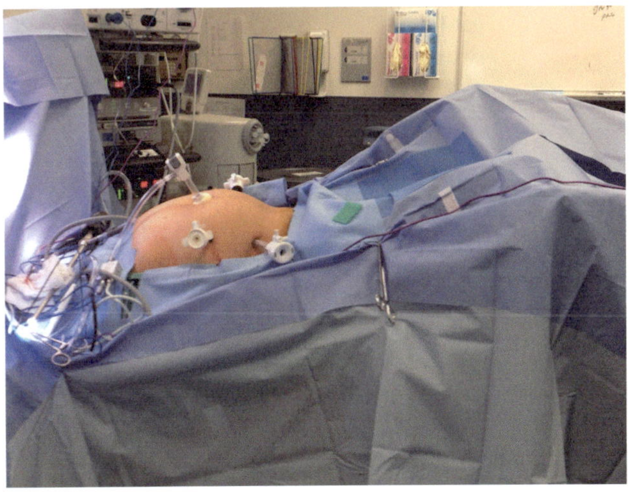

**Fig. 28.1** Steep reverse Trendelenburg may cause problems with physiology in the elderly

**Table 28.5** Physiologic effects of pneumoperitoneum

| Parameter | Change | |
|---|---|---|
| Respiratory | | |
| Functional residual capacity | Decrease | |
| Alveolar dead space | Increase | |
| Peak airway pressures | Increase | |
| Pulmonary compliance | Decrease | |
| FEV-1 | Decrease | |
| Force vital capacity | Decrease | |
| Peak expiratory flow | Decrease | |
| *Hemodynamic* | *With hypercarbia* | *With increased abdominal pressure* |
| Heart rate | Increase | Increase |
| Mean arterial pressure (MAP) | Increase | Increase or decrease[a] |
| Central venous pressure | Increase | Increase or decrease[a] |
| Stroke volume | Increase | Decrease |
| Cardiac output | Increase | Increase or decrease[a] |
| *Renal* | | |
| Urine output | Decrease | |
| Glomerular filtration rate | Decrease | |
| Renal blood flow | Decrease | |
| Serum creatinine | Increase or no change | |
| Vasopressin | Increase | |

[a]Increase or decrease depends on several factors. As preload falls, MAP may compensate as well as cardiac output. However, if continues or with large decrease in preload, cardiac output and MAP will decrease

### Acid/Base Effects

The most commonly used gas for insufflations is carbon dioxide ($CO_2$), which is very efficiently eliminated. $CO_2$ is absorbed through the peritoneum and eliminated by respiratory exchange in lungs. Insufflation increases $CO_2$ delivery to lungs by as much as 50 %, and an increase in minute ventilation of up to 16 % can be required to maintain normocarbia during pneumoperitoneum [28]. Elderly patients with severe chronic obstructive pulmonary disease, decreased cardiac output, or high metabolic and cellular metabolic rates (i.e., sepsis) may experience significant hypercarbia if the end-tidal $CO_2$ and arterial pH are not monitored [29].

### Pulmonary Effects

Abdominal insufflation during laparoscopy impedes diaphragmatic movement and results in decreased functional residual capacity (FRC) and an increase in alveolar dead space. Additionally, there is a rise in peak airway pressures with a decrease in pulmonary compliance [27]. Collectively, these factors can lead to significant hypoxemia, which can be minimized by controlled ventilation, which minimizes alveolar atelectasis and the potential resulting ventilation/perfusion mismatch [30]. Again, elderly patients with underlying pulmonary disease may be more prone to the deleterious effects of pneumoperitoneum on pulmonary volumes and oxygenation.

## Cardiovascular Effects

Pneumoperitoneum affects cardiovascular physiology, both due to the effects of hypercarbia and the direct effect of the increase in abdominal pressure on the thoracic cavity. At a $pCO_2$ of 55–70 mmHg, hypercarbia and acidosis cause hemodynamic changes due to myocardial depression and vasodilation, effects that are countered by a centrally mediated sympathetic stimulation that causes tachycardia and vasoconstriction, resulting in an increased heart rate, mean arterial pressure, cardiac output, and stroke volume [27]. In elderly patients with underlying pulmonary disease who have difficulty clearing the hypercarbia produced by $CO_2$ insufflation, these effects can be pronounced.

The hemodynamic effects attributed to the mechanical effect of increased intra-abdominal pressure are much more pronounced than the effects induced by hypercarbia. With decreased right atrial pressures, pneumoperitoneum compresses the inferior vena cava, leading to decreased venous return. With higher right atrial filling pressures, the vena cava is able to resist compression, and increased intra-abdominal pressure actually augments venous return [31, 32]. Additionally, increased intra-abdominal pressure results in compression of small capacitance vessels, further augmenting venous return. With hypervolemia, cardiac output is augmented by an elevated mean systemic pressure and increase in venous return. With euvolemia or hypovolemia, increased systemic pressure is outweighed by caval compression and decreased venous return, causing a decrease in cardiac output, the level which is directly related to the degree of increased abdominal pressure [33].

Certain considerations should be taken into account when considering laparoscopy in elderly patients with underlying cardiac disease. Increases in heart rate and afterload have the potential to increase ventricular wall tension and subsequent myocardial ischemia. Inadequate left ventricular reserve can lead to transient cardiac decompensation during abdominal insufflation, decreasing oxygen delivery and causing reflexive increases in pulmonary arterial pressure. In patients with underlying cardiac disease undergoing laparoscopy, additional intraoperative monitoring, including direct measurements of arterial and central venous pressure, may be considered.

## Renal Effects

Increased intra-abdominal pressure created by pneumoperitoneum decreases renal blood flow and glomerular filtration rate via a number of mechanisms. Decreased delivery of blood to the kidneys as a result of decreased cardiac output results in decreased renal blood flow. Animal studies have clearly demonstrated that increased intra-abdominal pressure resulting from insufflation of the abdominal cavity also results in decreased renal blood flow [34, 35], presumably due to vascular and parenchymal compression, though the exact mechanism by which this occurs has not been clearly elucidated. There is also evidence that pneumoperitoneum increases secretion of vasopressin, promoting water resorption and decreasing urine output. When performing laparoscopy on elderly patients with decreased baseline renal function, one should be mindful of maintaining adequate intravascular volume to promote renal blood flow. Fortunately, long-term deleterious effects of pneumoperitoneum on renal function are rare; transient changes in serum creatinine, glomerular filtration rate, and urine output tend to return to baseline fairly quickly postoperatively.

## Immune System Effects

Serum levels of several acute-phase reactants, proteins produced in response to tissue injury, have been shown to be elevated after laparoscopy. Probably the most widely studied of these is C-reactive protein (CRP), which rises 4–12 h after surgery, peaks at 24–72 h postoperatively, and remains elevated for about 2 weeks [36]; after laparoscopy, CRP levels do not reach the same degree of elevation as those seen after laparotomy. Interleukin-6 (IL-6) is the major cytokine responsible for the acute-phase protein response and is an early marker for tissue damage. As with CRP, elevations in IL-6 after laparoscopy are less pronounced than those seen after laparotomy [37]. Insufflation of the abdomen with $CO_2$ as opposed to room air has also been shown to be associated with a reduction in the IL-6 response. Similar associations have been seen with decreased release of TNF-α and IL-1 from cells incubated in $CO_2$ compared with room air or nitrogen [38], suggesting that there is a modulation of the proinflammatory response with $CO_2$ insufflation.

# Laparoscopic Surgery in the Elderly: Changes and Technical Points

The basic tenets of laparoscopy in general hold true when performing laparoscopic colorectal procedures on elderly patients—safe access to the peritoneal cavity, adequate visualization and exposure of target tissues, triangulation of trocars, and delicate tissue handling with appropriate traction/counter-traction are all paramount to successful laparoscopic surgery.

Many older patients have undergone prior open abdominal surgery, raising challenges with access and intra-abdominal adhesions. Gaining access via a Veress needle or optical laparoscopic visualization technique may risk inadvertent enterotomy if there are adhesions of bowel to the undersurface of the abdominal wall; in these circumstances a direct cutdown or Hasson technique may be preferred. In patients who have undergone previous abdominal surgery, extensive laparoscopic lysis of adhesions may be required in order to adequately visualize the target tissues. This can be very time-consuming and tedious, with risk of inadvertent enterotomy, which can be technically challenging to repair laparoscopically. In elderly patients with significant comorbidities, the benefits of laparoscopy must be weighed against the drawbacks of a prolonged operative time if extensive adhesiolysis is required.

The cardiopulmonary effects of pneumoperitoneum, as previously described, can be more pronounced in elderly patients due to underlying disease. Additionally, extreme positional changes are often utilized during advanced laparoscopic procedures to facilitate exposure, which can further compound the hemodynamic effects produced by pneumoperitoneum. Elderly patients may not be able to tolerate the physiologic changes induced by pneumoperitoneum and may require lower levels of insufflation to decrease intra-abdominal pressures. Patients with pulmonary hypertension or right-sided heart failure may not be able tolerate steep Trendelenburg position due to increased venous return to the heart. If abdominal insufflation or extreme positional changes create unsafe hemodynamics, one should consider converting to an open procedure.

Positioning is another very important factor. Baseline coagulopathies, medications, or platelet dysfunction, along with "frail" skin, may lead to increased bruising. Additional padding on the bony prominences, sacrum, (Fig. 28.2), and legs (Figs. 28.3 and 28.4) while in the modified lithotomy position is crucial.

Changes in the postoperative management in elderly patients undergoing laparoscopic procedures may also be

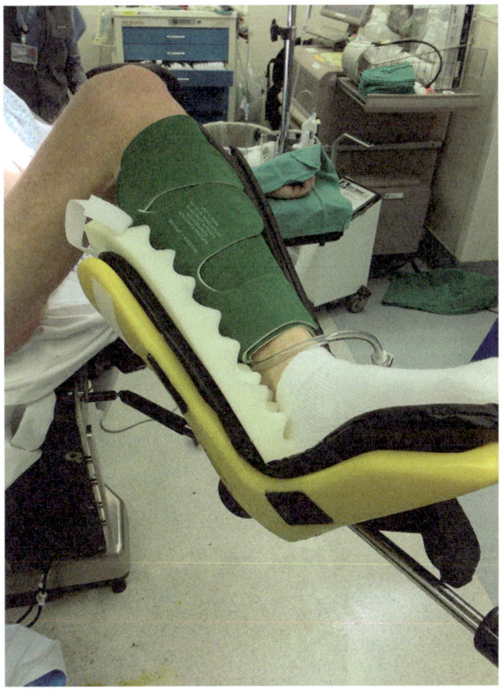

**Fig. 28.3** Added padding in the stirrups

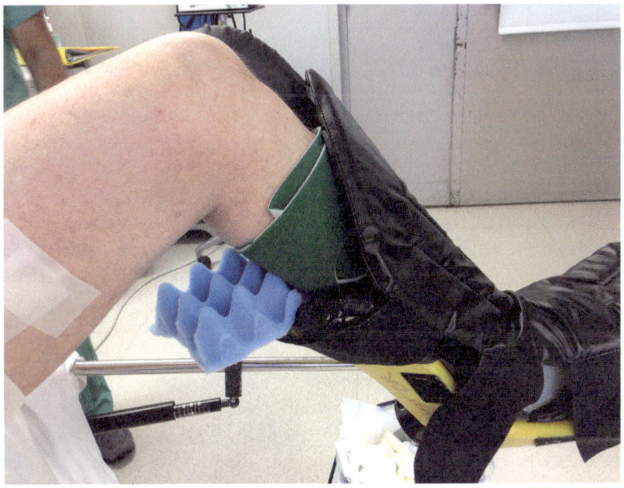

**Fig. 28.4** Additional padding at the calf. Mechanical compression devices are in place

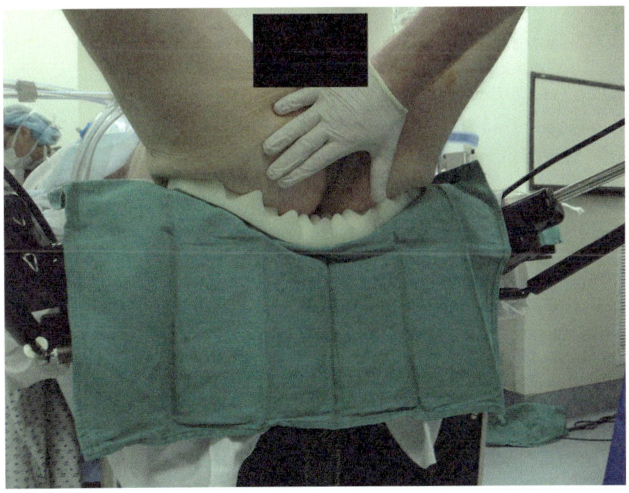

**Fig. 28.2** Additional padding on the sacrum

needed. The concept of early postoperative ambulation may be difficult to employ in this patient population, whose mobility may have been poor even preoperatively [24]. Early discontinuation of Foley catheters is often met with nursing resistance due to urinary incontinence or the need for reinsertion in elderly men with enlarged prostates or women with pelvic floor prolapse; Foley catheter reinsertion may increase the risk for postoperative urinary tract infections. Early enteral feeding post-laparoscopy should be employed judiciously in elderly patients, as this population may be more likely to have an aspiration event associated with episodes of nausea and vomiting, increasing the risk of pneumonia and need for mechanical ventilation.

## Conclusions

Management of the elderly patient with colorectal problems can be complex and may affect every aspect of the patients care. Every plan for operative intervention should begin with appropriate assessment of comorbidities and assessment for fitness for surgery. The use of laparoscopy, while previously a contraindication in the elderly, has emerged to provide significant advantages for the elderly patients similar to those in younger patients. The use of laparoscopy introduces unique and important physiologic changes perioperatively, of which the responsible colorectal surgeon must be aware, and must be taken into account in the context of common morbidities in the elderly. Nevertheless, with appropriate preoperative planning, laparoscopy seems to have proven advantages over open surgery in the elderly and may soon be considered standard of care.

## References


1. Fleisher LA, Beckman JA, Brown KA, Calkins H, Chaikof EL, Fleischmann KE, et al. ACC/AHA 2007 guidelines on perioperative cardiovascular evaluation and care for noncardiac surgery: executive summary: a report of the American College of Cardiology/ American Heart Association Task Force on Practice Guidelines (Writing Committee to Revise the 2002 Guidelines on Perioperative Cardiovascular Evaluation for Noncardiac Surgery) Developed in Collaboration with the American Society of Echocardiography, American Society of Nuclear Cardiology, Heart Rhythm Society, Society of Cardiovascular Anesthesiologists, Society for Cardiovascular Angiography and Interventions, Society for Vascular Medicine and Biology, and Society for Vascular Surgery. J Am Coll Cardiol. 2007;50(17):1707–32.
2. American College of Cardiology/American Heart Association Task Force on Practice Guidelines (Writing Committee to Revise the 2002 Guidelines on Perioperative Cardiovascular Evaluation for Noncardiac Surgery), American Society of Echocardiography, American Society of Nuclear Cardiology, Heart Rhythm Society, Society of Cardiovascular Anesthesiologists, Society for Cardiovascular Angiography and Interventions, et al. ACC/AHA 2007 guidelines on perioperative cardiovascular evaluation and care for noncardiac surgery: executive summary: a report of the American College of Cardiology/American Heart Association Task Force on Practice Guidelines (Writing Committee to Revise the 2002 Guidelines on Perioperative Cardiovascular Evaluation for Noncardiac Surgery). Anesth Analg. 2008;106(3):685–712.
3. American College of Cardiology Foundation/American Heart Association Task Force on Practice Guidelines, American Society of Echocardiography, American Society of Nuclear Cardiology, Heart Rhythm Society, Society of Cardiovascular Anesthesiologists, Society for Cardiovascular Angiography and Interventions, et al. 2009 ACCF/AHA focused update on perioperative beta blockade incorporated into the ACC/AHA 2007 guidelines on perioperative cardiovascular evaluation and care for noncardiac surgery. J Am Coll Cardiol. 2009;54(22):e13–118.
4. Taylor EF, Thomas JD, Whitehouse LE, Quirke P, Jayne D, Finan PJ, et al. Population-based study of laparoscopic colorectal cancer surgery 2006–2008. Br J Surg. 2013;100(4):553–60.
5. Peters WR, Fleshman JW. Minimally invasive colectomy in elderly patients. Surg Laparosc Endosc. 1995;5(6):477–9.
6. Reissman P, Agachan F, Wexner SD. Outcome of laparoscopic colorectal surgery in older patients. Am Surg. 1996;62(12): 1060–3.
7. Kang CY, Chaudhry OO, Halabi WJ, Nguyen V, Carmichael JC, Stamos MJ, et al. Outcomes of laparoscopic colorectal surgery: data from the Nationwide Inpatient Sample 2009. Am J Surg. 2012;204(6):952–7.
8. Sklow B, Read T, Birnbaum E, Fry R, Fleshman J. Age and type of procedure influence the choice of patients for laparoscopic colectomy. Surg Endosc. 2003;17(6):923–9.
9. Chautard J, Alves A, Zalinski S, Bretagnol F, Valleur P, Panis Y. Laparoscopic colorectal surgery in elderly patients: a matched case-control study in 178 patients. J Am Coll Surg. 2008;206(2): 255–60.
10. Roscio F, Bertoglio C, De Luca A, Frigerio A, Galli F, Scandroglio I. Outcomes of laparoscopic surgery for colorectal cancer in elderly patients. JSLS. 2011;15(3):315–21.
11. Akiyoshi T, Kuroyanagi H, Fujimoto Y, Konishi T, Ueno M, Oya M, et al. Short-term outcomes of laparoscopic colectomy for transverse colon cancer. J Gastrointest Surg. 2010;14(5):818–23.
12. Stocchi L, Nelson H, Young-Fadok TM, Larson DR, Ilstrup DM. Safety and advantages of laparoscopic vs. open colectomy in the elderly: matched-control study. Dis Colon Rectum. 2000; 43(3):326–32.
13. Stewart BT, Stitz RW, Lumley JW. Laparoscopically assisted colorectal surgery in the elderly. Br J Surg. 1999;86(7):938–41.
14. Law WL, Chu KW, Tung PH. Laparoscopic colorectal resection: a safe option for elderly patients. J Am Coll Surg. 2002;195(6): 768–73.
15. Vignali A, Di Palo S, Tamburini A, Radaelli G, Orsenigo E, Staudacher C. Laparoscopic vs. open colectomies in octogenarians: a case-matched control study. Dis Colon Rectum. 2005;48(11): 2070–5.
16. Feng B, Zheng MH, Mao ZH, Li JW, Lu AG, Wang ML, et al. Clinical advantages of laparoscopic colorectal cancer surgery in the elderly. Aging Clin Exp Res. 2006;18(3):191–5.
17. Frasson M, Braga M, Vignali A, Zuliani W, Di Carlo V. Benefits of laparoscopic colorectal resection are more pronounced in elderly patients. Dis Colon Rectum. 2008;51(3):296–300.
18. Lian L, Kalady M, Geisler D, Kiran RP. Laparoscopic colectomy is safe and leads to a significantly shorter hospital stay for octogenarians. Surg Endosc. 2010;24(8):2039–43.
19. Kirchhoff P, Dincler S, Buchmann P. A multivariate analysis of potential risk factors for intra- and postoperative complications in 1316 elective laparoscopic colorectal procedures. Ann Surg. 2008;248(2):259–65.
20. Fiscon V, Portale G, Frigo F, Migliorini G. Laparoscopic resection of colorectal cancer: matched comparison in elderly and younger patients. Tech Coloproctol. 2010;14(4):323–7.
21. Rogers JP, Dobradin A, Kar PM, Alam SE. Overnight hospital stay after colon surgery for adenocarcinoma. JSLS. 2012;16(2):333–6.
22. Senagore AJ, Madbouly KM, Fazio VW, Duepree HJ, Brady KM, Delaney CP. Advantages of laparoscopic colectomy in older patients. Arch Surg. 2003;138(3):252–6.
23. Wang Q, Suo J, Jiang J, Wang C, Zhao YQ, Cao X. Effectiveness of fast-track rehabilitation vs. conventional care in laparoscopic colorectal resection for elderly patients: a randomized trial. Colorectal Dis. 2012;14(8):1009–13.
24. Pawa N, Cathcart PL, Arulampalam TH, Tutton MG, Motson RW. Enhanced recovery program following colorectal resection in the elderly patient. World J Surg. 2012;36(2):415–23.
25. Clinical Outcomes of Surgical Therapy Study Group. A comparison of laparoscopically assisted and open colectomy for colon cancer. N Engl J Med. 2004;350(20):2050–9.

26. Cheung HY, Chung CC, Fung JT, Wong JC, Yau KK, Li MK. Laparoscopic resection for colorectal cancer in octogenarians: results in a decade. Dis Colon Rectum. 2007;50(11):1905–10.
27. Grabowski JE, Talamini MA. Physiological effects of pneumoperitoneum. J Gastrointest Surg. 2009;13(5):1009–16.
28. Brown DR, Fishburne JI, Roberson VO, Hulka JF. Ventilatory and blood gas changes during laparoscopy with local anesthesia. Am J Obstet Gynecol. 1976;124(7):741–5.
29. Safran DB, Orlando III R. Physiologic effects of pneumoperitoneum. Am J Surg. 1994;167(2):281–6.
30. Gutt CN, Oniu T, Mehrabi A, Schemmer P, Kashfi A, Kraus T, et al. Circulatory and respiratory complications of carbon dioxide insufflation. Dig Surg. 2004;21(2):95–105.
31. Diamant M, Benumof JL, Saidman LJ. Hemodynamics of increased intra-abdominal pressure: interaction with hypovolemia and halothane anesthesia. Anesthesiology. 1978;48(1):23–7.
32. Kashtan J, Green JF, Parsons EQ, Holcroft JW. Hemodynamic effect of increased abdominal pressure. J Surg Res. 1981;30(3):249–55.
33. Dexter SP, Vucevic M, Gibson J, McMahon MJ. Hemodynamic consequences of high- and low-pressure capnoperitoneum during laparoscopic cholecystectomy. Surg Endosc. 1999;13(4):376–81.
34. Chiu AW, Azadzoi KM, Hatzichristou DG, Siroky MB, Krane RJ, Babayan RK. Effects of intra-abdominal pressure on renal tissue perfusion during laparoscopy. J Endourol. 1994;8(2):99–103.
35. Shuto K, Kitano S, Yoshida T, Bandoh T, Mitarai Y, Kobayashi M. Hemodynamic and arterial blood gas changes during carbon dioxide and helium pneumoperitoneum in pigs. Surg Endosc. 1995;9(11):1173–8.
36. Vittimberga Jr FJ, Foley DP, Meyers WC, Callery MP. Laparoscopic surgery and the systemic immune response. Ann Surg. 1998;227(3):326–34.
37. Ure BM, Niewold TA, Bax NM, Ham M, van der Zee DC, Essen GJ. Peritoneal, systemic, and distant organ inflammatory responses are reduced by a laparoscopic approach and carbon dioxide versus air. Surg Endosc. 2002;16(5):836–42.
38. West MA, Hackam DJ, Baker J, Rodriguez JL, Bellingham J, Rotstein OD. Mechanism of decreased in vitro murine macrophage cytokine release after exposure to carbon dioxide: relevance to laparoscopic surgery. Ann Surg. 1997;226(2):179–90.
39. Delgado S, Lacy AM, García Valdecasas JC, Balagué C, Pera M, Salvador L, Momblan D, Visa J. Could age be an indication for laparoscopic colectomy in colorectal cancer? Surg Endosc. 2000;14(1):22–6.

# Laparoscopic Colectomy in the Obese Patient

29

Arida Siripong and H. David Vargas

**Key Points**

- Obese patients suffering from colorectal diseases requiring surgery are common in general and colon rectal surgical practice.
- Laparoscopic colectomy in the obese patient is associated with increased operative time and higher conversion rates, indicating increased technical difficulty and need for surgeon experience and expertise.
- Laparoscopic colectomy in the obese patient requires specific patient and surgeon preparation, unique technical strategies, and dedicated surgical instrumentation for safe and successful performance.
- Laparoscopic colectomy offers benefits to obese patients when successfully completed.

## Introduction

The obesity epidemic represents one of the greatest healthcare challenges of our generation. According to the Centers for Disease Control and Prevention, 37.5 % of adult Americans are obese, with an associated annual financial implication of 147 billion dollars [1]. Traditionally, obesity has been defined by body mass index (BMI), with a BMI greater than 30 kg/m$^2$ defined as obese and BMI greater than 40 kg/m$^2$ as morbidly obese. While BMI serves as a useful snapshot to stratify patients, it does not acknowledge several important factors, including adipose distribution, muscle mass composition, and differences across race and gender [2, 3]. Emerging evidence suggests that alternate definition of obesity, such as visceral abdominal fat (VAT) and waist-to-hip ratio (WHR), may provide more accurate representations of the physiologic changes that accompany obesity and its health consequences [4, 5].

For the surgeon, central obesity may represent the true challenge from both the technical and perioperative risk standpoints. Visceral adipose tissue (VAT), an alternate definition of obesity that uses CT imaging to measure central adipose tissue, plays a fundamental role in the development of multiple medical comorbidities, such as insulin resistance, diabetes, hypertension, cardiovascular disease, hyperlipidemia, and obstructive sleep apnea [4–7]. Various tools for measuring VAT have been described, including computed tomography (CT), ultrasonography (US), waist circumference (WC), and waist-to-hip ratio (WHR). WHR and WC are anthropometric markers that indirectly describe VAT [8–10]. In contrast, CT offers a more precise measurement but is costly, time-consuming, and associated with ionizing radiation exposure. Ultrasonography may be more practical and affordable with comparable measurements of VAT by CT but without having the associated risk of radiation [11–13]. Thus, the take-home message remains that measuring and defining obesity evolves and will potentially improve stratification of operative risk.

There exists variability in obese patients as well—"the healthy obese patient"—who tend to be younger and have yet to develop medical conditions so often associated with obesity. Despite this perceived appearance of well-being, however, surgeons must scrutinize any obese patient for medical comorbidities. Surgeons contemplating any colorectal operation in the obese patient must ensure optimal medical management for cardiovascular disease, pulmonary conditions, hypertension, and diabetes to reduce operative risk and potential medical complications related to abdominal surgery—especially when it may be occult. As a policy, you should have a low threshold for preoperative clearance and an active role of medical specialist during the perioperative period. This cannot be overstated nor overlooked.

In addition, the relationship between obesity and colorectal disease has been well described [14–16]. Obesity has been

**Electronic supplementary material:** Supplementary material is available in the online version of this chapter at 10.1007/978-1-4939-1581-1_29. Videos can also be accessed at http://www.springerimages.com/videos/978-1-4939-1580-4.

A. Siripong, M.D. • H.D. Vargas, M.D., F.A.C.S., F.A.S.C.R.S. (✉)
Department of Colon and Rectal Surgery, Ochsner Clinic,
1514 Jefferson Highway, New Orleans, LA 7021, USA
e-mail: aridasir@gmail.com; dvargas@ochsner.org

H.M. Ross et al. (eds.), *Minimally Invasive Approaches to Colon and Rectal Disease: Technique and Best Practices*,
DOI 10.1007/978-1-4939-1581-1_29, © Springer Science+Business Media New York 2015

linked to an increased incidence of colorectal neoplasia and adenoma formation, with insulin-like growth factors proposed as a mediator in the oncogenic process [14–16]. Recent data also suggests that obesity may be linked to more severe disease presentations of diverticular disease [17] and earlier presentation of inflammatory bowel disease [18].

The increasing prevalence of obesity and its impact on colorectal pathology means that surgeons are now more often faced with identifying the optimal operative approach in these patients. The laparoscopic technique is an accepted alternative to open resection for colorectal disorders in both obese and non-obese patients, with comparable oncologic results to open resection [19–21]. Data also suggests that the proven benefits of laparoscopy in non-obese patients, including accelerated recovery of bowel function, decreased postoperative pain, and shorter hospital stay, similarly apply in the setting of obesity [22–25]. The technical challenge of this patient population, however, is apparent given the associated longer operative times and higher conversion rates in obese patients undergoing minimally invasive colorectal procedures. The purpose of this chapter then is to provide readers with a systematic and rational approach to performing laparoscopic colectomy in the obese patient.

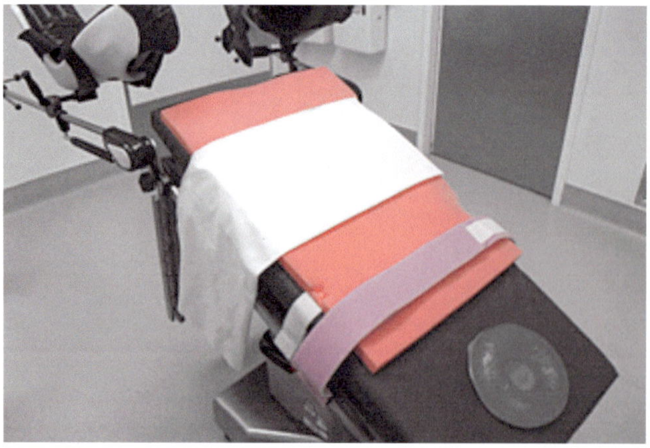

**Fig. 29.1** Pigazzi patient positioning system™. Notice the steep positioning that is required

**Table 29.1** Preoperative considerations

| |
|---|
| • Surgeon well experienced with laparoscopy |
| • Patient selection |
| • Preoperative expectations |
| – Increased likelihood for need for conversion |
| – Longer operative time |
| • Bowel prep |
| – May need longer bowel preparation |
| – When optimized, can improve exposure with decompressed bowel |
| • Antibiotic prophylaxis |
| – Appropriate weight-based dosing for preoperative administration |
| • Perioperative DVT prophylaxis |

## Technical Considerations

When contemplating laparoscopic colectomy in the obese patient, one must consider the pragmatic situation first and then the strategic. The "nuts and bolts" (so to speak) of the former includes those issues related to the implications of the size and weight of this patient cohort. Though mundane, you must first address the necessary tools that must be specifically designed. Thus, the realities of weight restrictions of operating tables and stirrups, potential need for longer ports and instruments, and means of stabilizing and protecting the obese patient in severe degrees of positioning must be accounted for prior to considering actual operative strategies (Fig. 29.1). While there can be no doubt of the importance of the details of this aspect of a technical discussion, the evolution of such technology continues. Given the increasing numbers of obese patients requiring colectomy, thoughtful and purposeful innovation can be anticipated and surgeons must be cognizant of such advances. We will attempt to intertwine these two facets—pragmatic and strategic—with the understanding that the emphasis of our discussion will favor operative strategies.

## Defining an Operative Plan and Precise Preoperative Localization of Pathology

A fundamental aspect of the preoperative phase of surgery involves developing the operative plan (Table 29.1). For an elective colectomy, this should include the preoperative diagnosis, the anticipated extent of resection, incision/port placement, exposure strategy, dissection and mobilization, vascular ligation, bowel resection, and anastomosis. Execution of the plan remains dependent upon the actual circumstances encountered at the time of operation. Surgeons must consider prior to surgery all of the potential variations that may be encountered and how such endeavors enable one to adapt and press on when the unexpected occurs. While it is impossible to anticipate every possible variation, reducing such variables improves operative efficiency.

One aspect of preoperative planning which requires additional consideration is the localization of the pathology to be resected and specifically when dealing with small tumors or polyps. In the case of inflammatory conditions, imaging will generally identify the segment of bowel to be resected. For polyps or tumors, we use preoperative colonoscopy. The colonoscopic description of location identifies the segment, while tattooing techniques enable intraoperative confirmation. Clearly, the experienced surgeon should maintain a healthy skepticism of the precision of colonoscopic descriptions, as inaccuracies persist irrespective of the experience and skill of the endoscopist. The tattoo is often viewed as the "fail-safe" alternative at operation. However, in the obese

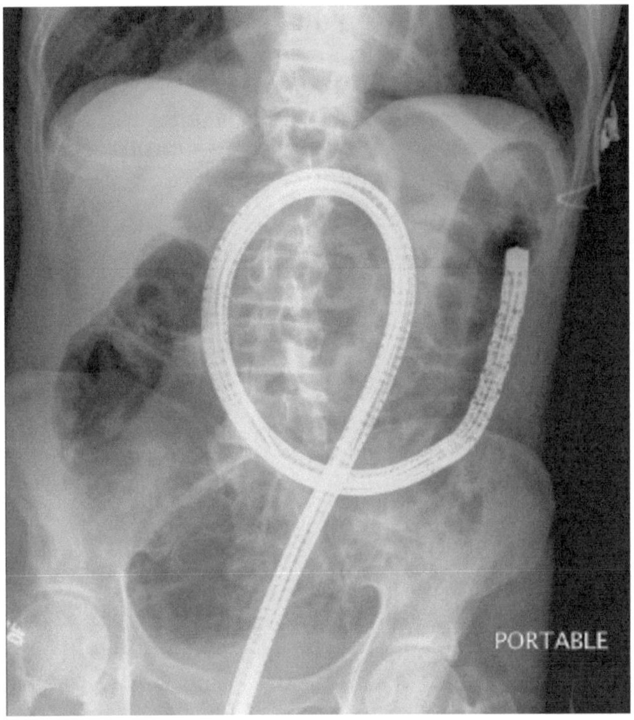


**Fig. 29.2** Localization of small tumor using radiograph with colonoscopy

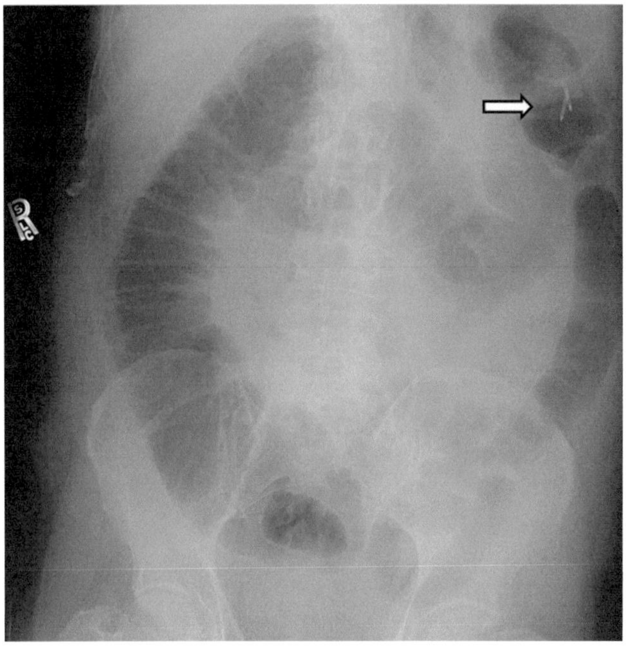

**Fig. 29.3** Localization of tumor by endoclip placement (*arrow*) and post-procedure radiograph

patient, failure to easily identify the lesion (even with preoperative marking) can become exasperating, and dissection may become paralyzed by the lack of confirmation of the target lesion. A large omentum, enlarged appendices epiploicae, and abundant retroperitoneal and mesenteric fat can all lead to the tattoo mark not being seen. This can be especially problematic when attempting to use a medial-to-lateral mobilization technique, which often involves initial proximal vessel ligation. One would be hesitant to perform this "point of no return" maneuver without first identifying the tattoo. Tattoos in the region between the hepatic flexure and the sigmoid colon are particularly at risk for such difficulties given the size and weight of the omentum in the obese patient. Intraoperative colonoscopy certainly is often available in most operating rooms, but this can be time-consuming, has potential drawbacks related to sterility, and any bowel distension in the obese patient will be disastrous. As such, the surgical team can expend considerable energy and time that otherwise could be invested later in the case where it is truly needed. If intraoperative colonoscopy is used to help localize the tattoo marking, we recommend $CO_2$ instead of air insufflation, as this will dissipate from the bowel and cause less bowel distention.

Techniques for localization prior to operation include both imaging and endoscopic means. As said, larger lesions can be seen on barium enema or on CT scan. The operating surgeon can also repeat the colonoscopy to confirm the lesion location, with two methods classically utilized for marking. First, an abdominal radiograph is taken with the tip of the scope at the lesion (Fig. 29.2). Second, an endoscopic clip can be placed at the lesion and abdominal films performed immediately after colonoscopy (Fig. 29.3).

Preoperative marking with abdominal radiographs also allows you to identify (prior to surgery) lesions that do not readily fit into standard segmental resections (i.e., right or sigmoid colectomy). This would include lesions between the hepatic flexure and the descending colon. In a challenging patient such as obese patients, this prepares the surgeon and the patient ahead of time and enhances the execution of the plan. Surgeons can also more accurately counsel patients both for what to expect in the operating room and potential changes in postoperative function. For example, if both are under the impression that a lesion is in the "sigmoid colon" and then to find it in the proximal descending colon or splenic flexure, this will demand an entirely new plan for resection which is technically much more difficult in the obese patient. In essence, the goal remains to pursue any means possible to reduce the likelihood of a preventable "surprise" at the time of operation that will impact the execution of the operative plan.

## Alterations of Anatomy and the Technical Challenge of the Obese Patient

The fundamental difference in obese patients is the loss of abdominal domain with laparoscopy and increased abdominal wall thickness. In male pattern obesity or central obesity, the former can be expected to be more of a problem. This is the result of the abundant retroperitoneal fat as well as intraperitoneal adipose tissue that diminishes the volume of space created by pneumoperitoneum and reduces overall laparoscopic perspective and visualization. The larger and heavier bowel along with its associated bulky mesentery proves much more difficult to manipulate and retract with the miniature end effectors of laparoscopic instrumentation. In addition, retraction of the small bowel proves much more problematic, with limited "room" in the abdomen and requires systematic and disciplined techniques, as simple positional changes and the effect of gravity are less effective. Mesenteric thickness makes dissection and control of vascular structures much more tedious and stressful, as major vessels are not only not readily identified but also more difficult to control if bleeding occurs. Mesenteric obesity also shortens effective bowel length and impacts various anastomotic techniques. Essentially, every aspect of surgery is made more challenging in the obese patient, and you must prepare specifically for such an endeavor.

One such way to overcome this is to increase the pneumoperitoneum and create a more "doming effect." Some have suggested using two insufflators to accomplish this. However, cardiopulmonary compromise, as indicated by hypercarbia or hypotension, can result due to decreased venous return. This must be anticipated and monitored closely by the surgical and anesthesia team with appropriate cardiovascular monitoring as indicated, taking into account underlying cardiopulmonary conditions, effect of bowel preparation, expected blood loss, and duration of surgery.

## Ergonomic Issues in Laparoscopic Colectomy in the Obese Patient

The man-machine environment of the laparoscopic operative suite presents certain ergonomic challenges for the operating surgeon and team. Design of instruments, monitor height and location, table height, and surgeon positioning and posture all affect the surgeon's experience and as a consequence, the technical conduct of the operation. During laparoscopic operations, surgeons suffer from high levels of mental and physical stress. After a certain time—~4 h—the so-called surgical fatigue syndrome may occur. This syndrome includes mental fatigue, degradation of manual dexterity, and importantly a reduced capacity for good judgment results [26]. This can be further exacerbated when operating on the obese patient.

To help overcome this, you must consider specific ramifications of the girth of the patient: alterations in the vertical height of the operating field (i.e., ventral surface of the patient), the increased lateral distance to the operative field, and the consequences for surgeon position and posture. Surgeons must consider step stools to return hand and wrist height to the more comfortable posture with optimal height at level of elbows [27]. As the ports will be further away from the surgeon's center of gravity, flexion and adduction of the shoulder occurs. This again reduces ergonomic efficiencies and exacts a physical toll. Seemingly trivial, these physical challenges will be magnified over the course of a longer operation. Fatigue and mental stress contributes to frustration and intolerance of additional procedural difficulties that are naturally expected to occur in a complex operation as laparoscopic colectomy. With obese patients, it is simply exacerbated. Therefore, as you prepare for this patient group, identifying means to reduce physical stress and improving ergonomics of surgical technique will enhance your comfort and physical experience, and as a consequence, improve patient surgical outcomes.

## Learning Curve for Laparoscopic Colectomy in the Obese Patient

Another concept to consider is a learning curve that is specific to complex operations—in this case the obese patient. In general, the learning curve for laparoscopic colectomy has been well described as being longer than that for other laparoscopic procedures, varying first by specific procedure (right vs. left vs. total colectomy) [28]. In regard to patient-related factors, obesity presents a greater technical challenge and results in a longer learning curve to achieve proficiency. Sarli et al. demonstrated that when operating on obese patients. Risk of conversion decreased with increased surgical team experience [29]. Yet the learning curve must also account for various pathologic conditions such as those related to inflammation (i.e., diverticulitis or Crohn's disease) as well as locally advanced cancer. Therefore, especially early in your practice experience and learning curve, it is imperative that you consider all factors which make an operation complex: (1) patient-related factors such as obesity or severe comorbid conditions; (2) disease-related factors such as severe inflammation complicated by phlegmonous masses or fistulas; (3) large neoplasms demonstrating local invasion; (4) complex resections such as left colectomy, extended resections, and total abdominal or proctocoloectomy; or (5) acute emergent presentation of disease such as perforation, hemorrhage, or large bowel obstructions. Such factors should each be considered into the decision to attempt laparoscopic colectomy.

Given that over 1/3 of our patient population now presents with BMI > 30, the young surgeon unfortunately cannot avoid (for long) performing laparoscopic colectomy in this challenging group. To that end, the senior author (HDV) strongly encourages that any laparoscopic colectomy in an obese patient, even when straightforward on all other accounts (i.e., right colectomy, benign disease without inflammation or fistula), should be scheduled as an early first case without a significant number of cases to follow, whenever possible. In addition, it would be advisable for skilled assistants to be present (preferably a more experienced laparoscopic surgeon or partner) for the duration of the procedure. Such assistance improves retraction and exposure, reduces surgeon stress, and undoubtedly leads to better intraoperative decision-making and clinical outcomes for patients.

## Operative Details (Table 29.2)

### Positioning and Securing the Obese Patient

The weight and proportions of the obese patient impact many practical issues of laparoscopic colectomy. The operating room bed and leg stirrups must accommodate the weight of the patient, as both components have specific weight restrictions, and manufacturers offer product models to accommodate extreme patient weights. The traditional tucking of the arms of the patient may not be possible due to the breadth of the torso, and arms may need to be placed outstretched and secured (Fig. 29.4). While arm sleds enable the arms to be placed alongside of the torso, such positioning forces the surgeon and assistants further away from the operative field and causes the aforementioned ergonomic difficulties for the operating team. Additionally, more padding and attention to proper securing to the arm boards is often required to reduce peripheral nerve injuries (Videos 29.1 and 29.2).

A system for fixation of the patient to the OR table must be reliable given the weight of the patient and the extremes of rotation and head down positioning of that must be performed to allow gravity to assist in intraperitoneal exposure (Fig. 29.5). The senior author prefers taping around the patient's chest and operating room table three times using 3-in. wide cloth or silk tape to provide fixation (Fig. 29.6). Others describe methods including beanbags and gel pads directly beneath the patient's torso. In any case, we suggest that, irrespective of the method, prior to prepping the patient and draping, the patient should be placed in the anticipated table positions (extreme rotation, Trendelenburg) in order for all OR personnel to observe for any movement of the patient's torso or extremities (Fig. 29.7).

**Table 29.2** Intraoperative considerations

| |
|---|
| • Patient positioning |
| – Predisposed to increased risk of intraoperative nerve injuries from compression or traction |
| – More prevalent nerve injuries due to stretch or pressure sores in obese |
| • Experienced first assistant(s) |
| • Additional trocar placement as needed |
| – 4 to 6 trocars to assist with retraction and exposure |
| • Longer ports and instruments |
| – Standard (100 cm) vs. longer versions (150 cm) |
| – Estimate by positioning the instruments on abdomen before actually making port site incisions |
| • Avoid umbilicus for hand port |
| – Umbilical location more caudal in obese population |
| • Early recognition for need for conversion |
| • Energy devices for intracorporeal vessel ligation |
| – Shortened, thickened mesentery |
| – EnSeal® or LigaSure® device |
| • Complete omental dissection as necessary to facilitate specimen extraction |
| • Low threshold to enlarge extraction site, due to larger specimen size |
| • Port site closure device |

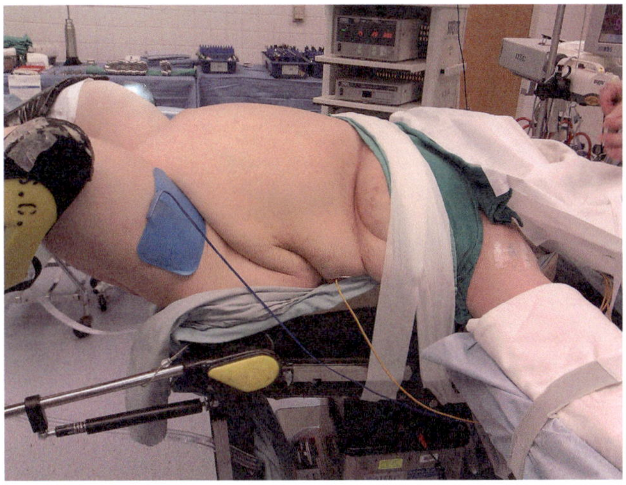

**Fig. 29.4** Positioning in a patient with a BMI of 55. (Courtesy of Conor Delaney, MD)

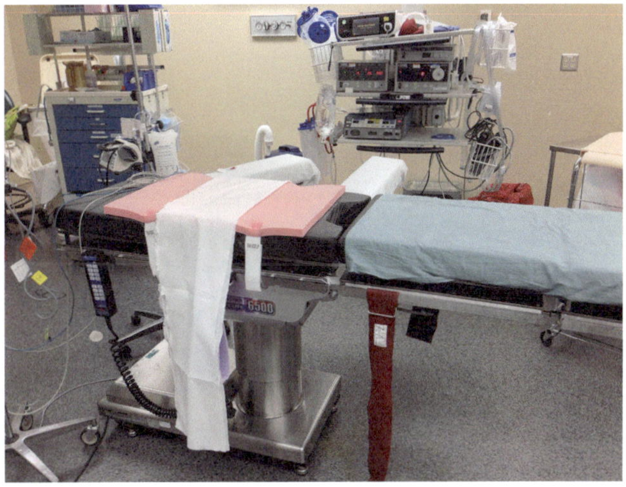

**Fig. 29.5** Preparing for operating table positioning with additional padding

### Ureteral Stent Insertion: Selective Use

On one hand, increased retroperitoneal adipose tissue may be protective of retroperitoneal structures such as the ureter;

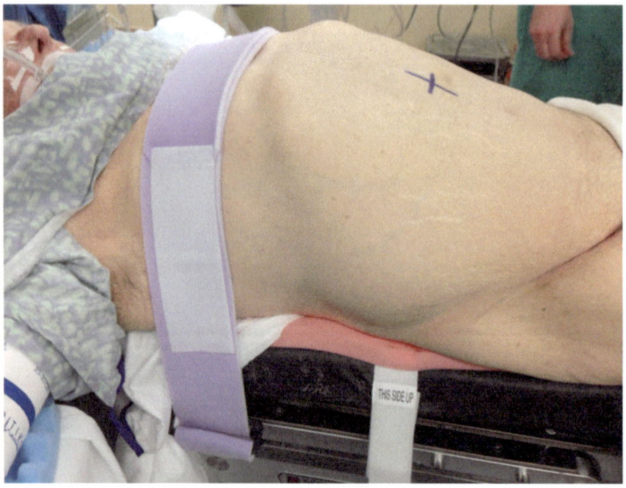

**Fig. 29.6** Chest Strap to secure the patient to the table. 3″ silk tape may be used as an alternative

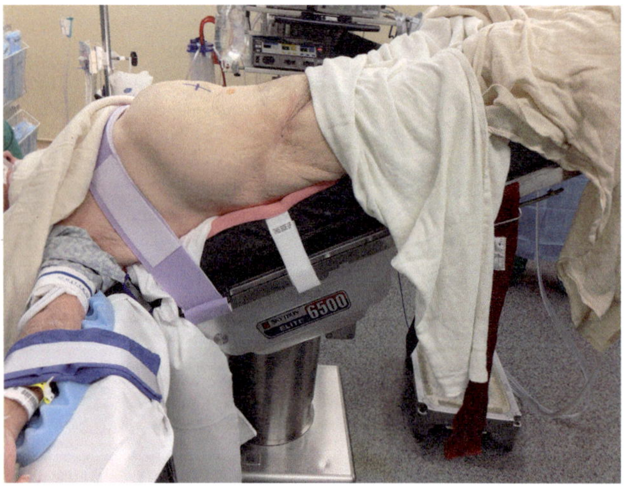

**Fig. 29.7** Reverse Trendelenburg demonstrating no shift in the patient with proper securing to the table

yet, excess layers may also make visual identification more challenging. Additionally, if dissection strays from the embryologic planes, meddlesome bleeding may occur obscuring the laparoscopic perspective. Generally, good practice dictates ureteral identification prior to division of the inferior mesenteric artery or superior hemorrhoidal artery. In the case of a hand-assisted colectomy, you can palpate the ureter. Ureteral stents can also be helpful in identifying the ureter, as well as noticing a ureteral injury (should it occur) intraoperatively, but have not been shown to prevent one. A trade-off exists then with either additional time inserting stents versus meticulous dissection to establish the proper planes and identify the ureter. We feel that insertion of ureteral stents should be considered optional; though early in your experience and learning curve, this may reduce stress regarding this critical step. Exceptions where you may more strongly consider stent insertion would be cases where inflammation can be identified adjacent to the path of the ureter and iliac vessels (e.g., Crohn's iliopsoas abscess, posterior type diverticular abscess). In the case of prior radiation, a previous left colectomy or history of pelvic surgery, you should anticipate distorted anatomy, dense adhesions, and an irregular course of the ureter. Lastly, in the case of a solitary kidney, you may be inclined to pursue preoperative ureteral stent insertion.

## Ports and Exposure Techniques

Port sites must take into account the alterations in the anatomic landmarks, specifically the umbilicus, in regard to port locations (Fig. 29.8). Due to the large pannus, the umbilicus may not correlate to the traditional mid-abdominal view you may be accustomed to in normal-sized patients. In fact, for morbidly obese patients, it is often best to ignore the umbilicus altogether. On the other hand, the bony prominences of the costal margin and the iliac crest, the symphysis pubis, and

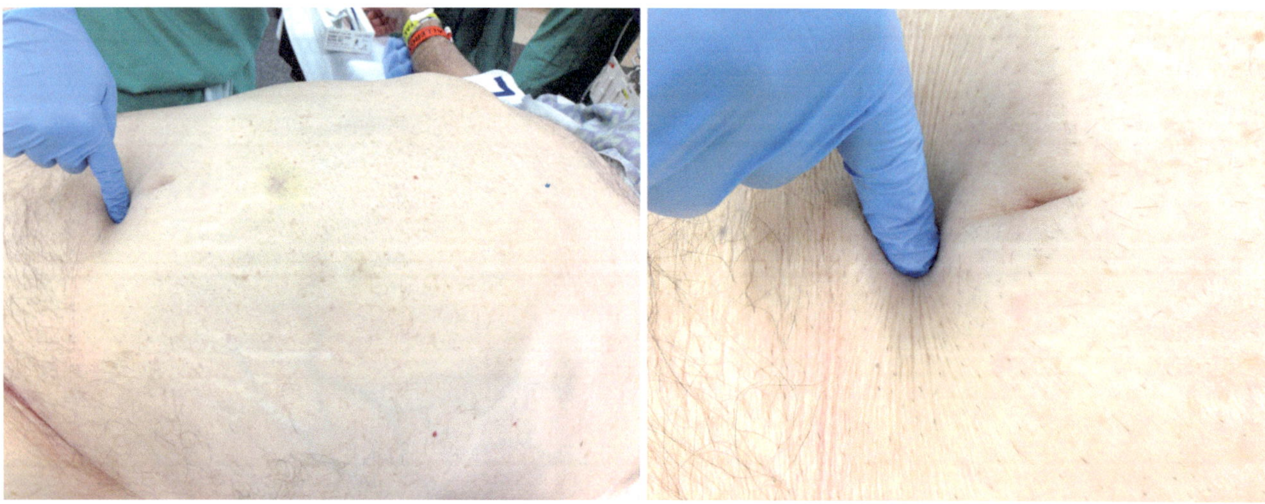

**Fig. 29.8** Low-lying umbilicus in the obese patient [Waist-to-hip Ratio (WHR) 1.2]

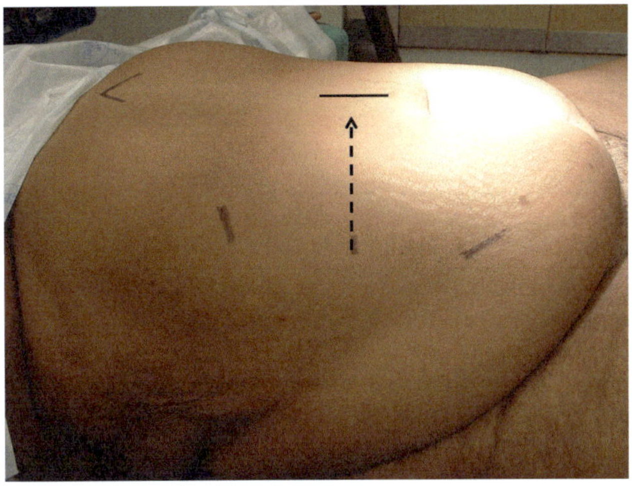

**Fig. 29.9** Wound extraction site (hand port) based on bony prominences. (*Arrow* indicates the distance between the lateral trocar site and the wound extraction site)

the xiphoid process will not vary with abdominal girth or body mass index and will better provide guidance as to the intra-abdominal structures of interest and the best means of exposing such (Fig. 29.9).

Care must also be taken when inserting ports to consider the trajectory and angle given the torque and levering phenomena required for visualizing and working in different quadrants of the abdomen. Such torque may result in enlargement of the fascial defect and must be considered when closing the abdomen, as they may be a source of subsequent hernias and bowel obstruction. The ports themselves may also need to be extra long, especially with the super-obese (BMI > 50) patient. Generally, standard ports are of adequate length. Lastly, prior to incision and insertion, you should sketch out the port sites considered and simulate reach and position of instruments. You can then anticipate the functionality of ports and determine whether or not you have adequate length of the instruments.

Generally, the number of ports will be greater when performing a colectomy in the obese patient. Due to the lessened effect of gravity and lack of intra-abdominal room, exposure and retraction of the small bowel and its mesentery require more instruments to keep the bowel out of the way. You should have a low threshold to place additional ports to accomplish retraction of the small bowel to avoid inadvertent enterotomies, worse visualization, longer operative times, and increased frustration. In the case of left colectomy, Leroy et al. employed five and six ports liberally with one port committed purely for retracting the small bowel mesenteric root [30]. In any case, five to six ports would indicate that perhaps as many as two assistants would be required to help the operating surgeon in the case of a left colectomy. Most would agree that left colectomies present a higher degree of complexity than the simpler right colectomy, and studies examining the respective learning curves comparing right to left validate this notion [28]. Thus, when considering performing a complex colectomy in a difficult patient, such as the obese patient, ensure adequate access and exposure.

Lastly, gravity and extreme patient positioning must be maximized and dynamic. One must constantly engage the anesthesia team to alter the table position facilitating the effects of gravity and exposure. The multiple quadrants of dissection and mobilization mandate continuous alterations in the table and patient position, and the team must anticipate such frequent changes along with the implications for other accessories such as Mayo stands, instrument tables, and video monitors and towers.

## Hand-Assisted Laparoscopic Colectomy (HALS)

Hand-assisted laparoscopic colectomy represents a distinct technical variation of laparoscopic surgery. This involves insertion of the surgeon's hand into the abdomen through an incision that ultimately serves as the wound for specimen extraction. The variation of this technique offers a pragmatic approach in the obese patient given the technical limitations and challenges described. Specifically, the surgeon's hand provides an efficient and atraumatic means of retraction and exposure. In the case of a thickened mesentery, return of palpation improves identification of critical structures and enables safe dissection of the mesentery. Lastly, palpation restores one's sense of proprioception and thus improves dissection in an abdominal cavity with diminished space and reduced visual cues. Difficult to validate and objectify, but perhaps the greatest attribute of the hand-assisted technique, it restores a surgeon's confidence and sense of control where typically the obese patient humbles and frustrates surgeons. Time motion analysis study and other studies [31–33] examining the hand-assisted effect using simulators [34] indicate technical advantages of this hybrid technique as compared to conventional laparoscopic colectomy technique.

In the obese patient, HALS may in fact be preferable, although data remains sparse regarding this specific patient group. The Cleveland Clinic compared HALS versus conventional multiport laparoscopic (LAP) colectomy, finding the HALS cohort experienced significantly fewer conversions to open (3.5 % vs. 12.7 %) [34]. Additionally, incision size was larger in the HALS group, but by only 1.3 cm (7.0 vs. 5.7 cm). Postoperative outcomes including length of stay, operative time, morbidity, and mortality did not differ between the two groups. Interestingly, patients converted to open experienced worse outcomes in terms of length of stay, blood loss, and OR time when compared to successfully performed HALS or traditional laparoscopy.

However, you must also realize that HALS is unique when compared to conventional multiport laparoscopic colectomy. Specific to the obese patient, nuances exist in regard to the optimal port locations and specifically the hand port that serves the additional purposes of specimen extraction and aid in performing the anastomosis. Most importantly, the surgeon's hand must be inserted in the most ergonomically efficient position thereby facilitating all aspects of operative technique: retraction, dissection, mesenteric isolation, and *all the while, preserving laparoscopic perspective*. One of the greatest criticisms of hand-assisted surgery involves the potential compromise of the laparoscopic perspective, and in the obese patient where loss of domain already reduces laparoscopic views, the configuration of hand port and laparoscopic camera location makes it all that more critical. For the occasional practitioner, hand-assisted laparoscopic colectomy can be foreign and frustrating at a baseline, and it would be inadvisable to only attempt to perform a new technique in one of the most challenging circumstances (i.e., obesity).

First, placement of the hand port should enable you to reach to all quadrants of the abdomen (Fig. 29.10). This is particularly imperative as the size of the pannus makes a Pfannenstiel site challenging and in those patients with central obesity (Fig. 29.11). Therefore, the senior author prefers the midline wound for hand port. Remember, the port must facilitate all aspects of the operation including exteriorization of the specimen, assessing the mesenteric blood supply, and ultimately anastomosis of the bowel. Remembering that the umbilicus inaccurately reflects intra-abdominal anatomic structures including mesenteric position craniocaudally, it is crucial that this port be placed cranial to the umbilicus. In the case of right colectomy, this enables exteriorization of both the proximal (terminal ileum) and distal (transverse colon) limbs to reach the wound for anastomosis. Placed too inferior, the middle colic and transverse colon mesentery will limit the reach of the transverse colon. You will thereby struggle and place on tension this part of the mesentery, which ultimately could prove disastrous and cause mesenteric venous bleeding. In the case of left colectomy, the midline wound again allows for an easier exteriorization of the entire left colon, including the splenic flexure, and again allows performance of all the important steps of assessing adequate perfusion of the marginal artery and the anastomosis. In the case of left-sided colectomy—including low anterior resection—I routinely divide the marginal artery with scissors *extracorporeally* and allow it to bleed freely verifying pulsatile flow. Attention to this detail assures well-perfused bowel for anastomosis.

The supraumbilical abdominal wall generally is the thinnest in the obese patient, and by placing the hand port in this location, you do not have to work against the heaviest aspect of the pannus. A standard hand port can also traverse the subcutaneous fat to enter the peritoneum to maintain a good seal. This location is also more versatile. In the event

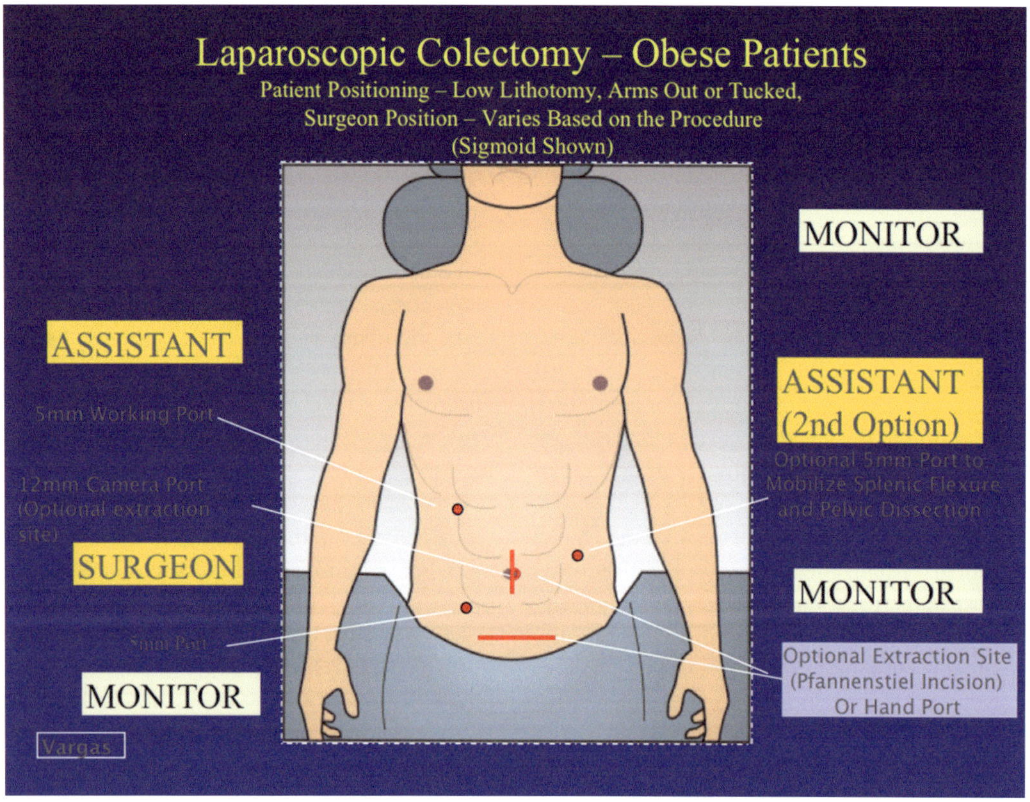


**Fig. 29.10** Trocar and hand port placement for colectomy in the obese patient

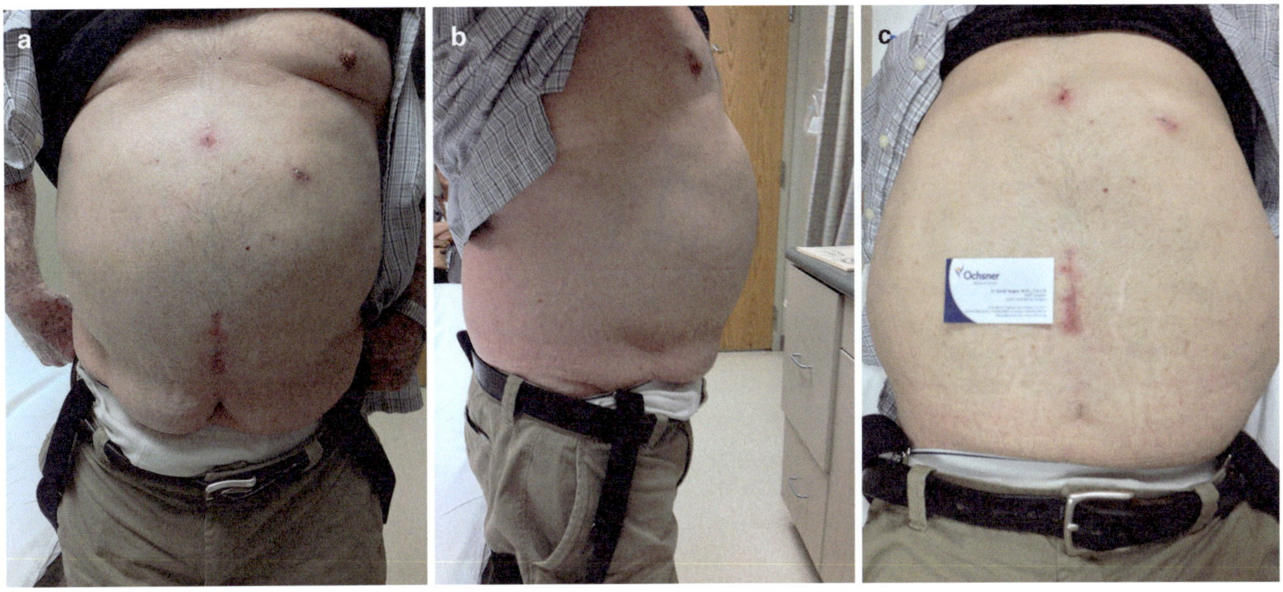


**Fig. 29.11** Central obesity

conversion occurs, extension of this wound can easily convert to a midline laparotomy. For all these reasons, I feel the midline wound for hand port placement facilitates all aspects of HALS colectomy and proves ergonomically efficient.

This is not to say that surgeons should attempt a new technique under challenging circumstances such as obesity. Too often, surgeons resort to HALS only after conventional laparoscopic techniques have foundered. Unfortunately, existing port sites have not been optimally placed for HALS colectomy, adding to the fatigue and frustrations. This failure to progress will (falsely) negatively influence impressions of the subsequent HALS portion of the procedure. For HALS to be successful, you must first be willing to explore and practice the technique under less difficult circumstances and then consider its use in more challenging conditions such as the obese patient. Then when you progress onto HALS use in the obese patient, I would strongly recommend starting the case with the hand in place (versus straight laparoscopy) in order to consciously place the ports and the hand port in the optimal positions.

## Dissection and Mobilization

In general, you must be familiar with the spectrum of mobilization approaches when operating on the obese patient. Specifically, medial-to-lateral exposure, in spite of potential for additional ports and assistants, may still be challenging and inaccessible. Thus, in the case of right colon mobilization, the inferior approach to the cecum and ileal mesentery may in fact be simpler. Similarly, lateral-to-medial dissection of the left colon often allows one to avoid the small bowel altogether, as the left colon mesentery acts as a shield. One must consider all mobilization techniques and assume that "one size does not fit all," and variations or combinations of mobilization techniques may be necessary.

Dissection with energy devices reduces troublesome minor bleeding that further diminishes exposure due to absorption of light. The senior author prefers ultrasonic dissection (Harmonic Scalpel, Ethicon, Cincinnati, OH), while others prefer the LigaSure (Covidien, Samford, CT) or EnSeal (Ethicon, Cincinnati, OH). These instruments, while costlier than scissors and cautery, reduce minor bleeding and provide value to the surgeon in regard to performing a cleaner, less bloody dissection and thus better visualization. In addition, they allow for both dissection and hemostasis, thus minimizing instrument exchange and increasing efficiency (Video 29.3).

Mobilization in the obese patient must be thorough and to a greater extent. You must be committed to "overmobilizing"—high ligation of vessels, complete mobilization back to the root of the mesentery, and dissection of more omentum off the transverse colon—as the obese patient's mesentery by virtue of its inherent thickness becomes foreshortened. Tension on the anastomosis, especially when performing left-sided resection, becomes a much greater potential issue when operating on the obese patient. In addition, performing extracorporealization of the specimen, as well as segments of bowel that are used for the anastomosis, through a thickened abdominal wall is much more difficult if adequate mobilization is not performed. This can result in poor visualization, inadvertent tearing of the mesentery in attempt to get the bowel to reach, and increased complications.

## The Omentum

The greater omentum becomes yet another repository for excess calories and increased adipose tissue. The mass, volume, and complexity of the layers of this organ will challenge even experienced surgeons. The omental enlargement and the technical difficulties one encounters when attempting to manipulate and dissect in these patients surprise and frustrate. Irrespective of the colectomy performed, right or left, you must confront and address the omentum. As usual, you must dissect the omentum off of the colon or divide the omentum during mobilization of the either of the flexures, with division of some portion of the omentum generally occurring during right colectomy given the fusion at the right side of the gastrocolic ligament. However, invariably, the omentum develops adhesions to the ascending colon, to descending colon, and to other aspects of the peritoneum. This often occurs without yet considering the potential presence of adhesions due to a specific pathologic condition serving as indication for operation. These additional adhesions generally are not particularly difficult to dissect but are more an issue of patience and persistence. Execution of the plan thus becomes the test of one's conviction and skill. Furthermore, simply placing the omentum over the top of the transverse colon into the upper abdomen is often a difficult, if not impossible, task simply due to the loss of domain overlying the stomach and liver.

Be aware that given the size of the specimen and the size of the omentum, it is very difficult to exteriorize the ensemble through a 6 cm incision; therefore, partial omentectomy is sometimes necessary just for the purpose of retrieving the specimen. It goes without saying that if the indication for surgery is neoplasia, you must perform en bloc resection and mandate enlargement of the incision. Lastly, if omentectomy is not the decision, you must be cognizant of preserving the blood supply to the remnant. The main blood supply for a pedicled omental graft should be based upon the left gastroepiploic artery.

In many respects, the intraoperative management of the omentum provides a microcosm of the entire endeavor of laparoscopic colectomy in the obese patient—surprisingly difficult and physically and mentally challenging—testing one's commitment and skill.

## Wound Extraction Site

The position of the specimen extraction wound should take into account the purpose of the wound. In addition to the retrieval of the specimen, this wound also enables some mesenteric division and anastomosis. While totally intracorporeal anastomosis has been described [35], the majority of surgeons still rely upon the wound extraction site to facilitate

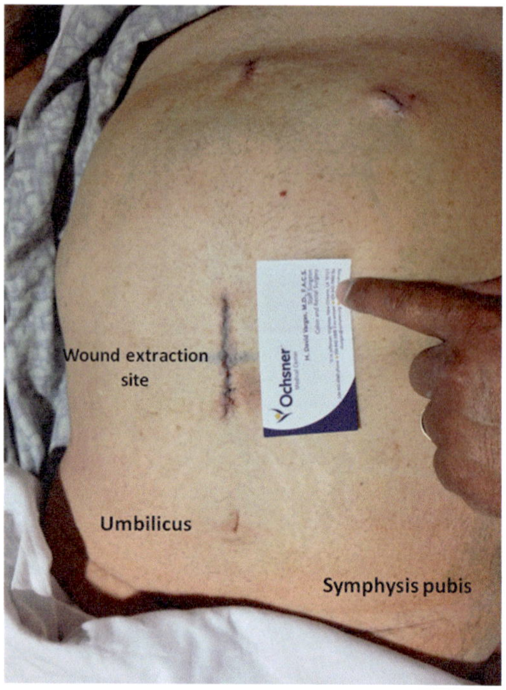


**Fig. 29.12** Hand port (and wound extraction) for a right colectomy

anastomosis, and thus, most exteriorize the mobilized bowel to be resected. This wound almost always will be larger in the obese patient merely because of the increased volume of the specimen (Fig. 29.12).

In the obese patient, it is unlikely that the wound will easily accommodate both the proximal and distal bowel and their thickened mesenteries for resection, as is often the case in right colectomy. To deal with this, you can either divide one end intracorporeally or deliver sequentially the proximal then distal aspects of the bowel to be divided. In the case of left colectomy, generally surgeons divide the distal bowel intracorporeally and then delivering the left colon is less of an issue.

Major vessels must be divided intracorporeally to avoid tearing of the shortened mesentery upon exteriorization. In addition, invariably there will be some portion of the mesentery (especially near the margin of the bowel) to be resected that still must be divided. Importantly, this can be divided within the extraction site if the bowel is mobilized adequately. In the case of right colectomy, full mobilization of the hepatic flexure with division of the right colic artery and the right branch of the middle colic artery will facilitate exteriorization and avoid the dreaded tearing of the mesentery, which, if it involves venous branches of the middle colic vein, proves catastrophic and often necessitates urgent conversion. In the case of left colectomy, we advocate full mobilization of the splenic flexure to the ligament of Treitz with high ligation of the IMA and often division of the IMV at the ligament of Treitz. Due to the shortened mesentery,

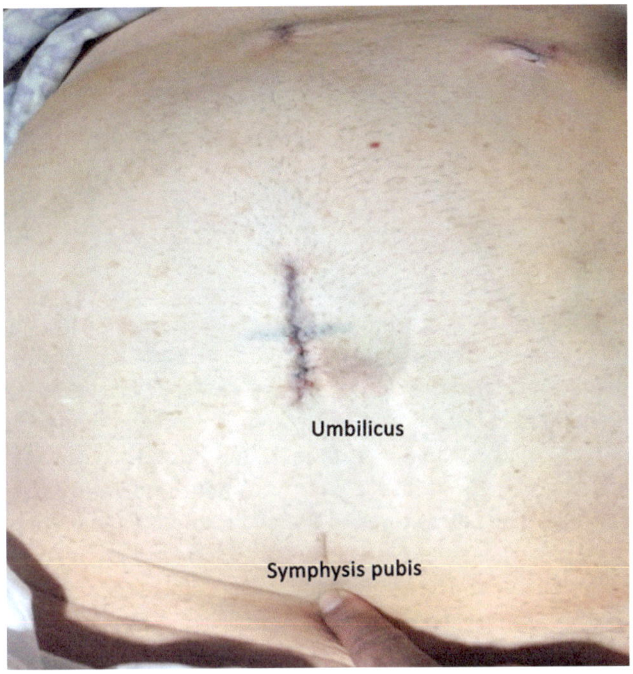


**Fig. 29.13** Notice the inferior umbilicus in this patient with a BMI 30 and WHR of 1.2

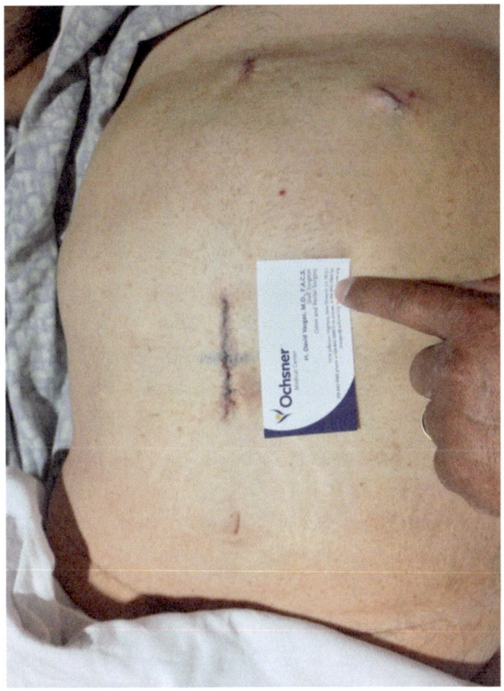

**Fig. 29.14** Hand-port incision superior to the umbilicus

"overmobilization"—i.e., more mobilization than what one would normally perform for a normal body habitus patient—often will reduce the possibility of any issues related to tension and subsequent need to further dissect and mobilize after the specimen has been removed.

Lastly, the most critical element of the operation—the anastomosis—must then be accomplished, and the specimen extraction wound usually again plays a role. In the case of right colectomy, the two ends of bowel are exteriorized and anastomosed by the technique of choice. Again, thoughtful consideration should take into account that the umbilicus tends to be lower due to the effects of the weight of the pannus (Fig. 29.13). Exteriorizing the transverse colon can therefore be difficult if the specimen extraction wound is too low. Surgeons will then be forced to extend the wound cephalad to effect exteriorization of the transverse colon for anastomosis. To avoid this, the author bases his extraction wound on bony prominences: the midpoint of the specimen extraction wound is the midpoint between the costal margin and the iliac spine in the anterior axillary line. This midline vertical wound will be positioned just caudal to the third portion of the duodenum facilitating exteriorization of the hepatic flexure and transverse colon in the case of right colectomy and serves the same purpose well for exteriorization of the splenic flexure and transverse colon in the case of left-sided resections. In the obese patient, the wound will tend to be cranial or cephalad to the umbilicus (Fig. 29.14). Undoubtedly, the wound is more conspicuous; however, issues related to cosmesis clearly remain secondary to the ultimate successful outcome of performing a complex operation with a small incision, which remains "dwarfed" by the size of the patient's girth.

## Pelvic Operations

### Essential Technical Adjustments

Pelvic dissections require additional exposure as the urachus, bladder, uterus, prostate, and lateral retroperitoneal fat all conspire to limit visualization. Clearly, additional ports enable insertion of graspers and fan retractors to facilitate traction and countertraction for clarification of the mesorectal fascial plane. Sling retraction of the uterus and bladder using suspension sutures placed percutaneously using heavy suture on a straight needle facilitates anterior visualization (Video 29.4). In addition, a 45° angle laparoscope also provides superior imaging of the deep pelvis anteriorly. These two simple maneuvers have proven critical to conducting deep dissection.

### Strategy for Deep Dissection

Generally, posterior dissection approaching the sacral promontory should be just dorsal to the superior hemorrhoidal artery, thereby avoiding traction and potential dissection of the superior hypogastric nerves. As one dissects onto the mesorectum, this plane can be followed into loose areolar tissue posteriorly that is more familiar to pelvic surgeons. The maximal dissection of this plane should be performed undermining the lateral aspects of the spheroid-shaped mesorectum. The anterior dissection should then be undertaken opening the cul de sac of the pouch of Douglas and identifying the mesorectal fascia anteriorly and dissecting between the leaves of Denonvilliers' fascia. The demonstration of the plane in a female can be enhanced by having an assistant go to the perineum and place an intestinal-sizer instrument into the vaginal vault and displace the vagina ventrally. Once the plane is established, the author prefers placing the fan retractor onto the posterior aspect of the vagina and then retracting the anterior mesorectum posteriorly (Video 29.5). The dissection can then be carried distally to the anorectal ring. In the male patient, the fan retractor is positioned onto Denonvilliers' fascia on the seminal vesicles and then subsequently the prostate gland.

Most importantly, the lateral aspects of the dissection are then undertaken using the planes developed anterior and posterior to guide the dissection. The lateral mobilization of the mesorectum often remains underestimated and arguably represents the most challenging plane to demonstrate due to the redundancy of the lateral tissues. The retroperitoneal adipose tissues displace the mesorectal plane and diminish efforts for appropriate traction and countertraction. The tendency is to dissect more laterally, which oncologically is not necessarily worse; however, such dissection brings into play the branches of the hypogastric artery and anterolaterally the nervi erigentes in a male and the uterine vessels in a female. For obvious reasons, this lateral dissection can prove consequential and potentially disastrous. As we know, the appropriate plane generally is bloodless. Nuisance bleeding suggests imprecise dissection and continued dissection will prove humbling. If this occurs, you should stop and redirect your dissection to another area to find the right plane (e.g., if bleeding occurs while dissecting anterior to posterior in the lateral aspect, change to posterior to anterior or vice versa). Dissection to the pelvic floor and into the hiatus should be confirmed by performing intraoperative digital rectal exam and palpating circumferentially. Overall, the pelvic dissection in an obese patient and especially an obese male with a narrow pelvis represents one of the truly most difficult operations. This demands patience, persistence, meticulous method, and capable and experienced assistants. The reward remains a bloodless field, an intact anal anastomosis and sphincter preservation.

## Wound Management

Wound infections remain the bane of operations in the obese patient. While laparoscopic colectomy reduces wound infections when compared to open colectomy, there remains a linear increase in wound infections seen with increasing body mass index and may still range as high as 20 % according to a recent NSQIP study [36]. Currently, means to reduce wound infections remain theoretic or anecdotal at best. The author utilizes wound protectors for the specimen extraction site and irrigates with pulse evac using a bacitracin-saline solution. The latter serves to debride necrotic fat and dilute bacterial contamination. Anecdotally, I have found a reduced infection rate and have noticed that when infections do occur, the magnitude appears much diminished. Wound abscess and dehiscences seem much more rare when this technique is employed. This is especially true of the obese patient with deep subcutaneous layer. While there is an increased cost of the bacitracin and the pulse evac device, wound infections remain costly and potential savings by avoiding infection easily will be avoided.

**Table 29.3** Postoperative considerations

| |
|---|
| • Early ambulation |
| • Perioperative DVT prophylaxis |
| • Atelectasis |
| • Wound infection |
| • Cardiovascular dysfunction |
| • Pulmonary toilet |

## Postoperative Care and Enhanced Recovery Pathways (ERP)

Generally, postoperative care of the obese patient undergoing laparoscopic colectomy follows standard algorithms (Table 29.3). Although there is no standardized universal pathway, most ERPs involve the following facets of postoperative care: minimally invasive surgical technique, reduced perioperative fluid resuscitation, strategies for reducing postoperative nausea and vomiting, multimodal pain management with reduction in narcotic use, early postoperative feeding and avoidance of nasogastric tubes, early ambulation, and deep venous thromboembolism prevention. Enhanced recovery pathways have been shown to improve postoperative outcomes of colectomy in regard to reduced ileus, postoperative complications, length of stay, and reduced cost [37]. Essentially, there are no contraindications for implementation of ERPs for obese patients and exceptions should be made on a case-by-case basis.

## Venous Thromboembolism (VTE) Prophylaxis

One controversial area of postoperative care that requires attention is duration of VTE prophylaxis. Obesity, malignancy, pelvic dissection, inflammatory bowel disease, and

**Table 29.4** Modified Caprini risk assessment model for VTE in general surgical patients

| 1 Point | 2 Points | 3 Points | 4 Points |
|---|---|---|---|
| • 41–60 years old | • 61–74 years old | • Age >75 years old | • Stroke (<month prior) |
| • Minor surgery | • Major open surgery (45 min) | • History of VTE | • Elective arthroplasty |
| • BMI >25 kg/m$^2$ | • Laparoscopic surgery (45 min) | • Family history of VTE | • Hip, pelvis, or leg fracture |
| • Sepsis (<1 month) | • Malignancy | • Factor V Leiden | • Acute spinal cord injury (<1 month) |
| • Severe lung disease, including pneumonia (<1 month ago) | • Immobile (>72 h) | • HITT history | |
| • Acute MI | • Central venous access | • Congenital hypercoagulable condition | |
| • Inflammatory bowel disease | | | |
| • Congestive heart failure | | | |

| Surgical risk category | Score | Estimated VTE risk in absence of pharmacologic or mechanical prophylaxis | Recommended prophylaxis regimen |
|---|---|---|---|
| Very low | 0 | <0.5 | • Early ambulation |
| Low | 1–2 | 1.5 | • IPC |
| Moderate | 3–4 | 3.0 | • LMWH (30 mg BID or 40 mg daily) |
| | | | • Or UFH (5,000 units subq TID) |
| | | | • Plus IPC |
| High | 5 or greater | 6.0 | • LMWH (extended duration)[b] and IPC |

Adapted from: Gould MK, Garcia DA, Wren SM, et al. Prevention of VTE in nonorthopedic surgical patients: antithrombotic therapy and prevention of thrombosis, 9th ed: American College of Chest Physicians evidence-based clinical practical guidelines. Chest 2012;141: e2275S

*VTE* venous thromboembolic disease, *BMI* body mass index, *MI* myocardial infarction, *HITT* heparin-induced thrombotic thrombocytopenia, *IPC* intermittent pneumatic compression, *LMWH* low molecular weight heparin

[a]Extended duration (3–4 weeks) after postoperatively

colorectal resections are well-described additive risk factors for the development of VTE. Furthermore, colorectal procedures have been associated with a 4–10 % risk of deep vein thrombosis and fourfold higher rate of pulmonary embolism compared to other surgical patients. Therefore, optimizing VTE prophylaxis in the obese colorectal surgery patient is imperative.

Current recommendations regarding VTE prophylaxis in surgical patients have been published by the American College of Chest Physicians (ACCP) and are based on the modified Caprini risk assessment model (Table 29.4). Based on this system, the majority of obese patients undergoing colorectal procedure are classified into the moderate or high-risk group. While these guidelines recommend the use of mechanical (pneumatic compression devices) and chemoprophylaxis (unfractionated heparin or low molecular weight heparin) pre- and postoperatively, there is little consensus regarding the optimal prophylactic regimen dosing and duration of prophylaxis in high-risk patients. ACCP guidelines suggest that high-risk factors, including previous history of VTE and abdominal or pelvic surgery for malignancy, are indications for extended VTE prophylaxis (4 weeks) [38–43]. However, the role of obesity as a high-risk feature is unclear.

Separate from the ACCP guidelines, the bariatric literature and American Society of Bariatric and Metabolic Surgery's (ASBMS) position statement highlight the lack of consensus and insufficient data available to provide recommendations for the duration of VTE prophylaxis in the setting of morbid obesity [44]. Recently published studies, however, suggest decreased VTE complications without increased risk of bleeding when extended VTE prophylaxis is administered after laparoscopic bariatric procedures [45–47]. Of note, definitions of therapy duration are inconsistent in the literature, ranging from 10 to 30 days after discharge. The bariatric population clearly represents those with the most severe form of obesity. Although the bariatric data cannot be directly extrapolated to the colorectal obese population, these results nonetheless highlight the controversial nature and evolving recommendations regarding VTE prophylaxis in the setting of obesity.

## Outcomes of Laparoscopic Colectomy in the Obese Patient

The perception persists that perioperative outcomes are worse among obese patients compared to non-obese patients. Unfortunately, this influences many surgeons' clinical decision-making. Such bias unfortunately often is reinforced by anecdotal experiences. In the case of laparoscopic colectomy, the obese patient in fact benefits from a minimally invasive approach over open colectomy. As is the case in non-obese patients, short-term perioperative outcomes such as return of bowel function, tolerance of a diet, pain, and complications are improved when laparoscopic colectomy is employed.

Yet, when comparing to non-obese population, as expected, outcomes are worse. In a recent systematic review, Makino et al. examined results of prospective comparative trials of laparoscopic colectomy in obese and non-obese patients [48]. The analysis of this collective experience indicates that laparoscopic colectomy in the obese patient represents a greater technical challenge requiring more ports, longer operative time and more often result in conversion to open laparotomy compared to non-obese patients.

In spite of such technical difficulty, the other perioperative outcomes pertaining to morbidity including blood loss, wound infection, anastomotic leak, and mortality were not conclusively shown to be higher in the obese patient population undergoing laparoscopic colectomy [48]. In part, this is a result of differences in the definition of obesity, heterogeneous cohorts, and a few randomized prospective trials. What consistently has been shown is that there is no increased mortality. Future studies hopefully will be designed with improved methodology and provide more conclusive evidence regarding the utility of laparoscopic colectomy in the obese patient and benefits validating the increased effort put forth by surgeons to perform this challenging operation in the obese patient.

## Pearls and Pitfalls

- Expect longer, more technically difficult operations with attendant-increased conversion.
- Special attention must account for changes in the ergonomics of laparoscopic colectomy in the obese patient.
- Bowel preparation reduces intestinal size and weight and should improve visualization and retraction.
- Reduced abdominal domain, along with larger and heavier organs, diminishes operative exposure requiring increased ports and skilled assistants to perform laparoscopic colectomy.
- In the obese patient, hand-assisted laparoscopic colectomy potentially offers the benefit of improved retraction, exposure, and dissection technique.
- Wounds remain at a high risk for infection mandating meticulous technique and decreased threshold to investigate their presence.
- Prolonged prophylaxis to prevent deep venous thrombosis should be considered.

## Conclusion

The obese patient represents a true technical challenge for the general and colorectal surgeon. Unfortunately, diseases often requiring colorectal surgery are impacted by the obese condition, and given the epidemic nature of obesity, you must anticipate increased frequency managing these patients. Laparoscopic colorectal surgery offers potential benefits for such patients. Increased technical difficulty, however, humbles even experienced laparoscopic surgeons. Specific preparation, additional skilled assistants, and operative strategies should be employed to enhance operative outcomes. Hand-assisted laparoscopic colectomy in particular offers practical technical advantages and should be considered part of the armamentarium of the surgeon attempting to apply a minimally invasive approach in those with increased BMI. Finally, it is important to keep in mind that despite the potential struggles, when the colectomy is completed using minimally invasive technique, the obese patient will benefit from improved outcomes.

## References


1. Ogden CL, Carroll MD, Kit B, Flegal KM. Prevalence of obesity in the United States, 2009–2010. NCHS Data Brief. 2012;82:1–8.
2. Deurenberg P, Yap M, van Staveren WA. Body mass index and percent body fat: a meta analysis among different ethnic groups. Int J Obes Relat Metab Disord. 1998;22:1164.
3. Razak F, Anand SS, Shanon H, et al. Defining obesity cut points in a multiethnic population. Circulation. 2007;115:2111–8.
4. Matsuzawa Y, Funahashi T, Nakamura T. The concept of metabolic syndrome: contribution of visceral fat accumulation and its molecular mechanism. J Atheroscler Thromb. 2011;18:629–39.
5. Scaglione R, Di Chiara T, Cariello T, et al. Visceral obesity and metabolic syndrome: two faces of the same medal? Intern Emerg Med. 2009;5:111–9.
6. Despres JP, Lemieux I. Abdominal obesity and metabolic syndrome. Nature. 2006;444:881–7.
7. Matheiu P, Poirer P, Pibarot P, et al. Visceral obesity: the link among inflammation, hypertension and cardiovascular disease. Hypertension. 2009;53:577–84.
8. Janssen I, Katzmarzyk PT, Ross R. Body mass index, waist circumference, and health risk: evidence in support of current National institutes of Health guidelines. Arch Intern Med. 2002;162:2074.
9. Chan DC, Watts GF, Barrett PHR, Burke V. Waist circumference, waist-to-hip ratio and body mass index as predictors of adipose tissue in compartments in men. Q J Med. 2003;96:441–7.
10. Onat A, Avci GS, Barlan MM, Uyarel H, Uzunlar B, Sansoy V. Measures of abdominal obesity assessed for visceral adiposity and relation to coronary risk. Int J Obes Relat Metab Disord. 2004;28(8):1018–25.
11. Armellini F, Zamboni M, Robbi R, et al. Total and intra-abdominal fat measurements by ultrasound and computerized tomography. Int J Obes Relat Metab Disord. 1993;17:209–14.
12. Suzuki R, Watanabe S, Hirai Y, et al. Abdominal wall fat index, estimated by ultrasonography, for assessment of the ratio of visceral fat to subcutaneous fat in the abdomen. Am J Med. 1993; 95:309014.
13. Shuster A, Patlas M, Pinthus JH, Mourtzakis M. The clinical importance of visceral adiposity: a critical review of methods for visceral adipose tissue analysis. Br J Radiol. 2012;85(1009):1–10.
14. Pischon T, Lahmann PH, Boeing H, et al. Body size and risk of colon and rectal cancer in the European prospective investigation into cancer and nutrition (EPIC). J Natl Cancer Inst. 2006;98:920–31.
15. Moghaddam AA, Woodward M, Huxley R. Obesity and risk of colorectal cancer: a meta-analysis of 31 studies with 70,000 events. Cancer Epidemiol Biomarkers Prev. 2007;16:2533–47.

16. Larson SC, Wolk A. Obesity and colon and rectal cancer risk: a meta-analysis of prospective studies. Am J Clin Nutr. 2007; 86:556–65.
17. Dobbins C, DeFontgalland D, Duthie G, et al. The relationship of obesity to the complications of diverticular disease. Colorectal Dis. 2005;8:37–40.
18. Bertin B, Desreumaux P, Dubuquoy L. Obesity, visceral fat, and Crohn's disease. Curr Opin Clin Nutr Metab Care. 2010;13:574–80.
19. Pikarsky AJ, Saida Y, Yamaguchi T, et al. Is obesity a high-risk factor for laparoscopic colorectal surgery? Surg Endosc. 2002; 16(5):855–8.
20. Senagore AJ, Delaney CP, Madboulay K, Brady KM, Fazio VW. Laparoscopic colorectal surgery in obese and non-obese patients: do differences in body mass indices lead to different outcomes? Surg Endosc. 2004;18(10):1452–6.
21. Dostalik J, Martinek L, Vavra P, Andel P, Gunka I, Gunkova P. Laparoscopic colorectal surgery in obese patients. Obes Surg. 2005;15(9):1328–31.
22. Zhou Y, Wu L, Li X, Wu X, Li B. Outcomes of laparoscopic colorectal surgery in obese and nonobese patients: a meta-analysis. Surg Endosc. 2012;26:783–9.
23. Kamoun S, Alves A, Bretagnol F, Lefebre JH, Valleur P, Panis Y. Outcomes of laparoscopic colorectal surgery in obese and non-obese patients: a case-matched study of 180 patients. Am J Surg. 2009;198(3):450–5.
24. Delaney CP, Pokala N, Senagore AJ, et al. Is laparoscopic colectomy applicable to patients with BMI>30? A case-matched comparative study with open colectomy. Dis Colon Rectum. 2005; 48(5):975–81.
25. Park JW, Lim SW, Choi HS, Jeong SY, Oh JH, Lim SB. The impact of obesity on outcomes of laparoscopic surgery for colorectal cancer in Asians. Surg Endosc. 2010;24(7):1679–85.
26. Cuschieri A. Whither minimally access surgery: tribulations and expectations. Am J Surg. 1995;169(1):9–19.
27. Berquer R, Smith WD, Davis S. An ergonomic study of the optimum operating table height for laparoscopic surgery. Surg Endosc. 2002;16(3):416–21.
28. Tekkis PP, Senagore AJ, Delaney CP, Fazio VW. Evaluation of the learning curve in laparoscopic colorectal surgery: comparison of right-sided and left-sided resections. Ann Surg. 2005;242(1):83–91.
29. Sarli L, Rollo A, Cecchini S, et al. Impact of obesity on laparoscopic-assisted left colectomy in different stages of the learning curve. Surg Laparosc Endosc Percutan Tech. 2009;19(2):114–7.
30. Leroy J, Ananian P, Rubino F, et al. The impact of obesity on technical feasibility and postoperative outcomes of laparoscopic left colectomy. Ann Surg. 2005;241:69–76.
31. Sjoerdsma W, Meijjer DW, Jansen A, den Boer KT, Grimbergen CA. Comparison of efficiencies of three techniques for colon surgery. J Laparoendosc Adv Surg Tech A. 2000;19(1):47–53.
32. Claus GP, Sjoerdsma W, Jansen A, Grimbergen CA. Quantitative standardized analysis of advanced laparoscopic surgical procedures. Endosc Surg Allied Technol. 1995;3(4):210–3.
33. Leblanc F, Senagore AJ, Ellis CN, Champagne BJ, Augestad KM, Neary PC, Delaney CP, Colorectal Surgery Training Group. Assessment of comparative skills between hand-assisted and straight laparoscopic colorectal training on augmented reality simulator. Dis Colon Rectum. 2010;53(9):1323–7.
34. Heneghan HM, Martin ST, Kiran RP, et al. Laparoscopic colorectal surgery for obese patients: decreased conversions with the hand-assisted technique. J Gastrointest Surg. 2013;17:548–54.
35. Iorio T, Blumberg D. Totally intracorporeal laparoscopic colectomy (TILC) is associated with similar surgical outcomes in high and low operative risk patients. Surg Laparosc Endosc Percutan Tech. 2013;23(2):154–8.
36. Mustain WC, Davenport DL, Hourigan JS, Vargas HD. Obesity and laparoscopic colectomy: outcomes from the ACS-NSQIP database. Dis Colon Rectum. 2012;55(4):429–35.
37. Stein SL, Delaney CP. Postoperative management. In: Beck DE, Roberts PL, Saclarides TJ, et al., editors. ASCRS textbook of colon and rectal surgery. 2nd ed. New York: Springer; 2011. p. 137–56.
38. Gould MK, Garcia DA, Wren SM, et al. Prevention of VTE in non-orthopedic surgical patient: antithrombotic therapy and prevention of thrombosis, 9th ed: American College of Chest Physicians Evidence-Based Clinical Practice Guidelines. Chest. 2012;141(2 suppl):e227S–77.
39. Rasmussen MS. Preventing thromboembolic complications in cancer patients after surgery: a role for prolonged thromboprophylaxis. Cancer Treat Rev. 2002;28:141.
40. Rasmussen MS, Jorgensen LN, Willie-Jorgensen P, et al. Prolonged prophylaxis with dalteparin to prevent late thromboembolic complications in patients undergoing major abdominal surgery: a multi-center randomized open-label study. J Thromb Haemost. 2006; 4:2384.
41. Kakkar VV, Balibrea JL, Martinez-Gonzalez J, et al. Extended prophylaxis with bemiparin for the prevention of venous thromboembolism after abdominal surgery for cancer: the ACANBESURE randomized study. J Thromb Haemost. 2010;8:1223.
42. Lyman GH, Khorana AA, Kuderer NM, et al. Venous thromboembolism prophylaxis and treatment in patients with cancer: American Society of Clinical Oncology clinical practice guideline update. J Clin Oncol. 2013;31:2189.
43. Aki EA, Terrenato I, Barba M, et al. Extended perioperative thromboprophylaxis in patients with cancer: a systematic review. Thromb Haemost. 2008;100:1176–80.
44. American Society for Metabolic and Bariatric Surgery Clinical Issues Committee. ASMBS updated position statement on prophylactic measures to reduce the risk of venous thromboembolism in bariatric surgery patients. Surg Obes Relat Dis. 2013;9(4):493–7.
45. Borkgren-Okonek MJ, Hart RW, Pantano JE, et al. Enoxaparin thromboprophylaxis in gastric bypass patients: extended duration, dose stratification and antifactor Xa activity. Surg Obes Relat Dis. 2008;4:625–31.
46. Hamad GG, Choban PS. Enoxaparin for thromboprophylaxis in morbidly obese patients undergoing bariatric surgery: findings of the prophylaxis against VTE outcomes in bariatric surgery patients receiving enoxaparin (PROBE) study. Obes Surg. 2005; 15(10):1368–74.
47. Raftoupoulos I, Martindale C, Cronin A, Steinberg J. The effect of extended post-discharge chemical thromboprophylaxis on venous thromboembolism rates after bariatric surgery: a prospective comparison trial. Surg Endosc. 2008;22(11):2384–91.
48. Makino T, Shukla PJ, Rubino F, Milsom JW. The impact of obesity on perioperative outcomes after laparoscopic colorectal resection. Ann Surg. 2012;255(2):228–36.

# Minimally Invasive Surgery in Crohn's Disease Patients

30

Chang Sik Yu

**Key Points**

- Running the entire small bowel is necessary to prevent omitting skip lesions. Manual examination after exteriorization of the bowel is preferable.
- Do not hesitate to convert to hand-assisted or open procedure in complex fistulous condition.
- Advanced procedures such as laparoscopic total proctocolectomy are associated with increased conversion rates and should be attempted only with increased experience and expertise.

## Introduction

Since the early 1990s, a laparoscopic approach to colorectal surgery incorporating various surgical procedures has been applied to many colorectal diseases. Crohn's disease (CD) is a good indication for laparoscopic surgery because it is a benign disease, meaning the challenges associated with oncological conditions, such as a proximal ligation of the vascular pedicle, lymphadenectomy, and direction of mesenteric dissection, do not apply. Furthermore, CD patients are usually young, socially active, and body-image conscious. Therefore, cosmesis and a rapid recovery and return to daily activities are crucial issues for this cohort.

CD is currently incurable, and more than half of surgically treated patients are destined to undergo further surgery. Minimally invasive (MI) surgery is an important consideration for the surgeon as well as the patient, as an MI approach can lead to less adhesion formation and faster recovery.

Although surgical procedures for CD patients are usually limited to reflect the extent and location of the inflammation, the most common laparoscopic procedures are ileocolic resection and stoma creation. A thickened mesentery, inflammatory mass or phlegmon, and enteric fistula can make laparoscopic surgery technically challenging (Fig. 30.1), with complex cases often regarded as relative contraindications. However, even these complex cases may be satisfactorily undertaken with surgical experience and expertise.

The short-term benefits of MI surgery have been shown in randomized controlled trials and meta-analyses, although most trials had a limited sample size and were mainly concerned with the surgical outcomes of ileocolic resections.

## Indications and Contraindications

Although the vast majority of laparoscopic procedures in CD patients are for ileocolic resection, a variety of procedures, including total proctocolectomy, have been successfully attempted. However, these MI procedures may be associated with a high rate of conversion to open procedures, with the presence of a complicated fistula or abscess and recurrent disease identified as risk factors for conversion.

Schmidt et al. [1] analyzed 45 cases of conversion (40 % conversion rate) and found that palpable mass, complicated fistula, preoperative malnutrition, extracecal colonic disease, and steroid administration were risk factors. Moorthy et al. [2], using multivariate analysis, found that surgery for recurrence and the presence of a clinical mass were risk factors for conversion to open procedures (Table 30.1).

Interestingly, the majority of studies on conversion showed comparable postoperative morbidity to surgeries that did not require conversion. This implies, for the experienced surgeon, that laparoscopic surgery can be applied for almost all procedures and comorbidities in patients with CD.

---

**Electronic supplementary material:** Supplementary material is available in the online version of this chapter at 10.1007/978-1-4939-1581-1_30. Videos can also be accessed at http://www.springerimages.com/videos/978-1-4939-1580-4.

C.S. Yu, M.D., Ph.D. (✉)
Department of Colon & Rectal Surgery, Asan Medical Center, University of Ulsan College of Medicine,
388-1 Poongnap-dong, Songpa-gu, Seoul 138-736, Korea
e-mail: csyu@amc.seoul.kr; csyu007@amc.seoul.kr

H.M. Ross et al. (eds.), *Minimally Invasive Approaches to Colon and Rectal Disease: Technique and Best Practices*,
DOI 10.1007/978-1-4939-1581-1_30, © Springer Science+Business Media New York 2015

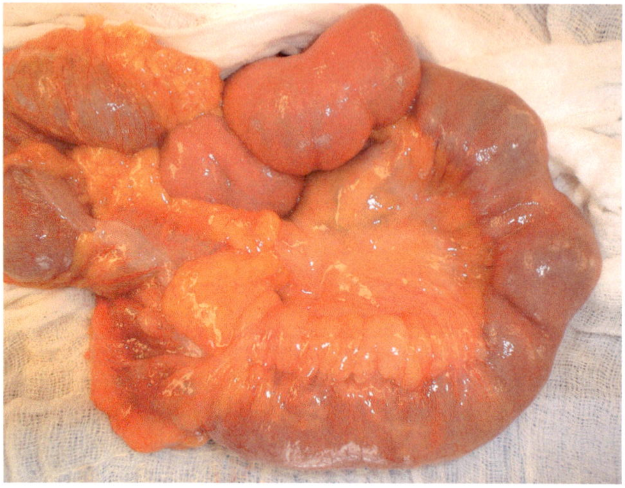

**Fig. 30.1** Crohn's disease of the terminal ileum

**Table 30.1** Risk factors for conversion

| Author | Year | No. of patients | Conversion rate (%) | Risk factors |
|---|---|---|---|---|
| Schmidt [1] | 2001 | 110 | 40 | Internal fistula, smoking, steroid administration extracecal colonic disease, malnutrition |
| Moorthy [3] | 2004 | 48 (26 recurrent vs. 22 primary) | 42.3 vs. 13 | Age, recurrent case, presence of a clinical mass |
| Alves [31] | 2005 | 69 | 30 | Recurrent medical episodes, intra-abdominal abscess or fistula |
| Okabayashi [21] | 2007 | 91 | 13.2 | Vienna classification B3L3/4 |

Obesity is a widely recognized challenge for both open and laparoscopic surgery. Canedo et al. [3] evaluated 213 laparoscopic surgery cases in patients with CD or ulcerative colitis and found a conversion rate of 18 % when the body mass index (BMI) was between 18.5 and 24.9 kg/m$^2$ and 22 % when the BMI was greater than or equal to 25 kg/m$^2$. This difference was not statistically significant. The authors also demonstrated comparable intergroup postoperative complication rates and hospital stays. This implies that being overweight or obese is not a contraindication for laparoscopic surgery for CD or ulcerative colitis.

## Evidence in the Literature

Since the introduction of laparoscopic colorectal surgery, many authors have reported on the short-term outcomes of laparoscopic surgery in patients with CD. However, most studies were conducted at a single center and were case controlled rather than randomized. Furthermore, the vast majority of these studies used ileocolic resection as the operation type in which laparoscopic and open approaches were compared. In this chapter, a review of high-quality studies and more recent evidence is presented.

## Laparoscopic vs. Open Surgery for Ileocolitis

There are only two randomized controlled trials (RCT) in the literature: Milsom's study [4] from the Cleveland Clinic and Maartense's study [5] from three centers in the Netherlands. In both studies, 60 patients were recruited: 31 laparoscopic vs. 29 open, and 30 laparoscopic vs. 30 open, respectively. Patients undergoing elective surgery with disease confined to the terminal ileum and cecum were included. Exclusion criteria were emergency or urgent surgery, multiple disease sites, a history of prior surgery, and obesity (BMI>32 kg/m$^2$). Both studies showed fewer complications and shorter hospital stays in the laparoscopic group. Also, Milsom et al. [4] found faster recovery of pulmonary function, and Maartense et al. [5] showed an earlier return to diet and lower cost in the laparoscopic group. However, there was no significant difference in the use of morphine or the Quality of Life Scale score.

The long-term outcomes of these two RCTs were reported by Stocchi et al. [6] and Eshuis et al. [7] with a median follow-up of 10.5 and 6.7 years, respectively. They concluded that open surgery was more likely to lead to incision hernia and small bowel obstruction. The recurrence rate was comparable between the groups. Eshuis et al. noted better body-image ratings and cosmesis in the laparoscopic group.

Recently, Dasari et al. [8] in their Cochrane review analyzed these RCTs exclusively and found no difference in the perioperative outcomes and reoperation rate for recurrence. They argued that no reliable conclusions could be drawn regarding the benefits of laparoscopic surgery probably because of the limited data available from these two small RCTs.

Other meta-analyses, however, reported faster recovery of bowel function and oral intake, shorter hospital stay, and lower complication rates, with one meta-analysis noting a lower surgical recurrence in laparoscopic patients (Table 30.2). Excluding Dasari's Cochrane review, which had limited inclusion criteria, the other meta-analyses showed a general consensus that there were short-term benefits associated with laparoscopic ileocecal resection for CD [8–12].

Lesperance et al. [13] analyzed Nationwide Inpatient Sample (NIS) data between 2000 and 2004. Among 49,609 resections in patients with CD, only 6 % were performed laparoscopically. They found that an age of less than 35 years old (OR 2.4), female gender (OR 1.4), ileocecal location

**Table 30.2** Meta-analysis of laparoscopic vs. open ileocolic resection for Crohn's disease

| Author | Years | No. of study | No. of patients | Op. time | Recovery of bowel function | Hosp. stay | Morbidity | Recurrence |
|---|---|---|---|---|---|---|---|---|
| Dasari [8] | 2011 | 2 | 120 | – | C | C | C | C |
| Tan [9] | 2007 | 14 | 881 | ↑ | ↓ | ↓ | ↓ | C |
| Polle [10] | 2006 | 14 | 729 | C | ↓ | ↓ | C | – |
| Tilney [11] | 2006 | 15 | 783 | ↑ | ↓ | ↓ | C | – |
| Rosman [12] | 2005 | 16 | 840 | ↑ | ↓ | ↓ | ↓ | ↓ |

C, comparable; ↑, longer; ↓, shorter or lesser; –, nothing stated

(OR 1.5), and undergoing the procedure in a teaching hospital (OR 1.2) were predictors of undergoing laparoscopic surgery for CD. Open surgery was an independent predictor of inpatient complications (OR 3.4).

Lee et al. [14] analyzed the National Surgical Quality Improvement Program (NSQIP) database (2005–2009). They identified 1,917 cases of ileocolic resections for CD, of which 644 (33.6 %) were performed laparoscopically. They found that laparoscopy was associated with a significantly lower rate of 30-day major and minor complications and a shorter hospital stay.

## Laparoscopic Colon Resections

Evidence in support of laparoscopic surgery for Crohn's colitis is lacking, and there are no RCTs for this condition. Instead, there are only a few limited retrospective case-control studies.

The largest series was conducted by Umanskiy and colleagues [15]. They analyzed the data of 125 prospectively collected cases, including 55 (44 %) laparoscopic procedures. The most common procedures were total colectomy and total proctocolectomy with ileostomy. Surprisingly, they reported a shorter mean operative time (212 vs. 286 min, $P=0.032$) in the laparoscopy group, which is a unique result. The authors suggested that this may be due to the high level of experience of the laparoscopic surgeons. Other short-term benefits of laparoscopy included less blood loss, early return of bowel function, and shorter hospital stay.

A case-matched study from the Cleveland Clinic [16] with 27 laparoscopic and 27 open colectomies showed that laparoscopy was associated with a longer operative time (240 vs. 150 min, $P=0.01$), but no other short-term benefits were demonstrated.

Nakajima et al. [17] evaluated 38 patients with Crohn's colitis who underwent subtotal or total colectomies divided into three groups (14 open, 18 hand assisted, and 6 laparoscopic). The operation time for the hand-assisted laparoscopic surgery (HALS) group was shorter than that for the laparoscopic group, but there was no difference in complication rates or blood loss.

The role of HALS in other diseases remains controversial. Orenstein et al. [18] reported favorable outcomes in a HALS group, while Cochrane review by Moloo et al. [19] showed only a decreased conversion rate in HALS groups.

There is no definitive evidence supporting the superiority of laparoscopic surgery or HALS in patients with Crohn's colitis. This may be due to the diversity of disease extent, complexity of surgical technique, and lack of surgical cases in a particular center to enable an RCT to be performed.

## Complex Crohn's Disease

Inflammatory conditions, such as abscess, phlegmon, or enteric fistulas, are frequently associated with CD and make laparoscopic surgery more challenging. Some surgeons have regarded these conditions as relative contraindications for laparoscopic surgery, due to the high conversion rate and postoperative morbidity.

Goyer et al. [20] reviewed 54 cases of laparoscopic Ileocolic resections for complex CD in which 43 % had fistula, 30 % abscess, and 27 % recurrent disease. They reported that the presence of complex CD was significantly associated with increased operation time (214 vs. 191 min, $P<0.05$), increased conversion rate (37 % vs. 14 %, $P<0.01$), and increased use of temporary stoma (39 % vs. 9 %, $P<0.001$). Postoperative morbidity and hospital stay were comparable.

Okabayashi et al. [21] investigated the association of Vienna classification with outcomes following 107 cases of laparoscopic surgery for CD. They found a significant association between conversions and more complicated types of CD (B3, L3/4). However, there was no difference in the rate of complications.

Recently, a case-match study was published by Beyer-Berjot et al. [22]. They compared 11 laparoscopic ileocecal resections for fistulizing CD with 22 matched controls. They found no significant difference in operation time (120 vs. 120 min), conversion rate (9 % vs. 0 %), postoperative morbidity (18 % vs. 32 %), and hospital stay (8 vs. 9 days).

Recurrent CD is found in approximately 50 % of surgically treated CD patients who have had the disease for over 10–15 years. Adhesion and the complex inflammatory condition of

**Table 30.3** Laparoscopic surgery for recurrent Crohn's disease (case-control study)

| Author | Year | Control group | No. of patients | Conversion (%) | Op. time (min) | Complication (%) |
|---|---|---|---|---|---|---|
| Holubar [26] | 2010 | Converted | 30 vs. 10 | 25 | 159 vs. 165 | 10 vs. 30 |
| Pinto [24] | 2011 | Primary laparoscopic | 50 vs. 80 | 32 vs. 18.7 | 201 vs. 182 | 40 vs. 36.2 |
| Chaudhary [25] | 2011 | Primary laparoscopic | 30 vs. 29 | 6.7 vs. 10.3 | 125 vs. 85 | 16.7 vs. 24.1 |
| Aytac [23] | 2012 | Open | 26 vs. 26 | 12 | 169 vs. 158 | 38.5 vs. 69.2 |

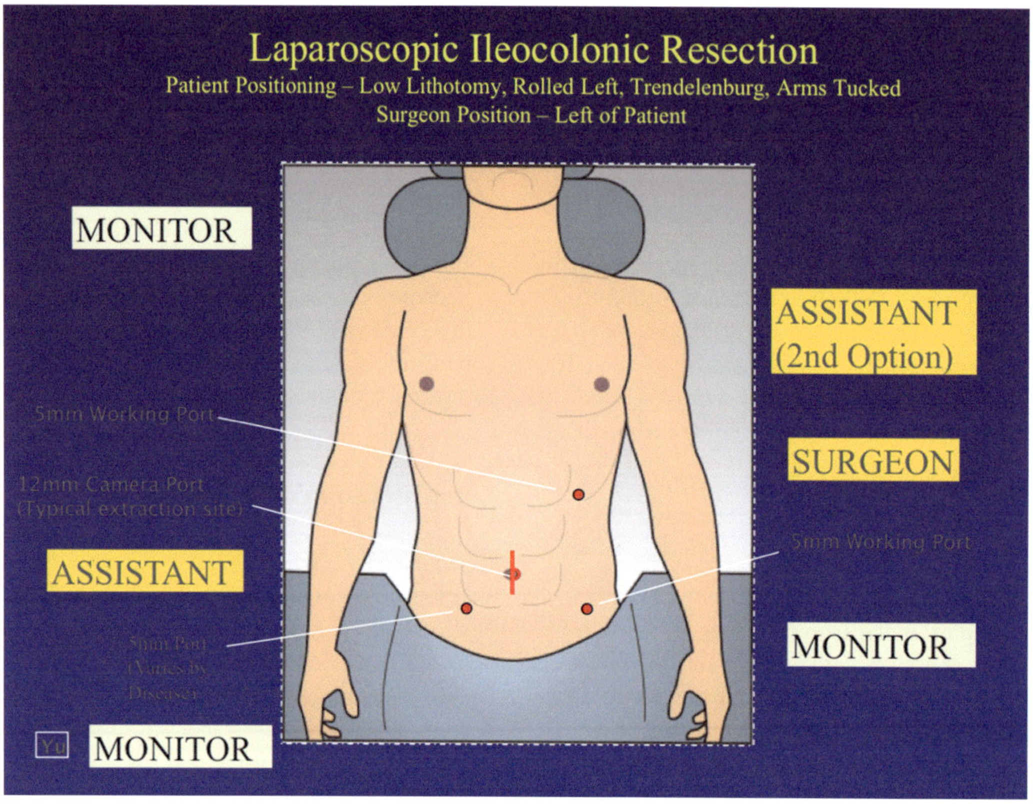


**Fig. 30.2** Trocar placement for a laparoscopic ileocolonic resection

the bowel make these reoperations more difficult, although many surgeons have tried to perform various laparoscopic surgeries for recurrent CD.

Aytac et al. [23] performed a case-matched study to compare the effectiveness of laparoscopic vs. open resection for recurrent CD. Twenty-six patients who underwent various laparoscopic procedures were compared with a matched control group. The conversion rate was 12 %, with adhesions cited as the primary cause. Comparable short-term results were reported except for a decreased wound infection rate in the laparoscopic group.

Pinto et al. [24] and Chaudhary et al. [25] compared primary and reoperative laparoscopy for CD and found similar perioperative and postoperative outcomes. They also found no intergroup differences in the effectiveness and feasibility of the resections. Holubar et al. [26] [27] reported a 20 % conversion rate in laparoscopic re-resection and no increased morbidity in converted cases (Table 30.3).

## Technical Considerations

### Basic Surgical Techniques for Ileocolic Resection

#### Number of Ports

The standard ports are one camera port at the umbilicus and two 5 mm ports at the left iliac fossa and the left flank. Another 5 mm port can be added at the right side for an assistant depending on the particular site of pathology (Fig. 30.2). Recently, single-port or single-incision laparoscopic surgery has been used successfully. The surgical outcomes of this single-incision technique will be discussed in a later section.

#### Running the Bowel (Video 30.1)

Despite the availability of contemporary preoperative imaging modalities, such as CT or MR enterography, thorough

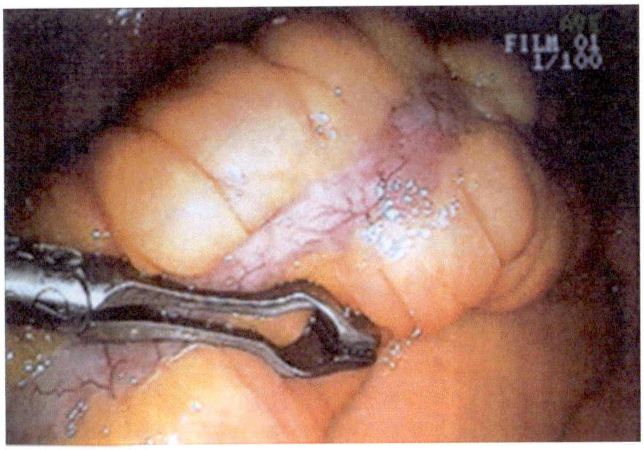


**Fig. 30.3** Laparoscopic view of Crohn's disease bowel with thickened mesentery

intraoperative examination of the entire small bowel, from the Treitz ligament to the ileocecal value, is mandatory for all cases.

The careful application of an atraumatic bowel grasper to the mesentery is strongly recommended in intracorporeal evaluation. However, I recommend extracorporeal manual examination along the mesenteric border after mobilization of the right colon, as this is the best way to prevent omission of a skipped lesion. In particular, careful examination of terminal ileum is needed to rule out an internal fistula.

### Mobilization of the Bowel

A lateral to medial dissection is preferable because of the thickened mesentery, abscess or phlegmon, and enteric fistula (Fig. 30.3). The extent of colonic mobilization should reflect that of the proposed colonic resection. Except for ileocecal resection, mobilization of the hepatic flexure is helpful for the anastomosis.

If the mesenteric thickening is not too severe, a traditional medial to lateral approach can be used without difficulty. Identification of the right ureter is important, especially in a complicated case with abscess or phlegmon.

### Mesenteric Division

It can be performed intracorporeally or extracorporeally, and a variety of energy devices can be used. Extracorporeal mesenteric division is exactly same with open method. Therefore, it is much easier to be performed when inflammatory condition of the mesentery is severe. We decide the appropriate device for vascular division according to size of the vessel and completeness of isolation.

Resection margin has to be minimized for bowel-saving surgery. Supple bowel wall and soft mesenteric border is the point of division. So, I would like to recommend extracorporeal anastomosis after meticulous palpation. Mesenteric or vascular division should be made near the bowel wall to prevent compromise of blood supply to the residual bowel.

### Anastomosis

The most popular methods of performing Ileocolic anastomosis are side to side and functional end to end using two linear staplers. They can be performed intracorporeally [27, 28] or extracorporeally. A seromuscular suture can be added where linear staple lines intersect. The mesenteric defect is left open.

### Complex Fistulous Cases (Video 30.2)

Several types of internal fistula such as entero-enteric and entero-colic are manageable laparoscopically without great difficulty. However, various kinds of internal or external fistulas or severe phlegmons are hard to handle with laparoscopic devices only. At this moment, the surgeon has to decide conversion to open or hand-assisted procedure. It is a wise way to make a decision at the beginning of laparoscopic exploration. Should you encounter a phlegmon with an abscess, it is beneficial to have the suction device readily available to have a large amount of spillage throughout the abdomen. Also, you should have the ability to intracorporeally suture should the need arise. With fistula and abscesses in Crohn's, you may inadvertently get into bowel (or require an enterotomy) to take down the fistula. Closing this (or marking it for extracorporeal closing/resection) is imperative to avoid future complications.

Simple enterovisceral fistulas can be treated by the removal of the diseased small bowel and simple suture closure of the victim organ, such as sigmoid colon or other segment of small bowel. The small opening of the bladder can be left open without suture. However, a Foley catheter remained in place for at least 7 days.

## Hand-Assisted Laparoscopic Surgery (HALS)

Its applicability and potential superiority in Crohn's colitis was described previously. Of note, it may reduce the conversion rate, especially in complex CD.

## Single-Incision Laparoscopic Colectomy (SILC)

Recently, MI surgery has evolved into a single-port laparoscopic surgery. Theoretically, such a minimal incision can provide improved cosmesis, less postoperative pain, and faster recovery. However, there is only limited evidence to support these benefits at this stage. Rijcken et al. [29] analyzed 34 SILC studies on surgical procedures for inflammatory bowel disease, including Ileocolic resections, sigmoid resections, total colectomies, and restorative proctocolectomies. They reported a similar overall complication profile.

Yang et al. [30] in a recent meta-analysis of comparative studies on SILC procedures including those performed for malignant disease compared 467 SILC cases to 539 conventional multiport laparoscopic colectomy (MLC) cases in 15 studies. The SILC group showed a significantly shorter length of stay, reduced incision length, and less blood loss, but there was no difference in postoperative complications. However, the authors stated that prospective randomized trials were needed to provide a higher level of evidence in support of SILC.

## Pearls and Pitfalls

- Be aware of the multiple fistulous connections in a Crohn's patient. What may appear to be straightforward disease may encompass more bowel than at first appearance.
- Run the entire bowel. Just because preoperative imaging did not demonstrate pathology does not mean it is not there.
- Ileo-sigmoid fistulas (or colonic) with disease in both locations may require concomitant resections.
- Do not hesitate to talk to your patients ahead of time about the need for diversion. Often these patients have poor nutrition, are on immunosuppressants, and are prone to poor healing. A temporary diversion, while not ideal, may avoid disastrous complications associated with a leak.

## Conclusion

Laparoscopic surgery for Crohn's disease is safe and feasible. However, its applicability has to be tailored to disease status and surgeon's competency. More randomized controlled trials are needed to determine appropriate selection criteria.

## References

1. Schmidt CM, Talamini MA, Kaufman HS, Lilliemoe KD, Learn P, Bayless T. Laparoscopic surgery for Crohn's disease: reasons for conversion. Ann Surg. 2001;233(6):733–9.
2. Moorthy K, Shaul T, Foley RJ. Factors that predict conversion in patients undergoing laparoscopic surgery for Crohn's disease. Am J Surg. 2004;187(1):47–51.
3. Canedo J, Pinto RA, Regadas S, Regadas FS, Rosen L, Wexner SD. Laparoscopic surgery for inflammatory bowel disease: does weight matter? Surg Endosc. 2010;24(6):1274–9.
4. Milsom JW, Hammerhofer KA, Böhm B, Marcello P, Elson P, Fazio VW. Prospective, randomized trial comparing laparoscopic vs. conventional surgery for refractory ileocolic Crohn's disease. Dis Colon Rectum. 2001;44(1):1–8.
5. Maartense S, Dunker MS, Slors JF, Cuesta MA, Pierik EG, Gouma DJ, et al. Laparoscopic-assisted versus open ileocolic resection for Crohn's disease: a randomized trial. Ann Surg. 2006;243(2):143–9. discussion 150–3.
6. Stocchi L, Milsom JW, Fazio VW. Long-term outcomes of laparoscopic versus open ileocolic resection for Crohn's disease: follow-up of a prospective randomized trial. Surgery. 2008;144(4):622–7. discussion 627–8.
7. Eshuis EJ, Slors JF, Stokkers PC, Sprangers MA, Ubbink DT, Cuesta MA, et al. Long term outcomes following laparoscopically assisted versus open ileocolic resection for Crohn's disease. Br J Surg. 2010;97(4):563–8.
8. Dasari BV, McKay D, Gardiner K. Laparoscopic versus Open surgery for small bowel Crohn's disease. Cochrane Database Syst Rev. 2011;1, CD006956.
9. Tan JJ, Tjandra JJ. Laparoscopic surgery for Crohn's disease: a meta-analysis. Dis Colon Rectum. 2007;50(5):576–85.
10. Polle SW, Wind J, Ubbink DT, Hommes DW, Gouma DJ, Bemelman WA. Short-term outcomes after laparoscopic ileocolic resection for Crohn's disease. A systematic review. Dig Surg. 2006;23(5–6):346–57.
11. Tilney HS, Constantinides VA, Heriot AG, Nicolaou M, Athanasiou T, Ziprin P, et al. Comparison of laparoscopic and open ileocecal resection for Crohn's disease: a metaanalysis. Surg Endosc. 2006;20(7):1036–44.
12. Rosman AS, Melis M, Fichera A. Metaanalysis of trials comparing laparoscopic and open surgery for Crohn's disease. Surg Endosc. 2005;19(12):1549–55.
13. Lesperance K, Martin MJ, Lehmann R, Brounts L, Steele SR. National trends and outcomes for the surgical therapy of ileocolonic Crohn's disease: a population-based analysis of laparoscopic vs. open approaches. J Gastrointest Surg. 2009;13(7):1251–9.
14. Lee Y, Fleming FJ, Deeb AP, Gunzler D, Messing S, Monson JR. A laparoscopic approach reduces short-term complications and length of stay following ileocolic resection in Crohn's disease: an analysis of outcomes from the NSQIP database. Colorectal Dis. 2012;14(5):572–7.
15. Umanskiy K, Malhotra G, Chase A, Rubin MA, Hurst RD, Fichera A. Laparoscopic colectomy for Crohn's colitis. A large prospective comparative study. J Gastrointest Surg. 2010;14(4):658–63.
16. da Luz MA, Stocchi L, Remzi FH, Geisler D, Hammel J, Fazio VW. Laparoscopic surgery for patients with Crohn's colitis: a case-matched study. J Gastrointest Surg. 2007;11(11):1529–33.
17. Nakajima K, Nezu R, Hirota M, Nishida T. The role of hand-assisted laparoscopic surgery in subtotal and total colectomy for Crohn's colitis. Surg Endosc. 2010;24(11):2713–7.
18. Orenstein SB, Elliott HL, Reines LA, Novitsky YW. Advantages of the hand-assisted versus the open approach to elective colectomies. Surg Endosc. 2011;25(5):1364–8.
19. Moloo H, Haggar F, Coyle D, Hutton B, Duhaime S, Mamazza J, et al. Hand assisted laparoscopic surgery versus conventional laparoscopy for colorectal surgery. Cochrane Database Syst Rev. 2010;10, CD006585.
20. Goyer P, Alves A, Bretagnol F, Bouhnik Y, Valleur P, Panis Y. Impact of complex Crohn's disease on the outcome of laparoscopic ileocecal resection: a comparative clinical study in 124 patients. Dis Colon Rectum. 2009;52(2):205–10.
21. Okabayashi K, Hasegawa H, Watanabe M, Nishibori H, Ishii Y, Hibi T, et al. Indications for laparoscopic surgery for Crohn's disease using the Vienna Classification. Colorectal Dis. 2007;9(9):825–9.
22. Beyer-Berjot L, Mancini J, Bege T, Moutardier V, Brunet C, Grimaud JC, et al. Laparoscopic approach is feasible in Crohn's complex enterovisceral fistulas: a case-match review. Dis Colon Rectum. 2013;56(2):191–7.
23. Aytac E, Stocchi L, Remzi FH, Kiran RP. Is laparoscopic surgery for recurrent Crohn's disease beneficial in patients with previous

primary resection through midline laparotomy? A case-matched study. Surg Endosc. 2012;26(12):3552–6.
24. Pinto RA, Shawki S, Narita K, Weiss EG, Wexner SD. Laparoscopy for recurrent Crohn's disease: how do the results compare with the results for primary Crohn's disease? Colorectal Dis. 2011;13(3): 302–7.
25. Chaudhary B, Glancy D, Dixon AR. Laparoscopic surgery for recurrent ileocolic Crohn's disease is as safe and effective as primary resection. Colorectal Dis. 2011;13(12):1413–6.
26. Holubar SD, Dozois EJ, Privitera A, Cima RR, Pemberton JH, Young-Fadok T, et al. Laparoscopic surgery for recurrent ileocolic Crohn's disease. Inflamm Bowel Dis. 2010;16(8):1382–6.
27. Bergamaschi R, Haughn C, Reed 3rd JF, Arnaud JP. Laparoscopic intracorporeal ileocolic resection for Crohn's disease: is it safe? Dis Colon Rectum. 2009;52(4):651–6.
28. Chang K, Fakhoury M, Barnajian M, Tarta C, Bergamaschi R. Laparoscopic right colon resection with intracorporeal anastomosis. Surg Endosc. 2013;27(5):1730–6.
29. Rijcken E, Mennigen R, Senninger N, Bruewer M. Single-port laparoscopic surgery for inflammatory bowel disease. Minim Invasive Surg. 2012;2012:106878.
30. Yang TX, Chua TC. Single-incision laparoscopic colectomy versus conventional multiport laparoscopic colectomy: a meta-analysis of comparative studies. Int J Colorectal Dis. 2013;28(1): 89–101.
31. Alves A, Panis Y, Bouhnik Y, Marceau C, Rouach Y, Lavergne-Slove A, Vicaut E, et al. Factors that predict conversion in 69 consecutive patients undergoing laparoscopic ileocecal resection for Crohn's disease: a prospective study. Dis Colon Rectum. 2005;48(12): 2302–8.

# Minimally Invasive Surgery in Ulcerative Colitis Patients

# 31

Marco E. Allaix and Alessandro Fichera

### Key Points

- Surgery is currently the gold standard for ulcerative colitis (UC) patients failing medical management or when dysplasia/cancer is diagnosed.
- A restorative proctocolectomy with ileal pouch-anal anastomosis (IPAA) is considered the standard of care for the surgical treatment of UC patients.
- Septic pouch-related complications are associated with adverse short-term and long-term functional outcomes.
- A staged approach has been proposed to reduce the risk of postoperative complications.
- Minimally invasive surgery, including laparoscopy, hand-assisted laparoscopic surgery (HALS), and single-incision laparoscopic surgery (SILS), has been introduced during the last two decades to reduce surgical trauma in this frail patient population.
- HALS combines the advantages of the open approach, i.e., tactile feedback, with those of laparoscopic surgery, i.e., small incisions.
- Restorative proctocolectomy can be safely offered to highly selected patients with early rectal cancer.

**Electronic supplementary material:** Supplementary material is available in the online version of this chapter at 10.1007/978-1-4939-1581-1_31. Videos can also be accessed at http://www.springerimages.com/videos/978-1-4939-1580-4.

M.E. Allaix, M.D.
Department of Surgery, University of Chicago Pritzker School of Medicine, 5841 S. Maryland Avenue, MC 5031, Chicago, IL 60637, USA
e-mail: meallaix@gmail.com

A. Fichera, M.D. F.A.C.S., F.A.S.C.R.S. (✉)
Department of Surgery, University of Washington Medical Center, 959 NE Pacific Street, Box 356410, Seattle, WA 98195, USA
e-mail: afichera@uw.edu

## Background

Over the last 10 years, significant improvements have been made in the medical treatment of patients with ulcerative colitis (UC), achieving increased remission rates and better symptom control [1]. However, surgery still remains the gold standard for those patients who fail medical management or when dysplasia or colorectal cancer is diagnosed [2].

A restorative proctocolectomy with ileal pouch anal anastomosis (IPAA) is currently considered the standard of care for the surgical treatment of UC patients with good anal sphincter function [3]. Yet, this operation is not without its own potential morbidity, with the most common postoperative complications including intestinal obstructions from adhesions, wound infection, and pouch leak [4]. To decrease the incidence of pouch-related complications, a staged surgical approach has been proposed [5]. Patients undergoing surgery for refractory UC are at high risk of postoperative complications in part due to immunosuppressive medical therapy, malnutrition, and the nature of the disease. Attempts at reducing surgical trauma and improving both short-term and long-term outcomes in this frail patient population have been made over the last two decades. One of the primary operative methods to achieve this has been the application of a minimally invasive approach to colorectal surgery, first reported in the early 1990s [6]. However, widespread adoption has been relatively slow, especially in ulcerative colitis patients. The long operative time related to the complexity of the surgical procedure and the intrinsic limitations of the total laparoscopic approach have recently promoted laparoscopic hand-assisted surgery (HALS), shown to be faster than the conventional laparoscopic surgery, while still offering the benefit of the minimally invasive approach [7]. More recently, though admittedly much more technically demanding, satisfactory short-term outcomes have been reported after single-incision laparoscopic surgery (SILS) [8].

H.M. Ross et al. (eds.), *Minimally Invasive Approaches to Colon and Rectal Disease: Technique and Best Practices*, DOI 10.1007/978-1-4939-1581-1_31, 

In our practice, a laparoscopic-assisted resection is currently the preferred approach to UC patients, with HALS being offered occasionally to the obese patient population.

To minimize complications, we have utilized a three-stage approach in patients with poor general condition and/or treated with aggressive medical therapy. This approach involves (1) total abdominal colectomy and end ileostomy, (2) restorative proctectomy with IPAA and diverting loop ileostomy, and (3) ileostomy takedown. Alternatively, a two-step approach that includes (1) restorative proctocolectomy with IPAA and diverting loop ileostomy and (2) ileostomy takedown is offered to healthier patients.

Today, controversies exist regarding (1) the best surgical approach (laparoscopic vs. HALS vs. SILS vs. open), (2) the surgical strategy (two vs. three stages), and (3) the management strategy in UC patients diagnosed with rectal cancer, where multidisciplinary therapy not only affects oncologic outcomes, but pouch function as well.

The following chapter describes the different surgical techniques and reviews the evidence coming from the literature regarding the optimal surgical approach to UC patients.

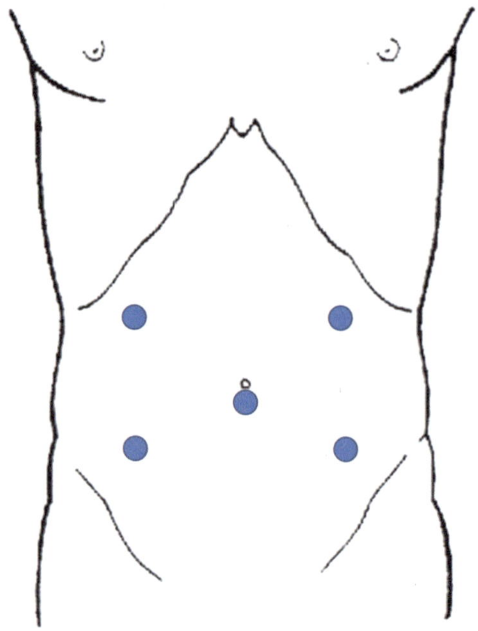

**Fig. 31.1** Trocar placement for a conventional laparoscopic-assisted procedure

## HALS and Conventional Laparoscopic Surgery

### Total Abdominal Colectomy with End Ileostomy

Regardless of the desired technique, a total abdominal colectomy with end ileostomy is the first step of our staged approach.

#### Step 1: Positioning of the Patient, Placement of Trocars, and Abdomen Exploration

After induction of general anesthesia and placement of all the monitoring devices, the patient is placed in the lithotomy position and secured to the bed. Both arms are tucked at the patient's side. A single dose of preoperative antibiotic and subcutaneous heparin are administered, as well as stress dose of corticosteroids, if needed. A urinary catheter is inserted and rectal irrigation with diluted iodine solution is completed. The patient is prepped and draped in standard fashion.

The monitors are placed initially at the head of the table. An open Hasson technique is used to insert the camera port just below the umbilicus. Pneumoperitoneum is established with $CO_2$, and it is maintained at 15 mmHg.

In case of a *conventional laparoscopic* procedure, after a brief exploration of the abdominal cavity, additional four 5-mm trocars are placed in each of the four abdominal quadrants (Fig. 31.1). A more thorough exploration of the abdominal cavity is then performed.

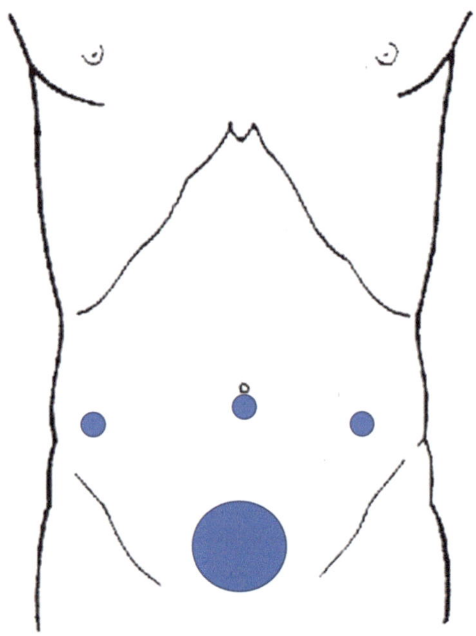

**Fig. 31.2** Trocar placement for a HALS procedure

When a *HALS* procedure is planned, only two 5-mm trocars are placed in the right and left lower quadrants. After feasibility of the laparoscopic approach is confirmed, a Pfannenstiel incision is performed two fingerbreadths above the pubis. The pneumoperitoneum is evacuated, and the hand-assisted device is inserted and secured in placed (Fig. 31.2). When feasible, the future ileostomy site is used as one of the port sites.

### Step 2: Mobilization of the Intra-Abdominal Colon

Pneumoperitoneum is reestablished and the patient is placed in reverse Trendelenburg and right lateral decubitus position. The surgeon stands between the patient's legs, with the camera operator being typically on the left side of the patient holding a 30° 5 mm scope. The ligament of Treitz is identified, and the small intestine is evaluated in its entirety, to rule out unexpected small bowel disorders or abnormalities that may preclude pouch construction. The small intestine is placed in the left upper quadrant away from the operating field, thus facilitating the initial mobilization of the ileocolic vascular pedicle. The surgeon moves to the patient's left side next to the camera operator, the assistant stands on the patient's left side, and the patient is placed in steep Trendelenburg and left lateral decubitus position to keep the small bowel out of the operating field. The ileocolic vascular pedicle is then identified, placed under tension, dissected, and divided with a vessel-sealing device. While we try to preserve the terminal ileal branches, we do not divide the ileocolic pedicle close to the bowel. Next, medial to lateral mobilization of the ascending colon is completed all the way up to the hepatic flexure in the submesenteric avascular plane. Attention is then directed to the lateral peritoneal attachments, which are taken down from the hepatic flexure to the cecum (Fig. 31.3). With the surgeon now on the patient's right side, the operating table is placed in reverse Trendelenburg and the transverse colon is mobilized from the hepatic to the splenic flexure by sequentially dividing the greater omentum just distal to the gastroepiploic arcade and the transverse mesocolon (Figs. 31.4, 31.5a, b and 31.6). The omentum is taken with the specimen, thus facilitating

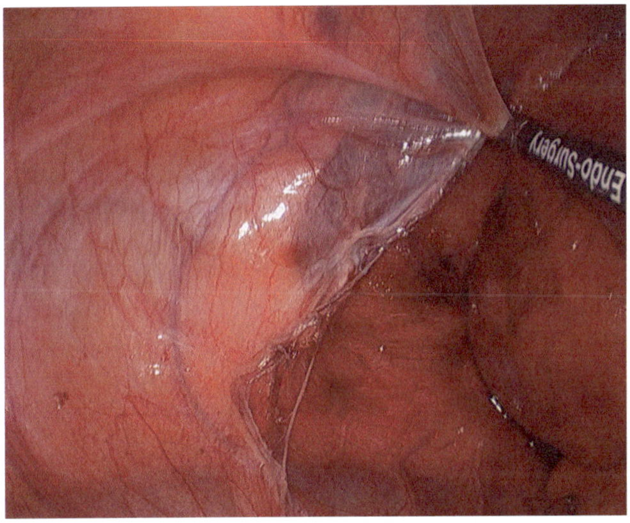


**Fig. 31.3** Mobilization of the ascending colon

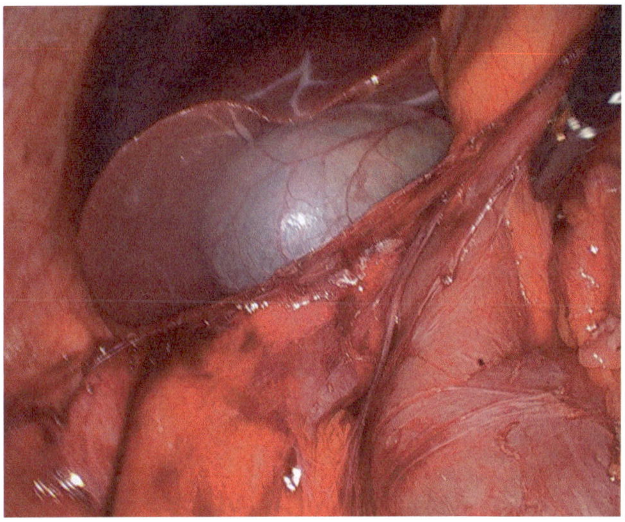

**Fig. 31.4** Mobilization of the hepatic flexure

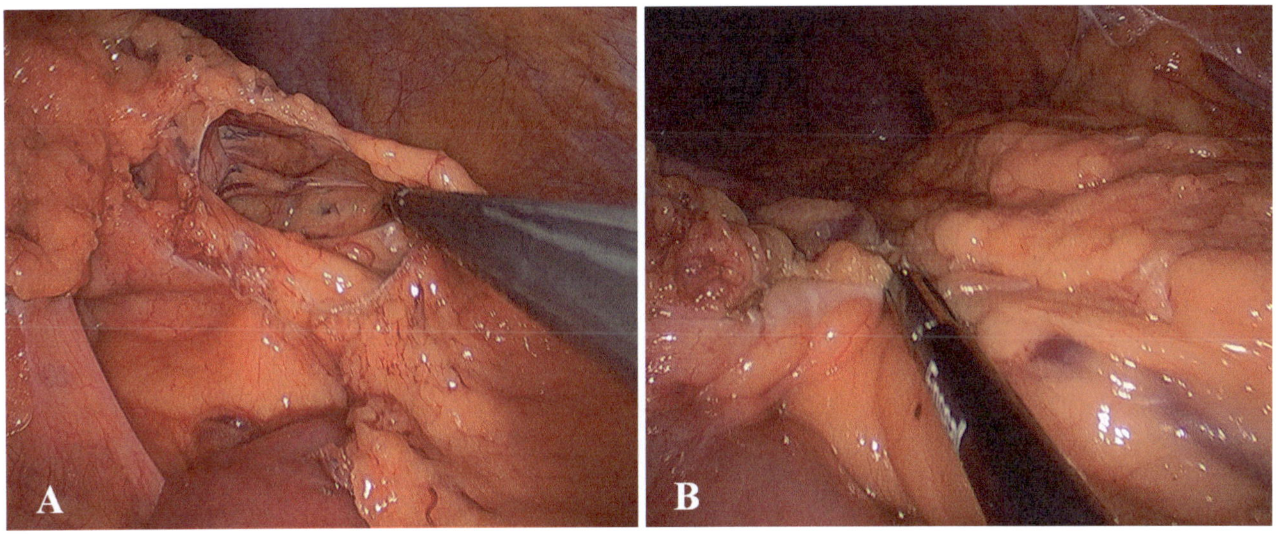


**Fig. 31.5** Mobilization of the transverse colon: (**a**) opening of the gastrocolic ligament; (**b**) division of the gastrocolic ligament

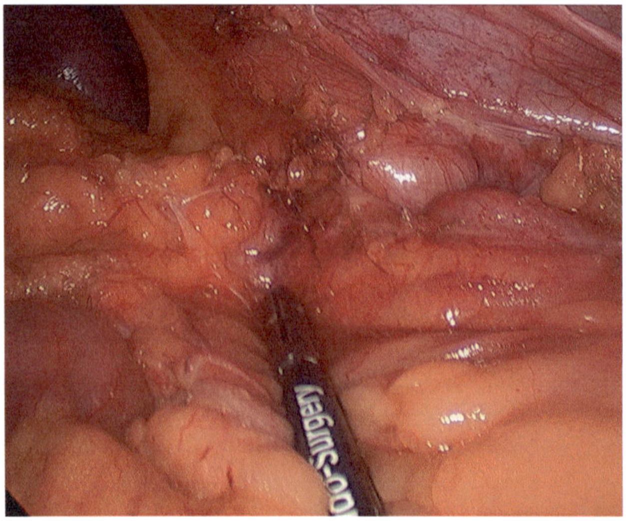

**Fig. 31.6** Takedown of the splenic flexure

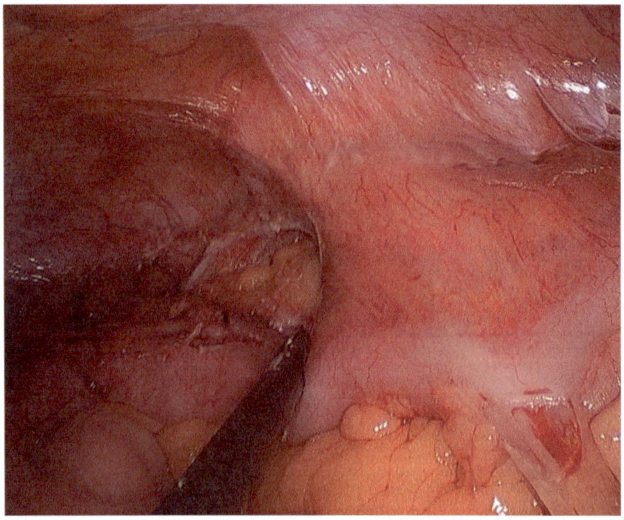

**Fig. 31.7** Mobilization of the descending colon

the dissection. The splenic flexure is taken down bluntly and sharply usually in an antegrade fashion, but in difficult cases, a combination of antegrade (from the transverse colon) and retrograde (from the descending colon) mobilization is sometimes needed. At this point, the surgeon is operating between the patient's legs. The descending colon is mobilized all the way to the level of the sigmoid colon by sequentially dividing and ligating the lateral attachments and the mesentery (Fig. 31.7). At this point, pneumoperitoneum is evacuated and the specimen is exteriorized through the Pfannenstiel incision with a wound protector in place. The terminal ileum is dissected off of the mesentery and divided with a GIA stapler. An end ileostomy is matured.

## Completion Proctectomy with IPAA

A completion proctectomy with IPAA and loop ileostomy is the second step of our staged approach.

### Step 1: Positioning of the Patient, Placement of Trocars, and Exploration

The positioning of the patient is the same as for a total abdominal colectomy.

A circular incision is made around the ileostomy. The ileum is separated from its attachments to the subcutaneous tissue and fascia. The most distal ileum is then transected with a GIA stapling device. Through the ileostomy site, a 12-mm port is placed.

After exploration of the abdominal cavity, additional four 5-mm trocars are placed in each of the four abdominal quadrants as for a laparoscopic-assisted total colectomy.

### Step 2: Mobilization of the Small Bowel Mesentery

With the surgeon typically between the patient's leg and with the table in reverse Trendelenburg, the root of the mesentery of the small intestine is lifted off the retroperitoneum all the way to the third portion of the duodenum to allow a tension-free ileoanal anastomosis (Video 31.1). The avascular plane is easily identified and developed.

### Step 3: Pelvic Dissection

The monitors are positioned at the foot of the table. The surgeon is on the patient's right side with the assistant on the opposite side retracting the rectum up and out of the pelvis.

The Hartmann's pouch is identified. The left and right ureters are identified and preserved. The superior rectal vessels are identified and divided with a vessel-sealing device. The hypogastric plexus is also identified and preserved. Only after these structures have been identified, a total mesorectal excision plane is then entered. Even for benign disease, we prefer to follow this plane of dissection because it allows for a precise and bloodless rectal mobilization. Care is taken to identify the *neurovascular bundles* bilaterally (Fig. 31.8). The dissection proceeds initially posteriorly, then laterally, finally anteriorly. Effort is made to dissect the rectum posteriorly all the way to the levators at the pelvic floor. Then, the lateral rectal stalks, often including the middle rectal artery, are divided all the way to the levators, and finally the anterior dissection is completed, in a male patient posterior to Denonvilliers' fascia. At this point, when the rectum is adequately mobilized distally, the pneumoperitoneum is evacuated. The rectum will be divided at the pelvic floor either with a stapler, in the case of a stapled IPAA, or sharply in case of mucosectomy and handsewn IPAA.

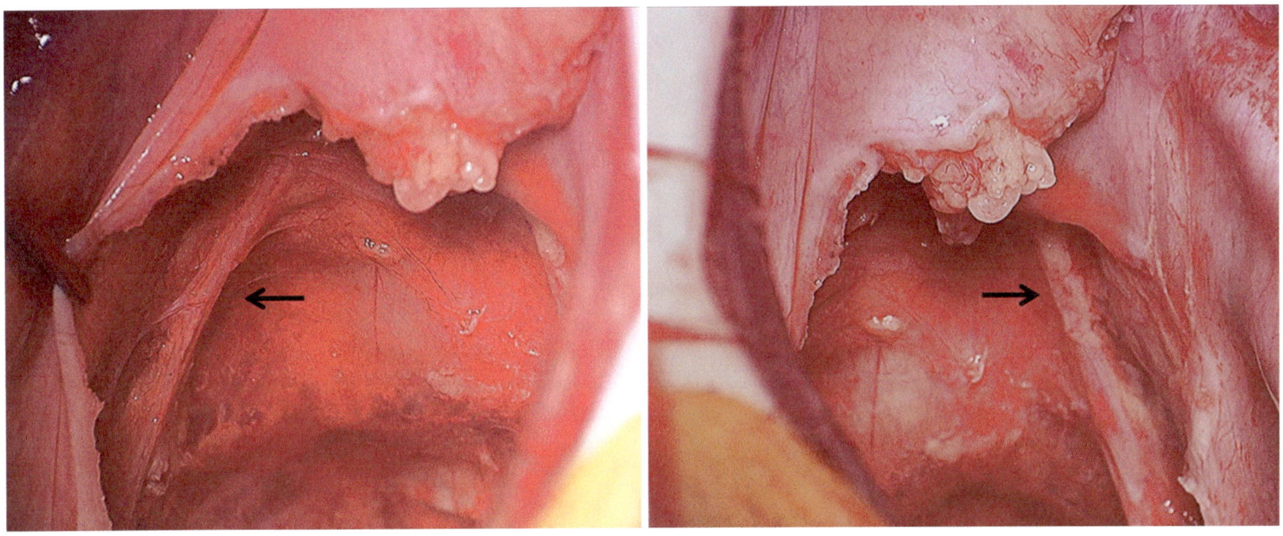

**Fig. 31.8** Hypogastric nerves

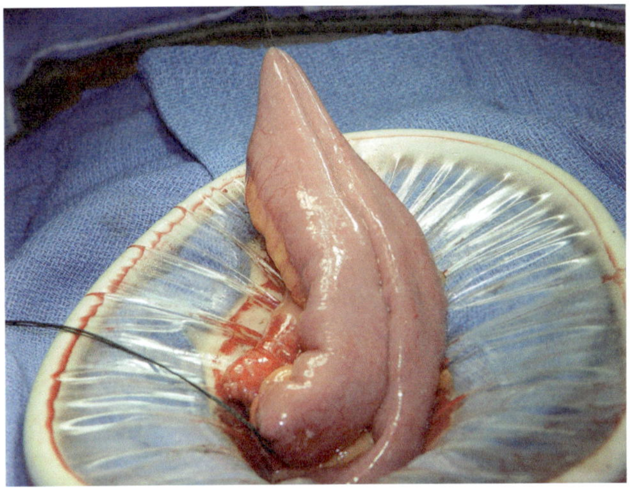

**Fig. 31.9** Marking of the apex of the pouch with silk suture

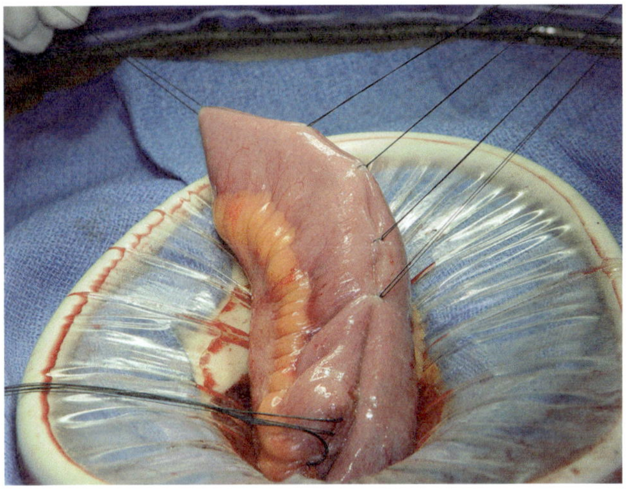

**Fig. 31.10** The two loops are approximated with Lambert sutures

## Step 4: Construction of the Ileoanal Pouch

Several pouch designs have been described, but it is our practice to perform a J-pouch. Handsewn IPAA with a transanal mucosectomy starting at the dentate line is reserved in our practice in case dysplasia is demonstrated by endoscopic biopsy irrespective of location and severity [9], while stapled IPAA is performed for the majority of patients without dysplasia.

The terminal ileal mesentery is then properly oriented and the most dependent loop of small bowel identified. A 3-0 silk 30-in. long suture is placed at the apex (Fig. 31.9), and the two loops are approximated with 4-0 nonabsorbable sutures (Fig. 31.10). The abdominal cavity is protected with moist laparotomy pads. and a bowel clamp is placed on the proximal small bowel. Enterotomies on the two loops are performed. The pouch is constructed as previously described [10]. Sequential fires of an 80-mm GIA stapler are applied through the enterotomies (Figs. 31.11 and 31.12), and the pouch is progressively everted as stapling progresses toward the apex of the pouch for accurate placement of the rows of staples as well as to achieve hemostasis (Fig. 31.13). When the pouch is completely constructed, it is inverted back (Fig. 31.14) and the two enterotomies are closed in layers. By using this technique, the apex of the pouch, the future site of the anastomosis, is not manipulated or traumatized. When performing a stapled ileoanal anastomosis, the anvil is placed at the apex of the pouch, and a standard double-stapled end-to-end anastomosis is constructed with an EEA stapler. For a

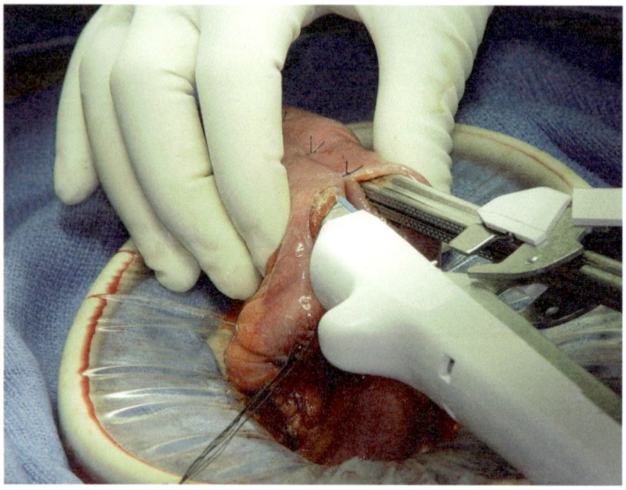

**Fig. 31.11** Pouch creation: application of sequential fires of an 80-mm GIA stapler through the enterotomies

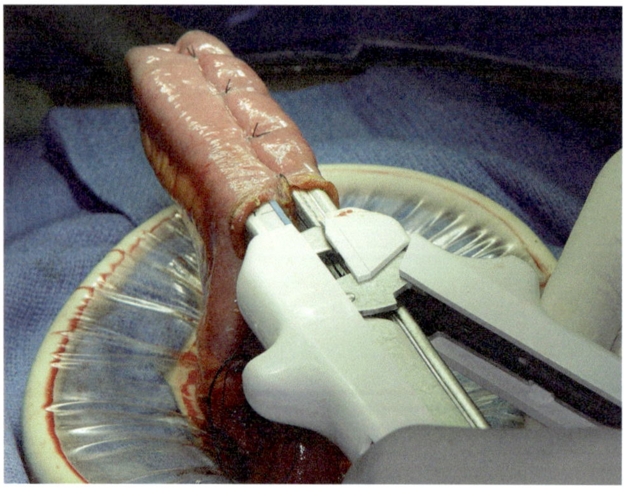

**Fig. 31.12** Pouch creation: application of sequential fires of an 80-mm GIA stapler through the enterotomies

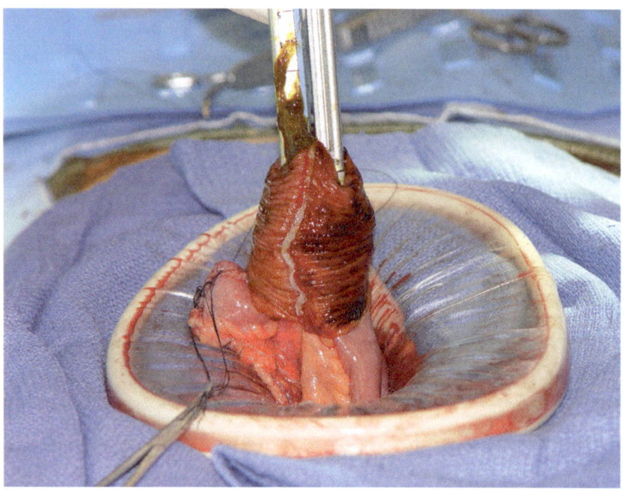

**Fig. 31.13** Pouch creation: progressive eversion of the pouch as the stapler progresses toward the apex of the pouch

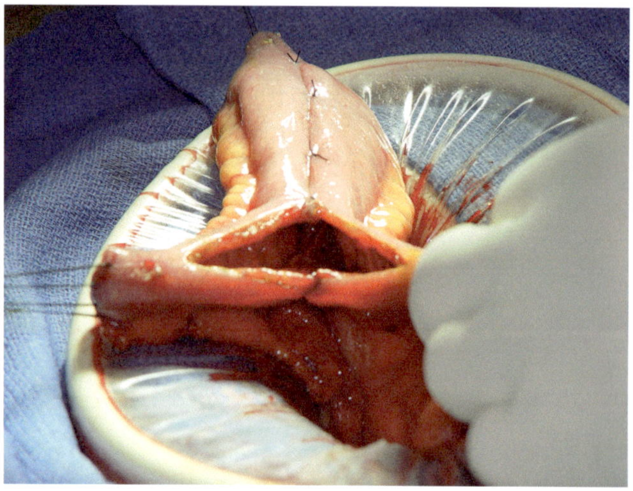

**Fig. 31.14** Pouch creation: inversion of the pouch and closure of the two enterotomies

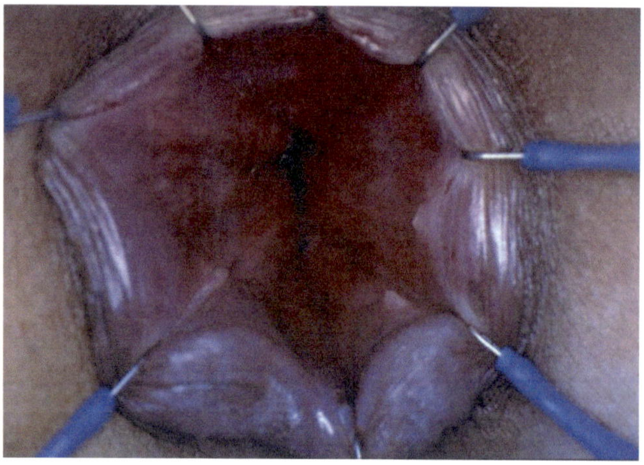

**Fig. 31.15** Exposure of the anal canal for mucosectomy

hand sewn IPAA, a completion mucosectomy is performed transanally. The submucosa of the residual distal rectum and anal transition zone is infiltrated with epinephrine containing local anesthetic solution to facilitate hemostasis. The circumferential mucosectomy is facilitated by placing a Lone Star™ (Lone star Co, Stafford, TX) retractor (Fig. 31.15). The internal sphincter is visualized and preserved circumferentially, and given the typically short remnant, there is no need for anal dilation or aggressive manipulation of the sphincter complex. The electrocautery is our preferred tool for a precise and hemostatic complete mucosectomy starting at the dentate line. The pouch is then carefully advanced to the pelvis (Fig. 31.16), and after adequate hemostasis, a two-layer interrupted pouch anal anastomosis is constructed (Fig. 31.17). The anastomosis is checked with a flexible sigmoidoscope for hemostasis and patency and a leak test of the anastomosis is performed. A pelvic drain is seldom necessary.

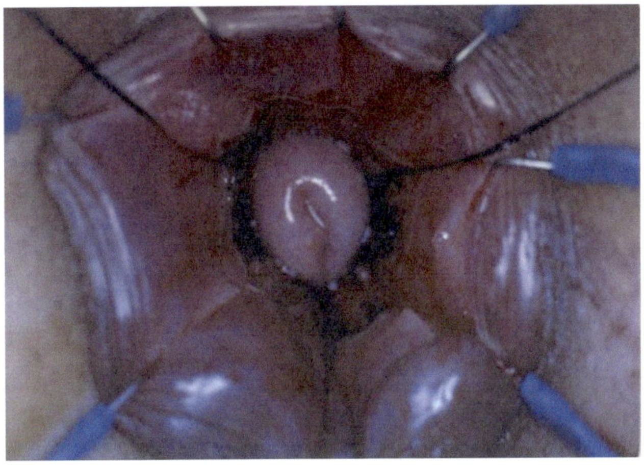

**Fig. 31.16** The pouch is delivered and visible at the level of the dentate line

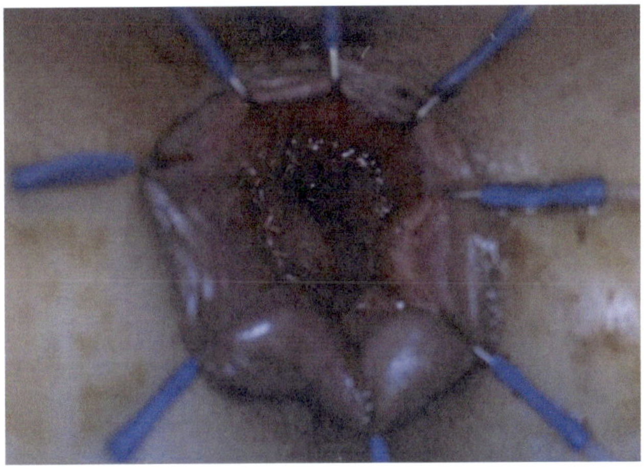

**Fig. 31.17** Two-layer handsewn ileoanal pouch anastomosis

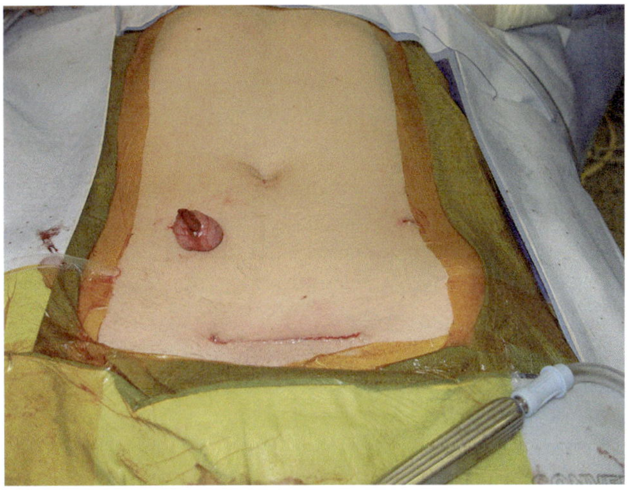

**Fig. 31.18** Patient after completion proctectomy and IPAA

After irrigation and hemostasis in the abdomen and pelvis, a suitable loop of small bowel is identified, and a 14-French red rubber catheter is placed through the mesentery. The loop is delivered through the previously developed ileostomy site and secured in place by suturing the red rubber catheter to the skin with nonabsorbable sutures. An anti-adhesive barrier is typically used to facilitate the subsequent takedown. The Pfannenstiel incision is closed in layers and the skin is closed with subcutaneous sutures. The incision is protected and the ileostomy matured in the standard Brooke fashion with 3-0 chromic interrupted sutures (Fig. 31.18).

An anastomosis between the ileal pouch and anal canal performed under tension is associated with increased risk of dehiscence with severe short-term and long-term sequelae [11].

Few studies have evaluated and compared several techniques for lengthening the small bowel mesentery, including complete small bowel mobilization to the origin of its mesentery, ileocolic vessel ligation close to their origin from the superior mesenteric pedicle, and transverse mesenteric relaxing incisions [12]. These strategies facilitate a tension-free IPAA in most cases.

We have had a very limited experience with these techniques, due to the frequent staged approach to these patients. By optimizing body weight, tissue characteristics, and general medical conditions, we have almost eliminated the need for mesenteric lengthening from our practice.

For patients with extremely short mesentery, an alternative strategy has been described by Goes et al. [13]. Multiple vascular ligations are performed between the right colon wall and the marginal vascular arcade, from the right branch of the middle colic artery that is preserved and provides the only blood supply to the ileal branch of the ileocolic artery. Right colic and ileocolic arteries at their origin and the superior mesenteric trunk at its distal third are divided.

This technique presents several drawbacks: (1) it is time consuming, (2) it is technically challenging, and (3) it can lead to pouch ischemia, but it offers additional length in the extreme situations.

## Total Proctocolectomy with IPAA

### Step 1: Positioning of the Patient, Placement of Trocars, and Abdomen Exploration

This step is the same as for a total abdominal colectomy.

### Step 2: Mobilization of the Intra-Abdominal Colon

The mobilization of the intra-abdominal colon follows the previously described steps of a total abdominal colectomy all the way to the pelvis.

### Step 3: Pelvic Dissection

The monitors that were placed at the head of the table are moved to the foot of the table. The surgeon is on the patient's right side with the assistant on the opposite side retracting the rectum up and out of the pelvis. Typically a medial to lateral approach to the mobilization of the inferior mesenteric artery is undertaken. The peritoneum overlying the sacral promontory is incised on the patient's right side, and the left ureter is clearly identified and mobilized off the operating field. The hypogastric plexus is also identified and preserved. Only after these structures have been identified, the inferior mesenteric artery is divided and ligated with a vessel-sealing device. The level of transection of the inferior mesenteric artery and vein follows the oncologic principles in presence of colorectal cancer. The total mesorectal excision plane is then entered, and this step of the procedure follows that already described for a proctectomy.

### Step 4: Construction of the Ileoanal Pouch

The IPAA construction follows the previously described steps for a proctectomy.

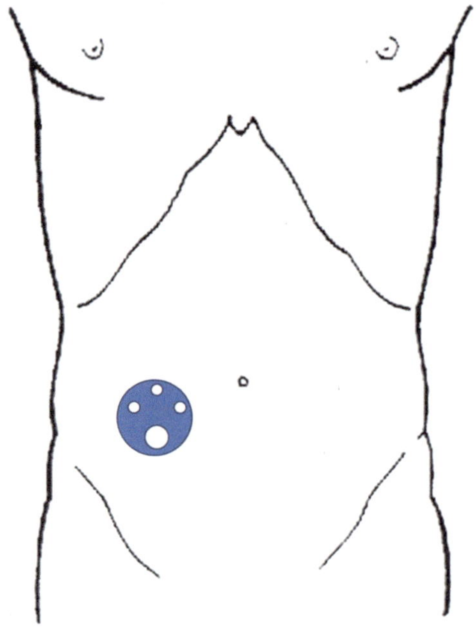

**Fig. 31.19** Trocar placement for a SILS procedure

## Single-Incision Laparoscopic Surgery (SILS)

### First Stage: Total Abdominal Colectomy with End Ileostomy

### Step 1: Positioning of the Patient, Placement of Trocars, and Abdomen Exploration

The positioning of the patient is the same as previously described for the other procedures.

The access to the peritoneal cavity is obtained by inserting a GelPOINT® Advanced Access Platform (Applied Medical, Rancho Santa Margarita, CA) through a circular incision at the future ileostomy site in the right lower quadrant. The GelSeal® cap provides additional working space and the ability to achieve triangulation with the instruments. One 12-mm and three 5-mm trocars are introduced through the gel platform (Fig. 31.19). The procedure is performed with conventional laparoscopic instruments, including a 12-mm 30° laparoscope and a 5-mm bipolar vessel-sealing device for tissue dissection and vascular resection. The Trendelenburg and side-to-side tilt positions dynamically vary during the procedure for optimal surgical field exposure [14].

The operation starts with the exploration of the abdominal cavity to evaluate the feasibility of the procedure. The most challenging part with higher risk of conversion is the initial dissection and division of the ileocolic vessels that are located right below the access site. Therefore, we start the dissection from the right colon, proceeding clockwise to the rectosigmoid junction.

### Step 2: Right Colon Dissection

The operating table is tilted to the left, and the patient is placed in Trendelenburg position. The surgeon is on the left side of the patient, and the GelPOINT® is oriented in order to have the optical port in medial position. The tissue sealing device is introduced thorough the cephalic trocar. The cecum is retracted upward and laterally by a grasper. The ileocolic vessels are now under tension. They are dissected and divided after visualization of right ureter and duodenum. Medial to lateral mobilization of the right colon is accomplished all the way up to the hepatic flexure, with blunt dissection down the avascular plane between the mesocolon and the Gerota's fascia.

### Step 3: Hepatic Flexure and Transverse Colon Dissection

The patient is placed in the reverse Trendelenburg position, with the surgeon standing between the patient's legs. The hepatic flexure is retracted by a grasper caudally and medially. After sharp division of the hepatocolic ligament, the table is tilted in a right lateral position to displace the small bowel, with the surgeon moving to the right side of the patient. The access device is turned 180°, and the transverse colon is fully mobilized by sequentially dividing the greater omentum, just distal to the gastroepiploic arcade and the transverse mesocolon. The omentum is then removed en bloc with the specimen in order to facilitate this step of the procedure.

### Step 4: Splenic Flexure and Left Colon Dissection

At this point the, GelPOINT® is rotated back 180°. The colon is retracted medially and toward the bottom in order to facilitate sharp dissection of the splenic flexure. Subsequently, the lateral attachments of the descending colon are taken sharply, and the avascular line of Toldt is bluntly dissected, with exposure of the left ureter.

### Step 5: Rectosigmoid Junction Section and Specimen Exteriorization

The patient is now placed in the Trendelenburg position with a slight left lateral tilt, and the access device is tuned again 180° to obtain a better sigmoid exposure. The inferior mesenteric vein and the branches of the sigmoid arteries are dissected and divided. At this point, we switch to a 5-mm laparoscope that is inserted through the cranial port. A laparoscopic stapler is then used to transect the rectosigmoid junction after dissection of the mesentery. The specimen is extracted through the access device, the terminal ileum is divided extracorporeally, and the ileostomy is matured. A large (20 F) red rubber rectal tube is routinely placed to decompress the rectal stump and kept in place with a nylon suture.

### Second Stage: Proctectomy and IPAA

At the beginning of the second procedure, the ileostomy is mobilized and the pouch is constructed extracorporeally. The anvil of the circular stapler is secured at the apex of the pouch. The pouch is then placed back into the abdominal cavity. Through the same ileostomy site, the GelPOINT® Advanced Access Platform (Applied Medical, Rancho Santa Margarita, CA) is inserted. One 12-mm and three 5-mm trocars are introduced into the gel platform, and the procedure is performed with conventional laparoscopic instruments. As for the total abdominal colectomy, we use a 12-mm 30° laparoscope and a 5-mm bipolar vessel-sealing device. The patient is in reverse Trendelenburg position for optimal exposure. The terminal ileal mesentery is mobilized back to the root at the level of the duodenum to minimize the tension on the IPAA. The proctectomy is then performed in the avascular mesorectal plane after identification of the left ureter in Trendelenburg position. The rectum is then mobilized all the way to the pelvic floor circumferentially and transected intracorporeally with multiple fires of a laparoscopic stapling device. The specimen is then removed through the access device. The IPAA is then constructed intracorporeally under laparoscopic vision. IPAA is protected with a diverting loop ileostomy.

## Surgical Approach to Ulcerative Colitis: Conventional Laparoscopy vs. HALS vs. SILS vs. Open Surgery

While laparoscopic surgery has gained wide acceptance for the treatment of several benign and malignant colorectal diseases, showing clear short-term benefits as compared to open surgery, the introduction of the laparoscopic approach to patients with UC has proceeded slowly, mainly due to the complexity of the procedure.

A laparoscopic approach to UC patients in the elective setting was first described by Peters et al. in 1992 [16]. Since then, several studies compared laparoscopic and open proctocolectomy and IPAA [15]. No significant differences were found in terms of short-term outcomes in terms of perioperative complications, reoperation and readmission rates, and early mortality, while higher level of satisfaction with cosmetic results and quality of life was reported after laparoscopic surgery. Few comparative studies have looked at long-term functional outcomes, reporting no differences between the laparoscopic and the open IPAA [16].

A laparoscopic approach has been also used for the surgical treatment of UC patients in the emergency setting, with better postoperative results compared to the open approach [17, 18].

The main shortcoming of laparoscopic surgery for UC is the significantly longer operative time. Considering the complexity of surgery, the HALS approach has been proposed, aimed at reducing the operative time while maintaining the benefit of the minimally invasive approach. Several small studies have compared HALS and conventional laparoscopy for both total colectomy and proctocolectomy in UC [19–24]. For instance, Marcello et al. [23] reported the results of the only prospective, randomized trial ever conducted in this field. Both groups of patients were similar in terms of age, gender, body mass index, and history of previous surgery. They found a significantly shorter operative time in favor of HALS, with no differences in terms of conversion rate to open surgery. Similar short-term postoperative outcomes were observed in both groups.

Fewer studies have compared HALS with open total colectomy or proctocolectomy [25, 26]. For instance, Maartense et al. [25] reported in 2004 the results of a randomized clinical trial comparing 30 HALS to 30 open proctocolectomies. HALS procedures took significantly longer than open surgery. No significant differences were found in terms of postoperative pain, complication rate, and postoperative hospital stay between the two groups. A trend toward higher costs for HALS was reported.

More recently, further efforts have been made to reduce the surgical trauma in UC patients, by applying a single-incision approach. Particularly for total abdominal colectomy, single incision represents a true "no scar" procedure, since the site of the temporary ileostomy is used as access point to the abdominal cavity. Initial results show that single-incision total abdominal colectomy is a feasible and safe procedure in expert hands, with similar perioperative results as compared with laparoscopic and HALS approaches [27]. Interestingly, some authors have reported shorter operative time of SILS total colectomy, mainly due to the limited time spent to close the only entry site [27]. Further large and randomized trials are needed to confirm these preliminary data regarding feasibility, safety, and efficacy of SILS in the surgical management of UC patients.

## Surgical Strategy

Anastomotic failure of the IPAA is a serious complication after restorative proctocolectomy for UC that adversely affects long-term functional outcomes [28]. To reduce the risk of pouch-related septic complications, thus minimizing the functional sequelae, a staged surgical approach has been proposed by us and several other authors in the literature [5]. To date few studies have specifically looked at the outcomes of minimally invasive surgery in a staged approach comparing 2- to 3-stage strategy. For instance, Pandey et al. [29] compared 68 consecutive UC patients undergoing a 2-stage approach with 50 consecutive UC patients treated with a 3-stage approach. Three-stage patients were more likely to have been receiving aggressive medical therapy than the 2-stage patients. Despite this difference, the overall complication rates were similar between the two groups (55 % for 2-stage patients vs. 52 % for 3-stage patients, $p=0.4$), while infectious complications were higher in the 2-stage group (38 vs. 21 %, $p<0.05$).

Several potential advantages are associated with a 3-stage strategy: (1) a temporary diverting loop ileostomy may mitigate the clinical significance of a IPAA leak, thus improving long-term pouch function in this frail patient population; (2) after total abdominal colectomy, the patient is weaned off medications; (3) the nutritional status is optimized in preparation for the complex stage of this surgical strategy that involves the IPAA construction; and (4) diagnostic questions may be answered with the examination of the specimen, since a postoperative diagnosis of Crohn's disease or indeterminate colitis is not infrequent after total colectomy for presumed UC. A multistep strategy allows planning the most appropriate and tailored restorative procedure according to the pathologic evaluation of the colon resected.

A staged laparoscopic approach has also been shown to be associated with (1) reduced waiting time between the first and the second step [30, 31] and (2) decreased intra-abdominal adhesion and therefore less intraoperative adhesiolysis during the second step after a total abdominal colectomy [31].

## Rectal Cancer and Ulcerative Colitis

The risk of developing colorectal cancer is increased in UC patients, and it correlates with the duration and the extent of disease [32]. UC-related colorectal cancers are often poorly differentiated and have a different genetic background compared to sporadic colorectal tumors. Today, limited data exist regarding clinical and oncologic outcomes and the best surgical approach to UC patients with rectal cancer. Radice et al. [33] reported in 1998 on 77 patients with colorectal cancer undergoing open IPAA: 56 colon, 17 rectal cancers, and four both. More than 70 % of patients had early stage disease (stage I or II). Mean follow-up was 6 (range, 2–15) years. Pouch failure occurred in 16 % of patients compared to 7 % for the overall IPAA registry. No differences between cancer and noncancer patients were observed in terms of operative complications, functional outcomes (median stool frequency, incontinence, pad usage, pouchitis), and oncologic results. The authors concluded that although pouch failure (largely due to postoperative radiation injury or disease progression) is more common, IPAA can be performed in colorectal cancer patients, with no significant impact on long-term IPAA function and oncologic outcomes.

In 2003, similar results were obtained by Remzi et al. [34] in 70 UC patients with colorectal cancer (26 rectal cancer patients), with a mean follow-up of 7.5 (range, 0.5–17) years. Cancer was incidentally diagnosed in 10 % of cases. Seventy-three percent of patients were diagnosed with stage I–II rectal cancer. No patient with a preoperative diagnosis of dysplasia or cancer within 8 cm from the anal verge was considered for a stapled IPAA; a mucosectomy with a handsewn anastomosis was performed in all of these cases. The authors concluded that restorative proctocolectomy with IPAA is a successful surgical approach for patients with coexisting rectal cancer in the setting of UC.

More recently, Merchea et al. [35] retrospectively reviewed 41 UC patients with rectal cancer. The tumor was preoperatively known in 83 % of patients. Eight cancers were in the proximal (>10 cm) rectum, 19 in the mid (5–10 cm) rectum, and 13 in the distal (<5 cm) rectum. The majority of patients (68 %) had stage I–II cancer. Interestingly, six (15 %) patients had undergone a previous subtotal colectomy with either an ileorectal anastomosis or end ileostomy and had developed cancer in the rectum. All these six patients previously had poor or no endoscopic surveillance after subtotal colectomy. Total proctocolectomy with end ileostomy was performed in 51 % of cases. Among the 11 (37 %) IPAA patients with diverting ileostomy, six had a double-stapled anastomosis, while five pouches were hand sewn. No patient who was treated with neoadjuvant chemoradiation therapy underwent IPAA. Postoperative morbidity was 10 %. Overall pouch failure rate was 18 %. Five (12 %) patients developed local recurrence, while distant metastases occurred in 22 % of cases. Almost 90 % of recurrences occurred in stage III–IV patients.

To the best of our knowledge, there are no studies to date that have specifically evaluated the impact of the laparoscopic approach on the oncologic outcomes in UC patients with rectal cancer. Based on the limited evidence currently available, we may conclude that (1) restorative proctocolectomy may be offered to highly selected patients with early rectal cancer, thus not requiring chemoradiation therapy. For locally advanced rectal cancer or very low lesions requiring an abdominoperineal resection, we do not offer IPAA;

(2) intense endoscopic surveillance is mandatory for early diagnosis of rectal cancer; (3) established oncologic principles should be observed in all cases with longstanding disease even if no cancer is preoperatively detected, since cancer can be incidentally found in the pathology specimen in up to 17 % of patients; and (4) neoadjuvant chemoradiation therapy may reduce the risk of recurrence and increase the disease-free survival in preoperative stage III disease, with similar short-term outcomes to that of rectal cancer in non-UC patients [36].

## Pearls and Pitfalls

- Restorative proctocolectomy with ileal pouch-anal anastomosis (IPAA) is the standard of care for the surgical treatment of ulcerative colitis (UC).
- Minimally invasive surgery is a valid alternative to open surgery in UC with excellent cosmetic and functional results.
- A staged approach has been proposed to reduce the risk of postoperative complications, such as septic pouch-related complications that are associated with poor short-term and long-term functional outcomes.
- The hypogastric nerves should always be visualized to avoid urinary and sexual dysfunction. Following the mesorectal plane, decrease bleeding and facilitate dissection.
- Full mobilization of the small bowel mesentery is mandatory to avoid excessive tension on the anastomosis.
- A restorative proctocolectomy may be offered to highly selected early rectal cancer patients, thus not requiring chemoradiation therapy. The authors favor a mucosectomy and handsewn anastomosis in the presence of dysplasia or cancer.

## Conclusion

Minimally invasive surgery reduces the surgical trauma in UC patients, a patient population at high risk of perioperative complications. While HALS combines the benefits of the open surgery with the advantages offered by the conventional laparoscopic surgery, it is offered selectively in our practice. Further studies are necessary to evaluate the real role of SILS in the management of UC patients. A minimally invasive staged strategy is associated with reduced postoperative complications and reduced time intervals between the different steps. However, studies are still needed to evaluate the impact of minimally invasive surgery on survival of UC patients diagnosed with rectal cancer.

**Acknowledgement** The authors declare no conflict of interest.

## References

1. Rutgeerts P, Sandborn WJ, Feagan BG, Reinisch W, Olson A, Johanns J, et al. Infliximab for induction and maintenance therapy for ulcerative colitis. N Engl J Med. 2005;353(23):2462–6.
2. Hancock L, Mortensen NJ. How often do IBD patients require resection of their intestine? Inflamm Bowel Dis. 2008;14 Suppl 2:S68–9.
3. Michelassi F, Lee J, Rubin M, Fichera A, Kasza K, Karrison T, et al. Long-term functional results after ileal pouch anal restorative proctocolectomy for ulcerative colitis: a prospective observational study. Ann Surg. 2003;238(3):433–41. discussion 442-5.
4. Heuschen UA, Hinz U, Allemeyer EH, Autschbach F, Stern J, Lucas M, et al. Risk factors for ileoanal J pouch-related septic complications in ulcerative colitis and familial adenomatous polyposis. Ann Surg. 2002;235(2):207–16.
5. Alves A, Panis Y, Bouhnik Y, Maylin V, Lavergne-Slove A, Valleur P. Subtotal colectomy for severe acute colitis: a 20-year experience of a tertiary care center with an aggressive and early surgical policy. J Am Coll Surg. 2003;197(3):379–85.
6. Peters WR. Laparoscopic total proctocolectomy with creation of ileostomy for ulcerative colitis: report of two cases. J Laparoendosc Surg. 1992;2(3):175–8.
7. Darzi A. Hand-assisted laparoscopic colorectal surgery. Surg Endosc. 2000;14(11):999–1004.
8. Fichera A, Zoccali M. Single-incision laparoscopic total abdominal colectomy for refractory ulcerative colitis. Surg Endosc. 2012; 26(3):862–8.
9. Fichera A, Ragauskaite L, Silvestri MT, Elisseou NM, Rubin MA, Hurst RD, et al. Preservation of the anal transition zone in ulcerative colitis. Long-term effects on defecatory function. J Gastrointest Surg. 2007;11(12):1647–52.
10. Michelassi F, Block GE. A simplified technique for ileal J-pouch construction. Surg Gynecol Obstet. 1993;176(3):290–4.
11. McMullen K, Hicks TC, Ray JE. Complications associated with ileal pouch-anal anastomosis. World J Surg. 1991;15(6):763–7.
12. Burnstein MJ, Schoetz Jr DJ, Coller JA, Veidenheimer MC. Technique of mesenteric lengthening in ileal reservoir-anal anastomosis. Dis Colon Rectum. 1987;30(11):863–6.
13. Goes RN, Nguyen P, Huang D, Beart RWJ. Lengthening of the mesentery using the marginal vascular arcade of the right colon as blood supply to the ileal pouch. Dis Colon Rectum. 1995; 38(8):893–5.
14. Fichera A, Zoccali M, Gullo R. Single incision ("scarless") laparoscopic total abdominal colectomy with end ileostomy for ulcerative colitis. J Gastrointest Surg. 2011;15(7):1247–51.
15. Wu XJ, He XS, Zhou XY, Ke J, Lan P. The role of laparoscopic surgery for ulcerative colitis: systematic review with meta-analysis. Int J Colorectal Dis. 2010;25(8):949–57.
16. Fichera A, Silvestri MT, Hurst RD, Rubin MA, Michelassi F. Laparoscopic restorative proctocolectomy with ileal pouch anal anastomosis: a comparative observational study on long-term functional results. J Gastrointest Surg. 2009;13(3):526–32.
17. Marcello PW, Milsom JW, Wong SK, Brady K, Goormastic M, Fazio VW. Laparoscopic total colectomy for acute colitis: a case-control study. Dis Colon Rectum. 2001;44(10):1441–5.
18. Bell RL, Seymour NE. Laparoscopic treatment of fulminant ulcerative colitis. Surg Endosc. 2002;16(12):1778–82.
19. Aalbers AGJ, Biere SSAY, van Berge Henegouwen MI, Bemelman WA. Hand-assisted or laparoscopic-assisted approach in colorectal surgery: a systematic review and meta-analysis. Surg Endosc. 2008;22(8):1769–80.
20. Nakajima K, Lee SW, Cocilovo C, Foglia C, Sonoda T, Milsom JW. Laparoscopic total colectomy: hand-assisted vs standard technique. Surg Endosc. 2004;18(4):582–6.

21. Rivadeneira DE, Marcello PW, Roberts PL, Rusin LC, Murray JJ, Coller JA, et al. Benefits of hand-assisted laparoscopic restorative proctocolectomy: a comparative study. Dis Colon Rectum. 2004; 47(8):1371–6.
22. Polle SW, van Berge Henegouwen MI, Slors FM, Cuesta MA, Gouma DJ, et al. Total laparoscopic restorative proctocolectomy: are there any advantages compared with the open and hand-assisted approach? Dis Colon Rectum. 2008;51(5):541–8.
23. Marcello PW, Fleshman JW, Milsom JW, Read TE, Arnell TD, Birnbaum EH, et al. Hand-assisted laparoscopic vs. laparoscopic colorectal surgery: a multicenter, prospective, randomized trial. Dis Colon Rectum. 2008;51(6):818–26.
24. Tsuruta M, Hasegawa H, Ishii Y, Endo T, Ochiai H, Hibi T, et al. Hand-assisted versus conventional laparoscopic restorative proctocolectomy for ulcerative colitis. Surg Laparosc Endosc Percutan Tech. 2009;19(1):52–6.
25. Maartense S, Dunker MS, Slors JF, Cuesta MA, Gouma DJ, van Deventer SJ, et al. Hand-assisted laparoscopic versus open restorative proctocolectomy with ileal pouch anal anastomosis: a randomized trial. Ann Surg. 2004;240(6):984–91.
26. Zhang LY. Hand-assisted laparoscopic vs. open total colectomy in treating slow transit constipation. Tech Coloproctol. 2006;10(2): 152–3.
27. Fichera A, Zoccali M, Felice C, Rubin DT. Total abdominal colectomy for refractory ulcerative colitis. Surgical treatment in evolution. J Gastrointest Surg. 2011;15(11):1909–16.
28. Heuschen UA, Allemeyer EH, Hinz U, Lucas M, Herfarth C, Heuschen G. Outcome after septic complications in J pouch procedures. Br J Surg. 2002;89(2):194–200.
29. Pandey S, Luther G, Umanskiy K, Malhotra G, Rubin MA, Hurst RD, et al. Minimally invasive pouch surgery for ulcerative colitis: is there a benefit in staging? Dis Colon Rectum. 2011;54(3):306–10.
30. Ouaïssi M, Lefevre JH, Bretagnol F, Alves A, Valleur P, Panis Y. Laparoscopic 3-step restorative proctocolectomy: comparative study with open approach in 45 patients. Surg Laparosc Endosc Percutan Tech. 2008;18(4):357–62.
31. Gu J, Stocchi L, Geisler DP, Kiran RP. Staged restorative proctocolectomy: laparoscopic or open completion proctectomy after laparoscopic subtotal colectomy? Surg Endosc. 2011;25(10): 3294–9.
32. Rutter MD, Saunders BP, Wilkinson KH, Rumbles S, Schofield G, Kamm MA, et al. Thirty-year analysis of a colonoscopic surveillance program for neoplasia in ulcerative colitis. Gastroenterology. 2006;130(4):1030–8.
33. Radice E, Nelson H, Devine RM, Dozois RR, Nivatvongs S, Pemberton JH, et al. Ileal pouch-anal anastomosis in patients with colorectal cancer: long-term functional and oncologic outcomes. Dis Colon Rectum. 1998;41(1):11–7.
34. Remzi FH, Preen M. Rectal cancer and ulcerative colitis: does it change the therapeutic approach? Colorectal Dis. 2003;5(5): 483–5.
35. Merchea A, Wolff BG, Dozois EJ, Abdelsattar ZM, Harmsen WS, Larson DW. Clinical features and oncologic outcomes in patients with rectal cancer and ulcerative colitis: a single-institution experience. Dis Colon Rectum. 2012;55(8):881–5.
36. Green S, Stock RG, Greenstein AJ. Rectal cancer and inflammatory bowel disease: natural history and implications for radiation therapy. Int J Radiat Oncol Biol Phys. 1999;44(4):835–40.

# Minimally Invasive Approaches to Colon and Rectal Diseases: Technique and Best Practices—Pediatrics

32

Eric J. Krebill and Daniel J. Robertson

## Abbreviations

| | |
|---|---|
| CD | Crohn's disease |
| IBD | Inflammatory bowel disease |
| IC | Indeterminate colitis |
| IPAA | Ileal pouch-anal anastomosis |
| LAARP | Laparoscopically assisted anorectal pull-through |
| MIS | Minimally invasive surgery |
| PSARP | Posterior sagittal anorectoplasty |
| PSARVUP | Posterior sagittal anorectovaginourethroplasty |
| UC | Ulcerative colitis |

### Key Points

- Abdominal entry, while similar to adults, needs to consider the thickness of the abdominal wall to avoid iatrogenic intra-abdominal and vascular injuries.
- Pediatric patients have much less "working space" within the abdomen compared to adults. This needs to be considered when choosing trocars and port sites.
- Insufflation pressures should take into consideration the weight/size of the child to avoid cardiopulmonary compromise.
- While many operations in pediatric patients are similar to adults, important differences remain that surgeons caring for this population need to be aware of.
- A mucosectomy and hand-sewn anastomosis are preferable for IPAA in pediatric patients.

E.J. Krebill, M.D.
Department of General Surgery Residency, Michigan State University, 221 Michigan St NE, Grand Rapids, MI 49503, USA
e-mail: eric.krebill@gmail.com

D.J. Robertson, M.D. (✉)
Department of Pediatric Surgery, Helen Devos Children's Hospital, 330 Barclay Ave NE Suite 202, Grand Rapids, MI 49503, USA
e-mail: daniel.robertson@helendevoschildrens.org

## Introduction

This chapter discusses the unique application of minimal access surgery in the pediatric patient with regard to colorectal diseases. Multiple barriers to earlier advancement and widespread acceptance in the field included a delay in the development of appropriately sized instrumentation, a relative paucity of minimally invasive skills among established pediatric surgeons at training institutions, and the fact that many complex colorectal conditions occur with comparatively low frequency in young children and neonates versus adult patients. As instrumentation became downsized and several early adopters became more facile with minimally invasive skills, the benefits of laparoscopic surgery in pediatric surgery became apparent, and the scope of procedures performed increased dramatically. The benefits of pediatric minimally invasive surgery (MIS) are similar to those in adults, including smaller incisions, decreased infection risk, greater surgical precision, magnified view without parallax between observers, reduced length of stay, and decreased cost of care. Unique to pediatric MIS is the small size of the operating space, which creates technical challenges and oftentimes a steeper learning curve. Despite the inherent mechanical and physiologic challenges of pediatric MIS, innovative operative techniques in the treatment of pediatric colorectal diseases have been substantial. We have chosen to highlight the technical departures from standardized adult MIS, the rationale for their modification, and their potential application in adult patients.

## History of Pediatric Minimally Invasive Surgery

The introduction and mainstream application of minimally invasive surgery in children lagged nearly a decade behind the first published description of laparoscopic cholecystectomy in 1985 by Eric Mühe [1]. While adult MIS was gaining

H.M. Ross et al. (eds.), *Minimally Invasive Approaches to Colon and Rectal Disease: Technique and Best Practices*, DOI 10.1007/978-1-4939-1581-1_32, © Springer Science+Business Media New York 2015

popularity in the late 1980s, most pediatric surgeons were slow to adopt this new technology. By default, they were handicapped by adult-sized instrumentation, energy devices, and trocars, requiring larger incisions for younger children and infants. This made it difficult for some surgeons to rationalize the use of relatively larger trocar incisions on already small patients through which an equivalent open surgery could be performed. They also made a rational, yet invalid, assumption that incisional morbidities were equivalent among open incisions and multiple small MIS incisions of equal length. Instead, the closing tension of a wound is proportional to the square of the incisional length [2]. In other words, total wound tension rises nonlinearly with increasing wound length. For comparison, the added closing tension of two 3-mm trocar incisions is still less than a 5-mm incision. This may be one factor that accounts for the observed decrease in laparoscopic incisional morbidities—less pain, smaller scars, and lower rates of infection, dehiscence, and herniation.

Technical factors also played a role in the delay in adopting minimally invasive techniques. Early instruments were too long and bulky and thus required large trocar incisions. Graspers were too traumatic for finer pediatric tissues and procedures. In addition, there is considerably less working space in the pediatric abdomen. For perspective, laparoscopy in a pediatric patient one-half as tall as an adult could present the surgeon with only 1/8 the working volume in the abdomen based on geometric scaling formulae. It has been estimated that the thoracoscopic anastomosis for esophageal atresia repair is performed in a 1 $cm^3$ space. The innovative contributions of early pioneers like Rothenberg, Georgeson, and Holcomb in the 1990s and early 2000s laid the groundwork for a new approach to many pediatric-specific diseases such as pyloric stenosis, appendicitis, and gastroesophageal reflux disease [3]. This groundwork led to the ability to apply these techniques to a wider array of more complex pediatric surgical diseases including neonatal colorectal diseases such as imperforate anus and Hirschsprung's disease.

## Patient Selection and Positioning

While the approach to pediatric laparoscopy is similar to adults, the equipment, patient positioning, and techniques must be modified. Many neonates and young children with congenital cardiopulmonary anomalies such as hypoplastic left heart or congenital diaphragmatic hernias with pulmonary dysplasia are poor candidates. They may not be able to compensate for the physiologic stress associated with a reduction in functional residual capacity (FRC) and the hypercarbia associated with gas insufflation. Other relative contraindications include previous open operations and small bowel obstruction, although laparoscopy can still often be used in selected cases.

Pediatric patients provide surgeons with multiple positioning options due to their small size. For some operations, like laparoscopic pull-through for imperforate anus repair, positioning the patient sideways on the operative table is beneficial. These patients can also be prepped circumferentially from nipples to toes and draped by passing the lower half of the baby through an adult extremity drape (Fig. 32.1). This allows access to the abdomen and perineum with a single prep. The head in babies is disproportionately larger than in older patients, and a "bump" under the body to lift the body can be useful, especially when operating deep in the pelvis. Alternatively, positioning patients at the foot of the table allows the surgeon to operate directly in-line with the upper abdomen, for instance, when operating on the stomach or esophageal hiatus. Many smaller patients do not require stirrups for dorsal lithotomy but can simply have their feet taped together over foam prior to positioning in "frog-leg" lithotomy. Patient positioning is also critical with regard to trocar sites. They are often much closer together than in adult-sized patients, and the child will need to be positioned on the table to allow appropriate access for the surgeon and all assistants.

The use of an adult extremity drape for circumferential lower body draping is demonstrated. This technique is useful

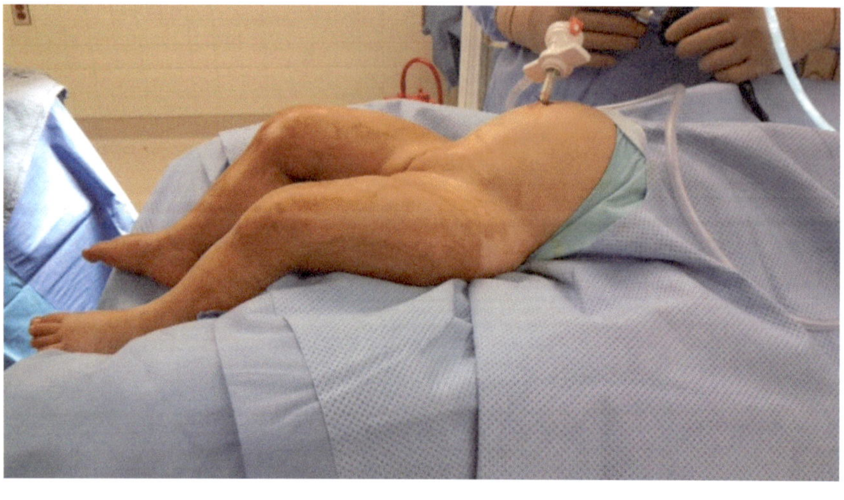

**Fig. 32.1** Patients can also be prepped circumferentially from nipples to toes and draped by passing the lower half of the baby through an adult extremity drape

when access to the perineum is required for laparoscopically assisted endorectal pull-through operations for Hirschsprung's disease or imperforate anus in small children and neonates (Fig. 32.1).

## Trocar Selection and Insertion Technique

The technology void created by the growth of pediatric laparoscopy was quickly filled by manufacturers as the demand for customized pediatric trocars, instrumentation, and energy devices grew. Appropriate trocar selection, placement, and insertion technique will avoid frustration associated with poor ergonomics, visibility, and longer operative times. Abdominal access techniques and pneumoperitoneum are achieved in a somewhat similar manner as in adult patients, with several notable caveats.

Most children (and many adults) have at least a small fascial opening at the base of the umbilicus which allows a very safe method for accessing the abdomen. The umbilicus is often not nearly as deep as in larger patients, and the authors usually perform a direct vertical skin incision at the very base of the umbilicus. A hemostat can then usually be placed directly into the peritoneum and subsequently replaced by the first trocar. This often takes less than 20 s. The traditional open Hassan technique can be useful in larger patients as well. The abdominal wall is significantly thinner and more compliant in neonates, toddlers, and young children compared to adolescents and adults. Due to the increased pliability of the abdominal wall, and especially without pneumoperitoneum established, optical entry techniques like the Visiport™, Covidien, Mansfield, MA, should typically be avoided. The insertion technique for the remaining trocars often requires a gentle "pop" in the proper direction as opposed to steady pressure, as it takes surprisingly little effort to push the abdominal wall flush against the retroperitoneum in smaller children, even with appropriate pneumoperitoneum. In fact, trocar insertion proves to be responsible for most catastrophic complications in pediatric MIS with an incidence of great vessel injury of only 0.05 %, but with an associated mortality of 20 % [4].

The bladder can often be emptied by manual lower abdominal compression (the Credé maneuver) in younger children prior to short procedures. Intraoperative Foley catheter drainage can be used for long cases and discontinued at the end of the procedure or in the early postoperative period. The Foley is often continued for 1 week after dividing a rectourethral fistula during laparoscopic imperforate anus repair in male infants prior to obtaining a voiding cystourethrogram (VCUG).

The abdominal wall of many pediatric patients is quite thin. This has both advantages and disadvantages. Transillumination of the abdominal wall during trocar placement can be quite helpful in avoiding blood vessels. Many trocars, however, are designed to capture or hold the abdominal wall in several different manners; these trocars work better when the abdominal wall is thicker. One such trocar used by many pediatric surgeons in larger patients or in the umbilicus is the radially expanding Step™ trocar (Covidien, Mansfield, MA). The device comes in lengths of 75 and 100 mm and has an expandable sleeve that starts at a diameter of 1.7 mm and is inserted with a Veress needle. Other trocars have plastic ribbing to grip the abdominal wall or balloons which can be insufflated and pulled back against the abdominal wall. However, these trocars do not perform as well in infants and smaller pediatric patients. The balloons may take up too much of the short distance between the trocar and the operative target. Other trocars don't grip the abdominal wall very well and have a tendency to slide out or become dislodged, especially when exchanging instruments. Therefore, the authors most often use reusable 2.7- and 3.5-mm trocars manufactured by Karl Storz (Tuttlingen, Germany), fitted with a short piece of 14-Fr catheter placed around the trocar at an appropriate (and adjustable) interval from the trocar exit as demonstrated in Fig. 32.2. This allows quite precise placement of the proper amount of intra-abdominal trocar length and allows the surgeon to suture the catheter to the skin to prevent unwanted movement. These trocars also have small heads which prevent them from colliding during instrument manipulation in an already crowded working environment.

Most surgeons do not close the fascial defect created by 5-mm trocars in adult patients. However, 5-mm port sites are at higher risk of trocar site herniation in children and are preferentially closed in pediatric patients [5, 6]. The use of stab incisions rather than traditional trocars for inserting laparoscopic instruments directly through the chest or abdominal wall is another maneuver used by some in pediatric

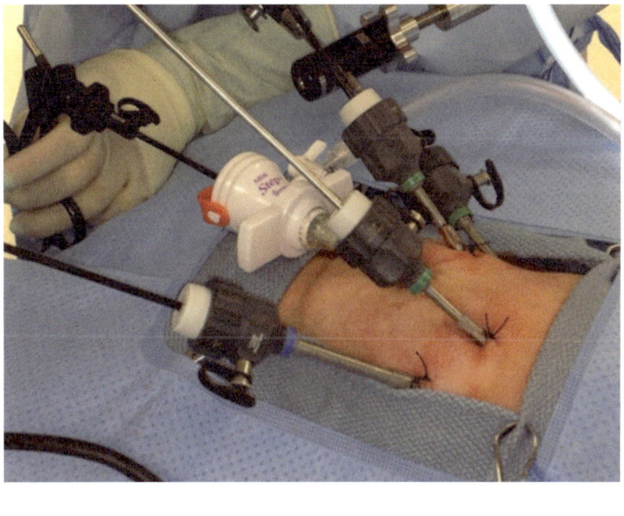

**Fig. 32.2** The Step™, radially expanding umbilical trocar, and the 3.5- and 2.7-mm reusable trocars are shown anchored to the skin with silk sutures tied to the clear, 14-Fr catheter used as a sleeve over the shaft of the trocar

MIS [7]. The authors use this technique for laparoscopic pyloromyotomy where instruments need to be changed out infrequently. We prefer small trocars for more complex operations that may require frequent exchanging of instrumentation, as it seems less traumatic to the abdominal wall.

## Pearls and Pitfalls

- The abdominal wall is very pliable in children, and extra care needs to be taken to avoid trocar injury to retroperitoneal structures.
- To avoid frustration with trocar displacement, choose trocars that can be secured well to the thin abdominal wall in children.

## Gas Insufflation

We know that pneumoperitoneum has the potential to cause pronounced physiologic changes in pediatric patients that can lead to complications. For instance, insufflation may cause an increase in end-tidal $CO_2$, cephalad displacement of the diaphragm, reduced pulmonary compliance, and increased airway resistance, which can be remedied by increasing the minute ventilation. Also, lower intra-abdominal pressures (IAP) of <10 mmHg increase venous return, leading to increased cardiac output and a 20–25 % increase in arterial pressures. On the other hand, if IAP is increased to 20 mmHg, the inferior vena cava becomes compressed, resulting in decreased venous return, decreased cardiac output, and decreased renal blood flow. Most children can tolerate an IAP of 15 mmHg during laparoscopy, but neonates less than 5 kg should be limited to pressures of 10–12 mmHg [8]. The authors prefer to select insufflation pressures based on patient size depicted in Table 32.1. Some insufflators may be too insensitive to the rapid pressure changes within the abdomen and may inadvertently result in over insufflation. Although attempts have been made to design pediatric insufflators that administer less volume or use a lower flow rate, we have not yet found one to be equivalent to the standard insufflators available.

**Table 32.1** Recommended pressure selection according to patient size in order to accomplish safe pneumoperitoneum in infants and young children during insufflation

| Patient size (kg) | Pressure of pneumoperitoneum (mmHg) |
|---|---|
| <5 | 10 |
| 5–10 | 12 |
| >10 | 15 |

## Pediatric Laparoscopic Instrumentation

Adult MIS instruments are frequently too long (32–36 cm) and too large in diameter (5–10 mm) for younger children, and especially neonates. Using adult-length instruments on small children may leave as much as 80 % of the instrument outside the patient which may lead to poor ergonomics, awkward manipulation, and imprecise movements. Ideally, two-thirds of an endoscopic instrument should be inside the body cavity with the other one-third outside the body to prevent motion parallax. In general, pediatric laparoscopic instrumentation has finer tips and the instruments come in varying lengths. The authors keep instruments in different sets based on patient size. Our infant tray generally has 2.7-mm instruments that are 20 cm in length. The adolescent tray has 5-mm instruments that are 30 cm. Our pediatric tray has a mixture of instruments ranging from 2.7 to 5 mm in diameter and from 25 to 30 cm in length. We similarly use a range of 0° and angled lens laparoscopes, ranging from a 20-cm, 2.7-mm-diameter scope to standard length 5-mm scopes. A small 70° scope is useful for performing contralateral inguinal exploration during inguinal hernia repair as well [9].

There are also multiple energy devices available for use in pediatric laparoscopy. Prior use and familiarity with any given energy device may be the best guide to follow when choosing instrumentation for a surgery, but it remains important to keep the active portion of the instrument visible on the screen and to use the lowest effective settings to avoid collateral damage and arcing potential.

Hand position is crucial when operating on smaller patients. Many pediatric surgeons operate when using trigger-handle instruments with their left hand inverted. The authors routinely do this, especially when operating on neonates as shown in Fig. 32.3. This allows a greater distance between the hand of the surgeon and that of the assistant in tight spaces. We prefer intracorporeal suturing and knot tying in order to use 2.7-mm instruments as opposed to automated devices such as the Endo Stitch™ by Covidien, which all require at least 5-mm ports. We manually bend or flatten small needles that are appropriate in size for the patient. We prefer an in-line, ring handle laparoscopic needle driver manufactured by Jarit (Integra, Plainfield, New Jersey).

The initial hesitancy to accept pediatric laparoscopy as a safe and effective surgical technique has quickly faded, and now, the question has changed from not whether minimally invasive surgery should be done for young children and infants, but for which conditions? As an example, thoracoscopic repair of infants with congenital diaphragm hernia has become a widespread technique, but recent data comparing it to standard open approaches show that the recurrence rate for thoracoscopic repair is unacceptably high.

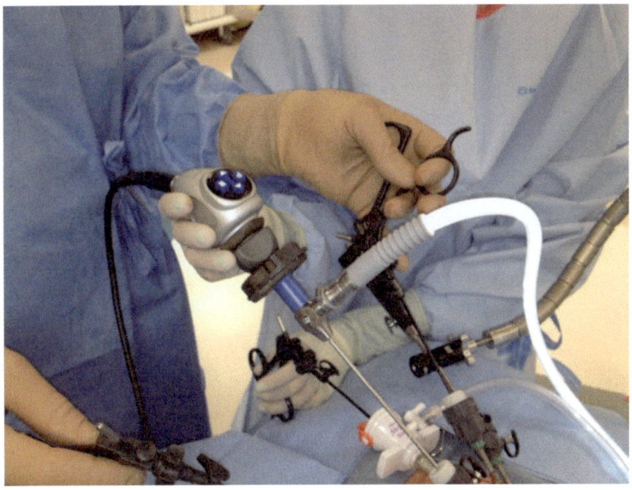

**Fig. 32.3** The surgeon is demonstrating the inverted, left hand technique with a standard trigger-handle laparoscopic instrument to allow enough space for the assistant's hands during instrument manipulation

The following sections will discuss a select number of pediatric colorectal diseases and our preferred therapeutic approach with minimally invasive techniques. Although certain diseases like Hirschsprung's disease and imperforate anus are fairly specific to pediatric surgery, the techniques described certainly translate to a number of adult colorectal diseases and disorders.

## Appendicitis

### Clinical Presentation and Indications

Appendicitis remains the most common surgical illness in children that is treated by both pediatric and adult general surgeons. It has an incidence of 70,000 pediatric cases per year with the highest rates occurring at 25 cases per 10,000 children per year between 10 and 17 years of age. Diagnosing acute appendicitis in children is very similar and perhaps more straightforward than in adults. A history of migrating abdominal pain in association with physical findings and leukocytosis remain accurate diagnostic clues for children and adults. For instance, migrating abdominal pain for acute appendicitis has a positive predictive value (PPV) of 94.2 % in children and 89.6 % in adults [10]. In the absence of classic signs and symptoms, diagnostic imaging can be a helpful adjunct. Given the increased awareness and risk of radiation exposure in children, ultrasound is usually the preferred modality, although certain clinical situations require CT imaging as well.

### Surgical Technique: Laparoscopic Appendectomy

Most commonly, pediatric laparoscopic appendectomy in the United States is performed through a three-port technique. We prefer to place a 12-mm port at the umbilicus and two additional working ports that range from 2.7 to 5 mm based on patient size. One is placed in the left lateral abdomen and another in the suprapubic region. In very small patients, the suprapubic port may be placed very low in the left lower abdomen to increase the distance between the trocar and the appendix. The surgeon stands to the left of the patient with the assistant initially on the patient's right. After trocar placement, the assistant moves to the patient's left as well in order to hold and manipulate the camera in-line with the working field. We prefer to use small graspers to sweep the bowel away from the operative field, taking care to avoid grasping and potentially injuring the bowel. We also avoid grasping the appendix where it is inflamed or visibly friable, grasping only the relatively healthy portion. Occasionally, a long Debakey grasper is needed for a very thick, inflamed appendix. We divide the mesoappendix with hook electrocautery regardless of patient size. Although residual bleeding is quite rare, a Maryland dissector can be used to grasp the area of concern to apply additional electrocautery. Other surgeons prefer various vessel-sealing devices for the mesoappendix such as the LigaSure™ (Covidien, Norwalk, CT) or Harmonic Scalpel (Ethicon, Cincinnati, OH), but we feel the added cost is unnecessary. Some surgeons also utilize an endostapler to control the mesoappendix, which often yields less than satisfactory results when there is significant inflammation. We prefer to use a 35-mm stapler with 2.5-mm staples to divide the appendix at its junction with the cecum. A cost-efficient, safe, and effective method has been validated using only electrocautery with a hook or Maryland dissector to divide the mesoappendix and three 0-PDS Endoloops (Ethicon Endo-Surgery, Cincinnati, OH) to ligate the base of the appendix with two proximal and one distal [11]. Although this gives the added advantage of a smaller 5-mm umbilical incision (the 12-mm incision is needed for the stapler), application of the Endoloops can be tedious and there can be a small amount of contamination when dividing an appendix with acute inflammation at the cecal junction. Furthermore, the appendix can usually be pulled out through the 12-mm trocar without needing a specimen retrieval bag.

Several early studies comparing open versus laparoscopic appendectomy were conflicted and resulted in little consensus among pediatric surgeons regarding the best operative approach. Other more recent studies suggest that laparoscopic appendectomy, in appropriately selected patients, can result in fewer postoperative complications. The rate of superficial wound infection is clearly reduced with laparoscopic appendectomy and patients may have slightly earlier discharge from the hospital [12–14]. Some earlier reports suggested that children with perforated appendicitis that underwent laparoscopic appendectomy had higher rates of abscess formation [15]. However, a recent study by Nadler and colleagues reported no difference in infectious complications and a lower overall rate of perioperative complications in their patients with perforated appendicitis treated with laparoscopy [16]. Pediatric subspecialty training also seems to have little impact on surgical outcomes with regard to readmission, wound infection, intra-abdominal infection, or mean hospital stay for appendicitis when compared against adult general surgeons and their outcomes [17]. These findings could be explained by the fact that laparoscopic appendectomy technique is similar across age groups, and most general surgeons are high-volume surgeons for adult appendectomy, even if they are low-volume for pediatric appendectomy.

## Pearls and Pitfalls

- Avoid grasping the appendix where it is very inflamed or gangrenous to avoid intraoperative rupture.
- In difficult cases, carefully mobilizing the cecum medially and off of the retroperitoneum can help discern the anatomy.

## Inflammatory Bowel Disease

### Clinical Presentation and Indications

There is an increasing frequency of inflammatory bowel diseases (IBD) such as ulcerative colitis (UC), Crohn's disease (CD), and indeterminate colitis (IC) in both pediatric and adult populations [18]. Ulcerative colitis and IC are most frequently diagnosed in children between the ages of 3 and 5, while CD increases during the adolescent years, peaking at 15 years of age. Pediatric surgeons become involved as the disease worsens and becomes refractory to medical management or when complications arise. The peak incidence of IBD occurs between the ages of 15 and 25 years, or a time when adolescents and young adults may traverse both pediatric and adult hospital settings when seeking surgical consultation [18]. Interestingly, a study by Jan et al. revealed that both hospital type and surgeon specialty within hospital type influenced the likelihood of surgical complications among adolescents and young adults with IBD requiring surgical intervention [19]. Despite higher complications among children's hospitals, pediatric surgeons had the lowest predicated probabilities of surgical complication or 30-day readmission (24 %) compared with general surgeons (39 %) and colorectal surgeons (35 %). The lifetime risk of surgery for IBD complications, such as extraintestinal manifestations, bowel obstruction, enteric fistulas, abscess formation, toxic megacolon, or massive hemorrhage, ranges from 40 to 70 % with a surgical complication rate of 13–55 % [20–24]. Other surgical indications unique to the pediatric population include more chronic symptoms such as delayed puberty or growth retardation as demonstrated by a failure to follow normal growth curves.

### Surgical Technique

Laparoscopic ileocecectomy for irreversible obstruction of the terminal ileum in patients with Crohn's disease can be performed through a four-trocar approach. A stapled intracorporeal or extracorporeal anastomosis can be performed through an enlarged right lower quadrant port incision depending on preference. We prefer extracorporeal anastomosis. Ileocecal resection for Crohn's disease is much less common in the pediatric population, but the adult experience has demonstrated this to be a safe technique with obvious cosmetic advantages, shorter length of stay, and fewer complications [25–27]. Therefore, additional instruction regarding operative technique will be deferred to the discussion found elsewhere in this text.

Surgery remains the definitive cure for patients with ulcerative colitis after failure of medical management or neoplastic degeneration. There are several notable differences in the surgical techniques that are usually applied to the pediatric patient. Patients usually undergo either a two-stage or a three-stage approach, depending on their clinical condition at the time of total abdominal colectomy. If patients are critically ill with toxic megacolon or on high-dose steroids, completion proctectomy and J-pouch creation are performed later in a staged approach with end ileostomy done at the time of the total abdominal colectomy. In patients who can tolerate it, we perform this laparoscopically in a manner quite similar to the adult operation (See Chap. 13). Although the specimen can be removed through the eventual ileostomy site, the specimen is often friable and dilated. The authors prefer to avoid making the ileostomy site incision any larger than required and alternatively use a relatively small transverse suprapubic incision for removal of the colectomy specimen.

The most notable disparity between typical adult and pediatric techniques involves the dissection and approach on the perineum. The ileal pouch-anal anastomosis (IPAA) is now commonly performed with a very low (end-to-end) EEA-stapled anastomosis in adults. This operation evolved after studies discovered that up to 50 % of patients undergoing endorectal mucosa resection and hand-sewn IPAA were left with early postoperative nighttime stool incontinence [28]. Despite preserving the richly innervated anal transition zone (ATZ), stapled IPAA has been shown to confer no early advantage with regard to decreased stool frequency or fewer episodes of fecal incontinence compared to hand-sewn IPAA [29]. Despite the results of a large meta-analysis that suggested stapled IPAA offered improved early nocturnal continence with coinciding higher anorectal resting and squeeze pressures, both procedures are acceptable with different benefits [30]. The stapled technique leaves several centimeters of anorectal mucosa at risk for the development of ulcerative colitis, polyposis, and in the long run, dysplastic conversion and malignant degeneration. Most practitioners recommend routine endoscopic surveillance for this cuff. Since most pediatric patients have significantly greater life expectancy, tedious surveillance of this at-risk mucosa can be avoided by performing a mucosectomy with a hand-sewn ileoanal anastomosis, with a reduced risk of eventual malignancy given that the life expectancy for these patients is longer.

A trans-abdominal low-anterior dissection of the rectum can be performed laparoscopically or via the small transverse suprapubic incision followed by the transanal mucosectomy on the perineum. For the mucosectomy, a circumferential incision is made just above the dentate line (Fig. 32.4), and multiple sutures are placed in this mucosal sleeve circumferentially to provide traction (Fig. 32.5). Pop-off sutures are preferred due to their ease of use and identical length. A Colorado needle-tip Bovie electrocautery is then used to dissect the muscularis layer proximally off of the mucosal sleeve (Fig. 32.6). At first, the plane can be somewhat difficult to create, but this often becomes easier and more apparent as the dissection is carried proximally. If the dissection becomes too facile at this stage, the surgeon may have inadvertently

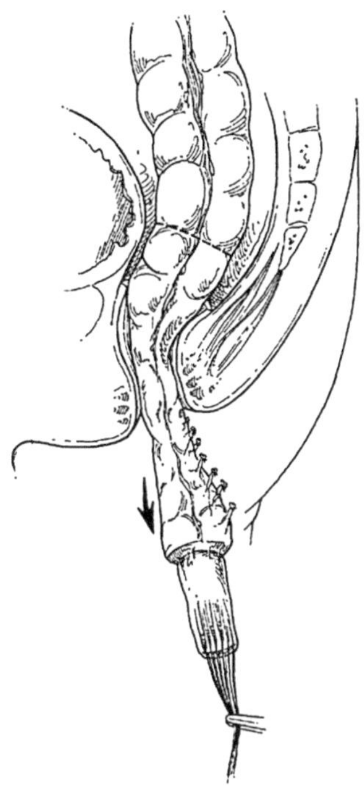

**Fig. 32.5** Rectum and colon pulled down in continuity, bringing transition zone through the anus (*Courtesy of Keith Georgeson, with permission*)

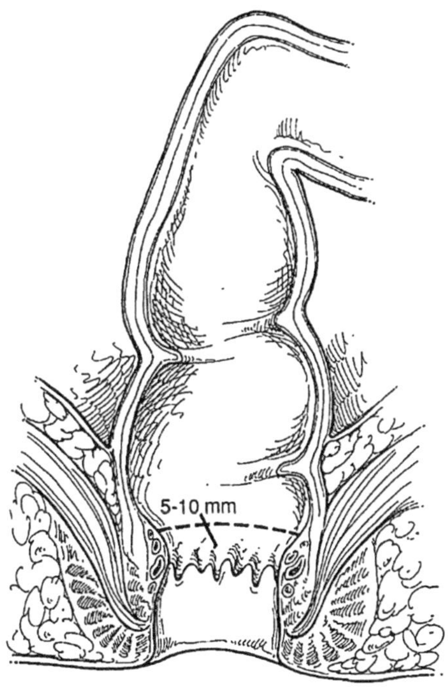


**Fig. 32.4** Mucosal incisions 5–10 mm above the pectinate or dentate line (*Courtesy of Keith Georgeson, MD, with permission*)

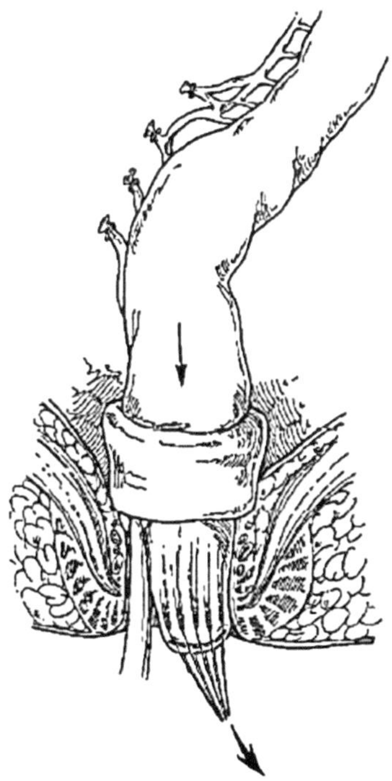

**Fig. 32.6** Placement of silk traction sutures into the rectal mucosa and development of the submucosal plane with blunt dissection (*Courtesy of Keith Georgeson, MD, with permission*)

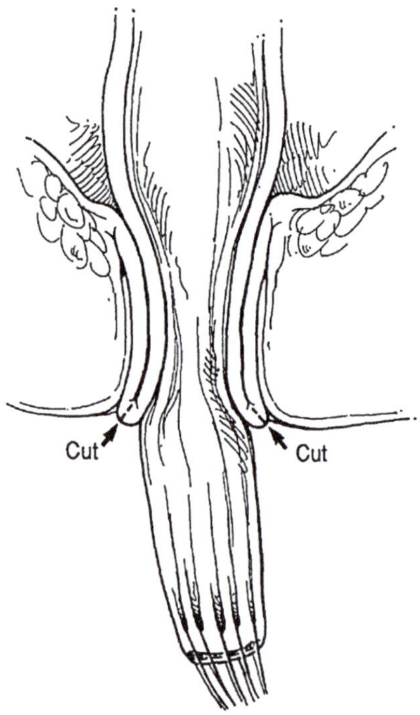


**Fig. 32.7** Transection of smooth muscle of rectum to join peritoneal dissection. Transection should begin posteriorly (*Courtesy of Keith Georgeson, with permission*)

created a full-thickness dissection instead of remaining in the submucosal plane. If any defects are created in the mucosal tube, sutures are placed to repair them. Unfortunately, this may plicate the mucosa, making it more difficult to get back into the right plane as the proximal dissection continues. Fine, cotton-tipped swabs can be used as pushers to help create the plane as well, although small bleeding vessels will require electrocautery.

Once the dissection is carried proximal enough, the muscular cuff itself will evert as depicted in Fig. 32.5. The muscular cuff is then incised circumferentially, converting the dissection to a full-thickness removal of the colon (Fig. 32.7). The muscular cuff is usually divided posteriorly and returned back to the anorectal canal flat to prevent it from causing obstruction. If the mesorectum was divided far enough distally in the abdomen the specimen can be freely removed from the field.

Obtaining the extra 5–6 cm of length on the J-pouch required for the hand-sewn ileoanal anastomosis can be challenging. Care must be taken to preserve enough mesenteric blood flow to the J-pouch from above when dividing the small sections of mesentery that are often needed to provide enough length. J-pouch ischemia can also be avoided while providing extra length by directly incising the peritoneum over the mesentery. The authors prefer not to open the apex of the J-pouch until it is through the pelvis and positioned for the anastomosis. We therefore staple the common wall between the limbs of the J-pouch from above, opening a corner of the stapled end, and making an enterotomy on the

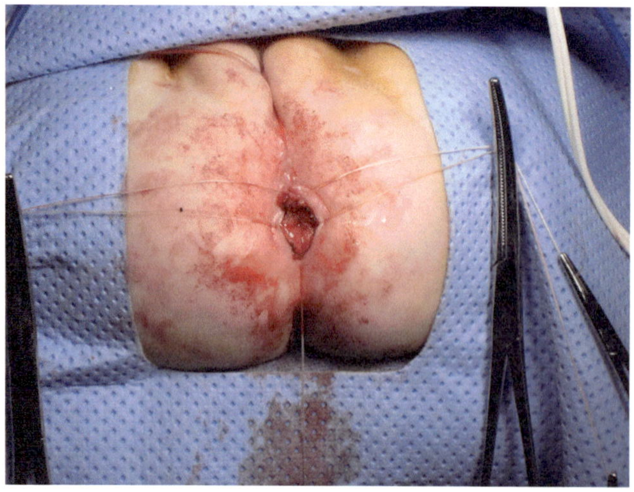

**Fig. 32.8** Creating the anastomosis of the neoanus

incoming limb to accommodate the stapler. We then close the common enterotomy with interrupted full-thickness sutures, to avoid narrowing of the incoming limb with the use of a stapling device.

Finally, the ileoanal anastomosis is completed by opening up the apex of the pouch and immediately placing stitches in four quadrants to fix it in place followed by intervening sutures taking big full-thickness bites of the J-pouch and healthy bites of the remaining cuff at the dentate line (Fig. 32.8). Given the extent of the pelvic dissection and the multiple suture/staple lines, we routinely protect the downstream anastomosis with a loop ileostomy. A loop ileostomy is preferred to a divided end ileostomy to prevent disruption of any mesenteric inflow to the J-pouch. We utilize the same ileostomy site as the end ileostomy which was taken down for the completion proctectomy.

## Pearls and Pitfalls

- When performing mucosectomy, especially when starting the dissection, if the dissection seems too easy, the plane is probably too thick, and the muscle is being left on the mucosal tube. Adjust the dissection to make the mucosal tube thinner.
- Ensure that the remaining muscular cuff is divided posteriorly and placed smoothly back along the wall of the anal canal to avoid obstruction of the pouch.
- Although with a stapled IPAA the apex of the J-pouch is opened to staple the limbs of the J-pouch together, it is preferable to staple the limbs together from above when performing mucosectomy. As it is difficult in some cases to get adequate length for hand-sewn IPAA, it is better to provide traction on the apex of the J-pouch prior to opening it in order to avoid tears at any point of the circumference of the eventual anastomosis.

## Hirschsprung's Disease

### Clinical Presentation and Indications

Hirschsprung's disease is a developmental disorder of the enteric nervous system that occurs in one out of 5,000 births [31]. It is characterized by a failure of ganglion cell migration through the neural crest during weeks 4–12 of gestation. This results in a functional obstruction due to a failure of distal colonic relaxation that is usually confined to the rectosigmoid region. The diagnosis should be considered in any newborn who fails to pass meconium in the first 24–48 h, or in children suffering from difficult bowel movements, poor feeding, poor weight gain, and progressive abdominal distension. The introduction of laparoscopic-assisted endorectal pull-through by Dr. Georgeson in the late 1990s revolutionized our surgical approach to this disease in neonates and young children [32]. Rarely does Hirschsprung's disease remain undiagnosed until adolescence or adulthood but must be considered in any adult with prolonged, refractory constipation [33]. A bedside rectal suction biopsy can be performed in infants less than 10 kg to detect hypertrophic nerve trunks and the absence of ganglion cells in the colonic submucosa, confirming the diagnosis, but not its extent. Older children and adults require full-thickness rectal biopsy in the operating room. The transition zone may be suggested by barium enema, but the extent of aganglionosis may be difficult to predict with accuracy, particularly in newborns. Surgical correction of Hirschsprung's disease requires removal of the aganglionic bowel and pull-through of ganglionated bowel to the level of the anus. Therefore, laparoscopic biopsies can be extremely useful to identify the proximal extent of resection.

### Surgical Technique: Laparoscopic-Assisted Endorectal Pull-Through

The most frequent pediatric diseases leading to laparoscopic colectomy and endorectal pull-through include ulcerative colitis, Hirschsprung's disease, and familial polyposis syndromes. We will describe the operation for Hirschsprung's disease as an example, while the mucosectomy is similar to that used for pediatric patients with ulcerative colitis.

The patient is positioned transversely at the foot of a shortened operating table with a blanket bump under the body. The patient's shoulders are taped to the side of the table where the feet are located as an extra precaution. The patient is prepped from the upper abdomen through the toes circumferentially and covered with an adult extremity drape through which the infant's body is passed as demonstrated in Fig. 32.1.

The first 5-mm radially expanding trocar is placed in the right mid-abdomen. The umbilicus can be used in larger patients, but the additional working distance gained from this port placement in infants is worth the tedious dissection through the layers of the rectus sheath (picking them up with hemostats and cutting between them). A left upper quadrant 2.7-mm trocar and a right lower quadrant 2.7-mm trocar are then placed under direct vision. A fine Maryland dissector is used to grasp a tiny amount of taeniae at the desired site for biopsy, and a fine scissors is used to take a seromuscular biopsy. After an initial cut, the biopsy is regrasped to lift it away from the colon, and the scissors are used to push the underlying mucosa away while taking tangential cuts until the specimen is free. It is important to angle the scissors tangential to the bowel to prevent inadvertent penetrance of the mucosa. Although uncommon, mucosal defects can be repaired with intracorporeal sutures. Biopsies are sent for frozen section to determine the level at which normal numbers of ganglion cells are present. Ideally, no biopsies will have been taken proximal to this level. In the 10 % of patients that do have long-segment Hirschsprung's disease, the colon can be mobilized laparoscopically for a pull-through as well. In patients with total colonic Hirschsprung's, we recommend waiting for permanent biopsies to confirm the diagnosis. The appendix can also be a useful biopsy to look for ganglion cells. We prefer to wait to perform a pull-through in these patients and instead perform ileostomy after the level of ganglion cells is confirmed (the aganglionosis can extend into the small bowel). A laparoscopic Duhamel procedure (i.e., leaving the aganglionic rectum in place and performing a retrorectal anastomosis with the rectum and normally innervated bowel) is then performed around 9 months of age, the technical details of which are described elsewhere.

After the level of normal, ganglionated bowel is defined by biopsy, laparoscopic division of the mesentery of the bowel to be resected is performed (Fig. 32.9). A Foley catheter placed on the sterile field may be required to decompress the bladder for a better view into the pelvis. Hook electrocautery works well to divide the mesentery in infants staying close to the colon and away from the retroperitoneum. The white line of Toldt can be mobilized if needed for extra length of the pull-through as well. Mucosectomy, as described in the above section on ulcerative colitis, is then performed. After the release of pneumoperitoneum, the infants' feet are wrapped in Kerlix and clipped to the drape above the head effectively placing the patient in dorsal lithotomy. Silk sutures are used to evert the anus and mucosectomy is then performed. The muscular cuff everts nicely after this dissection in infants and it can then be divided (Fig. 32.10). After the muscular cuff is divided, the specimen will typically drop out of the anorectal canal (Fig. 32.5). A marking suture at the level of the biopsy showing ganglion cells can be useful to determine where to make the anastomosis. If possible, the anastomosis should be performed proximal to the biopsy site to prevent problems from being too close to the transition zone. The anterior wall of the anastomosis is created first prior to completely dividing

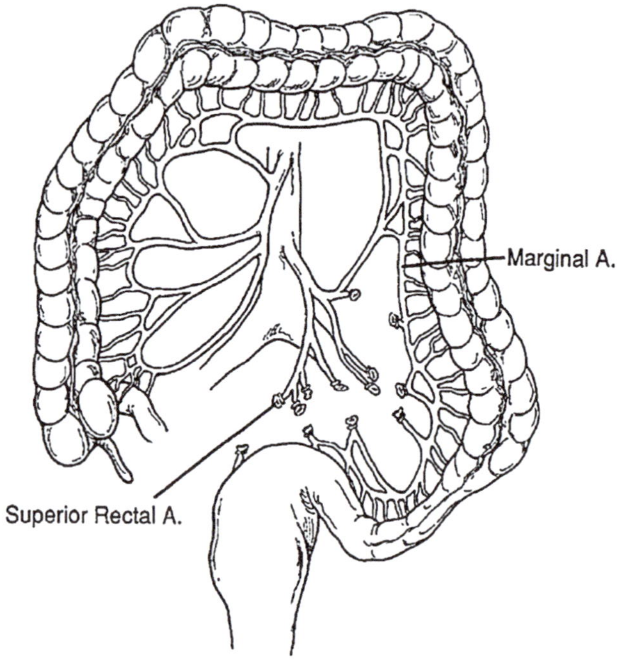


**Fig. 32.9** Anatomic depiction of the colorectal mesentery divided during the laparoscopic dissection of an endorectal pull-through operation (*Courtesy of Keith Georgeson, with permission*)

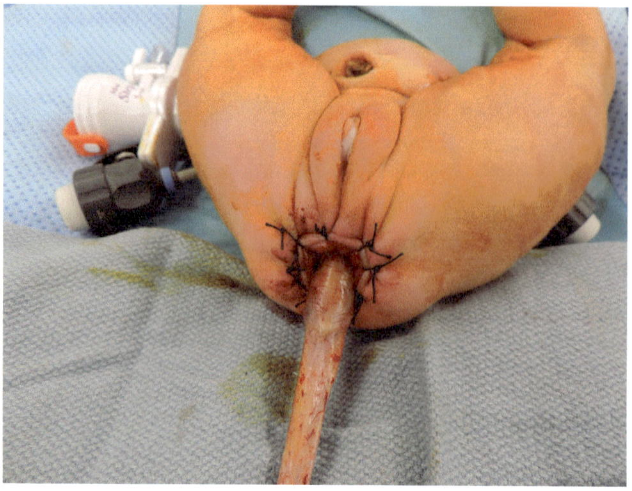

**Fig. 32.10** Eversion of the muscular cuff after mucosectomy in an infant undergoing pull-through for Hirschsprung's disease

the specimen. It is recommended to send the margin of the resected pull-through for a larger confirmatory frozen section biopsy. Figure 32.11 depicts the completed anastomosis with the resected pull-through segment passed off the field.

## Pearls and Pitfalls

- Mobilizing the mesentery of the sigmoid colon laparoscopically going into the pelvis greatly facilitates removal of the specimen from below. The specimen will literally drop right out of the anal canal.
- Ensure adequate mobility of the colon into the pelvis laparoscopically prior to commencing with perineal dissection. This often involves mobilizing the white line of Toldt and sometimes even the splenic flexure.
- In long-segment Hirschsprung's disease, it is valuable to await final pathology prior to committing to an extensive colectomy. Laparoscopic biopsies allow this without having to start with a perineal dissection. Even with experienced pediatric pathologists, calling ganglion cells on small samples by frozen section can be difficult.
- Try to create the anastomosis proximal to your last biopsy that showed ganglion cells to avoid problems with the transition zone.
- Always send the margin of the pull-through at the level of the anastomosis for frozen section to reconfirm that there are ganglion cells present.

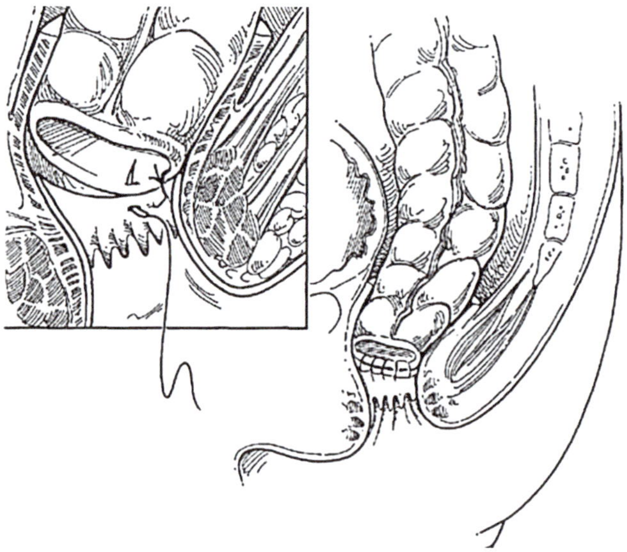

**Fig. 32.11** Securing neorectum to short anorectal cuff (*Courtesy of Keith Georgeson, with permission*)

## Anorectal Malformations or Imperforate Anus

Anorectal malformations describe a wide spectrum of defects in the development of the lower intestinal and urogenital tracts. An imperforate anus is usually discovered shortly after birth. While this term may accurately depict the patient's outward appearance, the malformation can involve a number of different but predictable patterns of fistulous connections between the rectum and urogenital structures or perineum. This created significant challenges for early pediatric surgeons as they attempted to repair these defects using a combination of abdominal, sacral, and perineal incisions. Today, the surgeon must determine which children should undergo primary repair in the neonatal period and which children require colostomy and definitive repair in a staged fashion. In 1982, Peña et al. reported the results of the modern open approach referred to as the posterior sagittal anorectoplasty (PSARP) or posterior sagittal anorectovaginourethroplasty (PSARVUP) [34]. Nearly two decades later, Georgeson et al. described the novel laparoscopically assisted anorectal pull-through (LAARP) for repair of high imperforate anus, utilizing minimal perineal dissection, preservation of the distal rectum, and accurate placement of the rectum within the levator ani and external anal sphincter muscle complex [35].

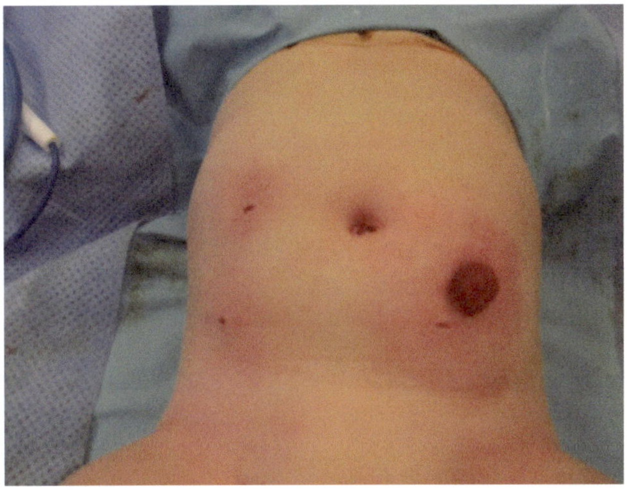

**Fig. 32.12** Incising the peritoneum to enter the pelvis to dissect out the rectum circumferentially. Note the position of the vas deferens which need to be preserved as dissection approaches the urethra

## Surgical Technique: Laparoscopic-Assisted Anorectal Pull-Through (LAARP)

A colostomy should be performed within 24–48 h of birth in children with complex malformations often grouped together as "high imperforate anus." These include rectourinary fistula in boys and rectovaginal fistula or cloaca in girls. Rectovestibular fistulas in girls are inside the vaginal introitus, but exterior to the hymen. Some pediatric surgeons repair this primarily with a perineal anoplasty, but the common wall between the vagina and rectum can be extensive, as can the dissection. Colostomy is often performed for this type as well. Definitive repair is then performed at 2–3 months of age. When creating the colostomy, the distal descending colon is divided at the junction with the sigmoid to maintain as much length as possible for the subsequent pull-through operation. A mucous fistula is also created. Subsequent contrast studies via this mucous fistula can help define the anomalous connections to the urethra or bladder in boys and to the vagina in girls. No fistula may be present in patients with trisomy 21. Loop colostomy is discouraged due to the possibility of spillover and the risk for urinary tract infection in those with urinary fistulae.

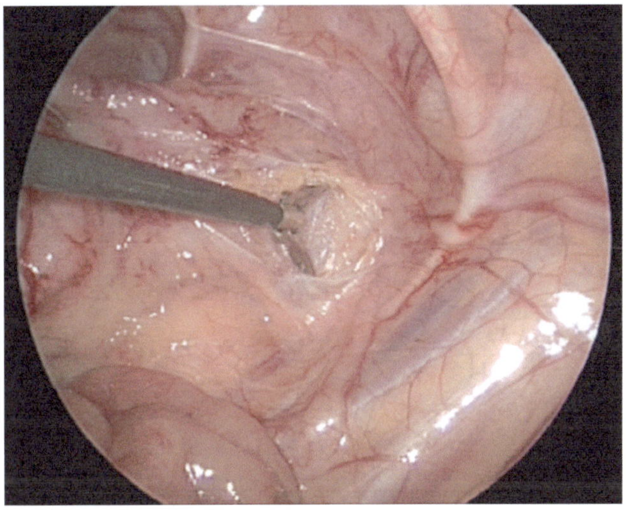

**Fig. 32.13** The rectum will extend toward the urethra anteriorly as dissection gets deep in the pelvis

LAARP is most useful in boys with rectourinary fistulas, although the authors have used it in females with no fistula and trisomy 21. In most females with high imperforate anus, the anatomy requires the open PSARP approach. For LAARP, the patient is positioned similar to that described in the above section on Hirschsprung's disease. Laparoscopic trocar placement is identical (Fig. 32.12). A Foley is placed sterilely on the field and left in place for 1 week postoperatively in those with urinary fistulas. The mucous fistula is located and dissection of the sigmoid colon is carried into the pelvis (Fig. 32.13). Care is taken to preserve the mesorectum to the rectourethral fistula (Fig. 32.14). Typically, there is considerable narrowing of the rectum as it gets closer to the urinary tract (Fig. 32.15). The surgeon must also be able to recognize and avoid injury to adjacent structures, including the ureters, vas deferens, and prostate depending on the level of the fistula. A fourth trocar is placed to provide traction on the fistula out of the pelvis for fistula ligation. It is important to ligate and divide the fistula close to the urethra (or bladder) to avoid leaving excess colonic mucosa on the stump (Fig. 32.16). This has been known to cause mucocele formation. While reports of post-LAARP complications are rare, a pediatric surgery group in Japan recommends routine MRI during follow-up to identify residual fistulae or cystic formations [37]. The authors ligate the fistula with silk ligatures and cut between them, although the use of clips has been described. In a very low fistula to the urethra at the level of the pelvic floor, the authors used a stapling device successfully. Endoloops (Ethicon Endo-Surgery, Cincinnati, OH)

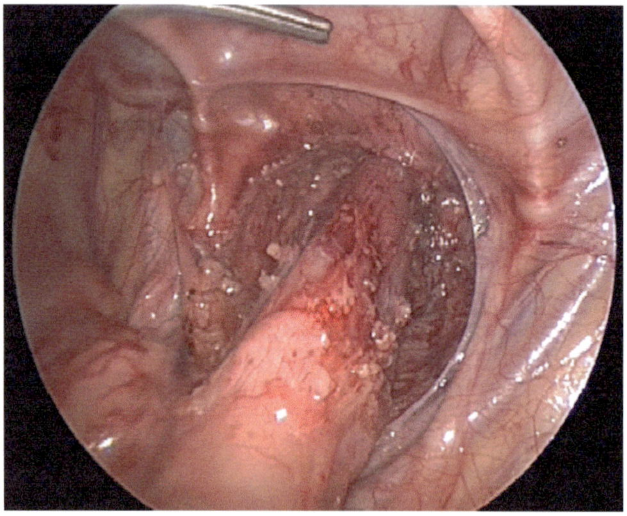

**Fig. 32.14** The rectum has been passed down to the perineum. This laparoscopic view demonstrates no twisting as it enters the pelvis

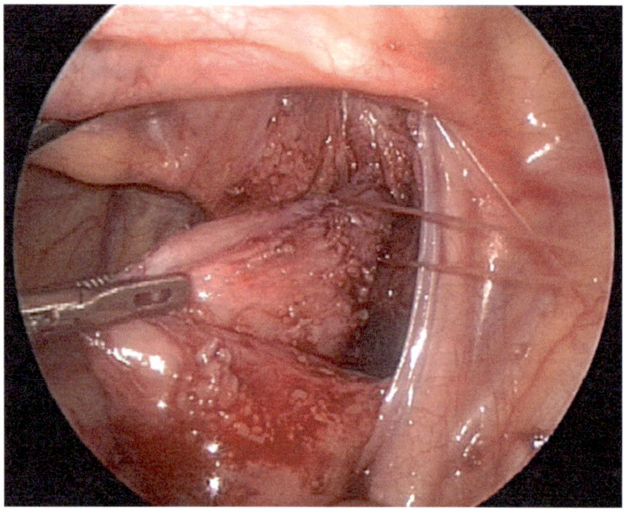

**Fig. 32.15** The actual rectourethral fistula often tapers down and becomes narrower at the junction with the urethra

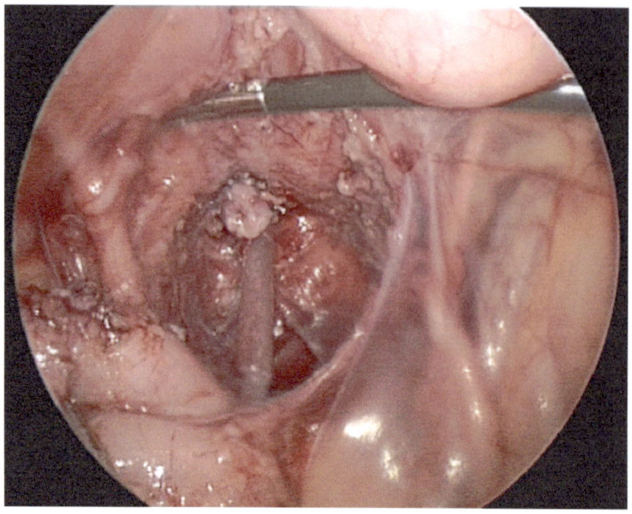

**Fig. 32.16** Anteriorly note the small stump of the fistula. Posteriorly the sheath from a trocar can be seen placed into the pelvis in the midline

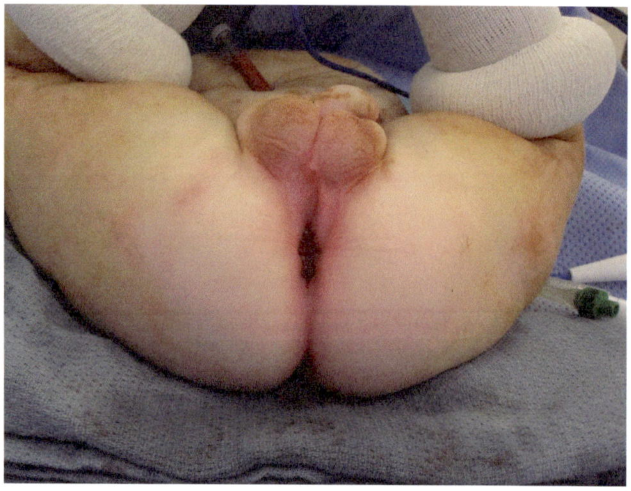

**Fig. 32.17** A completed anastomosis at the neoanus

can be used as well, but only after division of the fistula. Without traction on the rectum, after division the fistulous connection retracts deep into the pelvis making placement of the Endoloops more challenging.

After division of the fistula, the patient is placed into dorsal lithotomy (see section "Hirschsprung's Disease" for positioning). A Peña muscle stimulator is used to locate the point of maximal contraction of the external anal sphincter. A 12-mm skin ellipse is removed from this area in the midline on the perineum. While watching the pelvic floor laparoscopically (a quite unique view with no rectum in the pelvis), a 12-mm Step™ trocar sheath and a Veress needle are inserted between the two limbs of the puborectalis muscle in the midline and into the pelvis (Fig. 32.16). The trocar is placed through the sheath. The distal rectum is grasped with a laparoscopic grasper and brought out onto the perineum. If it will not pass through the canal made by the trocar, a large hemostat can be inserted through the tract instead and gently used to guide the rectum down to the perineum. A circumferential, single-layer anastomosis is then made between the distal rectal fistula and the dermis to create the neoanus (Fig. 32.17). The rectum can be grasped laparoscopically and retracted cephalad to deepen the anal dimple and lengthen the skin-lined portion of the anal canal.

Early postoperative studies have noted more favorable anorectal manometry findings and reliable indicators of potential continence in patients repaired with laparoscopic-assisted technique compared to PSARP. There is significantly earlier detection of a rectoanal relaxation reflex, lower resting rectal pressure, and improved rectal compliance in patients who underwent LAARP [36]. This translates to satisfactory defecatory function for patients with high or intermediate-type imperforate anus after LAARP that is at least as good as PSARP results [38]. Additional benefits of LAARP include shorter hospital stays and lower rates of rectum malposition based on magnetic resonance imaging [39].

## Pearls and Pitfalls

- When dividing the rectourethral fistula, ensure that the division is as close to the urethra as feasible, in order to prevent postoperative mucocele.
- Take care as the deep pelvic dissection commences to watch for and avoid injury not only to the ureters but also to the vas deferens and seminal vesicles as the urethra is approached.

## Fecal Incontinence

Many pediatric patients born with anorectal malformations, Hirschsprung's disease, spinal anomalies, and other congenital anomalies suffer from fecal incontinence that negatively impacts their emotional and social development. The goals of standard, nonsurgical management are to achieve regular bowel habits and stool consistency with a combination of diet modification, medication, and routine enemas to promote regular colonic emptying. Daily rectal enemas are easily administered in infants, but many children become intolerant or noncompliant. Historically, a diverting colostomy was necessary when nonoperative treatment failed, in which case the family is burdened with stoma care and the child incurs the additional social stress of having an ostomy. A permanent indwelling cecal tube can also be used to provide antegrade enemas at convenient times to flush out the colon. This is superior to enemas from below which may only partially evacuate the colon. The goal is to perform regular flushes at convenient times, which usually have rapid results, and to avoid incontinent "accidents" between flushes. Most patients are highly satisfied with antegrade enemas, and with titration, most can eliminate nearly all episodes of incontinence. The authors recommend titration to effect starting with a mixture of 100 ml of tap water and 20 ml of glycerin. Most patients flush once daily with success. Too much glycerin can result in cramping.

An alternative surgical procedure for fecal incontinence was introduced by Malone in 1990 [40]. He described a method in which the appendix is used as a conduit to administer an antegrade continence enema (ACE). In some patients who have undergone previous appendectomy, a neo-appendix can be fashioned with a tubularized cecal flap. Both have the advantage of creating a catheterizable channel so the patient does not require a permanent indwelling tube. The appendix is typically long enough and pliable enough that leakage is rare when the catheter is not stenting it, and most patients simply wear a Band-aid® or other adhesive bandage over the stoma between flushes. We prefer to bring the appendix up to the base of the umbilicus in most patients to hide it. In obese patients (some of whom are wheelchair bound), catheterizing deep in the umbilicus can be challenging, and alternative sites on the abdominal wall can be used, such as the right lower quadrant.

We only offer this procedure in patients who are emotionally and socially mature enough to voluntarily participate in the daily catheterizations.

## Surgical Technique: Laparoscopic-Assisted Appendicostomy

Trocar placement is identical to that described for laparoscopic appendectomy except a 10-mm trocar is placed at the umbilicus instead of a 12-mm trocar. The cecum and right colon are mobilized laterally so that the appendix tip will easily reach the umbilicus. Care is taken to preserve the mesoappendix. The appendiceal tip is then grasped with a laparoscopic trocar through the 10-mm trocar site, and the appendix is brought up to the umbilical skin, backing out the trocar in the process. Forceps are used to stabilize the appendix. Two 4–0 sutures are used to secure seromuscular bites of the appendix to the fascia. The tip of the appendix is excised with electrocautery, and a 10-Fr or 12-Fr Foley catheter is inserted all the way into the appendix prior to inflating the balloon which is drawn back to rest in the cecum at the appendiceal orifice. Circumferential 4–0 sutures are used to secure the appendiceal opening to the dermis. The Foley is secured with a suture to the skin to prevent inward migration, and the Foley itself is typically kept in for 4–6 weeks while the site heals. Small flushes daily are used to maintain patency for the first 2 weeks after which daily therapeutic flushes commence. The Foley can be removed after 4–6 weeks, but daily catheterization is required to prevent stricture formation at the skin level which is reported to occur in up to 20 % of patients. Some surgeons have reported using an umbilical V-Y appendicoplasty technique to decrease stricture rate, although we have found that daily compliance with an ACE program is most helpful in preventing this problem.

## Pearls and Pitfalls

- Patients must catheterize the channel every single day to minimize the risk of stomal stricture formation

## Summary

Minimally invasive surgery has now become almost universally a part of most pediatric surgery practices, and there are many applications in colorectal surgery. Smaller instrumentation and more widespread training for pediatric surgical techniques have been the primary factors in this development. The literature still lacks, and desperately needs, large, well-conducted prospective trials comparing laparoscopic with traditional open procedures to validate the presumed benefits of MIS. The appeal of smaller incisions, shorter hospital stays, and more rapid return to preoperative activities will continue to serve as the catalyst for the continued development of MIS.

## References


1. Mühe E. Long-term follow-up after laparoscopic cholecystectomy. Endoscopy. 1992;24(9):754–8.
2. Blinman T. Incisions do not simply sum. Surg Endosc. 2010; 24(7):1746–51.
3. Holcomb GW, Georgeson K, Rothenberg S. Atlas of pediatric laparoscopy and thoracoscopy. Philadelphia, PA: Saunder/Elsevier; 2008.
4. Roviaro GC, Varoli F, Saguatti L, et al. Major vascular injuries in laparoscopic surgery. Surg Endosc. 2002;16(8):1192–6.
5. Bax NMA, van der Zee DC. Complications in laparoscopic surgery in children. In: Bax NMA, Georgeson KE, Najmaldin A, Valla JS, editors. Endoscopic surgery in children. Berlin: Springer; 1999. p. 357–70.
6. Chen MK, Schropp KP, Lobe TE. Complications of minimal-access surgery in children. J Pediatr Surg. 1996;31(8):1161–5.
7. Ostlie DJ, Holcomb 3rd GW. The use of stab incisions for instrument access in laparoscopic operations. J Pediatr Surg. 2003; 38(12):1837–40.
8. Pennant JH. Anesthesia for laparoscopy in the pediatric patient. Anesthesiol Clin North America. 2001;19(1):69–88.
9. Bax NMA. Instrumentation in pediatric endoscopic surgery. In: Lobe TE, editor. Pediatric laparoscopy. Georgetown, TX: Landes Bioscience; 2002.
10. Lee SL, Ho HS. Acute appendicitis: is there a difference between children and adults? Am Surg. 2006;72(5):409–13.
11. Ponsky TA, Rothenberg SS. Division of the mesoappendix with electrocautery in children is safe, effective, and cost-efficient. J Laparoendosc Adv Surg Tech A. 2009;19 Suppl 1:S11–3.
12. Aziz O, Athanasiou T, Tekkis PP, et al. Laparoscopic versus open appendectomy in children: a meta-analysis. Ann Surg. 2006; 243(1):17–27.
13. Schmelzer TM, Rana AR, Walters KC, et al. Improved outcomes for laparoscopic appendectomy compared with open appendectomy in the pediatric population. J Laparoendosc Adv Surg Tech A. 2007;17(5):693–7.
14. Tsao KJ, St Peter SD, Valusek PA, et al. Adhesive small bowel obstruction after appendectomy in children: comparison between the laparoscopic and open approach. J Pediatr Surg. 2007;42(6):939–42 [discussion: 942].
15. McKinlay R, Neeleman S, Klein R, et al. Intraabdominal abscess following open and laparoscopic appendectomy in the pediatric population. Surg Endosc. 2003;17(5):730–3.
16. Nadler EP, Reblock KK, Qureshi FG, et al. Laparoscopic appendectomy in children with perforated appendicitis. J Laparoendosc Adv Surg Tech A. 2006;16(2):159–63.
17. Emil SG, Taylor MB. Appendicitis in children treated by pediatric versus general surgeons. J Am Coll Surg. 2007;204(1):34–9.
18. Loftus Jr EV. Clinical epidemiology of inflammatory bowel disease: incidence, prevalence, and environmental influences. Gastroenterology. 2004;126(6):1504–17.
19. Jan S, Slap G, Dai D, Rubin DM. Variation in surgical outcomes for adolescents and young adults with inflammatory bowel disease. Pediatrics. 2013;131:S81–9.
20. Munkholm P, Langholz E, Davidsen M, Binder V. Intestinal cancer risk and mortality in patients with Crohn's disease. Gastroenterology. 1993;105(6):1716–23.
21. Solberg IC, Vatn MH, Høie O, IBSEN Study Group, et al. Clinical course in Crohn's disease: results of a Norwegian population based ten-year follow-up study. Clin Gastroenterol Hepatol. 2007;5(12): 1430–8.
22. Wu XJ, He XS, Zhou XY, Ke J, Lan P. The role of laparoscopic surgery for ulcerative colitis: systematic review with meta-analysis. Int J Colorectal Dis. 2010;25(8):949–57.
23. Hurst RD, Molinari M, Chung TP, Rubin M, Michelassi F. Prospective study of the features, indications, and surgical treatment in 513 consecutive patients affected by Crohn's disease. Surgery. 1997;122(4):661–7. discussion 667–8.
24. Fichera A, Peng SL, Elisseou NM, Rubin MA, Hurst RD. Laparoscopy or conventional open surgery for patients with ileocolonic Crohn's disease? A prospective study. Surgery. 2007;142(4): 566–71. discussion 571.e1.
25. Laituri CA, Fraser JD, Garey CL, Aguayo P, Sharp SW, Ostlie DJ, Holcomb 3rd GW, St Peter SD. Laparoscopic ileocecectomy in pediatric patients with Crohn's Disease. J Laparoendosc Adv Surg Tech A. 2011;21(2):193–5.
26. Dutta S, Rothenberg SS, Chang J, Bealer J. Total intracorporeal laparoscopic resection of Crohn's disease. J Pediatr Surg. 2003; 38(5):717–9.
27. Milsom JW, Hammerhofer KA, Bohm B. Prospective, randomized trial comparing laparoscopic versus conventional surgery for refractory ileocolic Crohn's disease. Dis Colon Rectum. 2001; 44(1):1–8.
28. Johnston D, Holdsworth PJ, Nasmyth DG, et al. Preservation of the entire anal canal in consecutive proctocolectomy for ulcerative colitis: a pilot study comparing end-to-end ileo-anal anastomosis without mucosal resection with mucosal proctectomy and endo-anal anastomosis. Br J Surg. 1987;74:940–4.
29. Reilly WT, Pemberton JH, Wolff BG, et al. Randomized prospective trial comparing ileal pouch-anal anastomosis performed by excising the anal mucosa to ileal pouch-anal anastomosis performed by preserving the anal mucosa. Ann Surg. 1997;225(6): 666–77.
30. Lovegrove RE, Consantinides VA, Heriot AG, et al. A comparison of hand-sewn versus stapled ileal pouch-anal anastomosis (IPAA) following proctocolectomy: a meta-analysis of 4183 patients. Ann Surg. 2006;244(1):18–26.
31. Amiel J, Lyonnet S. Hirschsprung's disease, associated syndromes, and genetics: a review. J Med Genet. 2001;38:729–39.
32. Georgeson KE, Fuenfer MM, Hardin WD. Primary laparoscopic pull-through for Hirschsprung's disease in infants and children. J Pediatr Surg. 1995;30(7):1017–22.
33. Wheatley MJ, Wesley JR, Coran AG, Polley Jr TZ. Hirschsprung's disease in adolescents and adults. Dis Colon Rectum. 1990; 30:622–9.
34. Peña A, de Vries PA. Posterior sagittal anorectoplasty: important technical considerations and new applications. J Pediatr Surg. 1982;17(6):796–811.

35. Georgeson KE, Inge TH, Albanese CT. Laparoscopically assisted anorectal pull-through for high imperforate anus – a new technique. J Pediatr Surg. 2000;35(6):927–30.
36. Lin CL, Wong KK, Lan LC, Chen CC, Tam PK. Earlier appearance and higher incidence of the rectoanal relaxation reflex in patients with imperforate anus repaired with laparoscopically assisted anorectoplasty. Surg Endosc. 2003;17(10):1646–9.
37. Uchida H, Iwanaka T, Kitano Y, et al. Residual fistula after laparoscopically assisted anorectoplasty: is it a rare problem? J Pediatr Surg. 2009;44(1):278–81.
38. Wong KK, Wu X, Chan IH, Tam PK. Evaluation of defecative function 5 years or longer after laparoscopic assisted pull-through for imperforate anus. J Pediatr Surg. 2011;46(12): 2313–5.
39. Tong QS, Tang ST, Pu JR, Mao YZ, Wang Y, Li SW, Cao QQ, Ruan QL. Laparoscopically assisted anorectal pull-through for high imperforate anus in infants: intermediate results. J Pediatr Surg. 2011;46(8):1578–86.
40. Malone PS, Ransley PG, Kiely EM. Preliminary report: the antegrade continence enema. Lancet. 1990;336:1217–8.

# Laparoscopy in Pregnant Patients

# 33

Melissa M. Alvarez-Downing and David J. Maron

**Key Points**

- Laparoscopy can be performed safely in pregnancy.
- When addressing abdominal pain during pregnancy, the patient should be managed similarly to the nonpregnant patient.
- Consideration of the age of gestation and size of the gravid uterus is necessary to determine adequate port placement and surgical approach.
- Utilizing a strategy of expectant management is dangerous to the pregnant patient and fetus and should be avoided.

## Introduction

Approximately 1 in 500 to 1 in 635 women will require non-obstetrical abdominal surgery during pregnancy [1, 2]. While the most common non-obstetrical surgical emergencies include acute appendicitis, cholecystitis, and bowel obstruction, a wide range of operations performed in pregnancy have been reported.

The traditional approach to abdominal surgery during pregnancy has been via laparotomy in order to avoid injury to the gravid uterus and fetus. It was initially believed that laparoscopy was unsafe in pregnancy due to risks of $CO_2$ insufflation and instrumentation. Yet, as laparoscopy has gained popularity and experience, recent evidence has contradicted this initial belief and has shown that laparoscopy is indeed a safe surgical approach for a variety of conditions in the pregnant patient [3–5]. While most of the literature regarding laparoscopy in pregnancy pertains to appendicitis and cholecystitis, a few accounts of its use in the management of colorectal diseases have been reported [4]. Overall, when managing abdominal pain in the pregnant patient, the guiding principle is prompt diagnosis and treatment, which results in improved fetal outcome [6, 7].

## Overview of Changes in Physiology and Anatomy During Pregnancy

The physiologic changes that occur in pregnancy involve nearly every organ system of the expectant mother (Table 33.1). These changes, which occur slowly over time, are a response to the growing fetus and an internal shift of support, cumulatively accounting for drastic changes to the pregnant patient.

The cardiovascular system is affected by an increased plasma blood volume of 40–50 %. This triggers an augmented stroke volume and a 50 % increase in cardiac output [8]. Circulating increased progesterone levels cause a decrease in systemic vascular resistance and subsequent lower blood pressure with an increased heart rate by an average of 15 beats per minute. Additionally, there is a 20–30 % increase in red blood cell volume, which combined with increased plasma blood volume causes a purely dilutional decrease in the patient's hematocrit. Furthermore, increased hepatic production of coagulation factors causes a hypercoagulable state, which in addition to decreased activity can result in a significant risk for developing blood clots and emboli.

Changes in the respiratory system during pregnancy also take place. The enlarging uterus displaces the diaphragm cephalad and increases intra-abdominal pressure [9]. To compensate, relaxation of the rib-cage ligaments occurs with a resultant increase in chest wall size. While the total lung capacity (TLC) remains the same in pregnancy, there is a 20–30 % decrease in functional residual capacity (FRC) and its components: expiratory reserve volume (ERV) and residual volume (RV). A compensatory increase in inspiratory capacity (IC), through a 30–50 % increase in tidal volume (Vt), maintains the TLC. This maintenance of lung capacity

Electronic supplementary material Supplementary material is available in the online version of this chapter at 10.1007/978-1-4939-1581-1_33. Videos can also be accessed at http://www.springerimages.com/videos/978-1-4939-1580-4.

M.M. Alvarez-Downing, M.D. • D.J. Maron, M.D., M.B.A. (✉)
Department of Colorectal Surgery, Cleveland Clinic Florida, 2950 Cleveland Clinic Boulevard, Weston, FL 33331, USA
e-mail: marond@ccf.org

H.M. Ross et al. (eds.), *Minimally Invasive Approaches to Colon and Rectal Disease: Technique and Best Practices*, DOI 10.1007/978-1-4939-1581-1_33, © Springer Science+Business Media New York 2015

**Table 33.1** Physiologic changes to consider during pregnancy

| | |
|---|---|
| Cardiovascular | ↑Plasma blood volume (40–50 %) |
| | ↑SV |
| | ↑CO (50 %) |
| | ↓SVR |
| | ↓BP, ↑HR |
| Pulmonary | ↔TLC |
| | ↓FRC |
| | ↑IC |
| | ↑MV |
| Hematology | ↑RBC volume |
| | ↓Hct[a] |
| | ↑Hypercoagulable state |
| Gastrointestinal | ↓Gastric emptying |
| | ↓GEJ tone |
| | ↓Colonic motility |

*SV* stroke volume, *CO* cardiac output, *SVR* systemic volume resistance, *BP* blood pressure, *HR* heart rate, *TLC* total lung capacity, *FRC* functional residual capacity, *IC* inspiratory capacity, *MV* minute ventilation, *RBC* red blood cell volume, *Hct* hematocrit, *GEJ* gastroesophageal reflux
[a]Dilutional

**Table 33.2** Indications for laparoscopy during pregnancy

| What can wait | What can't wait |
|---|---|
| Small bowel obstruction (early) | Acute appendicitis |
| Acute uncomplicated diverticulitis | Acute cholecystitis, recurrent cholelithiasis |
| Inflammatory bowel disease exacerbation (mild) | Small bowel obstruction (late, complete) |
| | Acute complicated diverticulitis |
| | Incarcerated hernia |
| | Volvulus/necrotic bowel |
| | Peritonitis |
| | Inflammatory bowel disease exacerbation (severe) |
| | Colorectal cancer[a] |

[a]Stage II–III rectal cancer and stage IV colorectal cancer may be considered (as appropriate) for (neo)adjuvant chemoradiation therapy

is evident in spirometry testing (i.e., FEV1), which is not significantly different between pregnant and nonpregnant patients. Finally, there is an increase in minute ventilation, which is also attributed to an increased tidal volume. Clinically, 60–70 % of pregnant patients complain of dyspnea on exertion with 20 % of patients experiencing dyspnea at rest [10]. This dyspnea is attributed to the ventilatory stimulating effect of progesterone.

Gastrointestinal effects include delayed gastric emptying, decreased gastroesophageal tone and decreased colonic motility [11]. Clinically, patients are more prone to abdominal bloating, acid reflux, and constipation. All of these are important considerations when contemplating general anesthesia.

In addition to the physiologic changes that occur during pregnancy, significant anatomical alterations occur. Weight gain, which is expected to be between 25 and 35 lb during pregnancy [12], can vary drastically from patient to patient and may affect surgical approach. Additionally, the gravid uterus increases in size from 7.5 to 35 cm and enters into the abdominal cavity at the beginning of the second trimester, thus potentially affecting surgical approach and trocar placement.

## Indications for Laparoscopy

Indications for laparoscopy in pregnancy are the same as those in the nonpregnant patient (Table 33.2) [3]. Benefits of laparoscopy including less postoperative pain, decreased postoperative ileus, shorter length of hospital stay, and quicker return to work are similar in pregnant and nonpregnant patients [13]. Historical recommendations included delaying surgery until the second trimester as a strategy to avoid fetal loss during the first trimester. This has been challenged with reports that show that laparoscopy can be performed safely in any trimester [13, 14]. In fact, postponing surgery may result in increased maternal and fetal morbidity, as noted by Babler in 1908, who stated that the "the mortality of appendicitis complicating pregnancy is the mortality of delay" [15].

## What Can Wait?

### Small Bowel Obstruction (Early)

Small bowel obstruction secondary to adhesions in a pregnant patient can be managed expectantly as in the nonpregnant patient. Failed conservative management, complete bowel obstruction, worsening abdominal pain, fever, leukocytosis, or other signs of deterioration should prompt immediate surgical intervention.

### Acute Uncomplicated Diverticulitis

Acute diverticulitis can occur in young patients and may occur during pregnancy. If a patient presents with an episode of uncomplicated diverticulitis, i.e., mild abdominal pain and leukocytosis, without evidence of sepsis or free perforation, conservative management with IV or oral antibiotics and decreased po intake is acceptable. Inpatient observation should be considered to ensure the patient responds appropriately.

### Mild Inflammatory Bowel Disease Exacerbations

Inflammatory bowel disease (IBD) occurs most frequently in young adults during their reproductive years, making it a possible manifestation of abdominal pain in the pregnant patient. While the course of IBD is similar in the pregnant and nonpregnant patient, approximately one-third to one-half of patients with quiescent disease at the time of conception will relapse during the first trimester or postpartum period [11, 16, 17]. These exacerbations are more common in patients with active or uncontrolled disease at the time of conception [16]. Mild and moderate attacks should be managed medically with aminosalicylates, antibiotics, steroids, and, when necessary, immunosuppressive therapy. Variable effects on preterm labor and fetal outcome have been reported [11, 18]. It has been shown, however, that the majority of patients can be managed successfully with medical therapy and carry their fetuses to term [16]. In the setting of clinical deterioration or nonresponse to medical management, pregnant patients should be managed surgically as the nonpregnant patient.

## What Can't Wait?

### Acute Appendicitis

Appendicitis is the most common indication for non-obstetrical surgery during pregnancy with an incidence of 1:500 to 1:3,000 pregnancies [2, 19]. Acute appendicitis is considered a surgical emergency in pregnancy, with perforated appendicitis being the most common surgical cause of fetal loss [20]. While appendicitis during pregnancy was historically considered a contraindication to laparoscopy, many patients have been successfully treated with this procedure since it was first performed by Semm in 1981 [21]. Subsequently, multiple studies have shown that this approach offers similar advantages of shorter hospital stay, less postoperative pain, and faster return to daily activities over the open approach [22, 23]. Additionally, the ability to locate an ectopic appendix displaced by a gravid uterus, decreased manipulation of the uterus (which may result in decreased irritability and fetal loss), and an ability to explore the abdominal cavity for an alternate source of pain when a normal appendix is encountered are all benefits of laparoscopy [13, 22–24].

### Acute Cholecystitis and Symptomatic Cholelithiasis

Acute cholecystitis associated with repeated attacks, obstructive jaundice, gallstone pancreatitis, and peritonitis is an indication for cholecystectomy during pregnancy. Whether to perform cholecystectomy for symptomatic cholelithiasis during pregnancy has remained a controversial issue. Historically, nonoperative management was advocated. Yet, several studies have shown that conservative management results in higher morbidity and pregnancy-related complications [6, 7, 25]. In patients treated nonoperatively, the number of recurrent episodes of biliary symptoms, emergency department visits, and hospitalizations is higher. Additionally, early induction of labor is more common in these patients [6, 25]. In contrast, laparoscopic cholecystectomy performed in any trimester of pregnancy can be performed safely with a very low risk to the patient and fetus [13, 25]. These findings, combined with the ability to decrease morbidity from recurrent attacks, have made laparoscopic cholecystectomy the treatment of choice in pregnant patients, regardless of the trimester [3].

### Small Bowel Obstruction (Late, Complete)

While conservative management of bowel obstruction in pregnancy should be utilized as the first management strategy, bowel obstruction remains the third most common cause for non-obstetrical surgery in pregnancy. It is most common in the third trimester because of the enlarged gravid uterus and has increased in incidence as a greater number of patients undergo intestinal Roux-en-Y gastric bypass procedures. Surgical therapy is indicated when a patient fails conservative management with bowel rest and fluid and electrolyte replacement or when a complete bowel obstruction, intussusception, or internal hernia is present [26]. The use of laparoscopy to address bowel obstruction has been successfully reported during pregnancy regardless of the trimester [5, 27], although laparoscopy may be technically challenging due to the loss of abdominal domain from the enlarged gravid uterus and dilated bowel.

### Acute Complicated Diverticulitis

Acute complicated diverticulitis in pregnancy (i.e., free perforation, abscess, and/or sepsis) is a rare complication with only a few cases reported in the literature [4, 28, 29]. While there are no defined protocols for diagnosis and treatment in pregnancy, these patients should be managed in the same manner as the nonpregnant patient, with laparoscopic intervention utilized when possible. The use of laparoscopic lavage in selected patients with acute complicated diverticulitis has gained acceptance, and this may also be an option in the pregnant patient who presents with diverticulitis. One report of right-sided diverticulitis at 20 weeks gestation with localized rebound tenderness and low-grade fever demonstrated successful laparoscopic peritoneal drainage without complications to the fetus or resultant preterm labor [4].

## Peritonitis

Any pregnant patient presenting with an acute abdomen or clinical findings consistent with peritonitis warrants immediate surgical intervention. It is important to note that preterm labor associated with the inflammatory pathway is well established in the obstetrical literature. Inflammation is responsible for about a 10 % fetal loss in pregnant women with perforation and peritonitis [1]. Therefore, immediate surgical intervention, either via laparotomy or laparoscopy, is necessary for both improved maternal and fetal outcomes.

## Severe Inflammatory Bowel Disease Exacerbations

Inflammatory bowel disease (IBD) in pregnancy manifesting as fulminant colitis, toxic megacolon, perforation, obstruction, or hemorrhage warrants emergent surgical intervention. Some reports have demonstrated that surgery for IBD during the course of pregnancy is associated with a high rate of spontaneous abortions and stillbirths, yet other reports have contradicted these findings [11, 18]. In all, because surgery in pregnant patients with IBD exacerbation is reserved for extreme cases, the use of laparoscopy has not been described [18, 30].

## Colorectal Cancer (Video 33.1)

Colorectal cancer (CRC) in pregnancy is rare, with an incidence of 1 in 13,000 pregnancies reported in the literature [31]. Diagnosis of CRC during pregnancy can be challenging because of overlapping symptoms between malignancy and expected gestational changes [32]. Patients can present with nonspecific symptoms such as abdominal pain, nausea, vomiting, constipation, rectal bleeding, and back pain. As a result, a delay in diagnosis occurs and most colorectal cancers in pregnancy are detected at a later stage when compared to the nonpregnant patient. However, stage for stage, survival between pregnant patients and the general population is the same [32]. Additionally, CRC in pregnancy is often associated with tumors in the rectum compared to the more common colon cancers in the general population [32, 33]. In a series of 41 pregnant patients with colorectal cancer, 64 % of patients had a rectal carcinoma which was similar to 86 % of 205 pregnant patients previously reported in the literature [32].

Management of CRC during pregnancy requires an individualized approach and a multidisciplinary team with recommendations based on the gestational age of the fetus, cancer stage, colon vs. rectal primary, need for emergent vs. elective surgery, patient's desire for future fertility, and any complicating factors related to the tumor or pregnancy [11, 34]. Because radiation and chemotherapy have a limited role during pregnancy, surgical resection remains the most feasible treatment option. While limited data exists in patients with CRC who are less than 20 weeks gestation, successful surgical resection performed early in pregnancy with the birth of normal infants has been described [34]. If the diagnosis of CRC is made after 20 weeks gestation, resection may be delayed until delivery, but the delay should be minimized as much as possible. While no reports describing the use of laparoscopy for the resection of CRC in pregnant patients have been described in the literature, this approach can be utilized when appropriate.

It is important to note that timing of surgery and delivery is especially important when radiation and chemotherapy are required in the adjuvant setting. While radiation therapy must be postponed until delivery of the infant, chemotherapy can be administered in the second and third trimesters after the completion of organogenesis has occurred [35]. Termination of the pregnancy may be recommended in cases with advanced disease and/or complications, i.e., perforation or obstruction, or when the diagnosis is made during early pregnancy, which would significantly delay the administration of adjuvant therapy.

## Patient Positioning

Depending on the age of gestation, a pregnant mother will need to be placed in Trendelenburg with a slight left lateral position to avoid compression of the uterus on the inferior vena cava during the procedure. This is almost always necessary in woman over 20 weeks gestation. Lithotomy is not necessary in most procedures but, when utilized, should be done with standard precautions and padding. Similar to other laparoscopic procedures, patients should have all bony prominences well padded. As gravity still plays a major role in keeping the small bowel out of the operative view, patients need to be appropriately secured to allow for changes in the bed position (i.e., lateral and (reverse) Trendelenburg).

## Fetal Monitoring

Fetal monitoring during surgical intervention should be performed immediately before and after the procedure by the obstetrical team. Serial $PaCO_2$ measurements or continuous uterine and fetal monitoring during a procedure are not routinely employed [13, 14]. Continuous intraoperative $CO_2$ monitoring of the pregnant patient by capnography should be utilized [3].

## Instrumentation

There is no difference in the instrumentation necessary to perform laparoscopy in the pregnant patient.

## Trocar Placement

Trocar placement in the pregnant patient will depend on the surgical procedure to be performed and the size of the gravid uterus (Fig. 33.1). The most notable difference from standard laparoscopy is determining where to gain access to the peritoneal cavity. In patients who are in their first trimester, the uterus is still located in the pelvis and a standard open Hasson technique can be employed at the umbilicus [24, 36]. By the beginning of the second trimester (14 weeks), the gravid uterus is located intra-abdominally halfway to the umbilicus and eventually extends to the umbilicus by 20 weeks in most patients. This necessitates the need for alternative entry into the peritoneal cavity during the second and third trimester. The entry site should be far away from the gravid uterus to avoid risk of iatrogenic injury. The safest point of entry is in the left or right upper quadrant, midclavicular line, and two fingerbreadths below the costal margin.

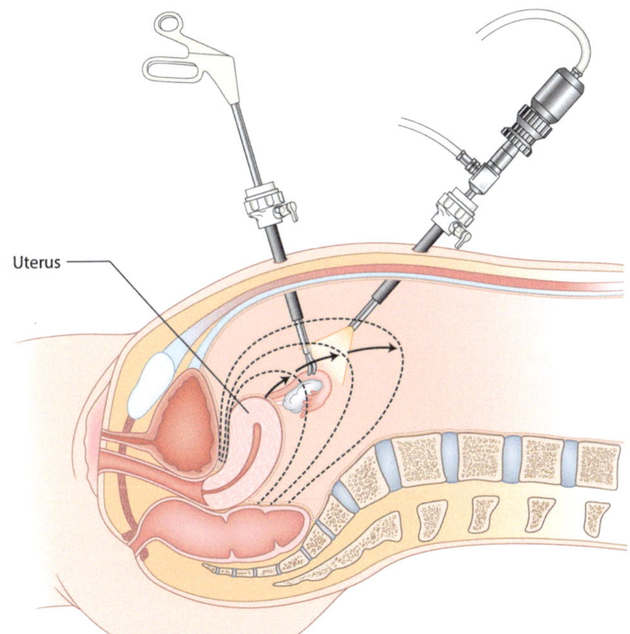


**Fig. 33.1** Relationship of gravid uterus depending on gestational age to trocar placement

An optical trocar (Optiview, Ethicon, Cincinnati, USA) or Veress needle is recommended to establish pneumoperitoneum [24, 37]. The remaining ports should be placed appropriately under direct visualization and in a location, which allows the procedure to be performed while taking into account the size of the gravid uterus.

## $CO_2$ Insufflation

Initial reluctance to perform laparoscopy in pregnant patients included concern over effects of $CO_2$ insufflation to the fetus. This was initially suggested by work performed by Hunter et al. on pregnant sheep in 1995 [38]. His data demonstrated that pneumoperitoneum with $CO_2$ to 15 mmHg caused a decreased pH in the mother and fetus, which could be reversed with either 30 min of steady-state insufflation or by hyperventilating the mother. Additionally, pneumoperitoneum with $CO_2$ caused tachycardia and hypertension in the fetus, both of which were returned to normal after $CO_2$ desufflation. None of these effects were identified with the use of nitrous oxide in this report. Yet, despite these initial findings, several recent studies have demonstrated no adverse effect on the fetus with a $CO_2$ insufflation of 10–15 mmHg [3, 24]. Therefore, guidelines developed by the Society of American Gastrointestinal Endoscopic Surgeons state that $CO_2$ insufflation of 10–15 mmHg can safely be used for laparoscopy in the pregnant patient [3].

## Tips and Tricks

### Pain

Pain in a pregnant patient should be addressed similarly as in a nonpregnant patient. Consideration of pregnancy-related conditions, e.g., round ligament strain, should be included in the differential diagnosis.

### Appendicitis

A diagnosis of appendicitis in the pregnant patient warrants immediate surgical intervention without delay. The use of laparoscopy may be beneficial in that it allows for easier visualization of a displaced appendix and adequate exploration of the remainder of the abdomen.

### Diverticulitis

Patients with acute diverticulitis during pregnancy should be treated conservatively. However, in the patient that requires exploration, peritoneal lavage and drainage may be of use. Any clinical deterioration requires standard operative/resectional intervention.

## IBD/Pouches

Total proctocolectomy, either with or without ileal pouch construction, should not be performed in the pregnant patient. In patients with fulminant colitis, toxic megacolon, perforation, obstruction, or hemorrhage who require surgical intervention, subtotal colectomy with end ileostomy is the procedure of choice, delaying reconstruction until after delivery.

## Technical Tips

### What Do or Should We Do Differently in Pregnancy?

The pregnant patient should be addressed in a similar manner to the nonpregnant patient with a detailed explanation of the risks and benefits of treatment options discussed with the patient. Pregnant patients should be placed in a slight left lateral decubitus position with extra care taken to avoid injury to the gravid uterus while entering the abdominal cavity.

### Useful Tricks in the Belly and Dealing with the Uterus

When performing a surgical procedure on a pregnant patient, it is important to minimize direct manipulation of the gravid uterus. Adequately securing the patient to the operating room table will allow steep reverse Trendelenburg or lateral decubitus so that gravity may move the uterus out of the field of view. If access to the pelvis is necessary to perform the desired procedure, the uterus can gently be elevated using a liver retractor device via a midline infraumbilical incision.

## References


1. Kammerer WS. Nonobstetric surgery during pregnancy. Med Clin North Am. 1979;63(6):1157–64.
2. Kort B, Katz VL, Watson WJ. The effect of nonobstetric operation during pregnancy. Surg Gynecol Obstet. 1993;177(4):371–6.
3. Pearl J, Price R, Richardson W, Fanelli R, Society of American Gastrointestinal Endoscopic Surgeons. Guidelines for diagnosis, treatment, and use of laparoscopy for surgical problems during pregnancy. Surg Endosc. 2011;25(11):3479–92.
4. Pelosi III MA, Pelosi MA, Villalona E. Right-sided colonic diverticulitis mimicking acute cholecystitis in pregnancy: case report and laparoscopic treatment. Surg Laparosc Endosc. 1999;9(1):63–7.
5. Gagne DJ, DeVoogd K, Rutkoski JD, Papasavas PK, Urbandt JE. Laparoscopic repair of internal hernia during pregnancy after Roux-en-Y gastric bypass. Surg Obes Relat Dis. 2010;6(1):88–92.
6. Othman MO, Stone E, Hashimi M, Parasher G. Conservative management of cholelithiasis and its complications in pregnancy is associated with recurrent symptoms and more emergency department visits. Gastrointest Endosc. 2012;76(3):564–9.
7. Muench J, Albrink M, Serafini F, Rosemurgy A, Carey L, Murr MM. Delay in treatment of biliary disease during pregnancy increases morbidity and can be avoided with safe laparoscopic cholecystectomy. Am Surg. 2001;67(6):539–42. discussion 42–3.
8. Guyton AC, Hall JE. Guyton and Hall textbook of medical physiology. 11th ed. Philadelphia: Saunders; 2005.
9. Hegewald MJ, Crapo RO. Respiratory physiology in pregnancy. Clin Chest Med. 2011;32(1):1–13. vii.
10. Milne JA. The respiratory response to pregnancy. Postgrad Med J. 1979;55(643):318–24.
11. Longo SA, Moore RC, Canzoneri BJ, Robichaux A. Gastrointestinal conditions during pregnancy. Clin Colon Rectal Surg. 2010; 23(2):80–9.
12. American College of Obstetricians Gynecologists. ACOG Committee opinion no. 548: weight gain during pregnancy. Obstet Gynecol. 2013;121(1):210–2.
13. Affleck DG, Handrahan DL, Egger MJ, Price RR. The laparoscopic management of appendicitis and cholelithiasis during pregnancy. Am J Surg. 1999;178(6):523–9.
14. Rollins MD, Chan KJ, Price RR. Laparoscopy for appendicitis and cholelithiasis during pregnancy: a new standard of care. Surg Endosc. 2004;18(2):237–41.
15. Babler EA. Perforative appendicitis complicating pregnancy. JAMA. 1908;51:1310–3.
16. Mogadam M, Korelitz BI, Ahmed SW, Dobbins III WO, Baiocco PJ. The course of inflammatory bowel disease during pregnancy and postpartum. Am J Gastroenterol. 1981;75(4):265–9.
17. Katz JA, Pore G. Inflammatory bowel disease and pregnancy. Inflamm Bowel Dis. 2001;7(2):146–57.
18. Dozois EJ, Wolff BG, Tremaine WJ, Watson WJ, Drelichman ER, Carne PW, et al. Maternal and fetal outcome after colectomy for fulminant ulcerative colitis during pregnancy: case series and literature review. Dis Colon Rectum. 2006;49(1):64–73.
19. Horowitz MD, Gomez GA, Santiesteban R, Burkett G. Acute appendicitis during pregnancy. Diagnosis and management. Arch Surg. 1985;120(12):1362–7.
20. Squires RA. Surgical considerations in pregnancy. Audio Dig Gen Surg. 1998;45:6.
21. Semm K. Endoscopic appendectomy. Endoscopy. 1983;15(2):59–64.
22. Kaplan M, Salman B, Yilmaz TU, Oguz M. A quality of life comparison of laparoscopic and open approaches in acute appendicitis: a randomised prospective study. Acta Chir Belg. 2009;109(3):356–63.
23. Lyass S, Pikarsky A, Eisenberg VH, Elchalal U, Schenker JG, Reissman P. Is laparoscopic appendectomy safe in pregnant women? Surg Endosc. 2001;15(4):377–9.
24. Lemaire BM, van Erp WF. Laparoscopic surgery during pregnancy. Surg Endosc. 1997;11(1):15–8.
25. Dhupar R, Smaldone GM, Hamad GG. Is there a benefit to delaying cholecystectomy for symptomatic gallbladder disease during pregnancy? Surg Endosc. 2010;24(1):108–12.
26. Herrington A, Gala R, Beck DE, Robichaux AG. Bowel obstruction in a pregnant patient with a restorative proctocolectomy and ileoanal j-pouch: a case report. Ochsner J. 2012;12(2):170–2.
27. Casey FE, Lau KN, Mesbah MC, Khalife ME. Use of laparoscopy for resolution of intussusception in the third trimester of pregnancy: a case report. J Reprod Med. 2009;54(11–12):712–4.
28. Sherer DM, Frager D, Eliakim R. An unusual case of diverticulitis complicating pregnancy at 33 weeks' gestation. Am J Perinatol. 2001;18(2):107–11.

29. Bodner J, Windisch J, Bale R, Wetscher G, Mark W. Perforated right colonic diverticulitis complicating pregnancy at 37 weeks' gestation. Int J Colorectal Dis. 2005;20(4):381–2.
30. Bohe MG, Ekelund GR, Genell SN, Gennser GM, Jiborn HA, Leandoer LJ, et al. Surgery for fulminating colitis during pregnancy. Dis Colon Rectum. 1983;26(2):119–22.
31. Girard RM, Lamarche J, Baillot R. Carcinoma of the colon associated with pregnancy: report of a case. Dis Colon Rectum. 1981; 24(6):473–5.
32. Bernstein MA, Madoff RD, Caushaj PF. Colon and rectal cancer in pregnancy. Dis Colon Rectum. 1993;36(2):172–8.
33. Mechery J, Ikhena SE. Cancer of the descending colon during pregnancy. J Obstet Gynaecol. 2007;27(3):311–2.
34. Walsh C, Fazio VW. Cancer of the colon, rectum, and anus during pregnancy. The surgeon's perspective. Gastroenterol Clin North Am. 1998;27(1):257–67.
35. Nesbitt JC, Moise KJ, Sawyers JL. Colorectal carcinoma in pregnancy. Arch Surg. 1985;120(5):636–40.
36. Hasson HM. A modified instrument and method for laparoscopy. Am J Obstet Gynecol. 1971;110(6):886–7.
37. Nezhat FR, Tazuke S, Nezhat CH, Seidman DS, Phillips DR, Nezhat CR. Laparoscopy during pregnancy: a literature review. JSLS. 1997;1(1):17–27.
38. Hunter JG, Swanstrom L, Thornburg K. Carbon dioxide pneumoperitoneum induces fetal acidosis in a pregnant ewe model. Surg Endosc. 1995;9(3):272–7. discussion 7–9.

# Economics of Laparoscopic Colectomy

# 34

Anthony J. Senagore

**Key Points**

- Laparoscopic colectomy utilization has approached ~50 % in the United States.
- A laparoscopic approach to colectomy ultimately is cost advantageous due to factors such as length of stay, reduced complications, diminished need for diagnostic studies due to reduced complications, and decreased readmissions.
- "Fast-track" or enhanced recovery pathways provide benefits for both open and laparoscopic colectomy.
- Reduced longer-term complications such as small bowel obstruction and hernia will likely contribute to further cost savings with a minimally invasive approach.
- Single-incision and robotic-assisted colectomy provide the potential for incremental advances in technique, but at significant cost increases related to devices required to perform the procedure.

## Introduction

The laparoscopic approach to colectomy has finally reached the tipping point, and upwards of 50 % of resections are now performed in this fashion, primarily as a result of the prospective randomized data regarding colorectal cancer [1–7]. This transition has been a long time in coming compared to other advanced laparoscopic procedures for a variety of reasons. First, there were initial concerns related to port-site recurrences in colorectal cancer, which ultimately were tied to refinements in skill and technical approach to the resection [8, 9]. Secondly, surgeons primarily doing colorectal surgery did not have access to "easy" operations to allow mastery of laparoscopic skills required for effective performance of this category of major abdominal surgery. Finally, access to a growing population of junior surgeons who have experienced laparoscopy as a normal component of the surgical armamentarium has significantly impacted the philosophical impediments to adoption of laparoscopic colectomy. The net result has been that the process around ascending the learning curve via better graduate training has created a larger pool of surgeon capable of delivering laparoscopic colectomy [10, 11]. Although from the beginning it was clear that there were significant improvements in patient care, it remained for refinements in both the technical components of the operation and perioperative care strategies to finally deliver the cost-effectiveness of laparoscopic colectomy [12–16]. We will explore the various issues that have impacted cost-efficiency of laparoscopic colectomy, as well as those issues that still require attention to realize the full benefits of this surgical approach.

## Advantages of Laparoscopic Colectomy

At the start of laparoscopic colorectal surgery, there were many concerns regarding the new complexities of technical difficulty, steep learning curve, need for specialized instrumentation and teams, and longer operating times. These issues did indeed increase the cost of colectomy initially; however, as mentioned above, it was clear that patients experienced a different recovery pattern that could be exploited for the benefit of the patient. The contemporaneous implementation of "fast-track" care for open colectomy patients originally blurred the source of benefits between laparoscopic and open colectomy; however, it is now confirmed that optimal clinical performance is achieved with adoption of enhanced recovery and laparoscopic resection [14, 17–20].

The sources of cost savings after adoption of a mature technical surgical team and the care plan components addressed above are multiple and are related to the index admission, cost of readmission, and long-term costs related complications such as both hernia and small bowel obstruction. It should be remembered that these benefits accrue to the patient and the health-care system, in conjunction with

A.J. Senagore, M.D., M.S., M.B.A. (✉)
Department of Surgery, Central Michigan University, School of Medicine, Saginaw, MI, USA
e-mail: anthony.senagore@cmich.edu

H.M. Ross et al. (eds.), *Minimally Invasive Approaches to Colon and Rectal Disease: Technique and Best Practices*,
DOI 10.1007/978-1-4939-1581-1_34, © Springer Science+Business Media New York 2015

equal or better outcomes related to the management of the illness predicating the resection. This was most clearly confirmed with respect to cancer surgery as was mentioned at the outset of this manuscript. Delaney et al. analyzed 150 matched patients undergoing surgery by the open or laparoscopic approach and clearly identified significantly lower total direct costs with the latter technique [18]. Interestingly, this article suggested benefits primarily in the postoperative phase that offset the higher intraoperative costs related to instrumentation due to reductions in hospital stay, bed and nursing utilization, and pharmacy, laboratory, and radiology services. These resource benefits were consistently reported early in the history of laparoscopic colectomy and have now been supported by more recent analyses of administrative databases [13, 21–23]. These articles highlight the reductions in wound complications, surgical site infections, postoperative ileus, and cardiopulmonary complications.

Although the data above are convincingly in favor of laparoscopic colectomy, all of the benefits would be for naught if readmissions or unplanned post-discharge visits increased as a result of delayed complications or overaggressive discharge plans [24–28]. The extant data are equally supportive of these mid-term benefits of laparoscopic colectomy related to costs for unplanned patient visits. The articulated benefits are associated with a reduction in many of the typical inpatient complications mentioned above, which occur with a higher frequency with open compared to laparoscopic resections. The data confirm that readmission rates are at least similar if not consistently reduced with the joint application of laparoscopic colectomy and enhanced recovery protocols [26–28]. Obrien et al. confirmed that not only is the risk of readmission not increased with laparoscopic surgery, but also, most importantly, even when complications warrant readmission, there is no delay or harm related to the management of any of these adverse outcomes [27]. These benefits also can accrue to the payer under a prospective payment system (DRG) because certain complications result in upward migration of the classification of a given patient under the plan. The net result of a relative reduction in a number of complications typically classified significant comorbidity/complications (CCs) is a reduction by almost 50 % in the allocation of patients to the more expensive DRG [29]. Therefore, the skilled laparoscopic team can demonstrate a significant reduction in initial costs to the payer with the implementation of an enhanced recovery protocol. This is accomplished with a net reduction in resources used during the index admission compared to open colectomy, as well as a total reduction in resources with the combination of both index and unplanned admissions for an episode of care. It is likely that the current focus on readmission will be refined to allow a separate review of truly preventable, potentially preventable, and truly unpreventable complications with an accurate appraisal of total resources consumed when managing a cohort of patients. This approach would truly reward efficient index care, safe reductions in length of stay for the majority of the patients, and effective management of the few patients who do develop adverse outcomes after the initial discharge.

The last area of cost benefit associated with laparoscopic colectomy is related to the risk and rate of long-term complications associated with laparotomy, namely, incisional hernia and small bowel obstruction [30–35]. These longer-term benefits have typically not been quantified at either the patient level or as the total cost to the health-care system, as previously they were both generally considered unavoidable risks of laparotomy. However, the compelling data associated with laparoscopy offer yet another set of patient satisfaction data, in addition to the risks and costs associated with the management of either small bowel obstruction or incisional hernia. There is no data available that reflects the patients' satisfaction with a delayed versus avoided readmission related to the choice of the index procedure. However, there are clearly risks and significant costs associated with medical readmission for small bowel obstruction and more importantly re-operative management. This is even more compelling with respect to the surgical management of an incisional hernia, which often requires the use of expensive prosthetic mesh.

The longer-term cost data will likely become more compelling as the concept of an expanded episode of care is appreciated by accountable care organizations that may become responsible for an individual patient for many years if not a lifetime.

## Economic Impact of Single-Port and Robotic-Assisted Laparoscopy

Advances in laparoscopic experience and skill have led to consideration of single-port access as a means of primarily reducing trauma to the abdominal wall and improving cosmesis [36–39]. The predominant conclusions based upon the available data are that the procedure can be done safely with an additional learning curve for a skilled laparoscopic surgeon and possibly a longer duration of surgery even after the curve is completed. The results are generally similar to multiport laparoscopic colectomy in terms of safety and disease management. However, one of the few prospective randomized trials evaluating single-port colectomy suggests not only longer surgical times, but also a higher conversion rate [39]. One concern based upon data from single-port cholecystectomy is the potential for an increased risk of both short- and long-term wound complications [40]. Further evaluation is needed to determine if the possibility of improved cosmesis is consistently achieved with single-port colectomy compared to multiport techniques without undue increase in incisional hernia. However, assuming that the

**Table 34.1** A comparison of outcomes for laparoscopic vs. robotic colectomy in recent literature

| Author | deSouza | Tyler | Park |
|---|---|---|---|
| Complications | 21 % vs. 20 % | 22 % vs. 22 % | NA |
| OR duration (minutes) | 118 vs. 158 | NA | 130 vs. 196 |
| LOS (days) | 5 vs. 5 | 5.7 vs. 5.5 | NA |
| Cost | $12,361 vs. $15,192 | $16,519 vs. $20,696 | $10,320 vs. $12,235 |

*NA* not available, *OR* operating room, *LOS* length of stay
The available data suggest overall similar outcomes in terms of complications and length of stay after surgery; however, the data are equally consistent in demonstrating increased operative time and cost of hospitalization

learning curve can be ascended so as to avoid significant increases in operative time, it is unlikely that single port will either detract or enhance the economic performance associated with minimally invasive colectomy.

Interest in robotic-assisted laparoscopic colectomy has experienced a resurgence after the initial evaluation of the first generation of the da Vinci (Intuitive Surgical, Sunnyvale, CA) robot [41]. The available data supports the fact that robotic-assisted laparoscopic colectomy is capable of delivering the same short-term surgical outcomes attained by standard human-guided laparoscopic techniques [42–44]. These data, however, also consistently demonstrate significant cost increases related to device acquisition and the requisite resposable devices required to perform the procedure. It is important to understand that these costs persist even after the learning curve is completed for robotic-assisted laparoscopy. There is some suggestion that deep pelvic dissections may be improved in terms of circumferential resection margins and pelvic nerve damage [45–48]. Given the paucity of data indicating reproducible advantages, it would seem that early performance of a high-quality prospective randomized trial would be beneficial in defining the cost-effectiveness of robotic-assisted proctectomy. It is unlikely that robotic-assisted colectomy will ever be able to demonstrate economic efficiency. Table 34.1 looks at three recent studies comparing laparoscopic and robotic colectomy.

## Conclusion

The available data clearly demonstrate that laparoscopic colectomy has evolved to the level that a skilled surgeon can reproducibly provide patient-centric, high-quality, cost-efficient care for their patients requiring colorectal resections. Importantly, this surgical advancement has reduced the complication rate compared to the best results achieved with open colorectal resection. Further advancements in laparoscopic colorectal surgery should be aimed at reducing conversion rates and improving closure of the extraction site and trocar sites as these issues present the greatest opportunities for further quality and cost improvement in laparoscopic colectomy.

## References


1. Lacy AM, Garcia-Valdecasas JC, Delgado S, et al. Laparoscopy assisted colectomy versus open colectomy for treatment of nonmetastatic colon cancer: a randomised trial. Lancet. 2002;359:2224–9.
2. Veldkamp R, Kuhry E, Hop WC, Colon Cancer Laparoscopic or Open Resection Study Group, et al. Laparoscopic surgery versus open surgery for colon cancer: short-term outcomes of a randomised trial. Lancet Oncol. 2005;6:477–84.
3. Guillou PJ, Quirke P, Thorpe H, et al. Short-term endpoints of conventional versus laparoscopic assisted surgery in patients with colorectal cancer (MRC CLASICC trial): multicentre, randomized controlled trial. Lancet. 2005;365:1718–26.
4. COST Study Group. A comparison of laparoscopically assisted and open colectomy for colon cancer. N Engl J Med. 2004; 350:2050–9.
5. Bardakcioglu O, Khan A, Aldridge C, Chen J. Growth of laparoscopic colectomy in the United States: analysis of regional and socioeconomic factors over time. Ann Surg. 2013;258(2):270–4.
6. Patel SS, Patel MS, Mahanti S, Ortega A, Ault GT, Kaiser AM, Senagore AJ. Laparoscopic versus open colon resections in California: a cross-sectional analysis. Am Surg. 2012;78(10):1063–5.
7. Surgical Care and Outcomes Assessment Program (SCOAP) Collaborative, Kwon S, Billingham R, Farrokhi E, Florence M, Herzig D, Horvath K, Rogers T, Steele S, Symons R, Thirlby R, Whiteford M, Flum DR. Adoption of laparoscopy for elective colorectal resection: a report from the Surgical Care and Outcomes Assessment Program. J Am Coll Surg. 2012;214(6):909–18.
8. Zanghì A, Cavallaro A, Piccolo G, Fisichella R, Di Vita M, Spartà D, Zanghì G, Berretta S, Palermo F, Cappellani A. Dissemination metastasis after laparoscopic colorectal surgery versus conventional open surgery for colorectal cancer: a metanalysis. Eur Rev Med Pharmacol Sci. 2013;17(9):1174–84.
9. Påhlman L. The problem of port-site metastases after laparoscopic cancer surgery. Ann Med. 1997;29(6):477–81.
10. Prakash K, Kamalesh NP, Pramil K, Vipin IS, Sylesh A, Jacob M. Does case selection and outcome following laparoscopic colorectal resection change after initial learning curve? Analysis of 235 consecutive elective laparoscopic colorectal resections. J Minim Access Surg. 2013;9(3):99–103.
11. Maitra RK, Acheson AG, Gornall C, Scholefield JH, Williams JP, Maxwell-Armstrong CA. Results of laparoscopic colorectal surgery from a national training center. Asian J Surg. 2013;37(1):1–7.
12. Delaney CP, Senagore AJ, Gerkin TM, Beard TL, Zingaro WM, Tomaszewski KJ, Walton LK, Poston SA. Association of surgical care practices with length of stay and use of clinical protocols after elective bowel resection: results of a national survey. Am J Surg. 2010;199(3):299–304. discussion 304.
13. Delaney CP, Chang E, Senagore AJ, Broder M. Clinical outcomes and resource utilization associated with laparoscopic and open colectomy using a large national database. Ann Surg. 2008;247(5): 819–24.
14. Senagore AJ, Delaney CP. A critical analysis of laparoscopic colectomy at a single institution: lessons learned after 1000 cases. Am J Surg. 2006;191(3):377–80.
15. Senagore AJ, Luchtefeld MA, Mackeigan JM. What is the learning curve for laparoscopic colectomy? Am Surg. 1995;61(8):681–5.
16. Senagore AJ, Luchtefeld MA, Mackeigan JM, Mazier WP. Open colectomy versus laparoscopic colectomy: are there differences? Am Surg. 1993;59(8):549–53. discussion 553–4.

17. Senagore AJ, Delaney CP, Brady KM, Fazio VW. Standardized approach to laparoscopic right colectomy: outcomes in 70 consecutive cases. J Am Coll Surg. 2004;199(5):675–9.
18. Delaney CP, Kiran RP, Senagore AJ, Brady K, Fazio VW. Case-matched comparison of clinical and financial outcome after laparoscopic or open colorectal surgery. Ann Surg. 2003;238(1):67–72.
19. Senagore AJ, Duepree HJ, Delaney CP, Brady KM, Fazio VW. Results of a standardized technique and postoperative care plan for laparoscopic sigmoid colectomy: a 30-month experience. Dis Colon Rectum. 2003;46(4):503–9.
20. Vlug MS, Wind J, Hollmann MW, Ubbink DT, Cense HA, Engel AF, Gerhards MF, van Wagensveld BA, van der Zaag ES, van Geloven AA, Sprangers MA, Cuesta MA, Bemelman WA. LAFA study group. Laparoscopy in combination with fast track multimodal management is the best perioperative strategy in patients undergoing colonic surgery: a randomized clinical trial (LAFA-study). Ann Surg. 2011;254(6):868–75.
21. Guller U, Jain N, Hervey S, Purves H, Pietrobon R. Laparoscopic vs open colectomy: outcomes comparison based on large nationwide databases. Arch Surg. 2003;138(11):1179–86.
22. Kemp JA, Finlayson SR. Outcomes of laparoscopic and open colectomy: a national population-based comparison. Surg Innov. 2008;15(4):277–83.
23. Steele SR, Brown TA, Rush RM, Martin MJ. Laparoscopic vs open colectomy for colon cancer: results from a large nationwide population-based analysis. J Gastrointest Surg. 2008;12(3):583–91.
24. Hansen CD, Fox CJ, Gross CP, Bruun LC. Hospital readmissions and emergency department visits following laparoscopic and open colon resection for cancer. Dis Colon Rectum. 2013;56(9):1053–61.
25. Hendren S, Morris AM, Zhang W, Dimick J. Early discharge and hospital readmission after colectomy for cancer. Dis Colon Rectum. 2011;54(11):1362–7.
26. Rona K, Choi J, Sigle G, Kidd S, Ault G, Senagore AJ. Enhanced recovery protocol: implementation at a county institution with limited resources. Am Surg. 2012;78(10):1041–4.
27. O'Brien DP, Senagore A, Merlino J, Brady K, Delaney C. Predictors and outcome of readmission after laparoscopic intestinal surgery. World J Surg. 2007;31(12):2430–5.
28. Kariv Y, Wang W, Senagore AJ, Hammel JP, Fazio VW, Delaney CP. Multivariable analysis of factors associated with hospital readmission after intestinal surgery. Am J Surg. 2006;191(3):364–71.
29. Senagore AJ, Brannigan A, Kiran RP, Brady K, Delaney CP. Diagnosis-related group assignment in laparoscopic and open colectomy: financial implications for payer and provider. Dis Colon Rectum. 2005;48(5):1016–20.
30. Reshef A, Hull TL, Kiran RP. Risk of adhesive obstruction after colorectal surgery: the benefits of the minimally invasive approach may extend well beyond the perioperative period. Surg Endosc. 2013;27(5):1717–20.
31. Burns EM, Currie A, Bottle A, Aylin P, Darzi A, Faiz O. Minimal-access colorectal surgery is associated with fewer adhesion-related admissions than open surgery. Br J Surg. 2013;100(1):152–9.
32. Lee L, Mappin-Kasirer B, Sender Liberman A, Stein B, Charlebois P, Vassiliou M, Fried GM, Feldman LS. High incidence of symptomatic incisional hernia after midline extraction in laparoscopic colon resection. Surg Endosc. 2012;26(11):3180–5.
33. Cobb WS, Carbonell AM, Snipes GM, Knott B, Le V, Bour ES, Scott JD, Lokey JS. Incisional hernia risk after hand-assisted laparoscopic surgery. Am Surg. 2012;78(8):864–9.
34. Duepree HJ, Senagore AJ, Delaney CP, Fazio VW. Does means of access affect the incidence of small bowel obstruction and ventral hernia after bowel resection? Laparoscopy versus laparotomy. J Am Coll Surg. 2003;197(2):177–81.
35. Samia H, Lawrence J, Nobel T, Stein S, Champagne BJ, Delaney CP. Extraction site location and incisional hernias after laparoscopic colorectal surgery: should we be avoiding the midline? Am J Surg. 2013;205(3):264–7. discussion 268.
36. Park JW, Sohn DK, Park S, Park SC, Chang HJ, Son HJ, Oh JH. Safety and efficacy of single-port colectomy for sigmoid colon cancer: a phase II clinical trial. J Laparoendosc Adv Surg Tech A. 2013;23(9):745–50.
37. Al Sabah S, Liberman AS, Wongyingsinn M, Charlebois P, Stein B, Kaneva PA, Feldman LS, Fried GM. Single-port laparoscopic colorectal surgery: early clinical experience. J Laparoendosc Adv Surg Tech A. 2012;22(9):853–7.
38. Fung AK, Aly EH. Systematic review of single-incision laparoscopic colonic surgery. Br J Surg. 2012;99(10):1353–64.
39. Champagne BJ, Lee EC, Leblanc F, Stein SL, Delaney CP. Single-incision vs straight laparoscopic segmental colectomy: a case-controlled study. Dis Colon Rectum. 2011;54(2):183–6.
40. Phillips MS, Marks JM, Roberts K, Tacchino R, Onders R, DeNoto G, Rivas H, Islam A, Soper N, Gecelter G, Rubach E, Paraskeva P, Shah S. Intermediate results of a prospective randomized controlled trial of traditional four-port laparoscopic cholecystectomy versus single-incision laparoscopic cholecystectomy. Surg Endosc. 2012; 26(5):1296–303.
41. Delaney CP, Lynch AC, Senagore AJ, Fazio VW. Comparison of robotically performed and traditional laparoscopic colorectal surgery. Dis Colon Rectum. 2003;46(12):1633–9.
42. Fung AK, Aly EH. Robotic colonic surgery: is it advisable to commence a new learning curve? Dis Colon Rectum. 2013;56(6):786–96.
43. Tyler JA, Fox JP, Desai MM, Perry WB, Glasgow SC. Outcomes and costs associated with robotic colectomy in the minimally invasive era. Dis Colon Rectum. 2013;56(4):458–66.
44. Park JS, Choi GS, Park SY, Kim HJ, Ryuk JP. Randomized clinical trial of robot-assisted versus standard laparoscopic right colectomy. Br J Surg. 2012;99(9):1219–26.
45. Fernandez R, Anaya DA, Li LT, Orcutt ST, Balentine CJ, Awad SA, Berger DH, Albo DA, Artinyan A. Laparoscopic versus robotic rectal resection for rectal cancer in a veteran population. Am J Surg. 2013;206:509–17.
46. Erguner I, Aytac E, Boler DE, Atalar B, Baca B, Karahasanoglu T, Hamzaoglu I, Uras C. What have we gained by performing robotic rectal resection? Evaluation of 64 consecutive patients who underwent laparoscopic or robotic low anterior resection for rectal adenocarcinoma. Surg Laparosc Endosc Percutan Tech. 2013; 23(3):316–9.
47. Halabi WJ, Kang CY, Jafari MD, Nguyen VQ, Carmichael JC, Mills S, Stamos MJ, Pigazzi A. Robotic-assisted colorectal surgery in the United States: a nationwide analysis of trends and outcomes. World J Surg. 2013;6.
48. Zawadzki M, Velchuru VR, Albalawi SA, Park JJ, Marecik S, Prasad LM. Is hybrid robotic laparoscopic assistance the ideal approach for restorative rectal cancer dissection? Colorectal Dis. 2013;15(8):1026–32.

# Outcomes of Laparoscopic Surgery

# 35

Jennifer Leahy and Rocco Ricciardi

## Key Points

- Laparoscopic-assisted surgery (LAS) can be performed with multiple ports, a single port, or a hand-assisted device.
- Outcomes for these techniques are fairly similar among each other but improved compared to open surgery.
- Further data are needed evaluating cost-effectiveness, patient-centered outcomes, and long-term outcomes.

## Background

In this chapter on outcomes, our aim is to present an unbiased assessment of traditional and patient-centered metrics of care for laparoscopic procedures of the colon and rectum. Fortunately, the literature has an abundance of studies comparing laparoscopy to conventional surgery as well as other hybrid techniques. In this chapter, we summarize these data while providing an understanding of the incremental value of laparoscopic surgery as compared to open approaches and the results of straight laparoscopy with a hand-assisted approach, one port, or multiple ports. We also evaluate outcomes of laparoscopy based on disease-, patient-, and surgeon-related factors with an attempt to identify populations of patients that might obtain the greatest benefit from laparoscopic techniques. Our approach will focus on those studies with the most robust data from well-conducted trials that are generalizable and reproducible, presenting a comprehensive review of present day metrics, while establishing a wish list of other, more patient-centered outcomes.

J. Leahy, B.A., M.S. • R. Ricciardi, M.D., M.P.H. (✉)
Department of Colon and Rectal Surgery, Lahey Clinic,
41 Mall Rd., Burlington, MA 01805, USA
e-mail: jennifer.leahy@lahey.org; Rocco.Ricciardi@lahey.org

## Conventional Open Surgery (OS) Versus Laparoscopic-Assisted Surgery (LAS)

### Outcomes

A large number of studies have sought to compare laparoscopic colorectal procedures with the conventional open techniques (Table 35.1) [1–18]. In total, 11,671 patients were evaluated in these studies and outcomes evaluated included procedure time, intraoperative blood loss, length of stay, and postoperative complications. Length of procedure is an important variable and at least seven manuscripts [1, 5, 8, 14–16, 18] demonstrated increased operative time with LAS as compared to open surgery. In addition, several studies [5–8, 10, 14–16, 18] demonstrated significantly shorter length of stay, reduced blood loss [6, 10, 18], and fewer transfusion requirements.

An evaluation of postoperative adverse events has been studied in depth with LAS as compared to open surgery. Four studies [9, 13, 14, 18] demonstrated significantly lower rates of surgical site infections, but no significant differences in anastomotic leak [10–13, 18], functional outcomes [1, 3, 7], aggregate postoperative complications [1, 2, 4–7, 11, 13, 16, 18], quality of life [3, 15], hospital readmission [1, 6, 7], reoperation [6, 7, 16], or mortality [2, 5, 11, 18]. In one of the largest studies, Kockerling et al. [11] provided a prospective 24-center study of 1,143 consecutive patients undergoing a laparoscopic or a laparoscopic-assisted operation over a 3-year period. The indication for the laparoscopic procedure was malignancy in almost half of all patients and a total of 64 procedures (5.6 %) were converted to OS. Compared to open surgery, the authors identified similar rates of intraoperative or postoperative complications, anastomotic leak, and mortality.

In addition to this large study, Larson et al. [16] prospectively compared the safety and 90-day outcomes of 100 laparoscopic versus 200 conventional ileal pouch-anal anastomoses with diverting loop ileostomy. While the operative time was

H.M. Ross et al. (eds.), *Minimally Invasive Approaches to Colon and Rectal Disease: Technique and Best Practices*,
DOI 10.1007/978-1-4939-1581-1_35, © Springer Science+Business Media New York 2015

**Table 35.1** Conventional open surgery (OS) versus laparoscopic-assisted surgery (LAS) outcomes

| | OS (references) | LAS (references) | Equivalent (references) |
|---|---|---|---|
| Shorter procedure time | [1, 5, 8, 14–16, 18, 49, 51, 53, 55–58] | – | – |
| Lower conversion rate | – | – | – |
| Decreased length of stay | – | [5–8, 10, 14–16, 18, 49, 50, 56–58, 60–62, 67, 71, 74–77, 80, 94–98, 100–102] | [64] |
| Fewer overall complications | – | [48, 51, 55, 56, 61, 62] | [1, 2, 4–7, 11, 13, 16, 18, 49–53, 57, 61, 64] |
| Less surgical site infections | – | [9, 13, 14, 18] | [16, 55–57, 62] |
| Shorter time to first bowel movement | – | [16, 56, 57, 60, 64, 73, 75–77, 80, 94, 96, 98] | [1, 3, 7, 54] |
| Decreased mortality | – | – | [2, 5, 8, 11, 18, 48–52, 61, 62] |

significantly longer in the laparoscopic group (103 min longer), the authors identified significant benefits for the laparoscopic-treated patients when compared to the open approach with respect to early postoperative recovery including earlier time to bowel movement, quicker time to regular diet, and reductions in length of stay by 3 days [16]. There were, however, no significant differences in the rate of other morbidity, readmission, or anastomotic leak. The authors' concluded that a laparoscopic approach for ileal pouch-anal anastomosis with diverting loop ileostomy was safe and feasible and resulted in postoperative recovery that is comparable, if not significantly better, than the open procedure.

## Conversion

Although many surgeons feel that open conversion for laparoscopy is a failure in technique, others consider conversion as a limit to the safety of laparoscopy [19]. However, most studies demonstrate a reduction in the benefits of minimally invasive techniques following conversion. Nine manuscripts [19–27] compared the outcomes of 889 converted laparoscopic procedures to those of nonconverted procedures and, in some cases, to conventional open colorectal procedures. In understanding these outcomes, the reader must understand that definitions for conversion vary [21]. Three studies [19, 20, 24] based their definition on length of incision, other studies described an unexpected extension of any original incision [22, 25, 26], and another [23] on removal of the trocars. Gervaz et al. noted that most studies failed to include a precise definition for conversion and that the rate of conversion was significantly higher if a standard definition was used [3].

Two studies [22, 23] found that converted patients had significantly more blood loss than those that were not converted. As expected, it was noted that converted procedures [19, 21, 23] were in the operating room longer than nonconverted cases; yet, other data have been less convincing [20, 22, 27]. Certainly, the benefits of a shorter length of hospital stay following laparoscopic procedures were less pronounced with conversion. In fact, four studies [19, 21–23] found that converted patients had a significantly longer length of stay than nonconverted patients. However, the reason for conversion may be one of the most important influencers of length of stay, which at this time has not been thoroughly investigated, though includes factors such as bleeding, adhesions, large or fixated tumor, and failure to progress.

Following surgery, several studies [22, 24, 26] identified no differences in complications or mortality [19, 22] for converted as compared to nonconverted laparoscopic procedures, while others [22] identified no differences with patients who had conventional open procedures. One study [23] identified a significantly higher rate of postoperative complications for converted patients. Also, surgical site infections were significantly higher for patients after converted procedures [23, 26], which may be secondary to length of incision or procedure complexity. These data imply that laparoscopic conversion is not associated with a significant detriment to the patients' postoperative outcome and recovery.

In summary, there is considerable evidence indicating decreased length of stay and perioperative blood loss for LAS when compared to OS. Assessments of morbidity and mortality have not overwhelmingly demonstrated a benefit for LAS although wound infections are certainly less likely with minimally invasive techniques. In addition, although conversion does not appear to significantly worsen outcomes, the benefits of LAS are certainly attenuated with conversion.

## Laparoscopic-Assisted Surgery (LAS) Versus Hand-Assisted Laparoscopic Surgery (HALS)

Several studies have compared hand-assisted laparoscopic surgery (HALS) with standard multiport laparoscopic-assisted surgery (LAS) [28–37], while two compared HALS with conventional open surgery (OS) (Table 35.2) [38, 39]. In most studies, outcomes were similar between HALS and LAS [30–33, 36, 38], but three studies noted that there were significantly lower conversions with HALS as compared to LAS [28, 30, 34]. Others also reported on length of procedure: four studies demonstrated that HALS had a significantly shorter length of procedure [28, 30, 33, 34], yet some

**Table 35.2** Laparoscopic-assisted surgery (LAS) versus hand-assisted laparoscopic surgery (HALS)

| | LAS (references) | HALS (references) | Equivalent (references) |
|---|---|---|---|
| Shorter procedure time | – | [28, 30, 33, 34] | [31, 35] |
| Lower conversion rate | – | [28, 30, 34, 84] | – |
| Decreased length of stay | – | [29, 30, 32, 36] | [28, 31, 33–35, 37] |
| Fewer overall complications | – | – | [30–33, 36] |
| Less surgical site infections | – | – | [29, 30, 34, 36] |
| Shorter time to first bowel movement | – | – | [28, 31, 33] |
| Decreased mortality | | – | – |

**Table 35.3** Single (SILS) versus multiport (MILS) laparoscopic surgery

| | MILS (references) | SILS (references) | Equivalent (references) |
|---|---|---|---|
| Shorter procedure time | – | – | [40, 42–46] |
| Lower conversion rate | – | – | [40, 42–47] |
| Decreased length of stay | – | [40, 42, 44, 45, 47] | – |
| Fewer overall complications | – | – | – |
| Less surgical site infections | – | – | [44, 45] |
| Shorter time to first bowel movement | – | – | – |
| Decreased mortality | – | – | [45] |

investigators noted no difference between HALS and LAS [31, 35]. The true benefit of HALS may be related to more complex procedures, where HALS operating times have been demonstrated to be significantly less [30]. In a meta-analysis of HALS studies recently published, no differences in blood loss for HALS and LAS [28] were observed. Yet, there was a significant advantage for HALS in operating time and conversion rate for segmental colectomies and in operating time for total proctocolectomy.

As stated earlier, there were no significant differences in overall morbidity in several studies comparing HALS and LAS or in the two studies comparing HALS and OS [38, 39]. For studies that reported on individual adverse events, there were no differences between HALS and LAS in surgical site infections [29, 30, 34, 36], incisional hernia [36], anastomotic leak [29, 34–36], postoperative bleeding [29, 30, 34], abscess [30, 34, 35], small bowel obstruction [36], prolonged postoperative ileus [30, 34], readmission [33, 35], and reoperation [33, 35, 36]. The low rate of surgical site infection may be secondary to the use of wound protectors and smaller incisions with HALS and LAS [31].

Postoperative recovery metrics evaluated include hospital length of stay, return to normal function (including gastrointestinal function and return to normal diet), and pain. Most studies found no difference in length of stay between HALS and LAS [28, 31, 33–35, 37] while some identified a significantly longer length of stay for HALS as compared to LAS [29, 30, 32, 36]. However, the longer length of stay for HALS may be due to significantly more complex cases in the HALS-treated group. With respect to return of bowel function, no differences in this time have been reported for HALS and LAS [31, 33], which was confirmed in a meta-analysis [28]. In comparing postoperative pain, three studies found no differences [28, 31, 33] between the HALS and LAS groups, and one study identified no differences in pain between HALS and OS [39]. An assessment of quality of life was also conducted in one study that demonstrated similar results between the HALS and LAS groups [31]. Overall, most postoperative metrics have been similar between HALS and LAS but a more thorough understanding of differences in hernia formation may help better inform this comparison.

## Summary

HALS and LAS have similar outcomes with the exception that HALS may reduce operative time (especially in more complex cases) and conversion to open. More data are needed regarding hernia formation and other patience-centered outcomes.

## Single Versus Multiport Laparoscopic Surgery

In comparing single-incision laparoscopic surgery (SILS) with more traditional multi-incision (trocar) laparoscopic surgery (MILS), high-quality studies are difficult to identify. Most of the comparisons are not scientifically rigorous given the patient and disease process selection of small tumors, lower body mass index, and significant surgeon experience for the SILS groups. In the studies performed, no significant differences in the rate of conversion were identified, yet one study [41, 42] noted that SILS had a more frequent rate of conversion. The four studies also noted no significant difference in the length of procedure. Three analyses [42, 44, 45] noted significantly less blood loss for the SILS group and one study demonstrating more blood transfusions with MILS (Table 35.3) [45].

In comparing adverse events, all the analyses demonstrated no difference in overall complication rates. Two studies [44, 45] found no significant differences between the SILS and MILS groups in regard to surgical site infection, ileus, and anastomotic leak, while others [45] noted no significant differences between the two groups in the rate of mortality, incisional hernia, intra-abdominal abscess, reoperation, readmission, renal failure, and events of a cardiovascular, pulmonary, thromboembolic, and urinary nature. Overall, the four meta-analyses noted that patients in the SILS group had a significantly lower length of stay; however, significant heterogeneity was noted in all the studies. Incision length was smaller for the SILS group [40, 44, 45] and one study [45] noted that the overall cosmetic score for the SILS group was significantly higher. Oncological outcomes and margin status have also been evaluated, but the data appear somewhat heterogenous and biased.

Two randomized controlled studies [43, 46] noted no difference in length of procedure and no difference in conversion to laparotomy. Poon et al. [43] also noted no statistical significant differences between the SILS and MILS groups for intraoperative complications and estimated blood loss [43]. In addition, in one study [43], significantly lower median wound pain scores were identified on postoperative days 1 and 2 and that the length of stay for SILS patients was significantly shorter than for those in the MILS group. However, resumption of oral intake was similar in both SILS and MILS groups [46]. In terms of oncological outcomes, both studies [43, 46] saw that the SILS and MILS groups had similar numbers of lymph nodes harvested. Ultimately, however, Huscher et al. noted that even in the hands of experienced surgeons, SILS was technically more challenging [46].

Papaconstantinou et al. compared SILS, MILS, and HALS in 87 patients, with 29 in each of the three groups [47]. There were no differences among the three groups when considering age, gender, previous abdominal surgery, and pathology. The results revealed no statistical differences between the groups with respect to conversion rate, length of procedure, estimated intraoperative blood loss, readmission rate, minor wound complication rates, and number of lymph nodes harvested. However, a significantly lower pain score was noted in the SILS group as compared to MILS and HALS groups on postoperative days 1 and 2, but this difference was not present at time of discharge [47]. Patients in the SILS group also had significantly shorter length of stay than both the HALS and MILS patients. Lastly, both of the SILS and MILS groups of patients had a significantly shorter length of incision when compared with the HALS group. All reports note the technical challenges in utilizing SILS for colorectal surgery.

### Summary

Although the quality of reviews and significant bias in patient selection limit direct comparison, perioperative outcomes are similar between SILS, LAS, and HALS. SILS remains more technically demanding but newer devices may reduce the technical demands of working through one port.

## Outcomes Based on Disease Pathology

### Diverticulitis

Six studies [48–53] evaluated the role of laparoscopy in the treatment of diverticulitis with a total of 13,875 patients, 6,150 of which were treated through a laparoscope. The studies demonstrated that laparoscopic procedures required significantly more time to perform [49, 51, 53] in diverticulitis patients, with one study [49] estimating an hour difference in operative time. No significant differences in intraoperative complications were noted between the LAS and OS groups, and only one study [50] commented on blood loss, noting that there was significantly less blood loss in LAS procedures without significant differences in transfusion requirements.

Morbidity was measured in several of the manuscripts reviewing diverticulitis surgery. Overall morbidity was significantly lower for the laparoscopic procedures in two studies [48, 51] but not in other studies [49–53]. In a large retrospective study, Mbadiwe et al. found that patients in the LAS group experienced significantly fewer postoperative complications, but no difference in a subgroup analysis of emergent cases [52]. Similarly, in a study evaluating long-term outcomes, Klarenbeek et al. identified no differences in the number of late complications after diverticulitis surgery [51]. Others have described no differences in the rates of anastomotic leak [48, 49, 53], anastomotic stricture [51, 53], anastomotic bleeding [48], enterocutaneous fistula [51], intra-abdominal abscess [48, 51], postoperative small bowel obstruction [48, 51], recurrent diverticulitis [51], reoperation, and incisional hernia [51, 53]. Although the data on surgical site infections has been mixed [48, 53], there are substantial data demonstrating no difference in mortality with either approach [48–52]. In addition, despite evidence in other studies that postoperative ileus is significantly reduced with a laparoscopic approach, others found no difference for diverticulitis patients treated either with open of laparoscopic techniques [48, 49].

Three studies [49, 50, 53] considered the effect of laparoscopic surgery for diverticulitis on postoperative pain. The data were somewhat mixed [49, 50, 53], but maximal pain levels were noted to be significantly less for patients with diverticulitis-treated laparoscopically [49] as was narcotic use [49, 50]. Given the reduction in narcotics, time to bowel activity was significantly lower for the LAS group [49] as well as length of stay [49, 50]. Quality of life is an important consideration and the data are somewhat mixed here as one study [50] revealed significant improvements in quality of life during the early postoperative period, while two studies [51, 53] identified similar outcomes for long-term postoperative quality of life.

In summary, outcomes following LAS in diverticulitis appear to be at least equivalent as OS, with operative times generally longer for LAS. In procedures for complications of diverticulitis, laparoscopy may be technically demanding.

## Inflammatory Bowel Disease

Both ulcerative colitis and Crohn's disease are conditions of younger people who are more likely to be interested in the aesthetic advantages as well as the traditional benefits of minimally invasive techniques [54]. For this reason, laparoscopic techniques are often sought out by these patients; however, both conditions can be challenging to treat with minimally invasive methods, particularly during the acute inflammatory phases. There are three meta-analyses [55–57] comparing LAS and OS in patients with Crohn's disease for a total of 1,515 patients, with 795 treated laparoscopically. Length of procedure was noted to be significantly longer for the LAS group in three studies [56, 57] and blood loss similar in one study [57]. Early postoperative complication rates were noted to be similar [57], while in two other studies [56] the overall complication rate was significantly lower for the LAS group. There was no difference between the LAS and OS in rates of surgical site infection [55–57], anastomotic leak [56, 57], abscess [56, 57], bowel obstruction [57], postoperative ileus [55], inflammatory bowel disease recurrence [56], and overall reoperation rates [55, 56]. Postoperatively, there was no significant difference in the use of narcotics [57] and two studies [56, 57] noted that bowel function returned more quickly in the LAS group. Most studies [56, 57] found that patients in the LAS group experienced a significantly shorter hospital stay.

Few randomized controlled trials [54, 58, 59] have sought to identify the value of laparoscopy in patients with Crohn's disease. These studies demonstrated significantly longer procedure times for the LAS group [54, 58], shorter incision length for LAS patients [54], and no difference in blood loss [59]. Postoperatively, there was no difference in pain scores [58] or narcotic use [54], time to passage of flatus [54], or to first bowel movement [54]. One study [58] revealed significantly longer length of hospital stay for open surgery patients; although the researchers estimated evidence of bias. In a study by Milsom et al. [54], the LAS patients experienced significantly fewer minor complications, but the LAS and OS groups experienced similar rates for major complications without differences in recurrence. In another follow-up study, Stocchi et al. [59] found that rates of anorectal disease, anorectal surgery, endoscopic or radiologic recurrence, medication, and average number of operations per patient were similar between LAS and open groups. However, patients in the open surgery group were significantly more likely to undergo multiple operations. Lastly, Maartense et al. [58] found that quality of life was no different between the two groups at 2 weeks.

There are a limited number of high-quality studies evaluating the outcomes of LAS for ulcerative colitis with small sample sizes [60–62]. Surgeries analyzed were restorative proctocolectomy with ileal pouch-anal anastomosis (IPAA) [16, 39, 60, 63, 64] and total colectomy [61, 62]. Three studies found that the length of procedure was significantly longer for patient who underwent LAS over OS [16, 60, 62]. There was no difference in postoperative morbidity for patients who underwent restorative proctocolectomy with IPAA in the LAS and OS groups [16, 61, 64] and in the HALS and OS groups [39]. Postoperative morbidity was noted to be significantly lower for laparoscopic colectomy [61, 62]. There was no difference in surgical site infection [16, 62], anastomotic leak [16, 62, 64], abscess [16, 62], bowel obstruction [62, 64], prolonged ileus [16, 64], pouch failure [64], reoperation [16, 61, 62], readmission [16], and mortality [61, 62]. Importantly, rate of incisional hernia was significantly lower for patients who underwent LAS as compared to OS [64].

In comparing LAS versus OS, patients who underwent laparoscopic restorative proctocolectomy with IPAA had significantly shorter time to return of oral intake [16, 61, 62, 64] and return of bowel function [16, 60, 64] over the open procedure, although the two meta-analyses noted similar time to bowel function between the LAS and OS groups [61, 62]. Four studies found that the length of stay was significantly shorter for patients in the LAS group than the OS groups [16, 60–62] while one noted no difference [64]. There was no difference in quality of life between the LAS and OS groups [63, 64] and between the LAS and HALS groups [39], although Polle et al. [63] found that cosmesis scores were significantly higher for patients who underwent LAS than OS, especially for females. There was no difference in long-term defecatory function between the LAS and OS groups [63, 64] and long-term morbidity between the LAS and OS groups [63]. In a study by Fichera et al. [64], the long-term benefits of laparoscopic restorative proctocolectomy with IPAA were significantly less liquid bowel movements, pad wearing during the daytime and nighttime, and perianal rash.

In summary, LAS and OS have equivalent outcomes for IBD patients. LAS seems to be associated with shorter length of stay, improved cosmesis, and lower rates of minor complications. See Chaps. 30 and 31 for additional information regarding minimally invasive approaches in Crohn's disease and ulcerative colitis, respectively.

## Cancer

The literature has an abundance of well-conducted studies evaluating cancer outcomes following laparoscopy. In this section, we focus on oncological results [65–80]. In the past, there was substantial concern for the use of laparoscopy in the treatment of colorectal cancer because of inferior oncological results [68]. The oncological data for laparoscopic colectomy has been shown to be excellent, yet it should be recognized that rectal cancer procedures are much more challenging when performed laparoscopically leading to increased potential for margin positivity. Concerns of margin status were raised by Medical Research Council CLASICC trial of LAS versus open surgery for colorectal cancer. An increased likelihood of positive circumferential margins (12 %) in rectal cancer was noted for LAS when compared with OS (6 %). Although long-term outcomes remained unchanged, many surgeons became cautious of laparoscopy for rectal cancer, which led to decreased adoption of the technique. Later, a meta-analysis reviewed the results of LAS for rectal cancer and demonstrated no differences in the extent of oncological clearance [69].

In other oncological results such as lymph nodes, resection margins, recurrence rates, disease-free survival, and overall survival, LAS has demonstrated equivalency to open surgery. Several studies [66, 67, 71, 73, 75, 78, 80] have identified minimal differences in the number of lymph nodes harvested. In addition, eight studies [66, 67, 71, 75–77, 79, 80] identified no differences in margin positivity between the LAS and OS groups, although one study [73] demonstrated significantly smaller resection margins for LAS when used in colon cancer. There was no difference between the LAS and OS groups with respect to overall recurrence rates [66, 72, 77, 78] and time to recurrence [66]. Furthermore, the 5-year follow-up of the Clinical Outcomes of Surgical Therapy (COST) Study Group study found no difference in recurrence rate by disease stage [72]. Conversion from laparoscopic to open surgery also did not impact recurrence [72]. There was no difference in local or distant recurrence rates at 3 years [68, 71], 5 years [70, 72, 79], and 10 years [70], for any stage of disease [70] or between converted, successful laparoscopic and open surgery patients [70]. Lastly, there was no difference in wound/port-site recurrences [78].

Survival analyses confirm equivalency for LAS in colorectal cancer. There was no difference in disease-free survival at 3 years [68, 71], 5 years [70, 72, 74, 77, 79], and 10 years [67, 70, 78] or for any stage of disease [68–70, 72, 58]. However, while the conventional versus laparoscopic-assisted surgery in colorectal cancer study noted no difference in disease-free survival for converted patients at the 5-year follow-up, a post 10-year follow-up study of converted patients demonstrated significantly worse disease-free survival than those with a planned open surgery [70]. In addition, converted patients had significantly worse overall survival at 5 years [72] and at 10 years [70]. However, disease and anatomic factors may account for both the need for conversion and the worse prognosis. Ultimately, these results imply that when considering the oncological outcomes of number of lymph nodes harvested, resection margins, recurrence rates, disease-free survival, and overall survival, LAS can be used safely in patients with colorectal cancers without a change in oncological outcomes [65–72, 74–78, 80].

In addition to the oncological outcomes presented above, more traditional outcomes have been investigated including length of procedure, adverse events, incision length, estimated blood loss, and number of patients requiring blood transfusions. Patients who underwent LAS had significantly lower analgesic needs [71, 75–77], significantly shorter time to oral intake [73, 75, 77, 79, 80], significantly less time to bowel function return [73, 75–77, 80], and significantly shorter hospital stay [67, 71, 74–77, 80]. In addition, while patients in the LAS treatment group generally had a higher quality of life on a short-term scale [67], in the long term, there were no differences in quality of life [67, 68].

In summary, LAS and OS have equivalent oncological outcomes for colorectal cancer patients. Concern for circumferential margin positivity in rectal cancer in one trial was not identified in subsequent studies or in a meta-analysis. LAS has multiple benefits in the areas of return of bowel function, length of stay, and analgesic needs.

## Patient Factors

### Body Mass Index (BMI)

There were 13 studies [81–93] analyzing the outcomes of LAS as related to body mass index. The aggregate number of patients studied was 30,521 of whom 17,305 were classified as obese. In their comparison of HALS versus LAS in obese patients, Heneghan et al. demonstrated that patients who underwent HALS were significantly less likely to have conversion to open surgery and significantly less blood loss [84]. In comparing the effect of BMI on conversion rates for LAS, two studies [90, 91] noted no difference and six studies [82, 85, 86, 89, 92, 93] found that obesity was a significant predictor of conversion. Length of procedure was found to be significantly longer with increased BMI [85, 86, 88, 90, 92], although no difference was found in procedure length for two studies [89, 91]. No differences were noted in complication rates [86, 90] and number of transfusions [86, 88], yet obese patients had significantly longer incision lengths [85, 86] and significantly higher estimated blood loss [85, 86, 90].

Analyses of the effect of BMI on operative adverse outcomes reveal disparate results with no outcomes difference for high BMI patients in some studies [82, 86, 90, 91] and four studies demonstrating an increase in morbidity for obese patients [85, 89, 92, 93]. Rates of surgical site infections were significantly greater with increased BMI in most studies [85, 88, 89, 93] and obese patients are more likely to have wound dehiscence [87, 88] and incisional hernia [86]. BMI does not appear to effect anastomotic leak [85, 86, 89–91, 93], abscess [85, 86, 89, 93], readmission [86, 92], reoperation [86, 88, 90, 91], or mortality [82, 86–88, 90, 93]. In addition, no differences were noted in pain scores [91], time to oral intake [86, 91], time to recovery of bowel function [85, 86, 90, 91], and length of stay [86–88, 90–93].

In summary, elevated BMI is associated with increased rates of conversion, longer operative times, and, in general, higher morbidity rates (especially wound complications). However, higher BMI is not a contraindication to LAS for colorectal surgery. For further information, Dr. Vargas provides a detailed look at the use of laparoscopy in the obese patient in Chap. 29.

## Age

Elderly patients have physiologic needs that might lend themselves to greater benefits of laparoscopic colorectal surgery than the younger patient [94]. There were nine studies [94–102] that evaluated the outcomes of LAS in comparison with OS. In a study by Frasson et al. [96], no differences were noted between older and younger patients who underwent LAS in rate of infection complications, surgical site infections, abscess, anastomotic leak, bleeding, and postoperative small bowel obstruction. Scheibach et al. [99] identified more cardiac events and higher mortality for elderly laparoscopic patients, yet no difference in reoperation rates. In a study by Allardyce et al. [95], there were significantly fewer elderly patients with complications, particularly for those who underwent successful LAS. The authors commented that the findings were more distinct for the elderly when compared with the young patients. There was no difference between elderly patients who underwent LAS or OS in rates of surgical site infection [96–98, 101], abscess [96, 98, 101], noninfectious complications [96], anastomotic leak [96–98, 101, 102], bleeding [96, 101], postoperative small bowel obstructions [96–98, 101], readmission [98, 100], and reoperation [98, 101].

Lastly, the effect of age on narcotics use, return to bowel function, time to oral intake, length of stay, and independence status has been evaluated in patients who undergo laparoscopic colorectal surgery as well. Elderly patients who underwent LAS, in comparison to OS, had significantly lower use of narcotics [94], significantly earlier return to bowel functions [94, 97, 98], earlier time to oral intake [97], and shorter length of stay [94–98, 100–102]. In addition, two studies [94, 102] demonstrated that significantly more elderly patients who underwent LAS were able to keep their independent status, a key advantage of LAS in the elderly.

In summary, LAS appears to be safe with at least equivalent and often improved perioperative outcomes for the elderly patient. The data seem to indicate less functional decline after LAS, but more data are needed. Drs. Kann and Bleier provide additional information regarding the use of a minimally invasive approach in the elderly in Chap. 28.

## Surgeon Factors

Laparoscopic-assisted surgery is technically complex, requires significant experience, and is associated with a steep learning curve [103–107] that is characterized by improved outcomes with more experience and a gradual achievement of a steady state. A number of manuscripts have studied the learning curve for LAS [103–113]. Experiences and definitions differed among these studies with some analyzing outcomes over the course of a surgeon's experience and noting steady improvements [105, 106, 108], while other studies [103, 104, 107, 109–111, 113] analyzing patients in groups based on year of surgery and compared these groups in early and late experiences. Two studies noted no difference with rate of conversions based on surgeon experience or surgeon operative volume [103, 109] while others demonstrated a significant decrease in number of conversions with increasing experience [105, 106, 111] at a range between 90 and 310 cases [104, 106, 111, 112]. All studies demonstrated reductions in length of procedure time with experience [104, 105, 107, 108, 111–113]. It is clear for many of these studies that the learning curve for LAS colorectal procedures is appreciably longer than for other non-colorectal laparoscopic operations [111]. Despite the improvements in procedure time, surgeon experience in laparoscopy was not significantly associated with reductions in postoperative adverse events in seven studies [103, 105–108, 110, 113].

In summary, while the actual number of laparoscopic cases is likely to be dependent on the individual surgeon experience and other patient-related factors, LAS is associated with a substantial learning curve for which conversion rates decrease and overall outcomes improve with time.

## Desirable Metrics

The vast majority of outcomes evaluated in the studies above focused on traditional and logistically easy to define and measure outcomes such as operative time, length of stay, morbidity, and mortality. However, the value of laparoscopy may be in the benefits to functional status, quality of life, patient satisfaction, and physiologic recovery. In addition, many of the outcomes reported are short-term rather than the long-term gains that might be achieved from smaller incisions through protection from incisional hernia development. Unfortunately, these outcomes are difficult to measure but may be more valuable to the patient than other more definable metrics. Thus, the value of laparoscopic procedures, the true benefit related to incremental technical costs, could be better defined with an eye toward assessing these nontraditional and longer-term outcomes.

## Conclusion

This review describes the outcomes of laparoscopy in colorectal surgery, which up to recently have focused on easy to define and measure outcomes. Despite the numerous advantages of laparoscopic techniques, the procedures remain challenging with limited applicability in some case and patient types. As techniques become better refined and newer instrumentation is developed, the role for laparoscopy will also expand. Ultimately, as part of enhanced recovery, laparoscopic and other minimally invasive procedures provide the patient with faster short-term recovery than many other open or traditional procedures with comparable oncological and disease results.

## References


1. Fajardo A, Dharmarajan S, George V, Hunt S, Birnbaum E, Fleshman J, Mutch M. Laparoscopic versus open 2-stage ileal pouch: laparoscopic approach allows for faster restoration of intestinal continuity. J Am Coll Surg. 2010;211:377–83.
2. Braga M, Pecorelli N, Frasson M, Vignali A, Zuliani W, Carlo V. Long-term outcomes after laparoscopic colectomy. World J Gastrointest Oncol. 2011;3:43–8.
3. Dunker M, Bemelman W, Slors J, van Duijvendijk P, Gouma D. Functional outcome, quality of life, body image and cosmesis in patients after laparoscopic-assisted and conventional restorative proctocolectomy: a comparative study. Dis Colon Rectum. 2001; 44:1800–7.
4. Braga M, Vignali A, Gianotti L, Zuliani W, Radelli G, Gruarin P, et al. Laparoscopic versus open colorectal surgery: a randomized trial on short-term outcome. Ann Surg. 2002;236:759–66.
5. Lezoche E, Feliciotti F, Guerrieri M, Paganini A, De Sanctis A, Campagnacci R, D'Ambrosio G. Laparoscopic versus open hemicolectomy. Minerva Chir. 2003;58:491–502.
6. Pokala N, Delaney C, Senagore A, Brady K, Fazio V. Laparoscopic vs open total colectomy: a case-matched comparative study. Surg Endosc. 2005;19:531–5.
7. Kariv Y, Delaney C, Casillas S, Hammel J, Nocero J, Bast J, et al. Long-term outcome after laparoscopic and open surgery for rectal prolapse: a case-control study. Surg Endosc. 2006;20:35–42.
8. Noblett S, Horgan A. A prospective case-matched comparison of clinical and financial outcomes of open versus laparoscopic colorectal resection. Surg Endosc. 2007;21:404–8.
9. Yamamoto S, Fujito S, Akasu T, Moriya Y. Wound infection after a laparoscopic resection for colorectal cancer. Surg Today. 2008; 38:618–22.
10. Siddiqui M, Sajid M, Baig M. Open vs laparoscopic approach for reversal of Hartmann's procedure: a systematic review. Colorectal Dis. 2010;12:733–41.
11. Kockerling F, Rose J, Schneider C, Scheidbach H, Scheuerlein H, Reymond M, et al. Laparoscopic colorectal anastomosis: risk of postoperative leakage. Results of a multicenter study. Laparoscopic Colorectal Surgery Study Group (LCSSG). Srug Endosc. 1999; 13:639–44.
12. Goriainov V, Miles A. Anastomotic leak rate and outcome for laparoscopic intra-corporeal stapled anastomosis. J Minim Access Surg. 2010;6(1):6–10.
13. Lumly J, Fielding G, Rhodes M, Nathanson L, Siu S, Stitz R. Laparoscopic-assisted colorectal surgery. Lessons learned from 240 consecutive patients. Dis Colon Rectum. 1996;39(2): 155–9.
14. Howard D, Datta G, Cunnick G, Gatzen C, Huang A. Surgical site infection rate is lower in laparoscopic than open colorectal surgery. Colorectal Dis. 2010;12(5):423–7.
15. El-Gazzaz G, Kiran R, Remzi F, Hull T, Geisler D. Outcomes for case-matched laparoscopically assisted versus open restorative proctocolectomy. Br J Surg. 2009;96:522–6.
16. Larson D, Cima R, Dozaois E, Davies M, Piotrowicz K, Barnes S, et al. Safety, feasibility, and short-term outcomes and laparoscopic ileal-pouch-anal anastomosis: a single institutional case-matched experience. Ann Surg. 2006;243(5):667–70.
17. Zmora O, Hashavia E, Munz Y, Khaikin M, Shabtai M, Ayalon A, et al. Laparoscopic colectomy is associated with decreased postoperative gastrointestinal dysfunction. Surg Endosc. 2009; 23(1):87–9.
18. Schwenk W, Haase ON, Muller J. Short term benefits for laparoscopic colorectal resection. Cochrane Database Syst Rev. 2005; (3):CD003145.
19. Belizon A, Sardinha C, Sher M. Converted laparoscopic colectomy: what are the consequences? Surg Endosc. 2006;20:947–51.
20. Casillas S, Delaney CP, Senagore AJ, Brady K, Fazio VW. Does conversion of a laparoscopic colectomy adversely affect patient outcome? Dis Colon Rectum. 2004;47:1680–5.
21. Gervaz P, Pikarsky A, Utech M, Secic M, Efron J, Belin B, et al. Converted laparoscopic colorectal surgery. Surg Endosc. 2001; 15(8):827–32.
22. Gonzalez R, Smith C, Mason E, Duncan T, Wilson R, Miller J, Ramshaw B. Consequences of conversion in laparoscopic colorectal surgery. Dis Colon Rectum. 2005;49(2):197–204.
23. Marusch F, Gastinger I, Schneider C, Scheidbach H, Kondradt J, Bruch HP, et al. Importance of conversion for results obtained with laparoscopic colorectal surgery. Dis Colon Rectum. 2001;44(2):207–14.
24. Rotholtz NA, Laporte M, Zanoni G, Bun ME, Aued L, Lencinas S, Mezzadri NA. Predictive factors for conversion in laparoscopic colorectal surgery. Tech Coloproctol. 2008;12(1):27–31.
25. Schwander O, Schiedeck TH, Bruch H. The role of conversion in laparoscopic colorectal surgery: do predictive factors exist? Surg Endosc. 1999;13(2):151–6.
26. Tan P, Stephen J, Rieger N, Hewett PJ. Laparoscopically assisted colectomy, a study of risk factors and predictors in open conversion. Surg Endosc. 2008;22(7):1708–14.
27. Chan AC, Poon JT, Fan J, Lo SH, Law WL. Impact of conversion on the long-term outcome in laparoscopic resection of colorectal cancer. Surg Endosc. 2008;22:2625–30.
28. Aalbers A, Biere S, vanBerg Henegouwen M, Bemelman W. Hand-assisted or laparoscopic-assisted approach in colorectal surgery: a systematic review and meta-analysis. Surg Endosc. 2008;22:1769–80.
29. Chen W, Dinj W, Cui L. Hand-assisted laparoscopic versus laparotomy in total proctocolectomy with ileal pouch-anal anastomosis: a clinical controlled trial. Chinese J Gastrointest Surg. 2012;15:1077–9.
30. Cima R, Pattana-arun J, Larson D, Dozois E, Wolff B, Pemberton J. Experience with 969 minimal access colectomies: the role of hand-assisted laparoscopy in expanding minimally invasive surgery for complex colectomies. J Am Coll Surg. 2008;206: 946–50.

31. HALS Study Group. Hand-assisted laparoscopic surgery vs standard laparoscopic surgery for colorectal disease: a prospective randomized trial. Surg Endosc. 2000;14(10):896–901.
32. Hassan I, You Y, Cima R, Larson D, Dozois E, Barnes S, Pemberton J. Hand-assisted versus laparoscopic-assisted colorectal surgery: practice patterns and clinical outcomes in a minimally-invasive colorectal practice. Surg Endosc. 2008;22(3):739–43.
33. Marcello P, Fleshman J, Milsom J, Read T, Arnell T, Birnbaum E, et al. Hand-assisted laparoscopic vs. laparoscopic colorectal surgery: a multicenter, prospective, randomized trial. Dis Colon Rectum. 2008;51(6):818–26.
34. Moloo H, Haggar F, Coyle D, Hutton B, Duhaime S, Mamazza J, et al (2010) Hand assisted laparoscopic surgery versus conventional laparoscopy for colorectal surgery. Cochrane Database Syst Rev. 2010;(10):CD006585.
35. Ozturk E, Kiren R, Geisler D, Hull T, Vogel J. Hand-assisted laparoscopic colectomy: benefits of laparoscopic colectomy at no extra cost. J Am Coll Surg. 2009;209(2):242–7.
36. Sonoda T, Pandey S, Trencheva K, Lee S, Milsom J. Long-term complication of hand-assisted versus laparoscopic colectomy. J Am Coll Surg. 2009;208(1):62–6.
37. Targarona E, Gracia E, Garriga J, Martinez-Bru C, Cortes M, Boluda R, et al. Prospective randomized trial comparing conventional laparoscopic colectomy with hand-assisted laparoscopic colectomy: applicability, immediate clinical outcome, inflammatory response, and cost. Srug Endosc. 2002;16(2):234–9.
38. Kang J, Chung M, Chao P, Yeh C, Hsiao C, Lee T, Jao S. Hand-assisted laparoscopic colectomy vs open colectomy: a prospective randomized study. Surg Endosc. 2004;18(4):577–81.
39. Maartense S, Dunker M, Slors J, Cuesta M, Gouma D, van Deventer S, et al. Hand-assisted laparoscopic versus open restorative proctocolectomy with ileal pouch anal anastomosis. Ann Surg. 2004;240(6):984–92.
40. Maggiori L, Gaujoux S, Tribillon E, Bretagnol F, Panis Y. Single-incision laparoscopy for colorectal resection: a systematic review and meta-analysis of more than a thousand procedures. Colorectal Dis. 2012;14(10):e643–54.
41. Fung A, Aly E. Systematic review of single-incision laparoscopic colonic surgery. Br J Surg. 2012;99:1353–64.
42. Lv C, Wu S, Wu Y, Shi J, Su Y, Fan Y, et al. Single-incisions versus traditional multiport laparoscopic colorectal surgery—a cumulative meta-analysis and systematic review. Int J Colorectal Dis. 2013;28(5):611–21.
43. Poon J, Cheung C, Fan J, Lo O, Law W. Single-incision versus conventional laparoscopic colectomy for colonic neoplasm: a randomized controlled trial. Surg Endosc. 2012;26(10):2729–43.
44. Yang T, Chua T. Single-incision laparoscopic colectomy versus conventional multiport laparoscopic colectomy: a meta-analysis of comparative studies. Int J Colorectal Dis. 2013;28(1):89–101.
45. Zhou Y, Wu L, Zhao Y, Xu D, Li B. Single-incision versus conventional laparoscopy for colorectal disease: a meta-analysis. Dig Dis Sci. 2012;57:2103–12.
46. Huscher C, Mingoli A, Sgarzini G, Mereu A, Binda B, Brachini G, Trombetta S. Standard laparoscopic versus single-incision laparoscopic colectomy for cancer: early results of a randomized prospective study. Am J Surg. 2012;204(1):115–20.
47. Papaconstantinou H, Sharp N, Thomas J. Single-incision laparoscopic right colectomy: a case-matched comparison with standard laparoscopic and hand-assisted laparoscopic techniques. J Am Coll Surg. 2011;213(1):72–82.
48. Cirocchi R, Farinella E, Trastulli S, Sciannameo F, Audisio R. Elective sigmoid colectomy for diverticular disease. Laparoscopic vs open surgery: a systematic review. Colorectal Dis. 2012;14:671–83.
49. Gervaz P, Inan I, Perneger T, Schiffer E, Morel P. A prospective, randomized, single-blind comparison of laparoscopic versus open sigmoid colectomy for diverticulitis. Ann Surg. 2010;252:3–8.
50. Klarenbeek B, Veenhof A, Bergamaschi R, van deer Peet D, van dev Broek W, de Lange E, et al. Laparoscopic sigmoid resection for diverticulitis decreases major morbidity rates: a randomized control trial. Ann Surg. 2009;249(1):39–44.
51. Klarenbeek BR, Bermagaschi R, Veenhof AA, van der Peet D, van den Brock W, de Lange E, et al. Laparoscopic versus open sigmoid resection for diverticular disease: follow-up assessment of the randomized controlled Sigma trial. Surg Endosc. 2011;25:1121–6.
52. Mbadiwe T, Obirieze A, Cornwell E, Turner P, Fullum T. Surgical management of complicated diverticulitis: a comparison of the laparoscopic and open approaches. J Am Coll Surg. 2013; 216(4):782–8.
53. Raue W, Paolucci V, Asperger W, Akbrecht R, Buchlet M, Schwenk W. Laparoscopic sigmoid resection for diverticular disease has no advantage over open approach: midterm results of a randomized controlled trial. Langenbecks Arch Surg. 2011; 396(7):973–80.
54. Milsom J, Hammerhofer K, Bohm B, Marcello P, Elson P, Fazio V. Prospective, randomized trial comparing laparoscopic vs. conventional surgery for refractory ileocolic Crohn's disease. Dis Colon Rectum. 2001;44(1):1–8.
55. Dasari B, McKay D, Gardiner K. Laparoscopic verses open surgery for small bowel Crohn's disease (Review). Cochrane Database of Syst Rev. 2011;19(1)
56. Tan J, Tjandra J. Laparoscopic surgery for Crohn's disease: a meta-analysis. Dis Colon Rectum. 2007;50(5):576–85.
57. Tilney H, Constantinides V, Heriot A, Nicolaou M, Athanasiou T, Ziprin P, et al. Comparison of laparoscopic and open ileocecal resection for Crohn's disease: a meta-analysis. Surg Endosc. 2006;20(7):1036–44.
58. Maartense S, Dunker M, Slors J, Cuesta M, Pierik E, Gouma D, et al. Laparoscopic-assisted versus open ileocolic resection for Crohn's disease. Ann Surg. 2006;243(2):143–9.
59. Stocchi L, Milsom J, Fazio V. Long-term outcomes of laparoscopic versus open ileocolic resection for Crohn's disease: follow-up of a prospective randomized trial. Surgery. 2008;144(4):622–7.
60. Marcello P, Milsom J, Wong S, Hammerhofer K, Goormastic M, Church J, Fazio V. Laparoscopic restorative proctocolectomy: case-matched comparative study with open restorative proctocolectomy. Dis Colon Rectum. 2000;43(5):604–8.
61. Tan J, Tjandra J. Laparoscopic surgery for ulcerative colitis-a meta-analysis. Colorectal Dis. 2006;8(8):626–36.
62. Wu X, He X, Zhou X, Ke J, Lan P. The role of laparoscopic surgery for ulcerative colitis: systematic review with meta-analysis. Int J Colorectal Dis. 2010;25(8):949–57.
63. Polle S, Dunker M, Slors J, Sprangers M, Cuesta M, Gouma D, Bemelman W. Body image, cosmesis, quality of life, and functional outcome of hand-assisted laparoscopic versus open restorative proctocolectomy: long-term results of a randomized trial. Surg Endosc. 2007;21(8):1301–7.
64. Fichera A, Silvestri M, Hurst R, Rubin M, Michelassi F. Laparoscopic restorative proctocolectomy with ileal pouch anal anastomosis: a comparative observational study on long-term functional results. J Gastrointest Surg. 2009;13:526–32.
65. Kuhry E, Schwenk W, Gaupset R, Romild U, Bonjer H. Long-term outcomes of laparoscopic surgery for colorectal cancer: a Cochrane systematic review of randomized controlled trials. Cancer Treat Rev. 2008;34(6):498–504.
66. Neudecker J, Klein F, Bittner R, Carus T, Stroux A, Schwenk W. Short-term outcomes from a prospective randomized trial comparing laparoscopic and open surgery for colorectal cancer. Br J Surg. 2009;96(12):1458–67.
67. Braga M, Frasson M, Vignali A, Zuliani W, Civelli V, Di Carlo V. Laparoscopic vs. open colectomy in cancer patients: long-term complications, quality of life, and survival. Dis Colon Rectum. 2005;48:2217–23.

68. Jayne D, Guillou P, Thorpe H, Quirke P, Copeland J, Smith A, et al. Randomized trial of laparoscopic-assisted resection of colorectal carcinoma: 3-year results of the UK MRC CLASICC Trial Group. J Clin Oncol. 2007;25(21):3061–8.
69. Aziz O, Constantinides V, Tekkis PP, et al. Laparoscopic versus open surgery for rectal cancer: a meta-analysis. Ann Surg Oncol. 2006;13:413–24.
70. Green B, Marshall H, Collinson F, Quirke P, Guillou P, Jayne D, Brown J. Long-term follow-up of the Medical Research Council CLASICC trial of conventional versus laparoscopically assisted resection in colorectal cancer. Br J Surg. 2013;100(1):75–82.
71. Clinical Outcomes Surgical Therapy Group. A comparison of laparoscopically assisted and open colectomy for cancer. N Eng J Med. 2004;350(20):2050–9.
72. Fleshman J, Sargent D, Green E, Anvari M, Stryker S, Beart RJ, et al. Laparoscopic colectomy for cancer is not inferior to open surgery based on 5-year data from the COST Study Group trial. Ann Surg. 2007;246:655–62.
73. Hewett P, Allardyce R, Bagshaw P, Frampton C, Frizelle F, Rieger N, et al. Short-term outcomes of the Australasian randomized clinical study comparing laparoscopic and conventional open surgical treatments for colon cancer: the ALCCaS trial. Ann Surg. 2008;248(5):728–38.
74. Bagshaw P, Allardyce R, Frampton C, Frizelle F, Hewett P, McMurrick P, et al. Long-term outcomes of the Australasian randomized clinical trial comparing laparoscopic and conventional open surgical treatments for colon cancer: the Australasian Laparoscopic Colon Cancer Study Trial. Ann Surg. 2012; 256:915–9.
75. Veldkamp R, Kuhry E, Hop W, Jeekel J, Kazamier G, Bonjer H, et al. Laparoscopic surgery versus open surgery for colon cancer: short-term outcomes of a randomized trial. Lancet Oncol. 2005;6(7):477–84.
76. van der Pas M, Haglind E, Cuesta M, Furst A, Lacy A, Hop W, Bonjer H. Laparoscopic versus open surgery for rectal cancer (COLOR II): short-term outcomes of a randomized, phase 3 trial. Lancet Oncol. 2013;14(3):210–8.
77. Leung K, Kwok S, Lam S, Lee J, Yiu R, Ng S, et al. Laparoscopic resection of rectosigmoid carcinoma: prospective randomized trial. Lancet. 2004;363:1187–92.
78. Ng S, Leung K, Lee J, Yiu R, Li J, Hon S. Long-term morbidity and oncologic outcomes of laparoscopic-assisted anterior resection for upper rectal cancer: ten-year results of a prospective, randomized trial. Dis Colon Rectum. 2009;52(4):558–66.
79. Lujan J, Valero G, Hernandez Q, Sanchez A, Frutos M, Parilla P. Randomized clinical trial comparing laparoscopic and open surgery in patients with rectal cancer. Br J Surg. 2009;96(9):982–9.
80. Liang X, Hou S, Liu H, Li Y, Jiang B, Bai W, et al. Effectiveness and safety of laparoscopic resection versus open surgery in patients with rectal cancer: a randomized, controlled trial from China. J Laparoendosc Adv Surg Tech A. 2011;21(5):381–5.
81. Delaney C, Pokala N, Senagore A, Casillas S, Kiran R, Brady K, Fazio V. Is laparoscopic colectomy applicable to patients with body mass index >30? A case-matched comparative study with open colectomy. Dis Colon Rectum. 2005;48:975–81.
82. Denost Q, Quintane L, Buscail E, Martenot M, Laurent C, Rullier E. Short- and long-term impact of body mass index on laparoscopic rectal cancer surgery. Colorectal Dis. 2013;15:463–9.
83. Hardiman K, Chang E, Diggs B, Lu K. Laparoscopic colectomy reduces morbidity and mortality in obese patients. Surg Endosc. 2013;27(8):2907–10.
84. Heneghan H, Martin S, Kiran R, Khoury W, Stocchi L, Remzi F, Vogel J. Laparoscopic colorectal surgery for obese patients: decreased conversion with the hand-assisted technique. J Gastrointest Surg. 2013;17(3):548–54.
85. Khoury W, Stocchi L, Geisler D. Outcomes after laparoscopic intestinal resection in obese versus non-obese patients. Br J Surg. 2011;98(2):293–8.
86. Krane M, Allaix M, Zoccali M, Umanskiy K, Rubin M, Villa A, et al. Does morbid obesity change outcomes after laparoscopic surgery for inflammatory bowel disease? Review of 626 consecutive cases. J Am Coll Surg. 2013;216(5):986–96.
87. Merkow R, Bilimoria K, McCarter M, Bentrem D. Effect of body mass index on short-term outcomes after colectomy for cancer. J Am Coll Surg. 2009;208(1):53–61.
88. Mustain W, Davenport D, Hourigan J, Vargas H. Obesity and laparoscopic colectomy: outcomes from the ACS-NSQIP database. Dis Colon Rectum. 2012;55(4):429–35.
89. Pikarsky A, Saida Y, Yamaquchi T, Martinez S, Chen W, Weiss E, et al. Is obesity a high-risk factor for laparoscopic colorectal surgery? Surg Endosc. 2002;16(5):855–8.
90. Poulsen M, Ovesen H. Is laparoscopic colorectal cancer surgery in obese patients associated with an increased risk? Short-term results from a single center study of 425 patients. J Gastrointest Surg. 2012;16(8):1554–8.
91. Schwandner O, Farke S, Schiedeck T, Bruch H. Laparoscopic colorectal surgery in obese and nonobese patients: do difference in body mass indices lead to different outcomes? Surg Endosc. 2004;18(10):1452–6.
92. Senagore A, Delaney C, Madboulay K, Fazio V. Laparoscopic colectomy in obese and nonobese patients. J Gastrointest Surg. 2003;7(4):558–61.
93. Zhou Y, Wu L, Li X, Wu X, Li B. Outcome of laparoscopic colorectal surgery in obese and nonobese patients: a meta-analysis. Surg Endosc. 2012;26(3):783–9.
94. Stocchi L, Nelson H, Young-Fadok T, Larson D, Ilstrup D. Safety and advantages of laparoscopic vs. open colectomy in the elderly. Dis Colon Rectum. 2000;43(3):326–32.
95. Allardyce R, Bagshaw P, Frampton C, Frizelle F, Hewett P, Rieger N, et al. Australasian Laparoscopic Colon Cancer Study shows that elderly patients may benefit from lower postoperative complication rates following laparoscopic versus open resection. Br J Surg. 2010;97:86–91.
96. Frasson M, Braga M, Vignali A, Zuliani W, Di Carlo V. Benefits of laparoscopic colorectal resection are more pronounced in elderly patients. Dis Colon Rectum. 2008;51:296–300.
97. Law W, Chu K, Tung P. Laparoscopic colorectal resection: a safety option for elderly patients. J Am Coll Surg. 2002;195(6): 768–73.
98. Lian L, Kalady M, Geisler D, Kiran R. Laparoscopic colectomy is safe and leads to a significantly shorter hospital stay for octogenarians. Surg Endosc. 2010;24(8):2039–43.
99. Scheidbach H, Schneider C, Hugel O, Yildirim C, Lippert H, Kockerling F. Laparoscopic surgery in the old patient: do indications and outcomes differ? Langenbecks Arch Surg. 2005;390(4): 328–32.
100. Senagore A, Madbouly K, Fazio V, Duepree H, Brady K, Delaney C. Advantages of laparoscopic colectomy in older patients. Arch Surg. 2003;138(3):252–6.
101. She W, Poon J, Fan J, Lo O, Law W. Outcome of laparoscopic colectomy for cancer in elderly patients. Surg Endosc. 2013; 27(1):308–12.
102. Stewart B, Stitz R, Lumley J. Laparoscopically assisted colorectal surgery in the elderly. Br J Surg. 1999;86(7):938–41.
103. Chen G, Liu Z, Han P, Li J, Cui B. The learning curve for the laparoscopic approach for colorectal cancer: a single institution's experience. J Laparoendosc Adv Surg Tech A. 2013;23:17–21.
104. Park I, Choi G, Lim K, Kang B, Jun S. Multidimensional analysis of the learning curve for laparoscopic resection in rectal cancer. J Gastrointest Surg. 2009;13(2):275–81.

105. Tekkis P, Senagore A, Delaney C, Fazio V. Evaluation of the learning curve in laparoscopic colorectal surgery: comparison of right-sided and left-sided resections. Ann Surg. 2005;242(1):83–91.
106. Li J, Lo A, Hon S, Nq S, Lee J, Leung K. Institution learning curve of laparoscopic colectomy-a multi-dimensional analysis. Int J Colorectal Dis. 2012;27(4):527–33.
107. Schlachta C, Mamazza J, Seshadri P, Cadeddu M, Gregoire R, Poulin E. Defining a learning curve for laparoscopic colorectal resections. Dis Colon Rectum. 2001;44(2):217–22.
108. Agachan F, Joo J, Weiss E, Wexner S. Intraoperative laparoscopic complications. Are we getting better? Dis Colon Rectum. 1996;39:S14–9.
109. Bennett C, Stryker S, Ferreira M, Adams J, Beart R. The learning curve for laparoscopic colorectal surgery. Preliminary results from a prospective analysis of 1194 laparoscopic-assisted colectomies. Arch Surg. 1997;132:41–4.
110. Evans J, Poritz L, MacRae H. Influence of experience on laparoscopic ileocolic resection for Crohn's disease. Dis Colon Rectum. 2002;45:1595–600.
111. Marush F, Gastinger I, Schneider C, Scheidbach H, Konradt J, Bruch H, Laparoscopic Colorectal Surgery Study Group, et al. Experience as a factor influencing the indications for laparoscopic colorectal surgery and the results. Surg Endosc. 2001; 15(2):116–20.
112. Miskovic D, Ni M, Wyles S, Tekkis P, Hanna G. Learning curve and case selection in laparoscopic colorectal surgery: systematic review and international multicenter analysis of 4852 cases. Dis Colon Rectum. 2012;55(12):1300–10.
113. Yasunaga H, Matsuyama Y, Ohe K, Japan Surgical Society. Effect of hospital and surgeon volumes on operating times, postoperative complications, and length of stay following laparoscopic colectomy. Surg Today. 2009;39:955–61.

# Part VI

# Conclusions

# Future Directions in Minimally Invasive Surgery

# 36

Howard M. Ross and Matthew Miller Philp

**Key Points**

- Surgical advancements do not always proceed in a linear fashion.
- Advancements in care can result when surgeons partner with industry and each listens and learns from one another.
- Continued advances in robotic technology will transform minimally invasive approaches to colon and rectal disease.
- Occasionally, the quest to develop a novel technology will yield progress in unintended, but highly valuable, areas.
- The continual drive to improve patient outcomes impacts all areas of patient care, including perioperative management.

The valuable insight provided by the authors of this textbook has allowed all of the editors to review the evolution of minimally invasive surgery and its current application to colon and rectal disease. From the very beginning, the surgeon's desire to repair a structural problem through increasingly smaller incisions has been laudable, although progress has not always been linear. "Lufttamponade" therapy was an attempt in the early 1900s to treat upper gastrointestinal hemorrhage by increasing intra-abdominal pressure via air pumped through a tube placed in the abdominal cavity. Georg Kelling became the first "laparoscopist," when in an effort to understand why filling the abdominal cavity with air did not tamponade upper gastrointestinal bleeding, he peered into a dog's abdominal cavity through an eyepiece placed on a tube, calling it "celioscopy." It was this "Celioscopy" eventually led to laparoscopy as we know it today. Similarly, we have seen how devices designed to allow single incision laparoscopic colectomy are better applied to trans-anal surgery. These single incision devices placed trans-anally have revolutionized the ability to resect superficial cancers and polyps from the rectum.

The combination of a desire to improve surgical care with advances in technology, along with "out of the box" thinking, will likely continue to propel the steady march of progress in the realm of minimally invasive surgery. On the other hand, economic pressures threaten to limit innovation, and the cost of new technologies must always be carefully considered. Currently, robotic approaches to abdominal colectomy have not proven to have an outcome advantage over laparoscopic approaches, yet they are increasingly utilized despite the high costs of the "robot," service package, and instrumentation. What should our stance therefore be? Should we stand up and "tell the emperor he is not wearing clothes"? Perhaps. Any surgeon having actually trained with current robotic technology, however, will universally tout the remarkable, almost magical, ability to maneuver miniaturized instruments that move like your hand while being viewed in three dimensions.

As educators we have adopted the stance that all technologies must be carefully and objectively evaluated on many fronts. These include, but are not limited to, economic, procedural, and short- and long-term recovery benefits. Further, we feel obliged to educate interested practitioners, as creative thinking may otherwise lead to a use that does reveal reliable objective patient benefit. Surgeon partnership with industry is another facet of surgical progress that should not be underestimated. The history of surgical innovation is notable for the many successful pairings that have changed our world. The surgical stapler would likely not exist if Dr. Humer Hutel did not reach out to fifth-generation instrument

**Electronic supplementary material:** Supplementary material is available in the online version of this chapter at 10.1007/978-1-4939-1581-1_36. Videos can also be accessed at http://www.springerimages.com/videos/978-1-4939-1580-4.

H.M. Ross, M.D., F.A.C.S., F.A.S.C.R.S. (✉)
Division of Colon and Rectal Surgery, Department of Surgery, Temple University Health System, 3401 North Broad St., Philadelphia, PA 19140, USA
e-mail: Howard.Ross@tuhs.temple.edu

M.M. Philp, M.D.
Division of Colon and Rectal Surgery, Department of Surgery, Temple University Hospital, Temple University Health System, 7500 Central Ave., Physicians Office Building, Suite 210, Philadelphia, PA 19111, USA

H.M. Ross et al. (eds.), *Minimally Invasive Approaches to Colon and Rectal Disease: Technique and Best Practices*, DOI 10.1007/978-1-4939-1581-1_36, © Springer Science+Business Media New York 2015

manufacturer Victor Fischer in 1908 Hungary. The pairing of Dr. Mark Ravitch with Leon Hirsch from US Surgical Co. facilitated the development of our readily obtainable, reliable, reloadable, disposable, and simple-to-use surgical stapler of today.

The continued quest to develop technologies has encouraged surgeons to look closely at all aspects of patient care and recovery. Regimented "fast-track" care of the colon and rectal surgery patient is the direct result of the movement to shorten hospital stay and a by-product of the laparoscopic revolution. Surgeons in the mid-1990s recognized that patients who underwent laparoscopic colectomy appreciated an enhanced recovery with regard to return of bowel function and length of stay. Careful analysis revealed, however, that behaviors of these "laparoscopic" surgeons included the routine withholding of nasogastric tubes, early postoperative feeding and ambulation, and an effort to decrease opiate use. When these care paradigms were applied to all colectomy patients, regardless of the approach, enhanced patient recovery was also seen.

The future of minimally invasive surgery clearly involves the application of robotics. In the current versions of robotic colectomy, providers essentially have just switched out the standard ports and instruments utilized for laparoscopic colectomy for robot arms and instruments. Since the operations on the inside are the same, it is not surprising that outcomes are similar. The future may bring approaches where through a single incision multiple arms can enter the abdominal cavity and perform the entire resection and anastomosis. Even further, perhaps where we end up with robotic colectomy will bear little resemblance to how we currently approach the surgical treatment of colon and rectal disease. Whatever the future holds, technological advances will surely continue to allow miniaturization of instruments combined with better optics and maneuverability. We will be able to better assess tissue perfusion and anastomotic integrity. Individual surgeon outcomes will be more transparent, variability between providers will be diminished, and greater knowledge of the dynamic interplay between surgeon, tissue, and technology will be applied for what hopefully will result in measurable improvements in patient outcomes.

## Introduction

To understand where we are going, it's best to look at where we've come from. There have been tremendous advances in the field of laparoscopic colectomy since it was first reported nearly a quarter century ago in 1990 [1]. This was a natural progression of the minimally invasive revolution in general surgery occurring at the same time, as Mouret initially published on laparoscopic cholecystectomy in 1986 and subsequent use blossomed [2]. Unfortunately, experimental and early clinical reports raised concerns about the oncologic outcomes of laparoscopic colectomy [3], specifically higher rates of port site tumor recurrence. To address these concerns, several prospective randomized trials including the Clinical Outcomes of Surgical Therapy Study Group were initiated to compare the oncologic outcomes of laparoscopic colectomy with open laparotomy [4]. Not only was the oncologic equivalency between open and laparoscopic colectomy demonstrated, but also the additional benefits of decreased narcotic analgesic use and hospital length of stay were also identified. Confirmatory results were found in the European COLOR and CLASICC trials [5, 6].

Despite these results, and in contrast to laparoscopic cholecystectomy, laparoscopic colectomy has taken significantly longer to gain widespread adoption and still has not reached the same level of nationwide utilization. In 1991, 5 years after Mouret's publication, 52 % of cholecystectomies were being performed laparoscopically, and this increased to 75 % by 2000 [7]. In contrast, in 2009, approximately 5 years after the COST trial data was published, only 31 % of patients in a nationwide sample underwent attempted laparoscopic partial colectomy [8], and this represented a dramatic increase in laparoscopic colectomy rates. While the authors found several predictive factors for the use of a laparoscopic approach, including white race, hospital size, and geographic location, its overall use still paled in comparison. Rates were not much better in "specialized centers," as demonstrated by an additional study from 2008 to 2011 of academic medical centers showing a laparoscopic colectomy rate of 42 % [9].

Minimally invasive proctectomy, with its technical demands due to the narrow confines of the pelvis that make exposure and retraction more difficult, has even less use. The oncologic outcomes of laparoscopic proctectomy for resectable rectal cancer remain somewhat unclear. The CLASICC trial showed a statistically (albeit nonsignificant) trend towards increased circumferential radial margin positivity in patients undergoing laparoscopic low anterior resection. Since then, several other trials have demonstrated similar rates of short- and moderate-term outcomes. While laparoscopic proctectomy is gaining acceptance, it is missing the "push" that the COST trial did for laparoscopic use in colon cancer. This may come from the ACOSOG Z6051 trial [10], initiated in 2008, which is a phase III prospective trial comparing laparoscopic vs. open resection for tumors within 12 cm of the anal verge. The results of this important study and others like it may serve as an impetus to more widely expand the utilization of laparoscopy in rectal cancer surgery for those surgeons with the experience and expertise to become facile in its use.

## Expanding the Role of Minimally Invasive Colectomy

One of the reasons to explain the delay in widespread adoption of laparoscopic colectomy is the difficulty of the procedure. To overcome this, especially when struggling performing a "pure" or straight laparoscopic approach, hybrid techniques have been developed. Hand-assisted methods and laparoscopic mobilization only (followed by smaller incisions to complete the case) maintain more natural haptic feedback and use the same incisions as the specimen extraction site (Fig. 36.1a, b). Head-to-head comparisons of straight laparoscopic to hand-assisted techniques have shown no significant differences with respect to operative times, pain scores, narcotic use, and length of stay outcomes [11]. Furthermore, as Dr. Vargas points out in his chapter, patients with morbid obesity present a technical challenge for which hand-assisted techniques may allow for a greater proportion of these patients to receive the benefits of laparoscopic colectomy. Interestingly, however, a survey of general surgeons not currently offering laparoscopic colectomy showed that 74 % did not feel that hand-assisted devices would influence them to adopt laparoscopic colectomy [12].

## Equipment

The equipment available for laparoscopic colectomy continues to evolve and improve. Equipment in the early laparoscopic era was basic [2], and mesenteric vessels were divided with clips, ENDOLOOPS™ (Ethicon, Cincinnati, OH), or ligatures. The advent of advanced energy devices has made intracorporeal vessel division safe, rapid, and reliable. Surgeons now have at their disposal ultrasonic, bipolar, and combination devices that can seal vessels up to 7 mm in diameter [13]. Endoscopic stapling devices come in a variety of lengths, staple heights, and degree of articulation. Powered staplers have been introduced to reduce surgeon effort and provide uniform compression when stapling. This is not to say that everything is perfect. Rectal division after low anterior resection remains a challenge, as no available stapling device has true 90° articulation. While high-definition imaging has certainly provided a huge upgrade, cameras continue to fog up, and visualization can always be improved.

Needlescopic instrumentation is another promising area. Also referred to as minilaparoscopy, it involves the use of instruments 3 mm or less in diameter. These instruments have been used for multiple procedures including cholecystectomy, appendectomy, among others [14]. While they can obviate the need for standard 5 mm transfascial access ports and potentially result in reduced scarring and postoperative pain, their lack of rigidity results in durability issues, as well as poor control and tissue manipulation, especially in obese patients. Despite these disadvantages, needlescopic instruments continue to evolve. The percutaneous surgical set (Ethicon, Cincinnati, OH) allows for standard-size instrument heads to be placed on needlescopic shafts that can be assembled within the abdominal cavity. Although this is FDA approved, it is not yet commercially available, and generalized use will provide more insight into their ultimate utility [15].

## Limited Access Laparoscopy and Natural Orifice Surgery

As yesterday's laparoscopic pioneers pushed minimally invasive techniques over traditional open surgery, limited access laparoscopy and natural orifice transluminal surgery are being developed by tomorrow's generation of minimally invasive surgeons. Limited access laparoscopic surgery involves reducing the number of access sites used for a procedure.

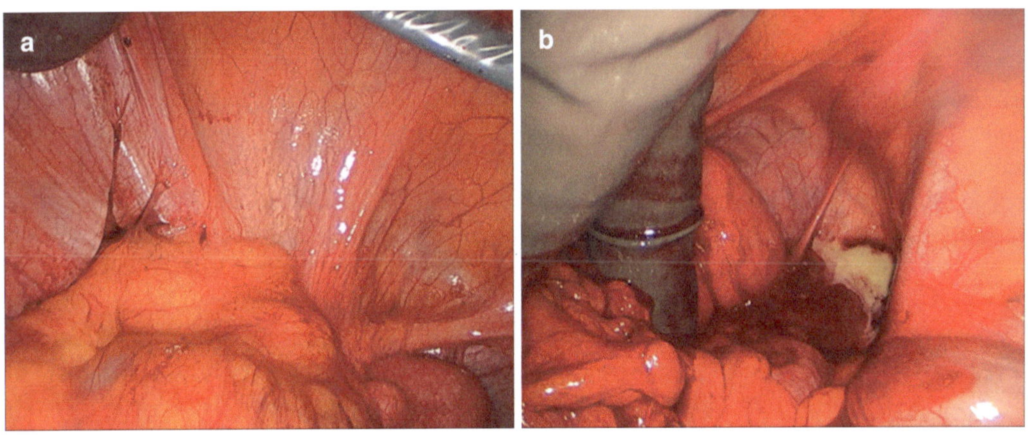

**Fig. 36.1** (**a**) Laparoscopic view of a colovesical fistula. (**b**) Hand-assisted laparoscopic techniques allow for takedown of the fistula and demonstration of the abscess cavity

In theory, this reduces a patient's pain and discomfort postoperatively. Reduction in the number of incisions provides the potential for improved cosmesis. Single-incision laparoscopic surgery (SILS) has been successfully used for a variety of colorectal procedures, including segmental colectomy, total colectomy, and even proctocolectomy [16–18]. The incision site is often chosen in the umbilicus or at a site of planned ostomy formation to minimize visible scar. Multiple trocars can be placed through a single fascial incision or one of the commercially available single-incision ports can be used. One of the difficulties with SILS colectomy is the loss of triangulation with traditional laparoscopy. Rather, in-line dissection and visualization must be performed. Various innovative technologies have been introduced to try and overcome some of these difficulties, including flexible tip cameras and curved instruments. Extracorporeal magnetic retraction has been used to make up for the lack of triangulation in retraction [19]. Despite the purported benefits of reducing the number of laparoscopic incisions, no randomized trial has shown any benefit of SILS colectomy over traditional laparoscopic colectomy, with the one notable exception of patient perceived cosmesis [20].

Unlike the appendix or gallbladder, one of the limiting factors in minimizing the invasiveness of laparoscopic colectomy is the need for specimen removal. Even when a true intracorporeal anastomosis is performed, often a bulky, diseased colon, mesentery, or tumor must be extracted through the abdominal wall, requiring an incision of several centimeters in length. Alternate anatomical sites have been described for specimen extraction, sometimes referred to as natural orifice specimen extraction (NOSE). These include the vagina, stomach, and anus [21–23]. Transvaginal access to the abdominal cavity has been performed for the longest period of time and is relatively safe. Transgastric access is a developing field and has been used successfully for "incisionless" cholecystectomy [24]. Concerns still remain regarding the safety of the gastrotomy closure and the potential consequences with a leak at the site. Transanal abdominal cavity access is interesting in that it is more easily achieved when performing low or left-sided colorectal anastomosis. Specimen extraction can then be performed via the rectal stump, obviating the need for abdominal extraction excisions. Yet, adding a colotomy for more proximal resections, similar to gastric extraction, provides an additional source of morbidity and risk to the procedure for an, as yet, unknown benefit.

Other more established techniques are witnessing expanded use in attempt to push the "scarless" surgery envelope. Transanal endoscopic microsurgery (TEM) was introduced by Buess in 1988 [25]. TEM allows for full-thickness rectal resections in locations more proximal than would be amenable to traditional transanal excision. Recently, transanal oncologic proctectomy using this same equipment, but accessing the presacral plane from below, has been reported [26]. While this is promising, challenges remain. Difficulties have been encountered dissecting proximal to the sacral promontory. Furthermore, mobilization of the splenic flexure to allow for a low-rectal anastomosis using current technology remains a significant challenge. Therefore, while the anus and rectum can be used as an extraction site in NOSE procedures and TEM used for rectal closure, technical and technological modifications are required to allow for more widespread adaption.

Furthermore, TEM setups consist of a rigid, operating proctoscope, binocular optics, insufflation, and multiple laparoscopic working ports. This specialized equipment comes with a high startup cost. Recently, commercially available, disposal laparoscopic transanal ports have become available. These devices allow for TEM procedures to be completed with standard laparoscopic equipment, at a fraction of the cost, which may increase its utilization more than any other factor.

Flexible endoscopy has been an indispensable tool for the colorectal surgeon for many years. Colonoscopy allows for diagnosis and treatment of a large number of colorectal diseases. Investigators have increasingly pushed the envelope on what types of colon lesions can be resected with an endoscope. Endoscopic polypectomy has evolved significantly from simple snare techniques [27]. More recently, large polyps can be removed en bloc with endoscopic mucosal resection techniques. Furthermore, borrowing techniques first developed from the upper GI tract, even larger masses and early cancers can be removed with endoscopic submucosal dissection. Hybrid laparo-endoscopic procedures have also been performed, where an abdominal surgeon assists an endoscopic surgeon in the removal of large polyps or performs wall closure after full-thickness colon resection. Newer techniques are being developed allowing for colonic wall closure after full-thickness resection using only the colonoscope [28]. Refinement in NOTES technology has included large, multichannel, operating endoscopes [29] that presumably could also be deployed for intracolonic dissections.

## Robotics

Another important potential influence on the future of minimally invasive colectomy is the emergence of robotic-assisted surgery (Fig. 36.2). Originally developed as voice-guided camera assistants for laparoscopy [30], modern surgical robotic platforms provide multiple surgeon-controlled arms with binocular vision [31]. They allow for wrist-like degrees of freedom during dissection and neutralize physiologic tremor. Robotic assistance has been applied to all areas of traditionally laparoscopic or open colon surgery, including segmental colectomy, single-incision colectomy,

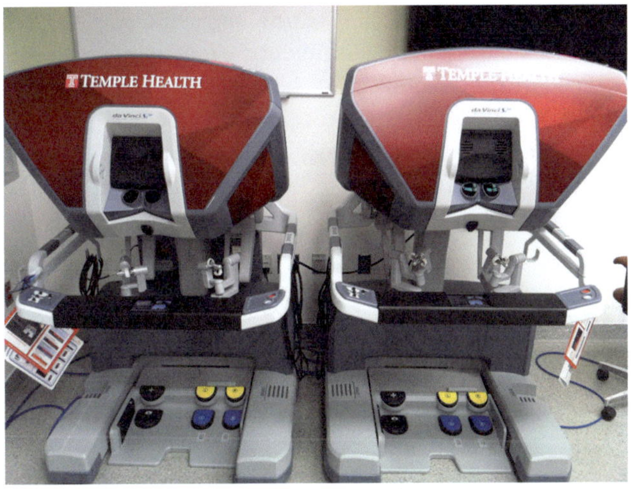


**Fig. 36.2** Dual console robotic equipment that can be used effectively for training

and even proctectomy [32–34], the latter of which may be the procedure that benefits the most from robotic assistance. The narrow confines of the pelvis magnify the benefits of improved visualization and precise dissection that robotic surgery allows. Some reports have suggested decreased rates of circumferential radial margin positivity with robotic-assisted proctectomy for cancer [35, 36]. In addition, technology to estimate the adequacy of perfusion to the bowel is available on the robotic platform (Video 36.1).

One of the major drawbacks of robotic-assisted surgery is the cost. A surgical robotics platform costs seven figures to obtain and has ongoing maintenance service contract costs. Dedicated, specially trained staff is needed to set up and assist in cases. Robots have space requirements and may necessitate OR facility modifications to allow for optimal deployment. The increased cost of robotic colectomy would be acceptable if associated increases in value were realized. However, no reports have yet to identify any consistent benefits of robotic-assisted colectomy over conventional laparoscopic colectomy. Multiple studies have confirmed the equivalence of robotic surgery to laparoscopic surgery, with respect to short-term complications and length of stay metrics, but at the expense of greater costs [37–40]. There is some data suggesting improved sexual function with robotic rectal surgery [35]; however, randomized clinical trials for confirmation are awaited. The ACOSOG Z6051 trial is including robotic proctectomy in its minimally invasive arm, and the ROLARR (robotic vs. laparoscopic resection for rectal cancer) trial [41] also aims to determine any potential advantages of robotic over laparoscopic surgery. Regardless, looking ahead, the robotic platforms of today likely are not the platforms of tomorrow. Transanal use, single-incision approaches, and smaller equipment profiles all will likely expand its horizons, along with increased use during residency training.

## Perioperative Care

Postoperative ileus (POI) is a major source of morbidity for patients undergoing laparoscopic colectomy. Ileus, although variably defined in clinical studies, is a delay in the return of gastrointestinal function after abdominal surgery. It has been estimated that managing prolonged ileus accounts for $1.46 billion in national healthcare costs for abdominal surgery. The incidence of prolonged ileus in laparoscopic colectomy patients is roughly 10 % [42, 43], and its development alone after colectomy increases hospitalization costs up to 15 % [44].

First proposed by Kehlet [45], fast-track, or enhanced recovery, protocols were developed to minimize ileus, decrease length of stay, and reduce complications. They encompass a wide range of preoperative, perioperative, and postoperative care measures with the focused goal of improving patient outcomes. Most protocols incorporate avoiding nasogastric tubes and drains, early feeding, and minimizing narcotics use, to name just a few components of care. Novel pharmaceutical agents have been developed to counteract the effects of narcotics on increasing POI [42, 46]. Fast-track protocols have been shown to reduce length of stay in the setting of laparoscopic colectomy [47]. Despite the technological advances in minimally invasive colectomy techniques, reduced incisions, and NOSE, POI will likely continue to cause morbidity and increase length of stay. Surgeons will have to continue to refine and improve their care protocols to maximize patient outcomes. When judged from the administrative perspective of cost and length of stay, even the most innovative surgical techniques will fail if the other important factors contributing to recovery are ignored.

## Healthcare Reform

The US healthcare system is currently in a period of great uncertainty. The Patient Protection and Affordable Care Act (PPACA) [48] signed into law by President Obama in 2010 is arguably the greatest change to our healthcare system since the origination of Medicare in 1965. While political brinkmanship and debate over the law continues, the Supreme Court has upheld the constitutionality of the individual mandate, so the numerous provisions of the PPACA seem likely to shape the face of medicine and surgery in the years to come. One of the major effects of the PPACA is expanding the availability of healthcare services to Americans. The law will accomplish this in various ways, including insurance exchanges, extended benefits for dependents, expansion of the Medicaid program, and financial disincentives for those to choose not to carry health insurance. With an aging population, and now with more patients eligible for healthcare benefits, one could expect the demand for minimally invasive treatments for colon and rectal diseases to dramatically increase.

A move away from traditional fee-for-service reimbursement will also affect the future of minimally invasive surgery. Accountable care organizations (ACOs) are groups, concentrated around primary care physicians, that assume responsibility for the total care of a cohort of patients [49]. In theory, costs savings are obtained through better integration and coordination of care within the ACO. Any potential cost savings are shared between the ACO and Medicare. This incentivizes high-quality healthcare delivery, over volume for profit. However, these cost savings may not be as relevant to inpatient services as they are to ambulatory ones [50]. The impact of ACOs on surgical care remains to be seen.

The expansion of minimally invasive colon surgery should fit well into the ideals of a high-quality procedure. Although there are slightly increased costs upfront, due to increased equipment cost, savings are realized by decreased hospital length of stay and infectious complications. ACOs could favor and promote the use of minimally invasive colectomy over open surgery in their networks, but only for properly selected patients.

Finally, as previously noted, implementation of laparoscopic colectomy in rural and smaller hospitals still lags behind larger or more urban institutions. Much of this is likely related to the practice preferences of surgical specialists trained in minimally invasive colectomy. There is clearly an opportunity for the role of minimally invasive colectomy to expand in these areas. As the next generation of surgeons enters the workforce, more experienced in a wide variety of minimally invasive surgery than their predecessors, there will likely be more practitioners offering laparoscopic colon surgery. Further measures have been implemented to increase the number of general surgeons in practice and direct them to geographic areas in need. The PPCA enacted a 10 % bonus payment to general surgeons in health provider shortage areas. Persistently unfilled residency training positions will be reallocated to primary care and general surgery positions.

## Pearls and Pitfalls

- Balance your eagerness to incorporate the "latest and greatest" technology with a thorough understanding of what it really has to offer, and ensure you know not only how it works, but also whether it is actually better.
- Innovation typically comes with higher costs, and you should be knowledgeable about them. However, while direct costs will likely always be greater, lower indirect costs could mean savings to your patient, the hospital, and the healthcare system.
- While improving outcomes for minimally invasive approaches to colorectal disease often focuses on individual aspects of care, it is truly the entire package that will ultimately make a difference. From appropriate preoperative evaluation and intraoperative technique to enhanced recovery protocols and technological advances that improve the entire process and lower costs, you need to be aware of all facets to lower morbidity and enhance your individual outcomes.

## Conclusion

The first quarter century of laparoscopic colectomy has seen dramatic changes. It has progressed from an investigational technique with questionable oncologic outcomes to a well-accepted minimally invasive operation with great benefits to patients and oncologic outcomes equivalent to open surgery. Robust, prospective clinical studies have been completed confirming its benefits. The surgical equipment for laparoscopic colectomy continues to evolve at a rapid rate, making procedures more efficient and reliable. The recent emergence of robotic colon surgery is clearly a triumph of engineering and medical science. However, its further adoption may be checked by the evolving nature of our healthcare system. Surgeons in the future will need to demonstrate high quality and value in their procedures to thrive; therefore, while robotic colectomy is currently not superior to well-established, lower-cost, high-value laparoscopic colectomy, the technology and its possibilities are too great to ignore.

Finally, the boundaries of minimally invasive colectomy have only been stretched and surgical investigators continue to push the envelope. The prospects of limited access laparoscopy, natural orifice surgery or specimen extraction, and robotics are exciting. What remains to be seen is whether these techniques are adopted on a large scale. There remains a great amount of work to be done in terms of getting "routine" laparoscopic colectomy implemented in many areas. Implementation of limited access laparoscopy or robotics presents even greater challenges. Cost and value will be important factors moving forward in our evolving healthcare climate, and robust clinical studies will be needed to demonstrate any advantages over standard laparoscopic techniques. While predicting the future is guaranteed to be flawed with inaccuracies, one surety is we are blessed to be witnesses and a part of exciting and rapidly evolving times that will (hopefully) ultimately improve outcomes in our patients with colorectal disease.

## References

1. Phillips EH, Franklin M, Carroll BJ, Fallas MJ, Ramos R, Rosenthal D. Laparoscopic colectomy. Ann Surg. 1992;216(6):703–7.
2. Spaner SJ, Warnock GL. A brief history of endoscopy, laparoscopy, and laparoscopic surgery. J Laparoendosc Adv Surg Tech A. 1997; 7(6):369–73.

3. Wexner SD, Cohen SM. Port site metastases after laparoscopic colorectal surgery for cure of malignancy. Br J Surg. 1995; 82(3):295–8.
4. Clinical Outcomes of Surgical Therapy Study Group. A comparison of laparoscopically assisted and open colectomy for colon cancer. N Engl J Med. 2004;350(20):2050–9.
5. Veldkamp R, Kuhry E, Hop WC, Jeekel J, Kazemier G, Bonjer HJ, et al. Laparoscopic surgery versus open surgery for colon cancer: short-term outcomes of a randomised trial. Lancet Oncol. 2005;6(7):477–84.
6. Guillou PJ, Quirke P, Thorpe H, Walker J, Jayne DG, Smith AM, et al. Short-term endpoints of conventional versus laparoscopic-assisted surgery in patients with colorectal cancer (MRC CLASICC trial): multicentre, randomised controlled trial. Lancet. 2005; 365(9472):1718–26.
7. Dolan JP, Diggs BS, Sheppard BC, Hunter JG. Ten-year trend in the national volume of bile duct injuries requiring operative repair. Surg Endosc. 2005;19(7):967–73.
8. Bardakcioglu O, Khan A, Aldridge C, Chen J. Growth of laparoscopic colectomy in the United States: analysis of regional and socioeconomic factors over time. Ann Surg. 2013;258(2):270–4.
9. Simorov A, Shaligram A, Shostrom V, Boilesen E, Thompson J, Oleynikov D. Laparoscopic colon resection trends in utilization and rate of conversion to open procedure: a national database review of academic medical centers. Ann Surg. 2012;256(3): 462–8.
10. Baik SH, Gincherman M, Mutch MG, Birnbaum EH, Fleshman JW. Laparoscopic vs open resection for patients with rectal cancer: comparison of perioperative outcomes and long-term survival. Dis Colon Rectum. 2011;54(1):6–14.
11. Marcello PW, Fleshman JW, Milsom JW, Read TE, Arnell TD, Birnbaum EH, et al. Hand-assisted laparoscopic vs. laparoscopic colorectal surgery: a multicenter, prospective, randomized trial. Dis Colon Rectum. 2008;51(6):818–26.
12. Moloo H, Haggar F, Martel G, Grimshaw J, Coyle D, Graham ID, et al. The adoption of laparoscopic colorectal surgery: a national survey of general surgeons. Can J Surg. 2009;52(6):455–62.
13. Tou S, Malik AI, Wexner SD, Nelson RL. Energy source instruments for laparoscopic colectomy. Cochrane Database Syst Rev. 2011;5, CD007886.
14. Krpata DM, Ponsky TA. Needlescopic surgery: what's in the toolbox? Surg Endosc. 2013;27(3):1040–4.
15. Press Announcements—FDA permits marketing of a new device for abdominal surgery [Internet]. [cited 2013 Oct 4]. Available from: http://www.fda.gov/NewsEvents/Newsroom/PressAnnouncements/ucm302561.htm
16. Ross H, Steele S, Whiteford M, Lee S, Albert M, Mutch M, et al. Early multi-institution experience with single-incision laparoscopic colectomy. Dis Colon Rectum. 2011;54(2):187–92.
17. Leblanc F, Makhija R, Champagne BJ, Delaney CP. Single incision laparoscopic total colectomy and proctocolectomy for benign disease: initial experience. Colorectal Dis. 2011;13(11): 1290–3.
18. Fichera A, Zoccali M, Felice C, Rubin DT. Total abdominal colectomy for refractory ulcerative colitis. Surgical treatment in evolution. J Gastrointest Surg. 2011;15(11):1909–16.
19. Uematsu D, Akiyama G, Magishi A, Nakamura J, Hotta K. Single-access laparoscopic left and right hemicolectomy combined with extracorporeal magnetic retraction. Dis Colon Rectum. 2010; 53(6):944–8.
20. Lee SW, Milsom JW, Nash GM. Single-incision versus multiport laparoscopic right and hand-assisted left colectomy: a case-matched comparison. Dis Colon Rectum. 2011;54(11):1355–61.
21. Uccella S, Cromi A, Bogani G, Casarin J, Serati M, Ghezzi F. Transvaginal specimen extraction at laparoscopy without concomitant hysterectomy: our experience and systematic review of the literature. J Minim Invasive Gynecol. 2013;20(5):583–90.
22. Dotai T, Coker AM, Antozzi L, Acosta G, Michelotti M, Bildzukewicz N, et al. Transgastric large-organ extraction: the initial human experience. Surg Endosc. 2013;27(2):394–9.
23. Franklin Jr ME, Liang S, Russek K. Natural orifice specimen extraction in laparoscopic colorectal surgery: transanal and transvaginal approaches. Tech Coloproctology. 2013;17 Suppl 1:S63–7.
24. Dallemagne B, Perretta S, Allemann P, Donatelli G, Asakuma M, Mutter D, et al. Transgastric cholecystectomy: from the laboratory to clinical implementation. World J Gastrointest Surg. 2010; 2(6):187–92.
25. Buess G, Kipfmüller K, Hack D, Grüssner R, Heintz A, Junginger T. Technique of transanal endoscopic microsurgery. Surg Endosc. 1988;2(2):71–5.
26. Sylla P. Current experience and future directions of completely NOTES colorectal resection. World J Gastrointest Surg. 2010; 2(6):193–8.
27. Steele SR, Johnson EK, Champagne B, Davis B, Lee S, Rivadeneira D, et al. Endoscopy and polyps-diagnostic and therapeutic advances in management. World J Gastroenterol WJG. 2013;19(27): 4277–88.
28. Agrawal D, Chak A, Champagne BJ, Marks JM, Delaney CP. Endoscopic mucosal resection with full-thickness closure for difficult polyps: a prospective clinical trial. Gastrointest Endosc. 2010;71(6):1082–8.
29. Dallemagne B, Marescaux J. The ANUBIS™ project. Minim Invasive Ther Allied Technol. 2010;19(5):257–61.
30. Jacobs LK, Shayani V, Sackier JM. Determination of the learning curve of the AESOP robot. Surg Endosc. 1997;11(1):54–5.
31. Freschi C, Ferrari V, Melfi F, Ferrari M, Mosca F, Cuschieri A. Technical review of the da Vinci surgical telemanipulator. Int J Med Robot. 2012;9(4):396–406.
32. Delaney CP, Lynch AC, Senagore AJ, Fazio VW. Comparison of robotically performed and traditional laparoscopic colorectal surgery. Dis Colon Rectum. 2003;46(12):1633–9.
33. Ragupathi M, Ramos-Valadez DI, Pedraza R, Haas EM. Robotic-assisted single-incision laparoscopic partial cecectomy. Int J Med Robot Comput Assist Surg MRCAS. 2010;6(3):362–7.
34. Peterson CY, McLemore EC, Horgan S, Talamini MA, Ramamoorthy SL. Technical aspects of robotic proctectomy. Surg Laparosc Endosc Percutan Tech. 2012;22(3):189–93.
35. D'Annibale A, Pernazza G, Monsellato I, Pende V, Lucandri G, Mazzocchi P, et al. Total mesorectal excision: a comparison of oncological and functional outcomes between robotic and laparoscopic surgery for rectal cancer. Surg Endosc. 2013;27(6): 1887–95.
36. Kang J, Yoon KJ, Min BS, Hur H, Baik SH, Kim NK, et al. The impact of robotic surgery for mid and low rectal cancer: a case-matched analysis of a 3-arm comparison—open, laparoscopic, and robotic surgery. Ann Surg. 2013;257(1):95–101.
37. Park JS, Choi G-S, Park SY, Kim HJ, Ryuk JP. Randomized clinical trial of robot-assisted versus standard laparoscopic right colectomy. Br J Surg. 2012;99(9):1219–26.
38. Deutsch GB, Sathyanarayana SA, Gunabushanam V, Mishra N, Rubach E, Zemon H, et al. Robotic vs. laparoscopic colorectal surgery: an institutional experience. Surg Endosc. 2012;26(4): 956–63.
39. Tyler JA, Fox JP, Desai MM, Perry WB, Glasgow SC. Outcomes and costs associated with robotic colectomy in the minimally invasive era. Dis Colon Rectum. 2013;56(4):458–66.
40. Fung AK-Y, Aly EH. Robotic colonic surgery: is it advisable to commence a new learning curve? Dis Colon Rectum. 2013; 56(6):786–96.
41. Collinson FJ, Jayne DG, Pigazzi A, Tsang C, Barrie JM, Edlin R, et al. An international, multicentre, prospective, randomised, controlled, unblinded, parallel-group trial of robotic-assisted versus standard laparoscopic surgery for the curative treatment of rectal cancer. Int J Colorectal Dis. 2012;27(2):233–41.

42. Delaney CP, Marcello PW, Sonoda T, Wise P, Bauer J, Techner L. Gastrointestinal recovery after laparoscopic colectomy: results of a prospective, observational, multicenter study. Surg Endosc. 2010;24(3):653–61.
43. Kronberg U, Kiran RP, Soliman MSM, Hammel JP, Galway U, Coffey JC, et al. A characterization of factors determining postoperative ileus after laparoscopic colectomy enables the generation of a novel predictive score. Ann Surg. 2011;253(1):78–81.
44. Iyer S, Saunders WB, Stemkowski S. Economic burden of postoperative ileus associated with colectomy in the United States. J Manag Care Pharm JMCP. 2009;15(6):485–94.
45. Basse L, Hjort Jakobsen D, Billesbølle P, Werner M, Kehlet H. A clinical pathway to accelerate recovery after colonic resection. Ann Surg. 2000;232(1):51–7.
46. Harbaugh CM, Al-Holou SN, Bander TS, Drews JD, Shah MM, Terjimanian MN, et al. A statewide, community-based assessment of alvimopan's effect on surgical outcomes. Ann Surg. 2013;257(3):427–32.
47. Vlug MS, Wind J, Hollmann MW, Ubbink DT, Cense HA, Engel AF, et al. Laparoscopy in combination with fast track multimodal management is the best perioperative strategy in patients undergoing colonic surgery: a randomized clinical trial (LAFA-study). Ann Surg. 2011;254(6):868–75.
48. Rangel C. H.R.3590—111th Congress (2009–2010)—Patient Protection and Affordable Care Act | Congress.gov | Library of Congress [Internet]. 2010 [cited 2013 Sep 27]. Available from: http://beta.congress.gov/bill/111th/house-bill/3590
49. Berwick DM. Making good on ACOs' promise—the final rule for the medicare shared savings program. N Engl J Med. 2011;365(19):1753–6.
50. Miller DC, Ye Z, Gust C, Birkmeyer JD. Anticipating the effects of accountable care organizations for inpatient surgery. JAMA Surg. 2013;148(6):549–54.

# Index


**A**
Abdomen
  anastomosis, 207–208
  bloody operative field, 208
  colonic length/mobilization, 206–207
  difficult splenic flexure, 202–205
  fatty mesentery, 209–210
  HALS, 202
  intraoperative colonoscopy, 210
  left-sided resection, 205–206
  patient positioning and restraining, 201–202
  precautions, 210
  preemptive conversion, 207
  reoperative surgery, 210
  right-sided resection, 205
  SRA, 208
  traction/countertraction, 202
  transverse colon, 205
  ureter, 208–209
Abdominoperineal resection (APR)
  anesthesia, prophylaxis, and positioning, 133
  biologic mesh, 139–140
  clinical trials, 131–132
  colon mobilization and division, 134
  indications, 131
  laparoscopic perineal approach, 138–139
  myocutaneous flaps, 139
  omentoplasty, 139
  ostomy creation, 136
  patient selection and preoperative considerations, 132–133
  perineal defect, reconstruction, 139
  perineal dissection, 137
  perioperative management and complications, 140–141
  port placement and entry into the abdomen, 133–134
  sigmoid colon division, 136
  TME, 132, 134–136
Accountable care organizations (ACOs), 404
Acute colonoscopic perforation, 304–306
Acute perforated diverticulitis, 306
Adhesiolysis and hernia reduction, 191–192
Adhesiolysis, laparoscopic. *See* Laparoscopic adhesiolysis
Air leak test, 116, 117
Airway problems, 243
American College of Chest Physicians (ACCP), 333
Anastomosis
  abdomen, 207–208
  bowel extraction and, 68
  coloanal, 116, 117
  colorectal, 116, 117
  creation
    colostomy after Hartmann's procedure, 184
    ileostomy with ileorectal anastomosis, 186
    laparoscopic rectopexy, 160–161
  exteriorization and, 59–60
  HALAR, 128
  ileocolic resection, CD patients, 341
  laparoscopic sigmoidectomy/left colectomy, 78–79
Anastomotic leak, 239–241
Anorectal malformations
  LAARP, 367–369
  modern open approach, 366
Anorectum division, 150
Antegrade continence enema (ACE), 369
Appendectomy, laparoscopic. *See* Laparoscopic appendectomy
Appendicitis
  acute, 375
  clinical presentation and indications, 361
  diagnosis, 377
  laparoscopic appendectomy, 361–362
  pregnant patients, 377

**B**
Benign polyps, 298
Bladder, 226
Bleeding, 238–239
Blood vessels, 226–227
Body mass index (BMI)
  LAS, 390–391
  obese patients, laparoscopic colectomy, 321
Bowel
  division, 78–79
  extraction and anastomosis, 68
  mobilization, 341
  obstruction
    malignant, 307–308
    postoperative small, 307

**C**
Cancer, disease pathology, 389–390
Celioscopy, 399
Cholecystitis, acute, 375
$CO_2$ insufflation, 377
Colectomy, laparoscopic. *See* Laparoscopic colectomy
Coloanal anastomosis, 116, 117
Colon anatomy, 43, 46
Colon and mesentery mobilization, 56–57
Colon cancer, 25
Colonic mesenteric vasculature
  gastrocolic trunk, 26–27
  ileocolic (ICA), 25, 26


H.M. Ross et al. (eds.), *Minimally Invasive Approaches to Colon and Rectal Disease: Technique and Best Practices*, DOI 10.1007/978-1-4939-1581-1, © Springer Science+Business Media New York 2015

Colonic mesenteric vasculature (*cont.*)
  right colic artery (RCA), 25
  superior mesenteric artery (SMA), 25–27
Colonic mobilization and vessel ligation, 279
Colon mesentery transection, 150–152
Colonoscopic-assisted laparoscopic wall excision, 297
Colon resections, laparoscopic. *See* Laparoscopic colon resections
Colorectal anastomosis, 116, 117
Colorectal cancer (CRC)
  pregnant patients, 376
  reoperative surgery, 230
Colorectal perforation
  acute colonoscopic perforation, 304–306
  acute perforated diverticulitis, 306
  postoperative anastomotic perforation, 306–307
Colostomy after Hartmann's procedure
  anastomosis creation, 184
  distal sigmoid colon resection, 183–184
  Hartmann's pouch and rectum mobilization, 183
  port placement, 180–182
  proximal colon mobilization, 182–183
Colostomy, laparoscopic. *See* Laparoscopic colostomy
Combined endo-laparoscopic surgery (CELS)
  benefits, 293
  clinical trials, 298
  colonoscopic-assisted laparoscopic wall excision, 297
  colon polyps, 293
  complications, 298
  endoscopy, 295
  indications, 294
  leak test, 297
  mobilization, 295, 296
  patient setup, 294–295
  polypectomy, 296–297
  polyp retrieval, 298
  port placement, 295
  postoperative care, 298
  precautions, 298–299
  preoperative planning, 294
Constipation, 156, 164. *See also* Fecal incontinence
Conventional open surgery (OS) *vs.* LAS
  clinical trials, 385–386
  conversion, 386
Conventional *vs.* laparoscopic-assisted surgery in colorectal cancer (CLASICC) trial
  APR, 131–132
  hand-assisted laparoscopic right colectomy, 62
  laparoscopic proctectomy, 400
Corticosteroids, 8–9
COST trial
  hand-assisted laparoscopic right colectomy, 62
  laparoscopic proctectomy, 400
Crohn's disease (CD)
  complex, 339–340
  ileocolic resection
    anastomosis, 341
    bowel mobilization, 341
    complex fistulous cases, 341
    extracorporeal manual examination, bowel, 340–341
    HALS, 341
    mesenteric division, 341
    SILC, 341–342
    standard ports, 340
  indications and contraindications, 337–338
  laparoscopic colon resections, 339
  laparoscopic proctocolectomy, 144–145
  laparoscopic *vs.* open surgery, ileocolitis, 338–339
  literature evidence, 338
  minimally invasive (MI) surgery, 337
  precautions, 342

**D**
da Vinci® system, 275–277
Deep dissection, 331–332
Descending colectomy, 46–47
Difficult splenic flexure
  abdomen, 202–205
  laparoscopic sigmoidectomy/left colectomy, 77–78
Distal sigmoid colon resection, 183–184
Diverticulitis
  acute
    complicated, 375–376
    conservative treatment, 377–378
    uncomplicated, 374
  disease pathology, outcomes, 388–389
  reoperative surgery, 230

**E**
Elderly patients, laparoscopy
  acid/base effects, 315
  aging, 309
  cardiovascular and physiologic risk stratification, 310
  cardiovascular effects, 316
  changes and technical points, 316–317
  clinical trials, 311
  early studies, 311–312
  enhanced recovery protocols, 314
  immune system effects, 316
  long-term outcomes, 314–315
  *vs.* open outcomes, 312–314
  patient factors, 309
  pneumoperitoneum physiology, 315
  preoperative risk assessment, 310–311
  pulmonary effects, 315–316
  renal effects, 316
  risk factors, 314
  *vs.* young, 312
Emergent laparoscopic colorectal surgery
  advantages and disadvantages, 303–304
  approach and abdominal entry, 304
  bowel obstruction
    malignant, 307–308
    postoperative small, 307
  colorectal perforation
    acute colonoscopic perforation, 304–306
    acute perforated diverticulitis, 306
    postoperative anastomotic perforation, 306–307
  precautions, 308
End ileostomy, 95–96
Endoscopy, 295
Enhanced recovery after surgery (ERAS), 10–11
Enhanced recovery pathways (ERP), 332
Enterotomy, 237–238
Extended right colectomy, 59
Exteriorization
  anastomosis and, 59–60
  laparoscopic sigmoidectomy/left colectomy, 78–79

**F**

Familial adenomatous polyposis (FAP), 145
Fatty mesentery, 209–210
Fecal incontinence, 369
Fetal monitoring, 376–377

**G**

Gas insufflation, pediatric MIS, 360
Gastrocolic trunk, 26–27
GI NOTES surgery, 264

**H**

Hand-assisted laparoscopic right colectomy
  bowel extraction and anastomosis, 68
  complication and solution, 68
  concept, 62–63
  COST trial and CLASSIC trial, 62
  hepatic flexure takedown, 66
  ileal mesentery mobilization, 66
  oncologic colon resection, 63
  patient positioning, 63–64
  port placement, 64–65
  postoperative care, 68
  retroperitoneal dissection and lateral attachments, 66
  surgeon, camera holder, and monitor, 65
  technical difficulty, 61
  vessel and mesentery division, 67
Hand-assisted laparoscopic surgery (HALS)
  abdomen, 202
  ileocolic resection, CD patients, 341
  *vs.* laparoscopic assisted surgery (LAS), 386–387
  obese patients, laparoscopic colectomy, 327–329
  TAC
    colonic mobilization, completion of, 106–107
    considerations, 109–110
    device placement, 104
    indications, 103
    mesenteric division, 107–108
    palm-down and palm-up techniques, 105
    partial colonic mobilization, direct vision, 105–106
    patient positioning, 104
    resection, specimen extraction and anastomosis, 108, 109
    surgical ports and energy devices, 104
  UC patients
    completion proctectomy with IPAA, 348–351
    total abdominal colectomy with end ileostomy, 346–348
    total proctocolectomy with IPAA, 351–352
Hand-assisted left colectomy
  complications, 87
  hand-port placement, 82–83
  indications, 81
  left colon dissection, 83–86
  patient setup, 82
  postoperative care, 86–87
  precautions, 87–88
  preoperative planning, 81
Hand-assisted low anterior resection (HALAR)
  anastomosis, 128
  bleeding, 128
  bowel injury, 129
  clinical trials, 129
  hand-access device placement, 129
  indications, 119
  mobilization, 122–124
  pelvic dissection, 130
  port placement and hand device, 121
  preoperative planning
    imaging and diagnostic studies, 120
    patient history and physical findings, 119
  resection, 127
  splenic flexure, 129–130
  surgical management
    patient positioning, 120, 121
    preoperative planning, 120
  TME, 124–127
  Trendelenburg position, 122
  ureteral injury, 128
  visualization, 129
  wound complications, 128
Hand-assist port, 228–229
Hartmann's procedure, 179, 180
Hasson (open) technique, 22
Healthcare Cost and Utilization Project (HCUP), 143
Hepatic flexure mobilization, 148
Hernia repair, 231
Hirschsprung's disease
  clinical presentation and indications, 365
  laparoscopic-assisted endorectal pull-through, 365–366
Hybrid approach *vs.* total robotic approach, 281

**I**

Ileal mesentery mobilization, 66
Ileal pouch-anal anastomosis (IPAA)
  completion proctectomy, 348–351
  stapled IPAA *vs.* mucosectomy and handsewn anastomosis, 145–146
  total proctocolectomy, 351–352
Ileoanal pouch formation and anastomosis, 152–153
Ileocolic artery (ICA), 25, 26
Ileocolic resection, CD patients
  anastomosis, 341
  bowel mobilization, 341
  complex fistulous cases, 341
  extracorporeal manual examination, bowel, 340–341
  HALS, 341
  mesenteric division, 341
  SILC, 341–342
  standard ports, 340
Ileorectostomy, 96–98
Ileostomy
  formation, 153
  with ileorectal anastomosis
    anastomosis creation, 186
    port placement, 184–185
    rectal resection, 186
    rectum mobilization, 185
  laparoscopic (*see* Laparoscopic ileostomy)
Imperforate anus. *See* Anorectal malformations
Inferior mesenteric artery (IMA)
  blood supply, 27, 28
  bowstring effect, 27
  embryologic surgical planes, 28–30
  gonadal vessels, 30
  innervation, 31–32, 34–35, 38–39
  pelvis, 30–31
  posterior and lateral compartments, 31, 33, 35–37
  splenic flexure, 28, 29
  superior rectal artery, 28
  ureter, 30–35

Inferior mesenteric vein (IMV), 44–46
Inflammatory bowel disease (IBD)
  clinical presentation and indications, 362
  disease pathology, outcomes, 389
  exacerbations
    mild, 375
    severe, 376
  reoperative surgery, 230–231
  surgical technique, 362–364
Insufflation and port placement, 191
International Classification of Diseases (ICD) code, 143
Intraoperative colonoscopy, 210
Ischemic ostomy, 170

**J**
J pouch, 250, 257, 259

**K**
Keyhole technique, 194–195

**L**
LAARP. *See* Laparoscopic-assisted anorectal pull-through (LAARP)
Laparoscopic adhesiolysis, 223
Laparoscopic anatomy. *See* Surgical anatomy
Laparoscopic appendectomy, 361–362
Laparoscopic-assisted anorectal pull-through (LAARP), 367–369
Laparoscopic-assisted appendicostomy, 369
Laparoscopic-assisted endorectal pull-through, 365–366
Laparoscopic-assisted surgery (LAS)
  *vs.* conventional open surgery (OS)
    clinical trials, 385–386
    conversion, 386
  desirable metrics, 391–392
  disease pathology, outcomes
    cancer, 389–390
    diverticulitis, 388–389
    inflammatory bowel disease (IBD), 389
  *vs.* HALS, 386–387
  patient factors
    age, 391
    body mass index (BMI), 390–391
  SILS *vs.* MILS, 387–388
  surgeon factors, 391
Laparoscopic colectomy, 381–382
Laparoscopic colon resections, 339
Laparoscopic colorectal surgery
  bowel preparation, 7
  elderly patients, 6
  iatrogenic ureteral injury, 10
  obese patients, 6
  preoperative evaluation, 5
  prevalence, 4
Laparoscopic colostomy, 174–176
Laparoscopic ileostomy, 171–174
Laparoscopic perineal approach, 138–139
Laparoscopic proctocolectomy
  epidemiology and economics, 143–144
  preoperative considerations
    Crohn's disease, 144–145
    familial adenomatous polyposis (FAP), 145
    patient positioning, 146
    site marking, 145
    stapled IPAA *vs.* mucosectomy and handsewn anastomosis, 145–146
    ulcerative colitis, 144
  technical approach
    anorectum division, 150
    colon mesentery transection, 150–152
    hepatic flexure mobilization, 148
    ileoanal pouch formation and anastomosis, 152–153
    ileostomy formation, 153
    left colon mobilization, 148
    precautions, 153
    rectal mobilization, 149–150
    right colon mobilization, 147–148
    splenic flexure mobilization, 148–149
    trocar placement, 146–147
Laparoscopic rectal resection, cancer
  colorectal/coloanal anastomosis, 116, 117
  indications, 111
  mesocolon and vascular pedicle dissection, 112–113
  operative technique, 112
  patient preparation, 111–112
  pelvic dissection, 114–116
  rectum division, 116
  splenic flexure and left colon mobilization, 113–114
  surgeon, assistant, and nurse positioning, 112
  TME, 111
Laparoscopic rectopexy
  anastomosis creation, 160–161
  clinical trials, 166
  complications, 165–166
  indications, 156
  patient setup, 157
  port placement, 157–158
  postoperative care, 165
  precautions, 166–167
  preoperative planning, 156–157
  rectum mobilization, 164
  redundant sigmoid colon, resection, 159–160
  sigmoid colon and rectum mobilization, 158–159
  transabdominal/transperineal approach, 155
  trocar placement, 162, 164
Laparoscopic sigmoidectomy/left colectomy
  bowel division, exteriorization, and anastomosis, 78–79
  contraindications, 71–72
  difficult splenic flexure, 77–78
  indications, 71
  lateral dissection, 77
  left ureter identification, difficulty, 76
  operative steps, 74
  port placement, 72–74
  positioning, 72
  positive leak test, 79–80
  preoperative planning, 72
  retromesenteric dissection, 76–77
  splenic flexure mobilization, 77
  surgery, 72
  vascular isolation and division, 74–76
Laparoscopic splenic flexure mobilization, 280
Laparoscopic visualization, 295, 317
Laparoscopy
  APR (*see* Abdominoperineal resection (APR))
  benefits of, 4–5
  conversions, 241–242
  elderly patients (*see* Elderly patients, laparoscopy)
  HALAR (*see* Hand-assisted low anterior resection (HALAR))

instrumentation
bipolar energy, 19–20
camera/laparoscope, 16–17
energy devices, 19
graspers, 17–18
hand-assisted devices, 20
insufflator, 17
monopolar energy, 19
scissors, 18
staplers, 18–19
trocars, 15–16
ultrasonic energy, 20
objectives, 55
PH repair (*see* Parastomal hernia (PH) repair)
physiologic effects of, 3
stoma reversal (*see* Stoma reversal, laparoscopic)
Lateral approach, right colectomy, 56
Lateral-to-medial mobilization, 38–41
Leak test, 297
Left colectomy
anterior resection and
descending colectomy, 46–47
inferior mesenteric vein and splenic flexure mobilization, 44–46
low anterior resection, 47–48
perineal dissection, 49
uterine retraction, 48–49
robotic surgery
laparoscopic splenic flexure mobilization, 280
medial-to-lateral dissection, left colon, 280
port placement, 279
positioning, 279
total mesorectal dissection, 280–281
Left colon
dissection, 83–86
mobilization, 148
Low anterior resection
left colectomy and anterior resection, 47–48
robotic surgery
laparoscopic splenic flexure mobilization, 280
medial-to-lateral dissection, left colon, 280
port placement, 279–280
positioning, 279
total mesorectal dissection, 280–281
Lufttamponade therapy, 399
Lumbar sympathetic nerve plexus, 101
Lysis of adhesions, 227–228

**M**
Malignant obstruction, 307–308
Medial approach
right colectomy, 55
sigmoid colon mobilization, 71
Medial-to-lateral mobilization
dissection, left colon, 280
mobilization, 35–38, 40–41
Mesenteric division, 341
Mesh securement, PH repair
keyhole technique, 194–195
Sugarbaker technique, 193–194
Mesocolon and vascular pedicle dissection, 112–113
Minimally invasive colectomy
equipment, 401
laparoscopy and natural orifice surgery, 401–402
Multi-incision laparoscopic surgery (MILS), 387–388
Myocutaneous flaps, APR, 139

**N**
Natural orifice specimen extraction (NOSE), 264–265
Natural orifice translumenal endoscopic surgery (NOTES)
GI NOTES, 264
initial clinical developments, 266–267
initial clinical pure transanal resection, 269
NOSE, 264–265
POEM, 264
precautions, 270
preclinical developments, 266
surgical paradigm, 263
taxonomy and abbreviations, 264
transanal rectosigmoid resection, 265–266
transanal TME (taTME) procedural steps, 267–269
Nerve damage, 218–219

**O**
Obese patients, laparoscopic colectomy
anatomy and technical challenge, 323–324
body mass index (BMI), 321
clinical trials, 333–334
definition, obesity, 321
dissection and mobilization, 329
ergonomic issues, 324
HALS, 327–329
learning curve, 324–325
omentum, 330
pelvic operations
deep dissection, 331–332
essential technical adjustments, 331
postoperative care and enhanced recovery pathways (ERP), 332
venous thromboembolism (VTE) prophylaxis, 332–333
wound management, 332
ports and exposure techniques, 326–327
positioning and securing, 325
precautions, 334
preoperative considerations, 322–323
prevalence, 322
technical considerations, 322
ureteral stent insertion, 325–326
visceral abdominal fat (VAT), 321
waist-to-hip ratio (WHR), 321
wound extraction site, 330–331
Omentoplasty, 139
Omentum, 242–243, 330
Oncologic colon resection, 63
Open stoma reversals, 186, 187
Ostomy
creation, APR, 136
marking, 7–8
reversal, reoperative surgery, 229–230

**P**
Palm-down and palm-up techniques, 105
Parastomal hernia (PH) repair
adhesiolysis and hernia reduction, 191–192
clinical trials, 196
complications, 195–196
incidence, 189
insufflation and port placement, 191
mesh measurement and preparation, 192–193
mesh securement
keyhole technique, 194–195
Sugarbaker technique, 193–194

Parastomal hernia (PH) repair (*cont.*)
patient setup, 191
postoperative care, 195
precautions, 196–197
preoperative planning, 190
risk factors, 189
stoma creation, 170
stomal relocation, 195
Sugarbaker technique, 189
Patient factors, LAS
age, 391
body mass index (BMI), 390–391
Patient Protection and Affordable Care Act (PPACA), 403–404
Pediatric minimally invasive surgery (MIS)
anorectal malformations/imperforate anus
laparoscopic-assisted anorectal pull-through (LAARP), 367–369
modern open approach, 366
appendicitis
clinical presentation and indications, 361
laparoscopic appendectomy, 361–362
fecal incontinence, 369
gas insufflation, 360
Hirschsprung's disease
clinical presentation and indications, 365
laparoscopic-assisted endorectal pull-through, 365–366
history, 357–358
inflammatory bowel disease (IBD)
clinical presentation and indications, 362
surgical technique, 362–364
laparoscopic instrumentation, 360–361
patient selection and positioning, 358–359
trocar selection and insertion technique, 359–360
Pelvic dissection
HALAR, 130
laparoscopic rectal resection, 114–116
Pelvis
accessing the abdomen/port configuration, 213–214
bleeding, 220
genitourinary structures, 219
inferior mesenteric vein division/splenic flexure mobilization, 217–218
lateral and anterior mobilization, rectum, 219
medial-to-lateral left colonic dissection, 214
nerve damage, 218–219
precautions, 220
rectal mobilization/bowel division, 218
rectum division, 220
retroperitoneal exposure/critical anatomy, 214–216
vascular pedicle division/proximal colonic mobilization, 216–217
Perineal approach, laparoscopic. *See* Laparoscopic perineal approach
Perineal defect, reconstruction, 139
Perineal dissection
APR, 137
left colectomy and anterior resection, 49
Perioperative assessment
cardiovascular effects, 3–4
elderly patients, 6
elective patients, evaluation
cardiac, 5–6
laboratory testing, 5
pulmonary, 6
emergency colorectal surgery patients, 6
ERAS, 10–11
intraoperative management
endoscopy availability, 10
gastric decompression, 10
patient monitoring, 9
patient positioning, 9–10
urinary drainage and ureteral stenting, 10
VTE prevention, 10
laparoscopy
benefits of, 4–5
physiologic effects of, 3
patient management
analgesic considerations, 9
antibiotics, 9
bowel preparation, 7
corticosteroids, 8–9
fasting, 7
informed consent, 9
lesion localization, 7
ostomy marking, 7–8
pulmonary effects, 4
renal effects, 4
reoperative surgery, 7
Peritoneal space
avoiding complications, 23
direct trocar insertion, 22
hand assist, 23
Hasson (open) technique, 22
laparoscopic entry techniques, 21
optical trocar, 22
reoperative surgery, 22
trocar positioning, 22
Veress needle, 21–22
Peritonitis, 376
Per-oral endoscopic myotomy (POEM), 264
Pneumoperitoneum
elderly patients, 315
obese patients, 243–244
Polypectomy, 296–297
Polyp retrieval, CELS, 298
Port placement
colostomy after Hartmann's procedure, 180–182
combined endo-laparoscopic surgery (CELS), 295
ileostomy with ileorectal anastomosis, 184–185
Positive leak test, 79–80
Postoperative anastomotic perforation, 306–307
Postoperative ileus (POI), 403
Postoperative small bowel obstruction, 307
Pregnancy
acute cholecystitis and symptomatic cholelithiasis, 375
acute diverticulitis
complicated, 375–376
conservative treatment, 377–378
uncomplicated, 374
appendicitis
acute, 375
diagnosis, 377
$CO_2$ insufflation, 377
colorectal cancer (CRC), 376
fetal monitoring, 376–377
IBD exacerbations
mild, 375
severe, 376
indications, 374
instrumentation, 377
pain, 377
patient positioning, 376
peritonitis, 376
physiology and anatomy, changes, 373–374

small bowel obstruction
early, 374
late and complete, 375
technical tips, 378
trocar placement, 377
Procidentia. *See* Laparoscopic rectopexy
Proctectomy with IPAA
HALS, 348–351
single-incision laparoscopic surgery (SILS), 353
Proctocolectomy, laparoscopic. *See* Laparoscopic proctocolectomy
Proximal colon mobilization, 182–183

**R**
Rectal prolapse. *See* Laparoscopic rectopexy
Rectal resection, 186. *See also* Laparoscopic rectal resection, cancer
Rectopexy, laparoscopic. *See* Laparoscopic rectopexy
Rectum
division, 116, 220
mobilization, 149–150, 164, 185
reoperative surgery, 227
Recurrence rates, 155, 156
Redundant sigmoid colon, resection, 159–160
Reoperative surgery
abdomen, 210
anatomy, 225–226
bladder, 226
blood vessels, 226–227
colorectal cancer, 230
complications, 221
conversion rate, 221, 222
conversion to open procedure, 229
diverticular disease, 230
enterotomy rates, 222
gaining access, 225
hand-assist port, 228–229
IBD, 230–231
laparoscopic adhesiolysis, 223
lysis of adhesions, 227–228
minimally invasive colorectal case, 222–223
ostomy reversal, 229–230
perioperative assessment, 7
peritoneal space, 22
preoperative evaluation, 223–225
prior hernia repair, 231
rectum, 227
timing of surgery, 224
ureter, 226
Resection
HALAR, 127
redundant sigmoid colon, 159–160
Restorative proctocolectomy, 131
Retromesenteric dissection, 76–77
Retroperitoneal exposure, 214–216
Right colectomy
clinical anatomy, 54–55
colon and mesentery mobilization, 56–57
complication and solution, 60
extended right colectomy, 59
exteriorization and anastomosis, 59–60
identification and division, vascular pedicles, 58
inferior approach, 55–56
lateral approach, 56
lateral-to-medial mobilization, 38–41
lesser sac, 41, 42
medial approach, 55
medial-to-lateral mobilization, 35–38, 40–41
objectives, laparoscopic procedure, 55
patient preparation, 53
patient setup, 53–54
procedure, 56
right colon attachments, division, 58–59
robotic surgery
patient positioning, 278
port placement, 278
procedure, 278–279
superior approach, 56
Right colic artery (RCA), 25
Right colon mobilization, 147–148
Robotics
assisted laparoscopy, 382–383
assisted surgery
drawbacks, 403
dual console equipment, 402–403
Robotic surgery
camera, 276
da Vinci® system, 275–277
disadvantages, 274
equipment, 275, 276
hybrid approach *vs.* total robotic approach, 281
indications, 275
instruments, 277
left colectomy/low anterior resection
laparoscopic splenic flexure mobilization, 280
medial-to-lateral dissection, left colon, 280
port placement, 279–280
total mesorectal dissection, 280–281
patient positioning, 277
port placement, 277–278
precautions, 281
procedure, 273, 274
right colectomy
patient positioning, 278
port placement, 278
procedure, 278–279

**S**
Sigmoid colon
division, 136
rectum mobilization and, 158–159
Sigmoidectomy, laparoscopic. *See* Laparoscopic sigmoidectomy
Single-incision laparoscopic colectomy (SILC), 341–342
Single-incision laparoscopic surgery (SILS)
*vs.* multi-incision laparoscopic surgery (MILS), 387–388
UC patients
proctectomy with IPAA, 353
total abdominal colectomy with end ileostomy, 352–353
Single-incision laparoscopy
clinical trials, 261
complications, 260–261
indications, 249–250
left colectomy
port at the umbilicus, 254–256
suprapubic location, 256–257
surgical procedure, 253
port types and port placement, 250
postoperative care, 260
precautions, 261
preoperative planning, 250
right hemicolectomy, 250–253
single-port surgery, 249

Single-incision laparoscopy (*cont.*)
  total proctocolectomy with ileal pouch anal anastomosis reconstruction
    colonic dissection, 258–259
    ileoanal anastomosis, 259
    ostomy, 259–260
    patient positioning, 258
    preparation and positioning, 258
    proctectomy, 259
    single-port multi-trocar access system placement, 258
    specimen extraction, 259
Single-port colectomy, 382–383
Small bowel obstruction
  early, 374
  late and complete, 375
  postoperative, 307
Splenic flexure
  HALAR, 129–130
  mobilization
    laparoscopic proctocolectomy, 148–149
    left colectomy and anterior resection, 44–46, 77
    left colon and, 113–114
Stapled IPAA *vs.* mucosectomy and handsewn anastomosis, 145–146
Stoma creation
  indications, 169
  ischemic ostomy, 170
  laparoscopic colostomy, 174–176
  laparoscopic ileostomy, 171–174
  mesenteric length, 176
  operating room setup and patient positioning, 171
  parastomal hernia, 170
  precautions, 176
  preoperative planning, 170
Stomal relocation, 195
Stoma reversal, laparoscopic
  colostomy after Hartmann's procedure
    anastomosis creation, 184
    distal sigmoid colon resection, 183–184
    Hartmann's pouch and rectum mobilization, 183
    port placement, 180–182
    proximal colon mobilization, 182–183
  complications, 186–187
  Hartmann's procedure, 179, 180
  ileostomy with ileorectal anastomosis
    anastomosis creation, 186
    port placement, 184–185
    rectal resection, 186
    rectum mobilization, 185
  outcome, 187–188
  patient setup, 180
  postoperative care, 186
  precautions, 188
  preoperative planning, 179–180
Straight laparoscopy. *See* Total abdominal colectomy (TAC)
Strictures, 241
Sugarbaker technique, 189, 193–194
Superior hemorrhoidal vessels, 134
Superior mesenteric artery (SMA), 25–27
Superior rectal artery (SRA), 208
Surgeon factors, LAS, 391
Surgical anatomy
  colonic mesenteric vasculature
    gastrocolic trunk, 26–27
    ileocolic (ICA), 25, 26
    right colic artery (RCA), 25
    superior mesenteric artery (SMA), 25–27
  inferior mesenteric artery (IMA)
    blood supply, 27, 28
    bowstring effect, 27
    embryologic surgical planes, 28–30
    gonadal vessels, 30
    innervation, 31–32, 34–35, 38–39
    pelvis, 30–31
    posterior and lateral compartments, 31, 33, 35–37
    splenic flexure, 28, 29
    superior rectal artery, 28
    ureter, 30–35
  left colectomy and anterior resection
    descending colectomy, 46–47
    inferior mesenteric vein and splenic flexure mobilization, 44–46
    low anterior resection, 47–48
    perineal dissection, 49
    uterine retraction, 48–49
  right colectomy
    lateral-to-medial mobilization, 38–41
    lesser sac, 41, 42
    medial-to-lateral mobilization, 35–38, 40–41
  transverse colectomy and middle colic vessels, 42–43
Surgical innovation, 399
Symptomatic cholelithiasis, 375

**T**

Thermal injury, 237–238
Total abdominal colectomy (TAC)
  abdomen and port placement, 90–91
  clinical trials, 100
  end ileostomy, 95–96
  hand-assisted (*see* Hand-assisted laparoscopic surgery (HALS))
  ileorectostomy, 96–98
  intraoperative complications, 99
  patient setup, 90
  postoperative care, 98
  postoperative complications, 99
  precautions, 100
  preoperative planning and decision making, 89–90
  right colon, 91
  sigmoid colon, left colon, and splenic flexure, 93–94
  specimen extraction, 94–95
  surgical indications, 89
  transverse colon and hepatic flexure, 91–93
Total abdominal colectomy with end ileostomy
  HALS, 346–348
  single-incision laparoscopic surgery (SILS), 352–353
Total lung capacity (TLC), 373–374
Total mesorectal dissection, 280–281
Total mesorectal excision (TME)
  APR, 132, 134–136
  HALAR, 124–127
  laparoscopic rectal resection, 111
  left colectomy, 279
Total proctocolectomy
  ileal pouch anal anastomosis reconstruction
    colonic dissection, 258–259
    ileoanal anastomosis, 259
    ostomy, 259–260
    patient positioning, 258
    preparation and positioning, 258
    proctectomy, 259
    single-port multi-trocar access system placement, 258
    specimen extraction, 259
  IPAA, 351–352

Transabdominal approach, 155
Transanal endoscopic microsurgery (TEMS), 283
Transanal minimally invasive surgery (TAMIS)
 indications, 284
 precautions, 289–290
 preoperative work-up, 284–285
 technique, 285–289
 TEMS, 283
Transanal rectosigmoid resection, 265–266
Transanal TME (taTME), 267–269
Transperineal approach, 155
Transverse colectomy and middle colic vessels, 42–43
Transverse colon
 abdomen, 205
 hepatic flexure and, 91–93
Trendelenburg position, HALAR, 122
Trocar placement
 laparoscopic proctocolectomy, 146–147
 laparoscopic rectopexy, 162, 164
 pregnant patients, 377
 prevention and management, 235–237

**U**

Ulcerative colitis (UC) patients
 conventional laparoscopy *vs.* HALS *vs.* SILS *vs.* open surgery, 353
 HALS and conventional laparoscopic surgery
  completion proctectomy with IPAA, 348–351
  total abdominal colectomy with end ileostomy, 346–348
  total proctocolectomy with IPAA, 351–352
 laparoscopic proctocolectomy, 144
 operative methods, 345
 precautions, 355
 rectal cancer and, 354–355
 SILS
  proctectomy with IPAA, 353
  total abdominal colectomy with end ileostomy, 352–353
 surgical strategy, 354
 treatment, 346
Ureter
 abdomen, 208–209
 reoperative surgery, 226
Ureteral stenting, 10
Urinary drainage, 10
Uterine retraction, 48–49

**V**

Vascular injury, 236
Vascular pedicles, 58
Venous thromboembolism (VTE)
 prevention, 10
 prophylaxis, obese patients, 332–333
Veress needle, peritoneal space, 21–22
Vessel and mesentery division, 67
Visceral abdominal fat (VAT), 321

**W**

Waist-to-hip ratio (WHR), 321
Wound extraction site, 330–331

MIX
Papier aus verantwortungsvollen Quellen
Paper from responsible sources
FSC® C105338

FSC
www.fsc.org

If you have any concerns about our products,
you can contact us on
**ProductSafety@springernature.com**

In case Publisher is established outside the EU,
the EU authorized representative is:
**Springer Nature Customer Service Center GmbH**
**Europaplatz 3, 69115 Heidelberg, Germany**

Printed by Libri Plureos GmbH
in Hamburg, Germany